PROFESSIONAL ISSUES
in
Speech-Language Pathology
and Audiology

Fifth Edition

PROFESSIONAL ISSUES
in
Speech-Language Pathology
and Audiology

Fifth Edition

Melanie W. Hudson, MA
Mark DeRuiter, PhD, MBA

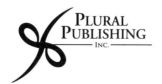

PLURAL
PUBLISHING
INC.

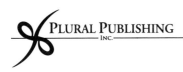

5521 Ruffin Road
San Diego, CA 92123

e-mail: information@pluralpublishing.com
Website: https://www.pluralpublishing.com

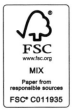

Typeset in 9/11 Adobe Garamond Pro by Flanagan's Publishing Services, Inc.
Printed in the United States of America by McNaughton & Gunn, Inc.

For permission to use material from this text, contact us by
Telephone: (866) 758-7251
Fax: (888) 758-7255
e-mail: permissions@pluralpublishing.com

Every attempt has been made to contact the copyright holders for material originally printed in another source. If any have been inadvertently overlooked, the publishers will gladly make the necessary arrangements at the first opportunity.

Library of Congress Cataloging-in-Publication Data

Names: Hudson, Melanie W., editor. | DeRuiter, Mark, editor.
Title: Professional issues in speech-language pathology and audiology /
  [edited by] Melanie W. Hudson, Mark DeRuiter.
Description: Fifth edition. | San Diego, CA: Plural, [2021] | Includes
  bibliographical references and index.
Identifiers: LCCN 2019029820 | ISBN 9781635502206 (paperback) | ISBN
  9781635502671 (ebook)
Subjects: MESH: Speech-Language Pathology | Audiology | Professional
  Practice
Classification: LCC RC423 | NLM WM 475 | DDC 616.85/5—dc23
LC record available at https://lccn.loc.gov/2019029820

Contents

6 Professional Accountability   131

Shelly S. Chabon, PhD and Becky Sutherland Cornett, PhD

7 International Alliances   141

Robert M. Augustine, PhD, Tina K. Veale, PhD, and Kelly M. Holland, MEd

Section III   Setting-Specific Issues

14   Health Care Legislation, Regulation, and Financing   279

18 Service Delivery Issues in Private Practice 361

Robin L. Edge, PhD

19 Strategically Promoting Access to Speech-Language Pathology and Audiology Services 381

Brooke Hallowell, PhD

Section IV Working Productively

20 Documentation Issues   401

21 Developing Leadership Skills   425

22 Safety in the Workplace   437

Foreword

In 1994, I returned to an academic environment at the University of Minnesota after a six-year hiatus in a setting where I was a researcher and clinical service provider. I was assigned to co-teach a revised version of a class called *Professional Issues* with a speech-language pathology colleague, Dr. Leslie Glaze. We had never met before, but we were united in the love of our two professions and one discipline. Previously we had taught as "subject-matter experts" in the areas of developmental and rehabilitative audiology and voice. From our own academic and clinical experiences, we knew that this more recent focus on the framework of being a professional in our disciplines was critical for our students as we prepared them for their future practice. We were very fortunate to use a new textbook edited by Rosemary Lubinski and Carol Frattali entitled *Professional Issues in Speech-Language Pathology and Audiology*. It guided our lectures, discussions, and writing assignments. I continued to teach that class for several more years, convinced more each time that this area was foundational for new (and not so new) practitioners.

It is with great pleasure that 25 years later, as I retire from the University of Minnesota, I have been asked to write this foreword for the fifth edition of *Professional Issues in Speech-Language Pathology and Audiology*, edited by Melanie Hudson and Mark DeRuiter. This volume reflects the fact that the impact and maturity of a discipline and, in our case, two professions cannot be measured by disciplinary expertise in speech-language pathology and audiology alone. Rather, the context in which we practice is just as important as what we practice. In fact, we cannot practice or do clinical research effectively without understanding the demands of culture, law, global influences, and the values and ethics of our own and other professions.

This volume contains 30 chapters written by 45 authors organized into four main sections—overview of the professions, employment issues, setting-specific issues, and working productively. This is a rare book, serving to enlighten students as they become professionals and to allow even experienced practitioners to learn about new trends in, and external pressures to, the discipline. It can be both a beginning textbook and a complex resource for individuals and groups as they grapple with professional practice and translational research in the twenty-first century. This volume contains the collective wisdom and experience of expert clinicians, scholars, and administrators from every practice setting, the academy, and professional associations. These authors have held a variety of national, state, and local leadership positions. I have worked with many of them directly and have listened to their thoughtful presentations. Seeing this volume today makes me want to teach *Professional Issues* again. There is no doubt that readers will have the highest quality experience that will assist them every day in their professions.

—Arlene Earley Carney, PhD, CCC-A

Arlene Earley Carney, PhD, CCC-A, is a Professor Emeritus in the Department of Speech-Language-Hearing Sciences at the University of Minnesota–Twin Cities. She has taught coursework in diagnostic and pediatric audiology, rehabilitative audiology, cochlear implants, and professional issues at Purdue University, University of Illinois at Urbana-Champaign, and the University of Minnesota. In addition, she had research and clinical appointments at Mailman Center for Child Development and Boys Town National Research Hospital. Currently, Arlene is the Vice President for Standards and Ethics in Audiology for the American Speech-Language-Hearing Association (ASHA), having served as editor for Hearing for the *Journal of Speech-Language-Hearing Research,* chair of the Standards Council and the Board of Ethics, and a member of the Council for Academic Accreditation. She is an ASHA Fellow and received the Honors of ASHA in 2015.

Reference

Lubinski, R., & Frattali, C. (Eds.) (1994). *Professional issues in speech-language pathology and audiology: A textbook*. San Diego, CA: Singular Publishing.

Preface

Welcome to the fifth edition of *Professional Issues in Speech-Language Pathology and Audiology*! Since the publication of the first edition over 25 years ago, the professions of audiology and speech-language pathology have continued to evolve. Our scopes of practice are regularly updated to reflect the dynamic growth and increasing complexity of our roles and responsibilities within our varied work settings. Our caseloads are more diverse than ever, and we must keep abreast of evidence-supported knowledge and skills that define best practices in our professions. Audiologists and speech-language pathologists continue to remain challenged and motivated to meet the demands of their professional environment.

This fifth edition of *Professional Issues in Speech-Language Pathology and Audiology* is intended to be a primary text for students and a resource for faculty and practicing clinicians seeking a comprehensive introduction to contemporary issues that influence our professions and our service delivery across settings. We aim to provide our readers with a better understanding that day-to-day clinical work, as well as personal professional growth and development, is influenced by political, social, educational, health care, and economic concerns. Your professional identity is enhanced when you understand the range of factors that define what you do, with whom, for how long, and at what cost. With this big-picture view of your profession, you will be better prepared to make informed decisions as you provide services, engage in advocacy efforts, and plan your career as an audiologist or speech-language pathologist.

How to Use This Text

This text is widely used in Communication Sciences and Disorders (CSD) programs, typically in professional issues courses or capstone seminars, but also as a general reference tool for faculty and practitioners. Table A provides a matrix of chapter content relevant to the Council for Clinical Certification (CFCC) standards for the ASHA Certificate of Clinical Competence (CCC). You should notice that certain topics are repeated in this table, as many are relevant to more than just one chapter's content. For instance, documentation is relevant to all work settings, as is ethical practice and technology, each warranting its own chapter. Evidence-based practice informs what we do as effective clinicians and is another persistent theme throughout the text, a topic also worthy of its own chapter, but referenced throughout the text.

This text should continue to serve as an excellent desk reference even after you complete your graduate education. Important topics such as the job search (and keeping your job!), ethical practice, accountability and documentation, leadership, cultural competence, economic issues, technology, research, and setting-specific issues will continue to be relevant as you grow professionally.

New to the Fifth Edition

The success of the first four editions of this text is attributed to the insightful and cutting-edge contributions made by each of the chapter authors, recognized experts in their respective subject areas. This fifth edition continues that tradition by including previous authors who have updated their chapters to reflect new issues and trends in audiology and speech-language pathology within their topic areas. In addition, there are several new chapters in this edition, including "Professional Accountability," by Shelly Chabon and Becky Cornett. This chapter discusses organizing and delivering superior health care services that are focused on effectiveness and efficiency. The reader is also reminded of the ethical commitments required to enable outcomes supporting communication and hearing. In "Safety in the Workplace," Donna Smiley and Cynthia Richburg address identification of threats and hazards, as well as the implementation of controls and policies to counter those threats/hazards in various work settings, including infection control and workplace violence.

Interprofessional education and interprofessional practice have become a major focus in graduate education programs and practice settings. Alex Johnson provides a rich overview of this topic that supports increasing the value of health care by providing evidence-based patient-centered care as part of an interdisciplinary team.

In Chapter 28, "Counseling," Michael Flahive provides a detailed discussion of the roles of audiologists and speech-language pathologists in supporting patients and family members who are dealing with some of the more challenging issues associated with communication and hearing disorders.

Tommie Robinson, a former ASHA President, and Janet Deppe, Director of State Affairs at ASHA, offer a dynamic discussion of how audiologists and speech-language pathologists may support advocacy efforts within their individual work settings and local communities and at the state and national levels.

This fifth edition also has new authors adding their expertise to the book, including Mark DeRuiter (also the co-editor), at the University of Arizona; Tricia Ashby, at the Washington Audiology and Imaging Center; Bob Augustine, Council of Graduate Schools; Stacy K. Betz, at Purdue University; Cathy DeRuiter, at Children's Clinics, Tucson; Robin Edge, at Jacksonville University; Mary Sue Fino-Szumski at Vanderbilt University; Susan Felsenfeld, at Buffalo State University; Liza Finestack, at

University of Minnesota; Carolyn Higdon, at University of Mississippi; Kelly M. Holland, Associate Director for International Partnerships, Global Experiences; Shirley Huang, at University of Colorado; Susan Ingram, at James Madison University; Marie Ireland, at Virginia Department of Education; Jeffrey Johnson, at VA Pittsburgh Healthcare System; Pui Fong Kan at University of Colorado; Lemmietta McNeilly, Chief Staff Officer for SLP at ASHA; Lissa Power de Fur, at Longwood University; Jeff Regan, Director of Government Affairs and Public Policy at ASHA; Gail Richard, former ASHA President; Steve Ritch, Manager of Associates Program at ASHA; Lisa Scott, at Florida State University, and Tina K. Veale, at Lewis University.

We have also updated the list of acronyms to include those that are referred to throughout this edition. This list is provided at the front of the book to use as a quick reference.

Professional issues always provide the basis for lively discussions among students and practitioners alike. As in past editions, we have included Critical Thinking questions at the end of each chapter to encourage discussion and reflection on the topics covered in that chapter.

Companion Website

PowerPoint lecture slides for each chapter have been made available for instructors on a PluralPlus companion website. Instructors can customize the slides to meet their needs. Please see the inside front cover of the text for access information.

A Final Thought

We hope that by reading this text, participating in class discussions, and engaging in critical reflection you will be motivated and inspired to explore more learning opportunities, become involved in your professional associations, and advocate for your professions and those you serve.

About the Editors

Melanie W. Hudson, MA, received her BS from James Madison University (VA) and her MA from George Washington University, with post-graduate studies at George Washington University and the University of Virginia. She is an ASHA Fellow, and Distinguished Fellow of National Academies of Practice (NAP). She served on ASHA's Board of Directors as Chair of the Speech-Language Pathology Advisory Council (2016-2018), the Board of Ethics, and the Board of Special Interest Group Coordinators. Melanie's publications include *Professional Issues in Speech-Language Pathology and Audiology, Fourth Edition* (Lubinski & Hudson; Delmar, Cengage Learning, 2013; Plural Publishing, 2018), and chapter author for "The Clinical Education and Supervisory Process in Speech-Language Pathology and Audiology," (McCrea & Brasseur, Slack, Inc., 2019). She served as President of the Georgia Speech-Language and Hearing Association and currently serves on the Georgia Board of Examiners for Speech-Language Pathology and Audiology. She worked as an SLP in Arlington (VA) Public Schools, in private practice, and as adjunct faculty. She is the National Director at EBS Healthcare and a frequent guest lecturer at universities and professional conferences.

Mark DeRuiter, PhD, MBA, is Clinical Professor and Associate Department Head for Clinical Education in the Department of Speech, Language, and Hearing Sciences at the University of Arizona. Mark earned his PhD and MBA degrees at the University of Minnesota and Augsburg University, respectively. Mark holds national certificates of clinical competence in audiology and speech-language pathology from the American Speech-Language-Hearing Association (ASHA). He is also a Fellow of ASHA and the American Academy of Audiology. Mark has a long history of service to the discipline. He has served ASHA as the Vice Chair for Speech-Language Pathology on their Council for Clinical Certification, chaired the national Speech-Language Pathology Scope of Practice document, and is a site visitor for ASHA's Council on Academic Accreditation. He has also served as President of the Council of Academic Programs in Communication Sciences and Disorders where he has held additional roles of Treasurer and Vice President for Professional Development.

Contributors

Tricia Ashby-Scabis, AuD
Director
American Speech-Language-Hearing Association
Audiology Practices
Chapter 13

Robert M. Augustine, PhD
Senior Vice President
Council of Graduate Schools
Washington, District of Columbia
Chapter 7

Fred H. Bess, PhD
Vickie and Thomas Flood Professor, Department of
    Hearing and Speech Sciences
Vanderbilt University School of Medicine
Director, National Center for Childhood Deafness and
    Family Communication
Vanderbilt Bill Wilkerson Center
Chapter 4

Stacy K. Betz, PhD
Associate Professor and Department Chair
Purdue University Fort Wayne
Fort Wayne, Indiana
Chapter 8

Corey Herd Cassidy, PhD
Professor and Associate Dean
Waldron College of Health and Human Services
Radford University
Radford, Virginia
Chapter 17

Shelly Chabon, PhD
Vice Provost for Academic Personal and Dean of
    Interdisciplinary General Education
Portland State University

Portland, Oregon
Chapter 6

Becky Sutherland Cornett, PhD
The Ohio State University Wexner Medical Center
    (retired)
Columbus, Ohio
Chapter 6

Janet Deppe, MS
Director, State Affairs
American Speech-Language-Hearing Association
Chapter 30

Cathy DeRuiter, MA
Speech-Language Pathologist
Children's Clinics and Rehabilitation Services
Tucson, Arizona
Minneapolis Public Schools
Minneapolis, Minnesota
Chapter 10

Mark DeRuiter, PhD, MBA
ASHA Fellow
Clinical Professor and Associate Department Head for
    Clinical Education
Department of Speech, Language, and Hearing
    Sciences
University of Arizona
Tucson, Arizona
Chapter 1 and Chapter 11

Judith Felson Duchan, PhD
Professor Emeritus
Department of Communication Disorders and Sciences
University at Buffalo
Buffalo, New York
Chapter 2

Carol C. Dudding, PhD
Associate Professor
Department of Communication Sciences and
   Disorders
James Madison University
Harrisonburg, Virginia
Chapter 27

Robin L. Edge, PhD
Associate Professor
Brooks Rehabilitation Department of Communication
   Sciences and Disorders
Jacksonville University
Jacksonville, Florida
Chapter 18

Susan Felsenfeld, PhD
Associate Professor and Department Chairperson
Department of Speech-Language Pathology
SUNY Buffalo State
Buffalo, New York
Chapter 2

Lizbeth H. Finestack, PhD
Associate Professor
Director of Graduate Studies
Department of Speech-Language-Hearing Sciences
University of Minnesota–Twin Cities
Chapter 8

Mary Sue Fino-Szumski, PhD, MBA
Assistant Professor and Director of Clinical
   Education
Department of Hearing and Speech Sciences
Vanderbilt University Medical Center
Nashville, Tennessee
Chapter 26

Michael Flahive, PhD
Retired Professor
Saint Mary's College
Notre Dame, Indiana
Chapter 28

Perry Flynn, MEd
Professor
Department of Communication Sciences and
   Disorders
University of North Carolina Greensboro
Consultant in Speech-Language Pathology
North Carolina Public Instruction
Chapter 16

Charlette McRay Green, MS
Executive Director Special Education
Cherokee County School District
Canton, Georgia
Chapter 16

Sue T. Hale, MCD
Associate Professor (retired)
Department of Hearing and Speech Sciences
Vanderbilt University School of Medicine
Nashville, Tennessee
Chapter 4

Brooke Hallowell, PhD
Dean, Health Sciences and Rehabilitation Studies
Professor, Communication Sciences and Disorders
Springfield College
Springfield, Massachusetts
Chapter 19

Jaynee A. Handelsman, PhD
EHDI Program Coordinator
Department of Otolaryngology
Michigan Medicine
Ann Arbor, Michigan
Chapter 5

Carolyn Wiles Higdon, EdD
Fellow of the American Speech-Language Hearing
   Association
Fellow of the National Academies of Practice
Licensed and Certified Speech-Language Pathologist
Professor, University of Mississippi
Professor, University of Guyana
Clinical Associate Professor, University of Mississippi
   Medical Center
CEO of Wiles Higdon and Associates, LLC
Oxford, Mississippi
Chapter 24

Kelly M. Holland, MEd
Associate Director
Institutional Partnerships
Global Experiences
Annapolis, Maryland
Chapter 7

Shirley Huang, MS
Doctoral Student
University of Colorado Boulder
Boulder, Colorado
Chapter 25

Melanie W. Hudson, MA
ASHA Fellow
Distinguished Fellow National Academies of Practice
National Director at EBS Healthcare
Atlanta, Georgia
Chapter 1, Chapter 12, and Chapter 26

Susan B. Ingram, PhD
Assistant Professor, Director of Clinical Education
Department of Communication Sciences and
    Disorders
James Madison University
Harrisonburg, Virginia
Chapter 27

Marie C. Ireland, MEd
Specialist
Virginial Department of Education
ASHA Vice President for SLP Practice 2018–2020
Chapter 16

Alex Johnson, PhD
Provost and Vice President for Academic Affairs
MGH Institute of Health Professions
Boston, Massachusetts
Chapter 15 and Chapter 23

Jeffrey P. Johnson, PhD
Geriatric Research Education and Clinical Center,
Audiology and Speech Pathology Service,
VA Pittsburgh Healthcare System
Pittsburgh, Pennsylvania
Chapter 15

Pui Fong Kan, PhD
Associate Professor
University of Colorado Boulder
Boulder, Colorado
Chapter 25

Raymond D. Kent, PhD
Professor Emeritus
Department of Communication Sciences and
    Disorders
Waisman Center
University of Wisconsin–Madison
Madison, Wisconsin
Chapter 9

Lemmietta G. McNeilly, PhD
Chief Staff Officer for Speech-Language Pathology
American Speech-Language-Hearing Association

Rockville, Maryland
Chapter 13

Barbara J. Moore, EdD
Director, Special Services
East Side Union High School District
San Jose, California
Chapter 20

Marva Mount, MA
Director
EBS Healthcare
Fort Worth, Texas
Chapter 12

Diane Paul, PhD
Director, Clinical Issues in Speech-Language
    Pathology
Speech-Language Pathology Professional Practices
American Speech-Language-Hearing Association
Chapter 13

Lissa Power-deFur, PhD
Professor, Chair
Department of Social Work and Communication
    Sciences and Disorders
Longwood University
Farmville, Virginia
Chapter 3

Jeffrey P. Regan, MA
Director of Government Affairs and Public Policy
American Speech-Language-Hearing Association
Chapter 14

Gail J. Richard, PhD
Professor Emeritus
Eastern Illinois University
Charleston, Illinois
Chapter 21

Cynthia McCormick Richburg, PhD
Professor and AuD Program Coordinator
Department of Communication Sciences and Disorders
Wichita State University
Wichita, Kansas
Chapter 22

Steven D. Ritch, CRMT
Manager, ASHA Associates Program
American Speech-Language-Hearing Association
Rockville, Maryland
Chapter 13

Tommie L. Robinson, Jr., PhD
Chief, Division of Hearing and Speech
Director, Scottish Rite Center
Children's National Health System
Associate Professor of Pediatrics
George Washington School of Medicine and Health
   Sciences
Washington, District of Columbia
Chapter 30

Lisa A. Scott, PhD
Director of Clinical Education
Florida State University
Tallahassee, Florida
Chapter 29

Donna Fisher Smiley, PhD
ASHA Fellow
Audiologist and Coordinator
Educational Audiology/Speech Pathology Resources
   for Schools (EARS) Program
Arkansas Children's Hospital
Little Rock, Arkansas
Chapter 22

Tina K. Veale, PhD
Professor and Program Director
Speech-Language Pathology
Lewis University
Romeoville, Illinois
Chapter 7

Table A

Matrix of Chapter Content Relevant to the Council for Clinical Certification Standards for the Certificates of Clinical Competence

Table A. Matrix of Chapter Content Relevant to the Council for Clinical Certification Standards for the Certificates of Clinical Competence

	Ch 1	Ch 2	Ch 3	Ch 4	Ch 5	Ch 6	Ch 7	Ch 8	Ch 9	Ch 10	Ch 11	Ch 12
Audiology Standards												
A9 Patient characteristics (ex. demographics)	X					X				X		
A15 Assistive technology												
A16 Cultural diversity	X					X				X		
A18 Principles of research								X	X			
A19 Legal and ethical practices		X	X	X	X	X					X	X
A20 Health care and education delivery	X					X	X					X
A21 Universal precautions												
A22 Oral and written communication											X	
A28 Business practices			X			X						
A29 Working with related professionals							X					X
C10 Preparing a report												
C11 Referring to others												
D2 Develop culturally approp. rehab plan						X	X					
D5 Collaboration EI, schools, etc.												
E1 Community education and advocacy							X					
E2 Consultation												
E3 Promoting access to care	X	X				X	X					
F1 Quality improvement		X				X						X
F2 Research and evidence-based practice		X				X	X	X	X			
F3 Implement research-based techniques		X				X		X	X			
F4 Administration and supervision			X			X						
F5 Program development						X	X					X
F6 Maintaining links with other programs			X			X						
Speech-Language Standards												
III-D Prevention, assessment, intervention						X	X					
III-E Ethical standards	X			X	X	X	X					X
III-F Research and evidence-based practice	X	X				X	X	X	X			
III-G Contemporary professional issues	X	X	X	X		X	X			X	X	X
III-H Certification and licensure	X		X	X		X				X	X	X
IV-B Oral and written communication											X	
IV-G.1f Reporting to support evaluation						X						
IV-G.1g Client referral												
IV-G.2f Reporting to support intervention						X						
IV-G.2g Client identification and referral												
IV-G.3a Communicate effectively					X	X					X	

Ch 13	Ch 14	Ch 15	Ch 16	Ch 17	Ch 18	Ch 19	Ch 20	Ch 21	Ch 22	Ch 23	Ch 24	Ch 25	Ch 26	Ch 27	Ch 28	Ch 29	Ch 30
			X			X				X		X					X
			X											X			
			X	X		X				X		X					
X		X	X	X	X		X	X	X	X		X	X	X	X	X	X
X	X	X	X			X			X			X		X			
								X	X								
			X				X	X	X	X		X	X		X	X	X
X			X				X		X					X			
X		X	X						X	X		X		X		X	
							X										
X		X	X			X				X					X		
			X									X					
X			X						X					X			
	X		X			X	X					X					X
		X	X				X	X									
X	X	X			X	X	X					X		X			X
			X	X		X						X					
			X	X					X			X		X			
			X														
X		X	X			X		X	X					X	X		
			X			X			X			X					
		X	X			X			X	X		X					X
			X				X			X		X		X			
X		X	X	X	X		X	X	X	X		X		X		X	
			X						X			X		X			X
X	X	X	X	X	X	X	X	X	X	X				X	X		X
X		X		X										X			
			X				X	X	X	X		X		X	X	X	X
	X						X							X			
										X				X	X		
							X			X							
	X	X	X				X			X				X	X		
X			X			X	X	X	X	X		X	X	X	X	X	X

Acronyms

AAA: American Academy of Audiology

AAC: Augmentative and Alternative Communication

AAO-HNS: American Academy of Otolaryngology – Head and Neck Surgery

AAPM: Advanced Alternative Payment Method

AAPPSLPA: American Academy of Private Practice in Speech-Language Pathology and Audiology

ABA: American Board of Audiology

ABC System: A (High Priority), B (Medium Priority), C (Low Priority)

ABER: Auditory Brainstem Evoked Response

ABIM: American Board of Internal Medicine

ABR: Auditory Brainstem Response

AC: Advisory Council

ACA: Patient Protection and Affordable Care Act

ACAE: Accreditation Commission for Audiology Education

ACE: Award for Continuing Education

ACE: American Council on Education

ACAE: Accreditation Commission for Audiology Education

ACEBP: Advisory Committee on Evidence-Based Practice

ACLU: American Civil Liberties Union

ACO: Accountable Care Organization

ACT: American College Testing Program

ADA: Americans with Disabilities Act

ADEA: Age Discrimination in Employment Act of 1967

ADL: Activity of Daily Living

AGREE: Appraisal of Guidelines for Research and Evaluation

AHRQ: Agency for Healthcare Research and Quality

AI: Artificial Intelligence

AIDS: Acquired Immune Deficiency Syndrome

AIHC: American Interprofessional Health Collaboration

ALS: Amyotrophic Lateral Sclerosis

AMA: American Medical Association

ANCDS: Academy of Neurologic Communication Disorders and Sciences

AAO-HNS: American Academy of Otolaryngology-Head and Neck Surgery

APD: Auditory Processing Disorders

APM: Alternative Payment Model

APR: Annual Performance Report

APS: Adult Protective Services

ARRA: American Recovery and Reinvestment Act of 2009

ASD: Autism Spectrum Disorder

ASHA: American Speech-Language-Hearing Association

AT: Assistive Technology

ATA: American Telemedicine Association

ATC: Assistive Technology for Cognition

AuD: Doctor of Audiology (Audiologist)

AUD: Audiology

AYP: Adequate Yearly Progress

BAA: British Academy of Audiology

BAAS: British Association of Audiological Scientists

BAAT: British Association of Audiologists

BBA: Balanced Budget Act

BBP: Bureau of Business Practice

BBRA: Balanced Budget Refinement Act

BCBSA: Blue Cross Blue Shield Association

BICS: Basic Interpersonal Communication Skills

BIPA: Benefits Improvement and Protection Act

BLS: Bureau of Labor Statistics

BOD: Board of Directors

BOE: Board of Ethics

BSHAA: British Society of Hearing Aid Audiologists

BSHT: British Society of Hearing Therapists

BYOD: Bring Your Own Device

CAA: Council on Academic Accreditation

CAE: Certified Association Executive

CACS: Cultural Awareness and Competence Scales

CALP: Cognitive Academic Language Proficiency

CAOHC: Council for Accreditation in Occupational Hearing Conservation

CAP: Computerized Accreditation Program

CAPCSD: Council of Academic Programs in Communication Sciences and Disorders

CAPD: Central Auditory Processing Disorders

CARF: Commission on Accreditation of Rehabilitation Facilities

CASLPA: Canadian Association of Speech-Language Pathologists and Audiologists

CCC: Certificate of Clinical Competence

CCC-A: Certificate of Clinical Competence in Audiology

CCC-SLP: Certificate of Clinical Competence in Speech-Language Pathology

CCI: Center for Cultural Interchange

CCI: Correct Coding Initiative

CCSPA: Council of University Supervisors in Speech-Language Pathology and Audiology

CCSS: Common Core State Standards

CCSSO: Council of Chief State School Officers

CDAL: Certified Director of Assisted Living

CDC: Centers for Disease Control and Prevention

CDCHU: Center on the Developing Child at Harvard University

CD-ROM: Compact Disc-Read-Only Memory

CDS: Communication Disorders and Sciences

CDSS: Clinical Decision Support System

CE: Continuing Education

CEC: Council for Exceptional Children

CEO: Chief Executive Officer

CF: Clinical Fellowship or Clinical Fellow

CFCC: Council for Clinical Certification in Audiology and Speech-Language Pathology

CFR: Code of Federal Regulations

CFSI: Clinical Fellowship Skills Inventory

CFY: Clinical Fellowship Year

CGC: Certified Genetic Counselor

CHEA: Council on Higher Education Accreditation

CHIP: Children's Health Insurance Program

CHW: Community Health Worker

CI: Confidence Interval

CIC: Completely in Canal

CIRRIE: Center for International Rehabilitation Research Information and Exchange

CISC: Cochlear Implant Specialty Certification

CLD: Cultural and Linguistic Diversity

CMHs: Certification Maintenance Hours

CMS: Centers for Medicare & Medicaid Services

CMV: Cytomegalovirus

COBRA: Consolidated Omnibus Budget Reconciliation Act

COE: Code of Ethics

COPs: Conditions of Participation

CORE: Collaboration, Observation, Reflection, and Evaluation

CORF: Comprehensive Outpatient Rehabilitation Facility

CoSN: Consortium for School Networking

CPLOL: Comité Permanent de Liaison des Orthophonistes/Logopèdes de l'Union Européenne

CPOP: Certificate Program for Otolaryngology Personnel

CPR: Cardiopulmonary Resuscitation

CPS: Child Protective Services

CPT: Current Procedural Terminology

CSC: Computer Sciences Corporation

CSD: Communication Sciences and Disorders

CSDCAS: Communication Sciences and Disorders Centralized Application Service for Clinical Education in Audiology and Speech-Language Pathology

CSEP: Center for the Study of Ethics in the Professions

CSSPA: Council of University Supervisors in Speech-Language Pathology and Audiology

CV: Curriculum Vitae

CWD: Child with a Disability

DDS: Doctor of Dental Surgery

DEU: Dedicated (Collaborative) Education Unit

DMD: Doctor of Dental Medicine

DO: Doctor of Osteopathic Medicine

DOE: U.S. Department of Education

DOTPA: Developing Outpatient Therapy Payment Alternatives

DPH: Doctor of Public Health

DPT: Doctor of Physical Therapy

DRA: Deficit Reduction Act

DRG: Diagnosis-Related Group

DSW: Doctor of Social Work

DTI: Diffusion Tensor Imaging

DVD: Digital Versatile/Video Disc

EBHC: Evidence-Based Health Care

EBP: Evidence-Based Practice

EBSR: Evidence-Based Systematic Review

ED: Department of Education

EdD: Doctor of Education

EDI: Electronic Data Interchange

EEG: Electroencephalography

EEO: Equal Employment Opportunity

EEOC: Equal Employment Opportunity Commission

EHA: Education for All Handicapped Children Act

EHB: Essential Health Benefits

EHDI: Early Hearing Detection and Intervention

EHR: Electronic Health Record

EI: Early Intervention

EIN: Employee Identification Number

ELL: English Language Learner

EMG: Electromyography

EMR: Electronic Medical Record

EMTALA: Emergency Medical Treatment and Labor Act

ENG: Electronystagmography

ENT: Ear, Nose, and Throat

EPC: Ethical Practices Committee

EPHI: Electronic Protected Health Information

EPSDT: Early Periodic Screening, Diagnosis, and Treatment

ERISA: Employee Retirement Income Security Act of 1974

ESEA: Elementary and Secondary Education Act

ESL: English as a Second Language

ESSA: Every Student Succeeds Act

ETS: Educational Testing Service

FAAP: Fellow of the American Academy of Pediatrics

FACS: Functional Assessment of Communication Skills for Adults

FAPE: Free Appropriate Public Education

FCM: Functional Communication Measure

FDA: Food and Drug Administration

FD&C Act: Federal Food, Drug and Cosmetic Act

FEES: Fiberoptic Endoscopic Evaluation of Swallowing

FERPA: Family Educational Rights and Privacy Act

FIM: Functional Independence Measure

FM: Frequency Modulated

fMRI: Functional Magnetic Resonance Imaging

FPCO: Family Policy Compliance Office

FRL: Free and Reduced Lunch

GAO: Government Accountability Office

GDP: Gross Domestic Product

GERD: Gastroesophageal Reflux Disease

GPA: Grade Point Average

GRE: Graduate Record Examination

HATS: Hearing Assistive Technology Systems

HBV: Hepatitis B Virus

HCA: Hearing Conservation Amendment

HCEC: Health Care Economics Committee

HCFA: Health Care Financing Administration

HCPCS: Healthcare Common Procedures Coding System

HES: Higher Education Data System

HHA: Home Health Agency

HHS: Health and Human Services

HIE: Health Information Exchange

HIPAA: Health Insurance Portability and Accountability Act of 1996

HIT: Health Information Technology

HIV: Human Immunodeficiency Virus

HMO: Health Maintenance Organization

HPSO: Healthcare Providers Service Association

HR: Human Resources

HSV: Herpes Simplex Virus

IALP: International Association of Logopedics and Phoniatrics

IASLT: Irish Association of Speech and Language Therapists

ICC: Infection Control Committee

ICC: Interagency Coordinating Council

ICD: International Classification of Diseases

ICF: International Classification of Functioning, Disability and Health

ICRA: International Collegium of Rehabilitative Audiology

IDEA: Individuals with Disabilities Education Act

IDEIA: Individuals with Disabilities Education Improvement Act

IEP: Individualized Education Program

IFSP: Individualized Family Service Plan

IIB: International Issues Board

IOM: Institute of Medicine

IOM: Internet-Only Manual

IP: Internet Protocol

IPA: Independent Practice Association

IPCP: Interprofessional Collaborative Practice

IPE: Interprofessional Education

IPEC: Interprofessional Education Collaboration

IPEC: Interprofessional Care Collaborative

IRB: Institutional Review Board

IRF-PAI: Inpatient Rehabilitation Facility-Patient Assessment Instrument

IRS: Internal Revenue Service

ISA: International Society of Audiology

ISA: Irish Society of Audiology

IST: Instructional Support Team

ITPA: Illinois Test of Psycholinguistic Abilities

JAAA: Journal of the American Academy of Audiology

JD: Juris Doctorate (law degree)

KASA: Knowledge and Skills Assessment

KT: Knowledge Translation

LAN: Local Area Network

LAST: Liberal Arts and Sciences Test

LCD: Local Coverage Determination

LCSW: Licensed Clinical Social Worker

LEA: Local Education Agency

LEP: Limited English Proficient

LLC: Limited Liability Company

LLD: Language Learning Disability

LLP: Limited Liability Partnership

LMS: Learning Management System

LOE: Levels of Evidence

LPAA: Life Participation Approach to Aphasia

LPC: Licensed Professional Counselor

LR: Likelihood Ratio

LRE: Least Restrictive Environment

LTACH: Long-Term Acute Care Hospital

LTC: Long-Term Care

LTCF: Long-Term Care Facility

MAC: Medicare Administrative Contractor

MACRA: Medicare Access and CHIP Reauthorization

MARC: Mentoring for Academic-Research Careers

MAT: Miller Analogies Test

MBP: Munchausen by Proxy

MC: Managed Care

MCO: Managed Care Organization

MD: Doctor of Medicine

MDAT: Multidisciplinary Assessment Team

MDS: Minimum Data Set

MedPAC: Medicare Payment Advisory Committee

MIPS: Merit-based Incentive Payment Model

MIPPA: Medicare Improvements for Patients and Providers Act

MMA: Medicare Prescription Drug, Improvement, and Modernization Act

MOA: Memorandum of Agreement

MOSAIC: Multiplying Opportunities for Services and Access to Immigrant Children

MOU: Memorandum of Understanding

MPFS: Medicare Physician Fee Schedule

MPH: Master of Public Health

MPPR: Multiple Procedure Payment Reduction

MRI: Magnetic Resonance Imaging

MRSA: Methicillin-Resistant Staphylococcus Aureus

MSDS: Material Safety Data Sheet

MTSS: Multi-Tiered Systems of Support

MUE: Medically Unlikely Edits

NACE: National Association of Colleges and Employees

NAEP: National Assessment of Educational Progress

NAFDA: National Association of Future Doctors of Audiology

NAFTA: North American Free Trade Agreement

NARF: National Association of Rehabilitation Facilities

NASEM: National Academies of Sciences, Engineering, and Medicine

NATS: National Association of Teachers of Speech

NCATE: National Council for Accreditation of Teacher Education

NCCP: National Center for Children in Poverty

NCELA: National Clearing House for English Language Acquisition

N-CEP: ASHA's National Center for Evidence-Based Practice in Communication Disorders

NCHS: National Center for Health Statistics

NCLB: No Child Left Behind Act

ND: No Date

NEA: National Education Association

NGA: National Governors Association Center for Best Practices

NGS: National Governmental Services

NHS: National Health Service

NICHD: National Institute of Child Health & Human Development

NICU: Neonatal Intensive Care Unit

NIDCD: National Institute on Deafness and Other Communication Disorders

NIH: National Institutes of Health

NIHL: Noise Induced Hearing Loss

NIRS: Near-Infrared Spectroscopy

NOMS: National Outcomes Measurement System

NPI: National Provider Identifier

NPO: Nothing by Mouth

NPV: Negative Predictive Value

NRH: National Rehabilitation Hospital

NSC: National Safety Council

NSOME: Nonspeech Oral-Motor Exercises

NSSE: National Survey of Student Engagement

NSSLHA: National Student Speech Language Hearing Association

NZAS: New Zealand Audiological Society

NZSTA: New Zealand Speech-language Therapists' Association

OAE: Otoacoustic Emission

OASIS: Outcome and Assessment Information Set

OBRA: Omnibus Reconciliation Act

OECD: Organization for Economic Cooperation and Development

OGET: Oklahoma General Education Test

OIG: Office of Inspector General

OPIM: Other Potentially Infectious Material

OPTE: Oklahoma Professional Teaching Exam

OSAT: Oklahoma Subject Area Test

OSEP: Office of Special Education Programs

OSERS: Office of Special Education and Rehabilitative Services

OSHA: Occupational Safety and Health Administration

OT: Occupational Therapy(ist)

OTD: Doctor of Occupational Therapy

OTO: Otologic Technician

OTR: Registered Occupational Therapist

PAHO: Pan-American Health Organization

P&P: Policy and Procedure

P2P: Peer-to-Peer File Sharing Program

PA: Physician Assistant

PAC: Post-Acute Care

PASC: Pediatric Audiology Specialty Certification

PCP: Primary Care Physician

PCMI: Patient-Centered Medical Home Model

PEP: Personalized Education Plan

PharmD: Doctor of Pharmacy

PhD: Doctor of Philosophy

PHI: Protected Health Information

PHR: Personal Health Record

PI: Performance Improvement

PICO: Patient, Intervention/Index Measure, Comparison, Outcome

PL: Public Law

PLOP: Present Level of Performance

PMPM: Per Member, Per Month Premium

PPACA: Patient Protection and Affordable Care Act

PPD: Purified Protein Derivative

PPE: Personal Protective Equipment

PPO: Preferred Provider Organization

PPS: Prospective Payment System

PQRI: Physician Quality Reporting Initiative

PQRS: Physician Quality Reporting System

PRI: Protected Research Information

PRN: Pro Re Nata—as the circumstances arise

PSAP: Personal Sound Amplification Products

PsyD: Doctor of Psychology

PT: Physical Therapy(ist)

PTA: Parent-Teacher Association

PTO: Paid Time Off

PV: Predictive Value

QCL: Quality of Communication Life

R0I: Research Project Grant

RAC: Recovery Audit Contractor

RAI: Resident Assessment Instrument

RBRVS: Resource-Based Relative Value Scale

RCCP: Registration Council for Clinical Physiologists

RCR: Responsible Conduct of Research

RCSLT: Royal College of Speech and Language Therapists

RCT: Randomized Controlled Trial

RDN: Registered Dietician Nutritionist

RFA: Request for Applications

RN: Registered Nurse

RPO: Related Professional Organization

RRT: Registered Respiratory Therapist

RSAC: ASHA Research and Scientific Affairs Committee

RtI or RTI: Response-to-Instruction/Intervention

RUC HCPAC: Resource Update Health Care Professionals Advisory Committee

RUC-IV: Resource Utilization Group, Version IV

RUG: Resource Utilization Group

RVU: Relative Value Unit

SAA: Student Academy of Audiology

SALT: Systematic Analysis of Language

SASLHA: South African Speech-Language-Hearing Association

SAT: Scholastic Aptitude Test

ScD: Doctor of Science

SCHIP: State Children's Health Insurance Program

SD: Spasmodic Dysphonia

SD: Standard Deviation

SEA: State Education Agency

SED: Survey of Earned Doctorates

SERTOMA: Service to Mankind

SGD: Speech Generating Device

SHRM: Society of Human Resources Management

SIG: Special Interest Group

SIGN: Scottish Intercollegiate Guideline Network

SITE: Society for Information Technology and Teacher Education

SLP: Speech-Language Pathologist

SLPA: Speech-Language Pathology Assistant

SLPCF: Speech-Language Pathology Clinical Fellowship

SLPD: Speech-Language Pathology Doctorate

SNF: Skilled Nursing Facility

SnNout: Sensitivity high, Negative result—rule out

SOAP: Subjective, Objective, Assessment, Plan

SPA: Speech Pathology Australia

SPAI: Supervisee Performance Assessment Instrument

SPP: State Performance Plan

SpPin: Specificity high, Positive result—rule in

SR: Systematic Review

SSR: Single Subject Research

SSW: Staggered Spondaic Word

STAR: State Advocates for Reimbursement

STATS: Short-Term Alternatives for Therapy Services

STEP: Student to Empowered Professional

STLD: Short-Term Limited-Duration Plan

SWOT: Strength, Weakness, Opportunity, Threat

TB: Tuberculosis

TCT: Teleaudiology Clinical Technician

tDCS: transcranial Direct Current Stimulation

TEFRA: Tax Equity and Fiscal Responsibility Act

TJC: The Joint Commission

TMS: Transcranial Magnetic Stimulation

TN: Trade NAFTA

TRHCA: Tax Relief and Health Care Act

TTY/TDD: Text Telephone/Telecommunications Device for the Deaf

UK: United Kingdom

USC: U.S. Code

VA: Veterans Administration

VEMP: Vestibular Evoked Myogenic Potential

VIA: Values in Action

VNG: Videonystagmography

VR/AR: Virtual Reality/Augmented Reality

WASP: Waveforms Annotations Spectograms and Pitch

WHO: World Health Organization

This text is dedicated to Dr. Rosemary Lubinski, whose commitment to the education and training of future speech-language pathologists and audiologists was the genesis and foundation of this text and its previous four editions. Her contributions to the professions are many and her work continues to inspire a generation of professionals.

◇◇◇

We would also like to include our chapter contributors who have shared their unique expertise and their wisdom with future audiologists and speech-language pathologists.

Finally, the editors would like to include their spouses, John Hudson and Cathy DeRuiter, respectively, and thank them for their ongoing encouragement and support.

SECTION I

Overview of the Professions

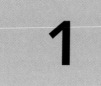

Professions for the Twenty-First Century

‹‹‹

Melanie W. Hudson, MA, and Mark DeRuiter, PhD, MBA

Introduction

You have chosen a dynamic profession, with substantial growth expected to continue in the coming years. According to the U.S. Department of Labor, the need for services provided by audiologists is expected to increase by 21 percent from 2016 to 2026, while the need for speech-language pathologists (SLPs) is expected to increase by 18 percent during the same time period (U.S. Bureau of Labor Statistics, n.d.). Even as we are writing this introductory chapter, there are changes occurring along with our growing numbers that will significantly impact the professions of audiology and speech-language pathology. As the demand for our services continues to grow, what are some of the major trends and issues impacting our professions?

Many factors have come into play in recent years that are transforming how we plan and carry out our work. Rapidly advancing technology, legislation in health care and education, demographic shifts that include an aging population and increasing levels of diversity, global economic changes, and new research are influencing how we deliver services. Even the influence of climate change is playing a role in how audiologists and SLPs make career decisions. Faced with these and other changes, how do we ensure that our clinical skills are state-of-the art, incorporating the latest technological advances? How do we provide services that are of the highest quality, yet cost-effective? What are the ripple effects of global economic changes and demographic shifts on our professional practice? And finally, what role does evidence play in our clinical decision making?

This chapter provides an overview of some of the most important trends and issues that are likely to affect your professional practice in the coming years: technology; trends in health care and education; economic influences; demographic shifts and globalization; and evidence-based practice. Each of these areas is addressed more fully in chapters specific to the topic, and within the appropriate context throughout the rest of the book. The information in this chapter will set the stage for advanced critical thinking and constructive dialogue. In this rapidly evolving professional climate, it is not enough to be performing only competently as a clinician. Today's audiologists and SLPs also need to be using analytical thinking and engaging in critical reflection when making decisions that affect the lives of others.

As you read this chapter, consider the scopes of practice in audiology and speech-language pathology. (See Appendix 1–A and 1–B at the end of the chapter for the current scopes of practice in audiology and speech-language pathology.) Remember that each of these practices is well defined and dynamic. Take time to reflect on how the trends and issues presented in this chapter influence your own decisions and plans for the future as we complete the first quarter of the twenty-first century.

Trends in Technology and the Digital Revolution

The future is an inevitable reality, . . . which we either adapt to or resist, but that we have the power to "envisage and take action to build alternative and desirable futures." (Facer & Sandford, 2010)

We are living in what is known as the Digital Revolution, also known as the Third Industrial Revolution, the change from mechanical and electronic technology to digital technology. Analogous to the Agricultural Revolution and Industrial Revolution, the Digital Revolution marked the beginning of the Information Age (Digital Revolution, 2019). Those born during the twenty-first century would not be able to imagine a world without computers, the internet, and personal electronic devices such as smartphones that enable instant communication with anyone, anywhere, any time. By 2015, around 50% of the world had constant internet connection, and ownership rates of smartphones and tablets has nearly surpassed those of home computers (Pariona, 2016).

These digital advances have made globalization possible, allowing businesses to operate more efficiently with increased opportunities to find and share information. We hold virtual meetings instead of traveling to conduct face-to-face business, and some of us even work from home as telecommuters. These advances have also had a significant impact on our individual lifestyles and daily routines. Instead of going to the shopping mall, or even the grocery store, we buy our goods from online retail merchants and order services from a company's online website. As a student reading this text, you may even have taken some, if not all, of your courses through an online university program. Advanced classroom technologies have enhanced learning opportunities for all students. Where digital technology saves us time and helps us stay connected and in touch, many people find it increasingly difficult to keep their personal and professional lives separate. This can lead to digital overload, causing stress and job burnout.

The advancing technological contributions to science are continually growing, notably in the areas of artificial intelligence and robot design. The evolution of three-dimensional (3D) printing and ongoing developments in computer design, such as Digital Twin (Newman, 2019), where providers and manufacturers can test the impact of potential change on the performance of a health care procedure by experimenting on a virtual version of the system (person or device), continue to change the landscape of the industrial sector.

As mentioned previously, artificial intelligence (AI) will play a major role in the health care industry due to the availability of big data and the drive to lower health care costs. Research firm Markets and Markets predicts that AI in health care will grow from $2.1 billion today to a $36 billion industry globally by 2025 (2019: Changes and Trends in Health Care, n.d.). Implications for practicing SLPs and audiologists include chat-based digital services in which users have a conversation with a chat-bot, software designed to understand and respond to natural language inputs. Through the use of coaching conversations, clinicians can provide an opportunity to apply their knowledge and skills together with AI to engage patients in meaningful conversations about their health.

The medical industry has also been impacted by the Digital Revolution. Genomic medicine, the use of genetic information for personalized treatment plans, will have long-lasting implications in the provision of health care. The use of simulated patients, virtual reality and augmented reality (VR/AR) to train health care professionals, the delivery of health care services through telepractice, and keeping sensitive information secure will certainly play important roles in the training of future health care providers.

New devices for hearing amplification and augmentative communication will be of special interest to SLPs and audiologists. Currently, audiologists are expressing concern regarding the future of the discipline as more hearing technologies are available to the public through smartphones and retail outlets. Although our patients may have increased access to better communication, there is a general concern that some patients may be at risk without the advice of a trained professional. The same is true for augmentative and alternative communication options that are readily available to patients and families on smartphone and tablet devices. What expertise is needed to guide these families? How can we be assured that they are being maximally used? What responsibility do we have as a profession to shape these various technologies and their availability? These are challenging times!

The positive and negative aspects of the impact of the Digital Revolution on human lives will continue to be discussed, explored, and analyzed as we move into the future. As audiologists and SLPs facing such challenges, we need to be well prepared to engage in critical thinking that supports our decision-making ability in a world of rapid technological advancement. Technology is discussed in more depth in Chapter 27.

Twenty-First Century Trends and Issues

Trends in Health Care

Health care in the United States is undergoing rapid transformation, a result of a range of reasons—political, demographic, and technological being among the key drivers. Recent health care legislation and regulation have created a shift in reimbursement policy, moving away from provider-centered payment models toward patient-centered models, with Medicare, Medicaid, and private health insurance being most relevant to practicing SLPs and audiologists. In addition, provider shortages, increasing costs paired with a lack of affordability, even for those with good insurance, and an aging population are changing the face of health care as we know it.

The costs associated with health care continue to increase while both public and private insurance reimbursement rates for providers fall below the actual cost of providing services. Many physicians view audiology and speech-language pathology as low priority services as they attempt to conserve limited financial resources. As a result, referrals and authorizations for evaluations and treatment are decreasing and jobs in physicians' offices and other health care facilities may be eliminated or reduced to an as-needed basis. See Chapter 19 for further discussion of access to services.

Another factor influencing reimbursement for health care services is that the age-old concept that "more care means better care" is no longer an accepted tenet in the evolving health care industry. The trend is moving in the direction of value-based reimbursement where quality of service is favored versus fee for service, which only rewards volume. Patient satisfaction surveys have more and more influence on insurance reimbursement and this has important implications for practitioners.

The number of health professionals working in home health care will continue to grow as the demand for treatment outside the traditional doctor's office is on the rise. A 2018 survey conducted by the Price Waterhouse Coopers Health Research Institute showed that 54 percent of respondents would prefer "hospital care at home if it cost less than the traditional option" (Price Waterhouse Coopers, n.d.). With the rise of home health care organizations, there is a corresponding decline in the occupancy of skilled nursing facilities (SNFs). In addition, providers and payers are pressuring SNFs to reduce

lengths of patient stays, so SNFs are looking at other services such as assisted living and adult day care, so that they can admit more clinically complex (therefore, more profitable) patients to increase their occupancy (2019: Changes and Trends in Healthcare, n.d.). These growing trends are changing job opportunities for service providers, including audiologists and SLPs.

Health information technologies (HITs) and electronic health records (EHRs) are other changes in health care that continue to shape what we do as audiologists and SLPs. Currently, there is a proliferation of different EHR and HIT options. Even though these systems are designed to increase reliability of access to records and clinician productivity, they can pose barriers as well. One challenge is the way we serve our patients. Many of us have experienced a health care provider who has spent more time looking at a computer screen than interacting with the patient. Additionally, records are not easily transferred across different EHR platforms, posing roadblocks to patients as they seek care, particularly from specialty providers.

One of our most important tasks as SLPs and audiologists is to ensure that our services are mandated and maintained at reasonable rates. As the population ages, we also need to ensure that our practices enable and prolong independent living, support access to needed services, support our patients' participation in decision making regarding their lives and care, and help them maintain a positive quality of life for as long as possible. We need to be not only skilled and knowledgeable clinicians but also ready to employ our skills as advocates on behalf of our patients. Chapters 15 and 19 provide further discussion of services in health care.

Trends in Education

The educational landscape continues to transform, with political influences and demographic shifts as major drivers. Federal, state, and local funding for schools influence the quantity and quality of services provided by school-based SLPs and audiologists. Government-mandated accountability with an emphasis on standardized testing to measure student achievement has provided data for important decision making, including systems used for teacher evaluations.

The paperwork burden and the demands that come with ever-increasing caseloads and responsibilities assigned to school-based service providers continue to be hot buttons and are the focus of advocacy efforts by professional organizations such as the American-Speech-Language Hearing Association (ASHA, n.d.-a). The use of multi-tiered systems of supports, such as Response to Intervention (RTI), the importance of using a variety of service delivery models, incorporating evidence-based practice (EBP), and engaging in interprofessional collaboration in the diagnosis and treatment of school-aged children have been noteworthy initiatives in the evolution of school-based services in recent years.

Many school districts have increased the hiring and use of paraprofessionals to ease the caseload burden and to support the work of school-based service providers. SLPs and audiologists will need to develop their knowledge and skills in supervision, particularly in the area of ethical accountability as they work with speech-language pathology assistants (SLPAs) and audiology assistants. You will find further discussion of support personnel in Chapter 13.

As in health care, technology continues to play a major role in education for SLPs and audiologists working in schools. Software programs designed specifically for special education documentation and record-keeping have become the norm. Technology tools that support oral, audio, and written skills allow students of all ages to express themselves beyond the capacity of their writing abilities. Much work with critical thinking can also be done in this manner when tools such as Seesaw blogs (https://web.seesaw.me/blogs/) and flipgrid (https://info.flipgrid.com/) are used to support learning.

Issues related to school safety and information and training on trauma-informed practices will continue to increase as education professionals seek resources for responding to traumatic events that affect children of all ages. Recent studies show that 25% of children under the age of 16 have experienced trauma in their lives (2019, National Child Traumatic Stress Network). Children bring their outside personal experiences with them to school, and educators are learning to adapt classroom management strategies, instructional supports, and school climate to support children who have experienced trauma to help them achieve success. Chapters 22 (Safety in the Workplace) and 28 (Counseling) will explore these issues more fully.

Audiologists and SLPs in the schools continue to play a major role in helping educators adopt more inclusive practices in education. Such practices are designed to enable special education students at all grade levels and with a wide range of needs to be involved in and make progress in the least restrictive environment (LRE). To that end, service delivery models that place an emphasis on working with students in their natural environment, in addition to interprofessional collaboration, are gradually taking the place of the more traditional medical (pull-out) model.

As educational trends continue to evolve, SLPs and audiologists will need evidence-based studies that demonstrate the quantitative and qualitative differences we make in students' lives. Practices that help students improve their ability to participate productively in education and employment will continue to be the focus

of school-based service providers as we move into the coming years. See Chapter 16 for further discussion of policy and service delivery in education.

Economic Trends

The United States is a highly developed nation, with the world's biggest economy in terms of gross domestic product (GDP), representing around one-fourth of the global GDP. At the time of this writing, economic indicators show that U.S. GDP growth will continue to slow from 2.1% in 2019 to 1.9% in 2020 and 1.8% in 2021. The projected slowdown in 2019 and beyond is a side effect of the trade war, a key component of the current administration's economic policies (Amadeo, 2019).

We have been experiencing a gradual economic recovery since the Great Recession of 2007–2009. The 2019 unemployment rate is 3.7% and is expected to be 3% in 2020 and 3.9% in 2021. It is of note that these statistics reflect a unique trait to this recovery, the fact that our basic structural unemployment has actually increased. Many workers are part-time but would prefer full-time work, and some have been out of work for so long that it is unlikely they will be able to return to the high-paying jobs they held previously. It led some workers to delay retirement or to come out of retirement and rejoin the labor force, while others retired earlier than planned (Bosworth & Burtless, 2016). In addition, most job growth is in low-paying retail and food service industries as opposed to the professional sector. As the labor force aged 55 to 64 is approaching retirement, their unemployment status can affect the financial security of future retirees, and this is an important consideration for those entering the workforce in the near future.

Inflation is 1.8% in 2019 and is expected to rise to 2% in 2020 and 2021 and is not considered to be a serious threat to the economy at the time of this writing (Amadeo, 2019).

In its occupational outlook report, the Bureau of Labor Statistics (BLS) predicts a full recovery from the recession in 2020, with 88% of all occupations expected to experience growth. A significant part of the growth is expected to occur in health care, and professions related to social assistance as the American population ages. Substantial increases are also expected to occur in education, technical, and scientific consulting, among others (U.S. Bureau of Labor Statistics, n.d.).

Employment prospects for SLPs and audiologists in all settings are excellent. According to the BLS, jobs for SLPs are expected to grow 18% from 2016 to 2026, while jobs for audiologists are expected to grow 21%. The average growth rate for all occupations is 7%. In 2018, the median pay for SLPs was $77,510 per year, or $37.26 per hour. For audiologists, it was $75,920 per year, or $36.50 per hour (U.S. Bureau of Labor

Statistics, n.d.). Chapters 10, 11 and 12 provide more detail on issues related to employment for audiologists and SLPs.

Demographic Trends and Globalization

The world's population is over 7 billion, with the largest populations in China and India (Current World Population, n.d.). The United States ranks third and its population continues to grow, in large part due to immigration. With an increase of 8.976 million in the past 5 years, the 2019 estimated population of the United States is 329.6712 million. According to a 2015 report, 8.5% of people worldwide (617 million) are aged 65 and over, and this group continues to grow at an unprecedented rate. This percentage is projected to jump to nearly 17% of the world's population (1.6 billion) by 2050 (He, Goodkind, & Kowal, 2016), outpacing the growth of the younger population over the next 35 years. In 2015, one in six people in the world lived in a more developed country, with more than a third of the world population aged 65 and older and over half of the world population aged 85 and older living in these countries. Among these older groups, there was a higher number of women than men.

Population aging, while due primarily to lower fertility rates, has created many new challenges, particularly in the health care arena. How many years can older people expect to live in good health? What are the chronic diseases that they may have to deal with? How long can they live independently? How many of them are still working? Will they have sufficient economic resources to last their lifetimes? Can they afford health care costs? (An Aging World, 2015).

Audiologists and SLPs working with this growing population will need to be prepared to face these challenges as they apply to their practice settings. As with all populations, providing the highest quality services that support hearing, communication, and swallowing will need to be the focus of continuing education as trends in best practices continue to evolve with this group. Finally, new graduates will need to be mindful of some of these challenges as they contemplate their own retirement years in planning their career paths.

The Census Report predicts that the foreign-born segment of the population of the United States will represent a substantial share of the general population growth, achieving 19% by 2060 (U.S. Population 2019, n.d.). English is the most commonly spoken language (83%), while 12% of the population speak Spanish and 0.69% speak Chinese. Growth of the Hispanic and Asian populations are expected to almost triple in the next 40 years. Additionally, according to the National Center for Education Statistics, bilingual/multilingual populations have a proportionately greater need for speech and language diagnostic and intervention services. (National Center for Education Statistics, 2015).

As our population becomes increasingly diverse in terms of age, spoken languages, race, ethnicity, religion, education, gender, sexual orientation, gender identity, and socio-economic factors, it is imperative that we demonstrate cultural competence in meeting the needs of those we serve. See Chapter 25, "Working with Culturally and Linguistically Diverse Populations," for further discussion.

Evidence-Based Practice

The foundations of best practices in audiology and speech-language pathology are rooted in evidence. EBP is the integration of: (a) clinical expertise/expert opinion, (b) external scientific evidence, and (c) client/patient/ caregiver perspectives (ASHA n.d.-b). What does this mean to the new clinician who wants to ensure the highest quality of services, yet lives in a world where "facts" are questioned, and empirical data is politicized?

The policymakers in both the insurance industry and government have implemented EBP requirements for reimbursement, making research in communication sciences and disorders (CSD) all the more important. Audiologists and SLPs can access sources for EBP guidance including bibliographies, evidence maps, and summaries of treatment efficacy in a wide range of clinical areas from ASHA (https://www.asha.org/) and the Academy of Neurologic Communication Disorders and Sciences (ANCDS; https://ancds.org), among others. ASHA and other organizations continue to build resources for professionals as the demands evolve for accountability and quality. See Chapter 8 for more discussion of EBP.

Summary

The professions of speech-language pathology and audiology are dynamic and diverse much like the patients that we work with. This chapter discussed some of the most dynamic changes, trends, and issues that are likely to affect your practices. Included in this discussion was information on technology and the digital revolution, trends in health care and education, economic influences, demographic shifts and globalization warranting cultural sensitivity and competency, and evidence-based practice needs. Knowledge of these topics is essential for applying analytical and critical reflection when making decisions that affect the lives of those we serve. It is the intention of this chapter and book, much like the overall goal of SLPs and audiologists to "optimally communicate" the present and projected practices that will shape our expertise and professional necessity long into the future.

Critical Thinking

1. Twenty-five years from now, what will professional historians say about the professions of audiology or speech-language pathology? What factors do you think will affect our development and our provision of services across settings and client groups?

2. Think about the geographical area in which you work or are likely to work. What comprises the demographics of this area? How have the demographics changed in the past 10 years? How should you prepare to work with the variety of client groups in your geographic area?

3. What technology do you use now in your clinical practice? How does it facilitate the quality and efficiency of what you do? What advances would you like to see in technology to help you provide better science for our professions or service to our clients?

4. How should our pre-professional and continuing education focus on social and economic changes in our society? How does knowledge about these areas improve your delivery of speech-language, swallowing, or hearing services?

5. What opportunities have you had for serving clients from diverse backgrounds? How well prepared do you feel to do this? What can you do to enhance your skills?

6. Why does keeping up on both domestic and worldwide current events help you as a professional audiologist or SLP?

7. How does globalization affect you as a clinician? What opportunities have you had to interact with professionals around the world? What might you do to develop such interactions?

References

2019: Changes and Trends in Health Care. (2019, April 30). Retrieved from https://casamba.net/regulatory-resources/2019-changes-and-trends-in-healthcare/

Amadeo, K. (2019, May 15). *U.S. economic outlook for 2019 and beyond.* Retrieved from https://www.thebalance.com/us-economic-outlook-3305669

American Speech-Language-Hearing Association. (n.d.-a). *Advocacy: Representing audiologists and speech-language pathologists.* Retrieved from https://www.asha.org/advocacy/

American Speech-Language-Hearing Association. (n.d.-b). *Evidence-based practice (EBP).* Retrieved from https://www.asha.org/research/ebp/evidence-based-practice/

Bosworth, B. P., & Burtless, G. (2016, July 28). *Impact of the Great Recession on retirement trends in industrialized countries.* Retrieved from https://www.brookings.edu/research/impact-of-the-great-recession-on-retirement-trends-in-industrialized-countries/

Current World Population. (n.d.). Retrieved from https://www.worldometers.info/world-population/

Digital Revolution. (2019, May 1). Retrieved from https://en.wikipedia.org/wiki/Digital_Revolution

Facer, K., & Sandford, R. (2010, January 12). *The next 25 years?: Future scenarios and future directions for education and technology.* Retrieved from https://onlinelibrary.wiley.com/doi/full/10.1111/j.1365-2729.2009.00337.x

He, W., Goodkind, D., & Kowal, P. (2016). An aging world: 2015. *International Population Reports.* Retrieved from https://www.census.gov/content/dam/Census/library/publications/2016/demo/p95-16-1.pdf

National Center for Education Statistics. (2015). Elementary and secondary education. *Digest of Education Statistics.* Available at https://nces.ed.gov/pubs2016/2016014_2.pdf

The National Child Traumatic Stress Network. (n.d.). Retrieved from https://www.nctsn.org/audiences/school-personnel

Newman, D. (2019, January 04). *Top 6 digital transformation trends in healthcare for 2019.* Retrieved from https://www.forbes.com/sites/danielnewman/2019/01/03/top-6-digital-transformation-trends-in-healthcare-for-2019/#2c6796986911

Pariona, A. (2016, November 1). *What was the digital revolution?* Retrieved from https://www.worldatlas.com/articles/what-was-the-digital-revolution.html

Price Waterhouse Coopers. (n.d.). U.S. PwC. Retrieved from https://www.pwc.com/

U.S. Bureau of Labor Statistics. (n.d.). Retrieved from https://www.bls.gov/

U.S. Population 2019. (n.d.). Retrieved from https://uspopulation2019.com/

Appendix 1–A

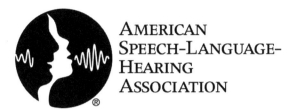

AMERICAN
SPEECH-LANGUAGE-
HEARING
ASSOCIATION

SCOPE OF PRACTICE IN AUDIOLOGY

AD HOC COMMITTEE ON THE SCOPE OF PRACTICE IN AUDIOLOGY

ABOUT THIS DOCUMENT

This scope of practice document is an official policy of the American Speech-Language-Hearing Association (ASHA) defining the breadth of practice within the profession of audiology. The *Audiology Scope of Practice* document has not been updated since 2004. The aim of this document is to reflect the current and evolving clinical practice in audiology. Such changes include, but are not limited to, telehealth, discussion of hearing technologies beyond traditional hearing devices (e.g., over-the-counter [OTC]), and personal sound amplification products (PSAPs). Additional updates in advancements in hearing device implantation, vestibular assessment and rehabilitation, hearing preservation, educational audiology, and interoperative monitoring practice are included.

This document was developed by the ASHA Ad Hoc Committee on the Scope of Practice in Audiology. Committee members were Julie Honaker (chair), Robert Beiter, Kathleen Cienkowski, Gregory Mannarelli, Maryrose McInerney, Tena McNamara, Jessica Sullivan, Julie Verhoff, Robert Fifer (board liaison), and Pam Mason (ex officio). This document was approved by the ASHA Board of Directors on August 20, 2018.

TABLE OF CONTENTS

- Introduction
- Definition of Terms
- Statement of Purpose
- Audiology Service Delivery Areas
- Additional Areas of Audiology Practice
- Works Cited
- Works Consulted
- Resources

INTRODUCTION

DEFINITION OF TERMS

Audiologist: By virtue of education, training, licensure, and certification, audiologists engage in professional practice in the areas of hearing and balance assessment, nonmedical treatment, and (re)habilitation. Audiologists provide patient-centered care in the prevention, identification, diagnosis, and evidence-based intervention and treatment of hearing, balance, and other related disorders for people of all ages. Hearing, balance, and other related disorders are complex, with medical, psychological, physical, social, educational, and employment implications. Treatment services require audiologists to know existing and emerging technologies, intervention strategies, and interpersonal skills to counsel and guide individuals and their family members through the (re)habilitative process. Audiologists provide professional and personalized services to minimize the negative impact of these disorders, leading to improved outcomes and quality of life. Audiologists are licensed and/or regulated in all 50 states and in the District of Columbia.

Scope of Practice in Audiology

Balance: Includes all aspects of equilibrium, specific to the balance and vestibular systems, both peripheral and central. This includes management of symptoms and signs consistent with both peripheral and central etiologies.

Hearing: Includes all peripheral and central functional components of sound reception and analytic processing. This also includes management of symptoms and sequelae of disorders of the auditory system such as tinnitus, hyperacusis, misophonia, and other auditory perceptual disorders.

Hearing, balance, and other related disorders: Throughout this document, the broad term hearing, balance, and other related disorders is used to reflect all areas of assessment and intervention within the audiology scope of practice.

IEP/IFSP/504 Plan: The *Individualized Education Plan* (IEP) is a written statement that guides the educational plan for a child, ages 3–21, in accordance with the Individuals with Disabilities Education Act of 2004 (IDEA). The *Individual Family Service Plan* (IFSP) guides the early intervention services for a child with disabilities and their family. The IEP and IFSP are developed, reviewed, and revised in accordance with federal law. Also, under the IDEA, a student with disabilities is ensured a Free and Appropriate Public Education (FAPE) as well as monitoring the student's progress. The parents/guardians play a central role in the IEP/IFSP progress (IDEA, 2004). A *504 Plan* is a plan developed to ensure that a child with a disability receives accommodations for a general education classroom.

Individuals: The term *individuals* is used throughout the document to refer to students, clients, patients, children, adults, families, and caregivers who are served by the audiologist.

Interprofessional collaborative practice (IPP): This term stems from the World Health Organization's (WHO) framework of looking at a health condition alongside a person's functional ability, social community, and personal goals, in concert with the perspective of other health care providers. Health care professionals must communicate and collaborate with each other and the individual receiving care, along with the individual's family or support system. This is called *interprofessional collaborative practice (IPP)*. The blending of skill sets results in better outcomes, improved quality of life, and greater satisfaction. It also minimizes the cost of care and improves the individual's safety and sense of well-being (Skevington, Lotfy, & O'Connell, 2004).

Management: This refers to the organization and coordination of activities in order to develop and provide relevant audiologic care for individuals. These activities include assessment techniques and treatment/intervention strategies. Appropriate management aids in the achievement of goals and objectives set forth for individuals with hearing and/or vestibular difficulties.

Other related disorders: This term is intended to reflect that audiologists with the appropriate training can use their skills and techniques to contribute to the knowledge, understanding, and overall care of individuals with other disorders outside the hearing and balance system. A few purely illustrative examples of this could include (a) performing a battery of facial nerve function tests on a patient with a facial paresis or (b) performing a battery of auditory tests on a patient with a developmental or cognitive delay. This type of care is increasingly used as a part of an interprofessional collaborative practice team.

Person-centered care: This approach considers the whole person, taking into account more than the physical symptoms of a specific, discreet disorder. It includes psychological, social, cultural, and environmental factors. Optimal outcomes are achieved when working collaboratively—along with

Scope of Practice in Audiology

input and accountability—with the individual, supportive family members and with fellow professionals.

Quality of life: WHO defines *quality of life* as an individual's perception of their position in life in the context of the culture and value systems in which they live and in relation to their goals, expectations, standards, and concerns. It is a broad-ranging concept affected in a complex way by the person's physical health, psychological state, personal beliefs, social relationships, and relationship to salient features of their environment (Skevington et al., 2004; WHOQOL Group, 1994).

Telehealth: the use of electronic information and telecommunications technologies to support long-distance clinical health care, patient and professional health-related education, public health, and health administration.

Working at the top of license: This is the concept that audiologists should engage in patient care activities that require their (i.e., the audiologists') specialized level of expertise and skill. Other less skilled tasks may be delegated to other individuals (e.g., assistants, automated systems, and/or individuals and family members; Burkhard and Trembath, 2015). This would greatly decrease the cost of achieving outcomes (and also increase family satisfaction by decreasing the inconvenience, cost, and overall burden of care; ASHA, 2013). Working at the top of the license is not meant to imply nor does it prohibit audiologists from completing tasks that are not at the top of the license.

Treatment/Intervention: These terms refer to the application of care given to an individual to directly address hearing and/or vestibular difficulties. *Management* (defined above) is the overall coordination of activities that address the needs of individuals. *Treatment/intervention* is one of those direct activities.

STATEMENT OF PURPOSE

The purpose of the *Scope of Practice in Audiology* is as follows:

1. Delineate areas of professional practice.
2. Inform others (e.g., health care providers, educators, consumers, payers, regulators, and the general public) about professional roles and responsibilities of qualified providers.
3. Support audiologists in the provision of high-quality, evidence-based services to individuals with hearing and balance concerns.
4. Support audiologists working at the top of their license.
5. Support audiologists in the conduct and dissemination of research.
6. Guide the educational preparation and professional development of audiologists to provide safe and effective services.
7. Inform members of ASHA, certificate holders, and students of the activities for which certification in audiology is required in accordance with the ASHA Code of Ethics (ASHA, 2016). Each practitioner evaluates his or her own experiences with pre-service education, practice, mentorship and supervision, and continuing professional development. As a whole, these experiences define the scope of competence for each individual. Audiologists should engage in only those aspects of the profession that are within her or his professional competence. ASHA members and ASHA-certified professionals are bound by the ASHA Code of Ethics (ASHA, 2016) to provide services that are consistent with the scope of their competence, education, and experience.

Scope of Practice in Audiology

By virtue of training and practice, audiology is a unique profession that specializes in and provides comprehensive diagnostic and nonmedical treatment services for hearing and balance disorders, and related impairments. These services are provided to individuals across the entire age span from birth through adulthood; these individuals include persons of different races, genders, religions, national origins, and sexual orientations. This position statement is not intended to be exhaustive; however, the activities described in this document reflect current practice within the profession. Practice activities related to emerging clinical, technological, and scientific developments are not precluded from consideration as part of the scope of practice of an audiologist. If the audiologist can document appropriate training for new and emerging clinical or technological procedures that fall under the heading of auditory, balance and other related disorders, then such innovations and advances may be incorporated into the *Audiology Scope of Practice*. Audiologists are trained in all areas of clinical service delivery; however, they commonly have one or more specific areas of specialization. ASHA also recognizes that credentialed professionals in related disciplines have knowledge, skills, and experience that could be applied to some areas within the Audiology Scope of Practice. Defining the scope of practice of audiologists is not meant to exclude other appropriately credentialed postgraduate professionals from rendering services in overlapping practice areas. Often, these partially overlapping skill sets can result in excellent opportunities for IPP.

Audiologists must achieve required competencies in ancillary professional areas. These areas are distinct from but contribute to diagnostic and nonmedical treatment activities. They are very important areas in which to maintain high standards of clinical service. Examples include cultural and linguistic competencies, IPP, patient- and family-centered care, supervision, and mentoring and knowledge of federal and state statutes and regulations.

This scope of practice does not supersede existing state licensure laws or affect the interpretation or implementation of such laws. It should serve, however, as a model for the development or modification of licensure laws.

The goals of this updated *Scope of Practice in Audiology* of the American Speech-Language-Hearing Association (ASHA) are as follows:

1. Revise the current scope of practice for audiologists based on new and evolving training, skills, technology, and literature within the profession.
2. Align our professional activities with the evolving best practice models in audiology within the overall health care field.
3. Serve as a resource for other agencies, professional organizations, and the general public (e.g., federal, state, nongovernmental organizations, licensing and credentialing bodies, etc.).
4. Provide a language and framework that is applicable for all audiologists, regardless of professional setting.

AUDIOLOGY SERVICE DELIVERY AREAS

Clinical service delivery areas include all aspects of hearing, balance, and other related disorders that impact hearing and balance, including areas of tinnitus, cognition, and auditory processing for individuals across the lifespan. Audiologists play critical roles in health literacy (https://www.asha.org/slp/healthliteracy); in the screening, diagnosis, and treatment of hearing, balance, and other related disorders; and in the use of the *International Classification of Functioning, Disability and Health* (ICF; WHO, 2014) to develop functional goals and collaborative practice. As technology and science advance, the areas of assessment and intervention related to hearing, balance,

Scope of Practice in Audiology

and other related disorders grow accordingly. Clinicians should stay current with advances in hearing and balance practice by regularly reviewing the research literature; regularly consulting the Practice Management (https://www.asha.org/practice/) section of the ASHA website, including the Practice Portal (https//www.asha.org/practice-portal/); and regularly participating in continuing education to supplement advances in the profession and to provide additional information that can inform the Scope of Practice in Audiology.

DIAGNOSTICS FOR HEARING, BALANCE, AND OTHER RELATED DISORDERS

Audiologists are responsible for the assessment of hearing, balance, and other related disorders, including tinnitus and auditory processing, across the lifespan that includes the following:

- Administration and interpretation of clinical case history.
- Administration and interpretation of behavioral, electroacoustic, and electrophysiologic measures of the peripheral and central auditory, balance, and other related systems.
- Administration and interpretation of diagnostic screening that includes measures to detect the presence of hearing, balance, and other related disorders. Additional screening measures of mental health and cognitive impairment should be used to assess, treat, and refer (American Academy of Audiology, 2013; Beck & Clark, 2009; Li et al., 2014; Shen, Anderson, Arehart, & Souza, 2016; Sweetow, 2015; Weinstein, 2017, 2018).

This assessment includes measurement and professional interpretation of sensory and motor evoked potentials, electromyography, and other electrodiagnostic tests for purposes of neurophysiologic intraoperative monitoring and cranial nerve assessment.

Diagnostic measures should be modified based on patient age and on cognitive and physical abilities of the individuals being assessed. Case findings of dementia, memory, vision, and balance (falling risk) should be used when difficulty in communication and or change of behavior is evident (Beck & Clark, 2009; Li et al., 2014; Shen et al., 2016; Sweetow, 2015; Weinstein, 2017; Weinstein, 2018). Assessment extends beyond diagnostic evaluation and includes informational counseling, interpretation of results, and intervention.

Assessment is accomplished using quantitative and qualitative measurements—including standardized testing, observations, and procedures and appropriately calibrated instrumentation—and leads to the diagnosis of abnormal audiologic and/or balance function. Interpretation of test results includes diagnostic statements as to the probable locus of impairment and functional ability within the hearing, balance, and other related systems under assessment.

Audiologists collaborate with other professionals and serve on care teams to help reduce the perceived burden of hearing, balance, and other related disorders and maximize quality of life for individuals.

TREATMENT FOR HEARING, BALANCE, AND OTHER RELATED DISORDERS

Audiologists provide comprehensive audiologic (re)habilitation services for individuals and their families across the lifespan who are experiencing hearing, balance, or other related disorders (e.g., tinnitus and auditory processing disorder). Intervention encompasses the following:

- Auditory training for sound identification and discrimination

Scope of Practice in Audiology

- Cerumen management
- Communication strategies (e.g., environmental manipulation, mode of communication)
- Counseling
- Manual communication
- (Re)habilitation related to auditory disorders
- Self-advocacy for personal needs or systems change
- Speechreading
- Strategies to address other related disorders (tinnitus, misophonia)
- Technology interventions
- Vestibular rehabilitation to include management of benign paroxysmal positional vertigo as well as peripheral and/or central vestibular disorders

In this role, audiologists

- design, implement, and document delivery of service in accordance with best available practice;
- screen for possible cognitive disorders;
- case-finding for dementia;
- provide culturally and linguistically appropriate services;
- integrate the highest quality available research evidence with practitioner expertise as well as with individual preference and values in establishing treatment goals;
- utilize treatment data to determine effectiveness of services and guide decisions;
- deliver the appropriate frequency and intensity of treatment utilizing best available practice;
- engage in treatment activities that are within the scope of the professional's competence; and
- collaborate with other professionals in the delivery of services to ensure the highest quality of interventions.

As part of the comprehensive audiologic (re)habilitation program, audiologists evaluate, select, fit, verify, validate, and monitor the performance of a variety of technologies interventions for hearing, balance, and other related disorders. Audiologists provide individual counseling and public education about the benefits and/or limitations of various different classes of devices. Treatment utilizing technology interventions include but are not limited to other emerging technologies:

- Auditory brainstem implants (ABIs)
- Assistive listening devices
- Balance-related devices
- Classroom audio distribution systems
- Cochlear implants
- Custom ear impressions and molds for hearing devices, hearing protection, in-ear monitors, swim plugs, communication devices, stenosis stents, and so forth
- Hearing aids
- Hearing assistive technology
- Hearing protection
- Large-area amplification systems
- Middle ear implants
- Over-the-counter (OTC) hearing aids

- Osseointegrated devices (OIDs),bone-anchored devices, and bone conduction devices
- Personal sound amplification products (PSAPs)
- Remote microphone systems
- Tinnitus devices (both stand-alone and integrated with hearing aids)

Treatment for children also includes developmental and educational interventions such as the following:

- Participation in the development and implementation of an IEP/IFSP for school-age children or implementation of an IFSP for children birth to 36 months of age
- Participation in the development and implementation of a 504 plan
- Measurement of noise levels in educational institutions and recommendations for noise reduction modification

EARLY HEARING DETECTION AND INTERVENTION (EHDI)

Audiologists provide screening, assessment, and treatment services for infants and young children with hearing-related disorders and their families. Services include the following:

- Apply Joint Committee on Infant Hearing (JCIH) protocols for early detection and intervention of infants and children with hearing loss (American Academy of Pediatrics, Joint Committee on Infant Hearing, 2007)
- Establish, manage, and/or review programs following the EHDI protocol
- Provide training and supervision to support personnel
- Monitor the program's outcome measures for quality assurance
- Perform audiological diagnostics to confirm or rule out the presence of a hearing loss
- Provide early intervention treatment for hearing loss to enhance communication and to improve cognitive and social skills
- Upon diagnosis of hearing loss, ensure that the child and family are enrolled in an appropriate early intervention program
- Provide comprehensive information about family support, training, and communication options
- Provide education to community/hospital personnel
- Collaborate with other professionals and with parent groups

EDUCATIONAL AUDIOLOGY

Audiologists in educational settings provide a full spectrum of hearing services to support academic and social achievement for school-age children, adolescents, young adults, and their families with hearing and related difficulties. Services include the following:

- Perform assessments and interpret the educational implications of the student's auditory needs. This also includes assessing and making appropriate recommendations as an advocate on behalf of students, ensuring least restrictive environments.
- Collect data from classroom assessments and from observations of students in various environments, and assess the impact of audiologic interventions on academic and social performance
- Collect data on classroom acoustics, and assess the impact on auditory perception

Scope of Practice in Audiology

- Ensure IPP with members of the school multidisciplinary team who facilitate listening, learning, and communication
- Collaborate with private sector/community-based audiologists and other professionals relative to the student's educational needs
- Provide instructional training for educators and staff for the development of skills needed in servicing students with hearing difficulties, which includes providing evidence and recommending support services and resources
- Provide (re)habilitative activities in collaboration with classroom teachers and other support personnel
- Monitor personal hearing instruments
- Recommend, fit, and manage hearing assistance technology
- Counsel children to promote personal responsibility, self-advocacy, and social awareness
- Counsel parents on management options, and provide resource information
- Assist with transitions between academic and vocational settings
- Manage school programs for the preservation of hearing and the prevention of hearing loss
- Manage and implement hearing screening programs

HEARING CONSERVATION AND PRESERVATION

The terms *hearing conservation* and *hearing preservation* are often used interchangeably. Both terms focus on preventing noise-induced hearing loss, whether from occupational or recreational sources. *Hearing conservation programs* are most often, although not exclusively, associated with occupational noise exposure and with U.S. Occupational Safety and Health Administration (OSHA) regulations (OSHA, 2002). In addition, hearing conservation programs have additional elements not found in hearing preservation programs: engineering controls for reducing environmental noise levels, administrative controls for monitoring hearing sensitivity levels, mandated use of hearing protection devices when needed, employee training about noise, the potential synergistic effects of chemical exposure combined with hazardous noise, and requirements for communication about hazards (e.g., warning signs, posting of signs in required hearing protection environments).

Hearing preservation programs focus on non-occupational settings and are most often intended to prevent hearing loss from occurring in individuals who enter the program with normal hearing sensitivity. Examples of hearing preservation programs may include (a) monitoring of auditory function for patients receiving chemotherapy or radiation therapy of the head or neck (University Health Network, 2018) or (b) providing education to students and young adults on the effects of recreational noise and methods to prevent hearing loss (see the Save Your Hearing Foundation at www.earpeacefoundation.org). Audiologists are uniquely qualified through education and training to design, establish, implement, and supervise hearing conservation programs for individuals of all ages in schools, in industry, and for the general public (Lipscomb, 1988).

Audiologists who engage in occupational hearing conservation must monitor current OSHA regulations (OSHA, 2002) regarding the impact of noise levels on hearing sensitivity. This extends to the distribution of, and instructions related to the use of, hearing protection devices.

Audiologists test hearing levels, determine functional hearing ability, measure noise levels, and assess the risk of incurring hearing loss from noise exposure from any source, including non-occupational and recreational noise (Franks, Stephenson, & Merry, 1996a, 1996b, 1996c).

Audiologists implement and manage all aspects of hearing conservation activities—including education, testing, and the determination of program effectiveness—and serve as the supervisor for OSHA and other U.S. government–mandated hearing conservation programs (Suter, 2003).

Audiologists educate the public and other professionals on how to recognize hazardous noise, ways of preventing noise-induced hearing loss, and the risks associated with reduced audibility when exposed to high-level sound.

TELEHEALTH

Telehealth, for audiology, is an alternative method of service delivery that encompasses both diagnostics and intervention services. Diagnostic services are provided using either synchronous or asynchronous protocols (i.e., *store and forward,* whereby data are collected, stored within a computer, and forwarded at a later time). Audiologists provide services using an evidence-based standard of care (American Telemedicine Association, 2017). When practicing via telehealth, audiologists provide care consistent with jurisdictional regulatory, licensing, credentialing and privileging, malpractice and insurance laws, and rules for their profession in both the jurisdiction in which they are practicing as well as the jurisdiction in which the patient is receiving care. The audiologists providing the service shall ensure compliance as required by appropriate regulatory and accrediting agencies (American Telemedicine Association, 2017).

Areas in which telehealth is a viable option include the following:

- Aural/auditory (re)habilitation
- Auditory evoked potentials
- Hearing aid and cochlear implant fitting/programming
- Hearing screening
- Otoacoustic emissions
- Otoscopy
- Pure-tone audiometry and speech recognition in noise
- Supervision of electrophysiology services (e.g., intraoperative monitoring and diagnostic examinations)
- Supervision of vestibular services (e.g., vestibular diagnostic examinations)
- Tympanometry
- Vestibular rehabilitation

COUNSELING

Audiologists counsel by providing information, education, guidance, and support to individuals and their families. Counseling includes discussion of assessment results and treatment options. Counseling facilitates decision making regarding intervention, management, educational environment, and mode of communication. The role of the audiologist in the counseling process includes interactions related to emotions, thoughts, feelings, and behaviors that result from living with hearing, balance, and other related disorders.

Audiologists engage in the following activities when counseling individuals and their families:

- Providing informational counseling regarding interpretation of assessment outcomes and treatment options
- Empowering individuals and their families to make informed decisions related to their plan of care
- Educating the individual, the family, and relevant community members
- Providing support and/or access to peer-to-peer groups for individuals and their families
- Providing individuals and their families with skills that enable them to become self-advocates
- Providing adjustment counseling related to the psychosocial impact on the individual
- Referring individuals to other professionals when counseling needs fall outside those related to auditory, balance, and other related disorders.

ADDITIONAL AREAS OF AUDIOLOGY PRACTICE

Audiology is a dynamic profession, and the fact that the audiology scope of practice overlaps with those of other professionals is a reality in rapidly changing health care, education, industrial, and other environments. Hence, audiologists in various settings work collaboratively with other academic and/or health care professionals to make appropriate decisions for the benefit of individuals with hearing, balance, and other related disorders. This is known as *interprofessional collaborative practice (IPP)* and is defined as "members or students of two or more professions associated with health or social care, engaged in learning with, from and about each other" (Craddock, O'Halloran, Borthwick, & McPherson, 2006, p. 237). Similarly, "interprofessional education [often referred to as "IPE"] provides an ability to share skills and knowledge between professions and allows for a better understanding, shared values, and respect for the roles of other healthcare professionals" (Bridges, Davidson, Soule Odegard, Maki, & Tomkowiak, 2011, para. 5). The advantage of using IPP/IPE is that it broadens the care teams' depth of knowledge and understanding of the individual being evaluated and/or treated. This type of collaboration improves outcomes, efficiency, and safety through person-centered care.

RESEARCH

Audiologists conduct and participate in basic and applied/translational research related to auditory, balance, and other related disorders. This research is undertaken as a facility-specific effort or is coordinated across multiple settings. Audiologists engage in activities to ensure compliance with Institutional Review Boards, federal regulations, and international laws pertaining to research. Audiologists also collaborate with other researchers and pursue research funding through grants.

ADMINISTRATION AND LEADERSHIP

Audiologists administer programs in education, higher education, schools, health care, private practice, and other settings. In this capacity, they are responsible for making administrative decisions related to fiscal and personnel management, leadership, program design, program growth and innovation, professional development, compliance with laws and regulations, and cooperation with outside agencies in education and health care. Their administrative roles are not limited to audiology, as they engage in program administration across departments and at different levels within an institution. In addition, audiologists promote effective and manageable workloads in school settings, provide appropriate services under the Individuals with Disabilities Education Improvement Act of 2004 (IDEA, and engage in program design and development.

EDUCATION

Audiologists serve as educators, teaching students in academic institutions and teaching professionals through continuing education in professional development formats. This more formal teaching is in addition to the education that audiologists provide to individuals, families, caregivers, decision makers, and policy makers, which is described in other domains. In this role, audiologists

- serve as faculty at institutions of higher education, teaching courses at the undergraduate, graduate, and postgraduate levels;
- mentor students who are completing academic programs at all levels;
- provide academic training to students in related disciplines and students who are training to become audiology assistants; and
- provide continuing professional education to audiologists and to professionals in related disciplines.

ADVOCACY AND OUTREACH

Audiologists focus on upholding person-centered care in our complex health care and educational systems. Audiologists advocate for hearing, balance, and other related disorders needs of the individuals and families whom they serve.

Audiologists advocate for the profession and for individuals through a variety of mechanisms, including community awareness, prevention activities, health literacy, academic literacy, education, political action, and training programs. Advocacy promotes and facilitates access to communication, including the reduction of societal, cultural, and linguistic barriers. Audiologists perform a variety of activities related to advocacy and outreach, including the following:

- Advising regulatory and legislative agencies about the continuum of care for hearing, balance, and other related disorders
- Engaging decision makers at the local, state, and national levels for improved administrative and governmental policies affecting access to services for the diagnosis and treatment of hearing, balance, and other related disorders
- Advocating at the local, state, and national levels for funding for services, education, and research
- Participating in associations and organizations to advance the audiology profession
- Promoting and marketing professional services
- Consulting with industry in the development of products and instrumentation related to hearing, balance, and other related disorders
- Helping to recruit and retain audiologists with diverse backgrounds and interests
- Collaborating on advocacy objectives with other professionals/colleagues regarding mutual goals
- Serving as expert witnesses, when appropriate
- Educating individuals about communication; development; disorders pertaining to auditory, balance, and other related systems; and audiology services

Scope of Practice in Audiology

- Advocating for fair and equitable services, including accessibility for all individuals, especially the most vulnerable
- Providing case management and serving as a liaison for individuals and their families in order to meet educational and vocational programming needs
- Consulting with individuals, their families, professionals, public and private agencies, and governmental bodies on technology intervention, hearing assistive technology, interpreting services, and other relevant assistive technology needed to enhance communication
- Consulting with state education agencies, local school districts, and interdisciplinary teams on direct service and IFSP, IEP, and 504 plan development
- Advocating for appropriate reimbursement of services

CULTURAL COMPETENCY

Audiologists serve diverse populations, and this includes persons of different races, ages, genders, religions, national origins, and sexual orientations. Audiologists' caseloads include individuals from diverse ethnic, cultural, and linguistic backgrounds as well as persons with disabilities. Culturally based family and community dynamics should be included in the development of an appropriate treatment plan that includes consideration of diversity and evidence-based practice guidelines.

CLINICAL SUPERVISION/PRECEPTING

Supervision is broadly defined as overseeing and directing the work of others. The terms *clinical supervisor* and *clinical supervision* are often used in reference to the training and education of student clinicians, recognizing that supervision is part of the training and education process. However, clinical supervisors do more than oversee the work of the student clinician. They teach specific skills, clarify concepts, assist with critical thinking, conduct performance evaluations, mentor, advise, and model professional behavior (Council on Academic Programs in Communication Sciences and Disorders [CAPCSD], 2013). Supervision is a distinct area of practice; is the responsibility of audiologists; and crosses clinical, administrative, and technical spheres. Audiologists are responsible for supervising clinical externs/trainees, audiology assistants, credentialed technical staff, and other professional and administrative support personnel. Audiologists also supervise colleagues and peers. Audiologists acknowledge that supervision is integral in the delivery of hearing, balance, and other related services and that supervision advances the profession. Supervision involves education, mentorship, encouragement, counseling, and support across all supervisory roles. In this role, audiologists

- possess service delivery and professional practice skills necessary to guide the supervisee;
- apply the art and science of supervision to all stakeholders (i.e., those supervising and being supervised), recognizing that supervision contributes to workplace efficiency;
- seek advanced knowledge in the practice of effective supervision;
- establish supervisory relationships that are collegial in nature; and
- establish supervisory relationships that promote growth and independence while providing support and guidance.

INTERPROFESSIONAL EDUCATION AND INTERPROFESSIONAL PRACTICE (IPE/IPP)

According to ASHA's definition, *interprofessional education* (IPE) is an activity that occurs when two or more professions learn about, from, and with each other to enable effective collaboration and improve outcomes for individuals and families whom we serve (ASHA, n.d.-b). Similarly, *interprofessional collaborative practice* (IPP) occurs when multiple service providers from different professional backgrounds jointly provide comprehensive health care or educational services by working with individuals and their families, caregivers, and communities to deliver the highest quality of care across settings. When both IPE and IPP are used, we refer to this combined term as *IPE/IPP*.

BUSINESS MANAGEMENT

Audiology is a service profession to which principles of business must be applied for success in educational, health care, and industrial settings. For a business entity (profit or nonprofit) to be successful, good business practices are essential. Providing high-quality services that are consistent in type and amount with a person's needs and with professional and ethical standards is good business practice. It is important that revenues collected for services cover and exceed all expenses (e.g., salary, benefits, overhead). Audiologists must understand their individual responsibility for adhering to practice standards that financially support their organization. Each audiologist's daily decisions (clinical and nonclinical) affect the financial viability of his or her organization. Audiologists must remain compliant and current on policy changes related to billing and coding.

LEGAL/PROFESSIONAL CONSULTING

Audiologists may be called upon to provide expertise to other professionals, business, industry, courts, attorneys, public and private agencies, and/or individuals in all areas related to the profession of audiology. Consulting services include but are not limited to

- recommendations for occupational and recreational hearing preservation and conservation, education, and advocacy for policy development;
- quality assessment and improvement; and
- expert witness testimony or second opinion and/or independent evaluation for educational, health, worker's compensation, or other legal purposes.

WORKS CITED

American Academy of Audiology. (2013). Medicare Publishes 2013 Policy Changes. Retrieved from https://www.audiology.org/practice_management/reimbursement/medicare/ medicare-publishes-2013-policy-changes

American Academy of Pediatrics, Joint Committee on Infant Hearing. (2007). Year 2007 position statement: Principles and guidelines for early hearing detection and intervention programs. Pediatrics, 120, 898–921.

American Speech-Language-Hearing-Association. (n.d.-a). Health literacy. Retrieved from https://www.asha.org/SLP/healthliteracy/

Scope of Practice in Audiology

American Speech Language-Hearing Association. (n.d.-b). Interprofessional Education/Interprofessional Practice (IPE/IPP). Retrieved from https://www.asha.org/practice/interprofessional-education-practice/

American Speech-Language-Hearing Association Ad Hoc Committee on Reframing the Professions. (2013). Reframing the professions of speech-language pathology and audiology. Rockville, MD: Author.

American Speech-Language-Hearing-Association. (2016). Code of ethics [Ethics]. Retrieved from https://www.asha.org/code-of-ethics/

American Telemedicine Association. (2017). Principles for delivering telerehabilitation services. Retrieved from http://hub.americantelemed.org/resources/telemedicine-practice-guidelines

Beck, D.L., & Clark, J.L. (2009). Audition matters more as cognition declines: cognition matters more as audition declines. Audiology Today, March/April, 48-59.

Bridges, D. R., Davidson, R. A., Soule Odegard, P., Maki, I. V., & Tomkowiak, J. (2011). Interprofessional collaboration: Three best practice models of interprofessional education. Medical Education Online, 16(1). doi:10.3402/meo.v16i0.6035

Burkard, R., & Trembath, S. (2015, March). Practicing at the top of the audiology license. Retrieved from https://www.asha.org/Articles/Practicing-at-the-Top-of-the-Audiology-License/

Council on Academic Programs in Communication Sciences and Disorders. (2013). White paper: Preparation of speech-language pathology clinical educators. Retrieved from http://scotthall.dotster.com/capcsd/wp-content/uploads/2014/10/Preparation-of-Clinical-Educators-White-Paper.pdf

Craddock, D., O'Halloran, C., Borthwick, A., & McPherson, K. (2006). Interprofessional education in health and social care: Fashion or informed practice? Learning in Health and Social Care, 5, 220–242. doi:10.1111/j.1473-6861.2006.00135

Franks, J. R., Stephenson, M. R., & Merry, C. J. (1996a). Personal hearing protection devices. In J. R. Franks, M. R. Stephenson, & C. J. Merry (Eds.), Preventing occupational hearing loss: A practical guide (pp. 35–40) [DHHS (NIOSH) Pub. No. 96-110]. Cincinnati, OH: National Institute for Occupational Safety and Health. Retrieved from https://www.cdc.gov/niosh/docs/96-110/pdfs/96-110.pdf

Franks, J. R., Stephenson, M. R., & Merry, C.J. (1996b). Program evaluation. In J. R. Franks, M. R. Stephenson, & C. J. Merry (Eds.), Preventing occupational hearing loss: A practical guide (pp. 49–51) [DHHS (NIOSH) Pub. No. 96-110]. Cincinnati, OH: National Institute for Occupational Safety and Health. Retrieved from https://www.cdc.gov/niosh/docs/96-110/pdfs/96-110.pdf

Franks, J. R., Stephenson, M. R., & Merry, C.J. (1996c). Record keeping. J. R. Franks, M. R. Stephenson, & C. J. Merry (Eds.), Preventing occupational hearing loss: A practical guide (pp. 46–48) [DHHS (NIOSH) Pub. No. 96-110]. Cincinnati, OH: National Institute for Occupational Safety and Health. Retrieved from https://www.cdc.gov/niosh/docs/96-110/pdfs/96-110.pdf

Individuals with Disabilities Education Act of 2004, 20 U.S.C. § 1400 et seq. (2004).

Scope of Practice in Audiology

Li, C.-M., Zhang, X., Hoffman, H. J., Cotch, M. F., Themann, C. L., & Wilson, M. R. (2014). Hearing impairment associated with depression in US adults, National Health and Nutrition Examination Survey 2005–2010. JAMA Otolaryngology–Head & Neck Surgery, 140, 293–302. doi:10.1001/jamaoto.2014.42

Lipscomb, D. M. (Ed.). (1988). Hearing conservation in industry, schools, and the military. Boston, MA: College-Hill.

Occupational Safety and Health Administration (OSHA). (2002). Hearing conservation [OSHA Publication No. 3074]. Retrieved from https://www.osha.gov/Publications/osha3074.pdf

Save Your Hearing Foundation. (2018). Ear peace: An epidemic of noise-induced hearing loss (NIHL) is currently sweeping the United States! Retrieved from www.earpeacefoundation.org

Shen, J., Anderson, M. C., Arehart, K. H., & Souza, P. E. (2016). Using cognitive screening tests in audiology. American Journal of Audiology, 25, 319–331. doi:10.1044/2016_AJA-16-0032

Skevington, S. M., Lotfy, M., & O'Connell, K. A. (2004). The World Health Organization's WHOQOL-BREF Quality of Life Assessment: Psychometric properties and results of the international field trial. A report from the WHOQOL group. Quality of Life Research, 13(2), 299–310.

Suter, A. H. (2003). Standards and regulations. In E. H. Berger, L. H. Royster, J. D. Royster, D. P. Driscoll, & M. Layne (Eds.), The noise manual (5th ed). Fairfax, VA: American Industrial Hygiene Association.

Sweetow, R. W. (2015, July). Screening for cognitive disorders in older adults in the audiology clinic. Audiology Today, 27(4), 38–43.

University Health Network – Hearing and Balance Center. (2018). Retrieved from http://www.uhn.ca/PatientsFamilies/Health_Information/Health_Topics/Documents/Hearing_Preservation_Program.pdf#search=hearing%20preservation%20programs

Weinstein, B. E. (2017). Preventive care for dementia and hearing loss. The Hearing Journal, 70(9), 18–20.

Weinstein, B. E. (2018). A primer on dementia and hearing loss. Perspectives of the ASHA Special Interest Groups, 3, 18–27. Retrieved from https://perspectives.pubs.asha.org/article.aspx?articleid=2681069

WHOQOL Group. (1994). Development of the WHOQOL: Rationale and current status. International Journal of Mental Health, 23(3), 24–56. Retrieved from https://www.tandfonline.com/doi/abs/10.1080/00207411.1994.11449286

World Health Organization. (2014). International Classification of Functioning, Disability and Health. Geneva, Switzerland: Author.

WORKS CONSULTED

Adams, M. E., Kileny, P. R., Telian, S. A., El-Kashlan, H. K., Heidenreich, K. D., Mannarelli, G. R., & Arts, H. A. (2011). Electrocochleography as a diagnostic and intraoperative adjunct in superior semicircular canal dehiscence syndrome. *Otology & Neurotology, 32,* 1506–1512. doi:10.1097/MAO.0b013e3182382a7c

Adams, M. E., Marmor, S., Yueh, B., & Kane, R. L. (2017). Geographic variation in use of vestibular testing among Medicare beneficiaries. *Otolaryngology-Head and Neck Surgery, 156,* 312–320. doi:10.1177/0194599816676450

Ahmed, M. F., Goebel, J. A., & Sinks, B.C. (2009). Caloric test versus rotational sinusoidal harmonic acceleration and step-velocity tests in patients with and without suspected peripheral vestibulopathy. *Otology & Neurotology, 30,* 800–805. doi:10.1097/MAO.0b013e3181b0d02d

American Academy of Audiology. (n.d.). *Position statement on the audiologist's role in the diagnosis & treatment of vestibular disorders.* Retrieved from https://www.audiology.org/publications-resources/document-library/position-statement-audiologists-role-diagnosis-treatment

American Academy of Audiology. (2010a). Audiology assistant task force report. *Audiology Today, 22*(3), 68–73. Retrieved from www.audiology.org/resources/audiologytoday/Documents/2010_05-06/AT%2022.3%20-%20LOW.pdf

American Academy of Audiology. (2010b). *Audiology assistants* [Position statement]. Retrieved from www.audiology.org/resources/documentlibrary/Documents/2010_AudiologyAssistant_Pos_Stat.pdf

American Academy of Audiology. (2013). *American Academy of Audiology clinical practice guidelines: Pediatric amplification.* Reston, VA: Author.

American Speech-Language-Hearing-Association. (2006). *Preferred Practice Patterns for the Profession of Audiology* [Preferred Practice Patterns]. Retrieved from https://www.asha.org/uploadedFiles/PP2006-00274.pdf

Anderson, D. G., Wierzbowski, L. R., Schwartz, D. M., Hilibrand, A. S., Vaccaro, A. R., & Albert, T. J. (2002). Pedicle screws with high electrical resistance: A potential source of error with stimulus-evoked EMG. *Spine, 27,* 1577–1581.

Aw, S. T., Todd, M. J., Aw, G. E., McGarvie, L. A., & Halmagyi, G. M. (2005). Benign positional nystagmus: A study of its three-dimensional spatio-temporal characteristics. *Neurology, 64,* 1897–1905.

Barker, F., MacKenzie, E., Elliott, L., & de Lusignan, S. (2015). Outcome measurement in adult auditory rehabilitation: A scoping review of measures used in randomized controlled trials. *Ear and Hearing, 36,* 567–573. doi:10.1097/AUD.0000000000000167

Beal-Alvarez, J., & Cannon, J. E. (2014). Technology intervention research with deaf and hard of hearing learners: Levels of evidence. *American Annals of the Deaf, 158,* 486–505.

Benecke, J. E., Calder, H. B., & Chadwick, G. (1987). Facial nerve monitoring during acoustic neuroma removal. *The Laryngoscope, 97,* 697–700.

Bentler, R. A., Niebuhr, D. P., Getta, J. P., & Anderson, C. V. (1993a). Longitudinal study of hearing aid effectiveness. I: Objective measures. *Journal of Speech and Hearing Research, 36,* 808–819.

Bentler, R. A., Niebuhr, D. P., Getta, J. P., & Anderson, C. V. (1993b). Longitudinal study of hearing aid effectiveness. II: Subjective measures. *Journal of Speech and Hearing Research, 36,* 820–831.

Scope of Practice in Audiology

Bhalodia, V. M., Schwartz, D. M., Sestokas, A. K., Bloomgarden, G., Arkins, T., Tomak, P., . . . Goodrich, I. (2013). Efficacy of intraoperative monitoring of transcranial electrical stimulation-induced motor evoked potentials and spontaneous electromyography activity to identify acute-versus delayed-onset C-5 nerve root palsy during cervical spine surgery. Journal of Neurosurgery: Spine, 19, 395–402. doi:10.3171/2013.6.SPINE12355

Bhalodia, V. M., Sestokas, A. K., Tomak, P. R., & Schwartz, D. M. (2008). Transcranial electric motor evoked potential detection of compressional peroneal nerve injury in the lateral decubitus position. Journal of Clinical Monitoring and Computing, 22, 319–326. doi:10.1007/s10877-008-9136-x

Bhattacharyya, N., Gubbels, S. P., Schwartz, S. R., Edlow, J. A., El-Kashlan, H., Fife, T., . . . Corrigan, M. D. (2017). Clinical practice guideline: Benign paroxysmal positional vertigo (update). Otolaryngology–Head and Neck Surgery, 156, S1–S47. doi:10.1177/0194599816689667

Blustein, J., & Weinstein, B. E. (2016). Opening the market for lower cost hearing aids: Regulatory change can improve the health of older Americans. American Journal of Public Health, 106, 1032–1035. doi:10.2105/AJPH.2016.303176

Bose, B., Sestokas, A. K., & Schwartz, D. M. (2004). Neurophysiological monitoring of spinal cord function during instrumented anterior cervical fusion. The Spine Journal, 4, 202–207.

Bose, B., Sestokas, A. K., & Schwartz, D. M. (2007). Neurophysiological detection of iatrogenic C-5 nerve deficit during anterior cervical spinal surgery. Journal of Neurosurgery: Spine, 6, 381–385.

Bose, B., Wierzbowski, L. R., & Sestokas, A. K. (2002). Neurophysiologic monitoring of spinal nerve root function during instrumented posterior lumbar spine surgery. Spine, 27, 1444–1450.

Calder, H. B., & White, D. E. (1996). Facial nerve EMG monitoring. American Journal of Electroneurodiagnostic Technology, 36, 28–46.

Calder, H. B., Mast, J., & Johnstone, C. (1994). Intraoperative evoked potential monitoring in acetabular surgery. Clinical Orthopaedics and Related Research, 305, 160–167.

Chisolm, T. H., Johnson, C. E., Danhauer, J. L., Portz, L. J., Abrams, H. B., Lesner, S., . . . Newman, C. W. (2007). A systematic review of health-related quality of life and hearing aids: Final report of the American Academy of Audiology Task Force on the Health-Related Quality of Life Benefits of Amplification in Adults. Journal of the American Academy of Audiology, 18, 151–183.

Chisolm, T. H., Noe, C. M., McArdle, R., & Abrams, H. (2007). Evidence for the use of hearing assistive technology by adults: The role of the FM system. Trends in Amplification, 11, 73–89.

Ciccia, A. H., Whitford, B., Krumm, M., & McNeal, K. (2011). Improving the access of young urban children to speech, language and hearing screening via telehealth. Journal of Telemedicine and Telecare, 17, 240–244. doi:10.1258/jtt.2011.100810

Clements, D. H., Morledge, D. E., Martin, W. H., & Betz, R. R. (1996). Evoked and spontaneous electromyography to evaluate lumbosacral pedicle screw placement. Spine, 21, 600–604.

Coe, J. D., Smith, J. S., Berven, S., Arlet, V., Donaldson, W., Hanson, D., . . . Shaffrey, C. I. (2010). Complications of spinal fusion for Scheuermann kyphosis: A report of the Scoliosis Research Society Morbidity and Mortality Committee. Spine, 35, 99–103. doi:10.1097/BRS.0b013e3181c47f0f

Scope of Practice in Audiology

Convery, E., Keidser, G., Seeto, M., & McLelland, M. (2017). Evaluation of the self-fitting process with a commercially available hearing aid. Journal of the American Academy of Audiology, 28, 109–118. doi:10.3766/jaaa.15076

Criter, R. E., & Honaker, J. A. (2013). Falls in the audiology clinic: A pilot study. Journal of the American Academy of Audiology, 24, 1001–1005. doi:10.3766/jaaa.24.10.11

Darden, B. V., Hatley, M. K., & Owen, J. H. (1996). Neurogenic motor evoked-potential monitoring in anterior cervical surgery. Clinical Spine Surgery, 9, 485–493.

Darden, B. V., Owen, J. H., Hatley, M. K., Kostuik, J., & Tooke, S. M. (1998). A comparison of impedance and electromyogram measurements in detecting the presence of pedicle wall breakthrough. Spine, 23, 256–262.

Darden, B. V., Wood, K. E., Hatley, M. K., Owen, J. H., & Kostuik, J. (1996). Evaluation of pedicle screw insertion monitored by intraoperative evoked electromyography. Clinical Spine Surgery, 9, 8–16.

Dennis, J. M. (1988). Intraoperative monitoring with evoked responses. Seminars in Hearing, 9, 89–164.

Dennis, J. M. (1992). Neurophysiological intraoperative monitoring. American Journal of Audiology, 1, 44–56. doi:10.1044/1059-0889.0103.44

Dennis, J. M., & Earley, D. A. (1988). Monitoring surgical procedures with the auditory brainstem response. Seminars in Hearing, 9, 113–124. doi:10.1055/s-0028-1091437

Department of Defense Hearing Center of Excellence. (2014). Vestibular clinical practice guidelines. Retrieved from https://hearing.health.mil/For-Providers/Standards-and-Clinical-Practice-Guidelines/Vestibular-Clinical-Practice-Guidelines

Department of Health, Western Australia. (2011). Clinical guidelines for paediatric cochlear implantation. Perth, Australia: Author. Retrieved from http://ww2.health.wa.gov.au/~/media/Files/Corporate/general%20documents/Health%20Networks/Neurosciences%20and%20the%20Senses/Clinical-Guidelines-for-Paediatric-Cochlear-Implantation.pdf

Devlin, V. J., Anderson, P. A., Schwartz, D. M., & Vaughan, R. (2006). Intraoperative neurophysiologic monitoring: Focus on cervical myelopathy and related issues. The Spine Journal, 6, S212–S224. doi:10.1016/j.spinee.2006.04.022

DiCindio, S., & Schwartz, D. M. (2005). Anesthetic management for pediatric spinal fusion: Implications of advances in spinal cord monitoring. Anesthesiology Clinics of North America, 23, 765–787. doi:10.1016/j.atc.2005.08.004

DiCindio, S., Theroux, M., Shah, S., Miller, F., Dabney, K., Brislin, R. P., & Schwartz, D. (2003). Multimodality monitoring of transcranial electric motor and somatosensory-evoked potentials during surgical correction of spinal deformity in patients with cerebral palsy and other neuromuscular disorders. Spine, 28, 1851–1855. doi:10.1097/01.BRS.0000083202.62956.A8

Domville-Lewis, C., Santa Maria, P. L., Upson, G., Chester-Browne, R., & Atlas, M. D. (2015). Psychophysical map stability in bilateral sequential cochlear implantation: Comparing current audiology methods to a new statistical definition. Ear and Hearing, 36, 497–504. doi:10.1097/AUD.0000000000000154

Donahue, A., Dubno, J. R., & Beck, L. (2010). Accessible and affordable hearing health care for adults with mild to moderate hearing loss. Ear and Hearing, 31, 2–6. doi:10.1097/AUD.0b013e3181cbc783

Earley, D. A., & Dennis, M. J. (1988). Application of somatosensory evoked potentials in the operating room. Seminars in Hearing, 9, 141–151.

Early Hearing Detection and Intervention Act H.R. 1539, S. 652 (2017).

Ecker, M. L., Dormans, J. P., Schwartz, D. M., Drummond, D. S., & Bulman, W. A. (1996). Efficacy of spinal cord monitoring in scoliosis surgery in patients with cerebral palsy. Journal of Spinal Disorders, 9, 159–164.

Educational Audiology Association. (2010a). Audiology services under 504 [School-Based Audiology Advocacy Series]. Pittsburgh, PA: Author. Retrieved from http://www.edaud.org/advocacy/11-advocacy-07-10.pdf

Educational Audiology Association. (2010b). Classroom audio distribution systems [School-Based Audiology Advocacy Series]. Pittsburgh, PA: Author. Retrieved from http://www.edaud.org/advocacy/12-advocacy-11-11.pdf

Educational Audiology Association. (2010c). Educational services under IDEA: Pertinent regulations. School-Based Audiology Advocacy Series. Pittsburgh, PA: Author. Retrieved from http://www.edaud.org/advocacy/9-advocacy-07-10.pdf

Edwards, B. M., & Kileny, P. R. (1996). Intraoperative monitoring. Current Opinion in Otolaryngology & Head and Neck Surgery, 4, 360–366.

Edwards, B. M., & Kileny, P. R. (1998, February). Audiologists in intraoperative neurophysiology monitoring. Seminars in Hearing, 19, 87–95.

Eikelboom, R. H., & Atlas, M. D. (2005). Attitude to telemedicine, and willingness to use it, in audiology patients. Journal of Telemedicine and Telecare, 11(Suppl. 2), S22–S25. doi:10.1258/135763305775124920

Eisenberg, L. S. (2009). Clinical management of children with cochlear implants. San Diego, CA: Plural Publishing.

Ekberg, K., Grenness, C. & Hickson, L. (2016). Application of the transtheoretical model of behaviour change for identifying older clients' readiness for hearing rehabilitation during history-taking in audiology appointments. International Journal of Audiology, 55(Suppl. 3), S42–S51. doi:10.3109/14992027.2015.1136080

Eshraghi, A. A., Nazarian, R., Telischi, F. F., Martinez, D., Hodges, A., Velandia, S., . . . Lang, D. (2015). Cochlear implantation in children with autism spectrum disorder. Otology & Neurotology, 36, e121–e128. doi:10.1097/MAO.0000000000000757

Scope of Practice in Audiology

Falowski, S. M., Celii, A., Sestokas, A. K., Schwartz, D. M., Matsumoto, C., & Sharan, A. (2011). Awake vs. asleep placement of spinal cord stimulators: A cohort analysis of complications associated with placement. Neuromodulation, 14, 130–135.

Fan, D., Schwartz, D. M., Vaccaro, A. R., Hilibrand, A. S., & Albert, T. J. (2002). Intraoperative neurophysiologic detection of iatrogenic C5 nerve root injury during laminectomy for cervical compression myelopathy. Spine, 27, 2499–2502. doi:10.1097/01.BRS.0000031313.90883.29

Feldman, A. S., & Grimes, C. T. (Eds.) (1985). Hearing conservation in industry. Baltimore, MD: Williams & Wilkins.

Ferguson, M. A., Kitterick, P. T., Chong, L. Y., Edmondson-Jones, M., Barker, F., & Hoare, D. J. (2017). Hearing aids for mild to moderate hearing loss in adults. Cochrane Database of Systematic Reviews, 2017(9), 1–9. doi:10.1002/14651858.CD012023.pub2

Fife, T. D., Tusa, R. J., Furman, J. M., Zee, D. S., Frohman, E., Baloh, R. W., . . . Eviatar, L. (2000). Assessment: vestibular testing techniques in adults and children. Report of the Therapeutics and Technology Assessment Subcommittee of the American Academy of Neurology. Neurology, 55, 1431–1441. doi:10.1212/WNL.55.10.1431

Fischer, M. E., Cruickshanks, K. J., Wiley, T. L., Klein, B. E., Klein, R., & Tweed, T. S. (2011). Determinants of hearing aid acquisition in older adults. American Journal of Public Health, 101, 1449–1455. doi:10.2105/AJPH.2010.300078

Folmer, R. L., Theodoroff, S. M., Casiana, L., Shi, Y., Griest, S., & Vachhani, J. (2015). Repetitive transcranial magnetic stimulation treatment for chronic tinnitus: A randomized clinical trial. Journal of the American Medical Association Otolaryngology Head Neck Surgery, 141, 716–722. doi:10.1001/jamaoto.2015.1219

Folmer, R. L., Carroll, J. R., Rahim, A., Shi, Y., & Hal Martin, W. (2006). Effects of repetitive transcranial magnetic stimulation (rTMS) on chronic tinnitus. Acta Oto-Laryngologica, 126(Suppl. 556), 96–101. doi:10.1080/03655230600895465

Fuller, T. E., Haider, H. F., Kikidis, D., Lapira, A., Mazurek, B., Norena, A., . . . Cima, R. F. (2017). Different teams, same conclusions? A systematic review of existing clinical guidelines for the assessment and treatment of tinnitus in adults. Frontiers in Psychology, 8, 206. doi:10.3389/fpsyg.2017.00206

Gearhart, J. P., Burnett, A., & Owen, J. H. (1995). Measurement of pudendal evoked potentials during feminizing genitoplasty: Technique and applications. The Journal of Urology, 153, 486–487. doi:10.1097/00005392-199502000-00067

Gifford, R. H. (2013). Cochlear implant patient assessment: Evaluation of candidacy, performance, and outcomes. San Diego, CA: Plural Publishing.

Gundlapalli, S., Anand, R. S., Schwartz, D. M., Wierzbowski, L. R., Cohen, D. E., & Cook-Sather, S. D. (2006). Neurophysiological monitoring under anesthesia to position a child with extreme lumbar spine flexion for MRI and CT scan. Paediatric Anaesthesia, 16, 195–199. doi:10.1111/j.1460-9592.2005.01635.x

Guthmann, D. S., Mathos, K., & Richter, J. (2017). Interdisciplinary collaboration to ensure the well-being of deaf and hard of hearing students with complex needs. JADARA, 51(1), 34–52. Retrieved from http://repository.wcsu.edu/jadara/vol51/iss1/

Hafner, H., & Martin, W. H. (1996). Intraoperative neurophysiologic monitoring: Clinical importance and applications. Electroencephalography and Clinical Neurophysiology, 99(2), P13.

Hang, A. X., Roush, P. A., Teagle, H. F., Zdanski, C., Pillsbury, H. C., Adunka, O. F., & Buchman, C. A. (2015). Is "no response" on diagnostic auditory brainstem response testing an indication for cochlear implantation in children? Ear and Hearing, 36, 8–13. doi:10.1097/AUD.0000000000000072

Hawkins, D. B. (2005). Effectiveness of counseling-based adult group aural rehabilitation programs: A systematic review of the evidence. Journal of the American Academy of Audiology, 16, 485–493.

He, S., Grose, J. H., Teagle, H. F., Woodard, J., Park, L. R., Hatch, D. R., . . . Buchman, C. A. (2015). Acoustically evoked auditory change complex in children with auditory neuropathy spectrum disorder: A potential objective tool for identifying cochlear implant candidates. Ear and Hearing, 36, 289–301. doi:10.1097/AUD.0000000000000119

Health Resources & Service Administration (HRSA). Telehealth programs. Retrieved from https://www.hrsa.gov/rural-health/telehealth/index.html

Henderson, D. (1985). Effects of noise on hearing. In A. S. Feldman & C.T. Grimes (Eds.), Hearing conservation in industry. Baltimore, MD: Williams & Wilkins.

Henry, J. A., Thielman, E. J., Zaugg, T. L., Kaelin, C., Schmidt, C. J., Griest, S., . . . Carlson, K. (2017). Randomized controlled trial in clinical settings to evaluate effectiveness of coping skills education used with progressive tinnitus management. Journal of Speech, Language, and Hearing Research, 60, 1378–1397. doi:10.1044/2016_JSLHR-H-16-0126

Hickson, L., Meyer, C., Lovelock, K., Lampert, M., & Khan, A. (2014). Factors associated with success with hearing aids in older adults. International Journal of Audiology, 53(Suppl. 1), S18–S27. doi:10.3109/14992027.2013.860488

Hilibrand, A. S., Schwartz, D. M., Sethuraman, V., Vaccaro, A. R., & Albert, T. J. (2004). Comparison of transcranial electric motor and somatosensory evoked potential monitoring during cervical spine surgery. The Journal of Bone and Joint Surgery, 86, 1248–1253.

Hoffman, H. T., Brunberg, J. A., Sullivan, M. J., Winter, P., & Kileny, P. R. (1991). Arytenoid subluxation: Diagnosis and treatment. The Annals of Otology, Rhinology & Laryngology, 100(1), 1–9. doi:10.1177/000348949110000101

Humes, L. E., Kinney, D. L., Brown, S. E., Kiener, A. L., & Quigley, T. M. (2014). The effects of dosage and duration of auditory training for older adults with hearing impairment. The Journal of the Acoustical Society of America, 136, EL224–EL230. doi:10.1121/1.4890663

Humes, L. E., Rogers, S. E., Quigley, T. M., Main, A. K., Kinney, D. L., & Herring, C. (2017). The effects of service-delivery model and purchase price on hearing-aid outcomes in older adults: A randomized double-blind placebo-controlled clinical trial. American Journal of Audiology, 26, 53–79. doi:10.1044/2017_AJA-16-0111

Scope of Practice in Audiology

Isaacson, B., Kileny, P. R., & El-Kashlan, H. K. (2005). Prediction of long-term facial nerve outcomes with intraoperative nerve monitoring. Otology & Neurotology, 26, 270–273.

Isley, M. R., Pearlman, R. C., & Wadsworth, J. S. (1997). Recent advances in intraoperative neuromonitoring of spinal cord function: Pedicle screw stimulation techniques. American Journal of Electroneurodiagnostic Technology, 37, 93–126.

Jackson, E. M., Schwartz, D. M., Sestokas, A. K., Zarnow, D. M., Adzick, N. S., Johnson, M. P., . . . Sutton, L. N. (2014). Intraoperative neurophysiological monitoring in patients undergoing tethered cord surgery after fetal myelomeningocele repair. Journal of Neurosurgery: Pediatrics, 13, 355–361. doi:10.3171/2014.1.PEDS11336

Jacobson, G. P., McCaslin, D. L, Grantham, S. L., & Piker, E. G. (2008). Significant vestibular system impairment is common in a cohort of elderly patients referred for assessment of falls risk. Journal of the American Academy of Audiology, 19, 799–807. doi:10.3766/jaaa.19.10.7

Kai, Y., Owen, J. H., Lenke, L. G., Bridwell, K. H., Oakley, D. M., & Sugioka, Y. (1993). Use of sciatic neurogenic motor evoked potentials versus spinal potentials to predict early-onset neurologic deficits when intervention is still possible during overdistraction. Spine, 18, 1134–1139.

Kemink, J. L., LaRouere, M. J., Kileny, P. R., Telian, S. A., & Hoff, J. T. (1990). Hearing preservation following suboccipital removal of acoustic neuromas. The Laryngoscope, 100, 597–602. doi:10.1288/00005537-199006000-00009

Khan, A., Pearlman, R. C., Bianchi, D. A., & Hauck, K. W. (1997). Experience with two types of electromyography monitoring electrodes during thyroid surgery. American Journal of Otolaryngology, 18, 99–102. doi:10.1016/S0196-0709(97)90095-8

Kileny, P. R., & Edwards, B. M. (1997, March). Intraoperative cranial nerve monitoring. In S. K. Samra (Ed.), Seminars in Anesthesia, Perioperative Medicine and Pain (Vol. 16, No. 1, pp. 36–45). Philadelphia, PA: WB Saunders.

Kileny, P. R., & Zwolan, T. A. (2004). Pre-perioperative, transtympanic electrically evoked auditory brainstem response in children. International Journal of Audiology, 43(Suppl. 1), S16–S21.

Kileny, P., Dobson, D., & Gelfand, E. T. (1983). Middle-latency auditory evoked responses during open-heart surgery with hypothermia. Electroencephalography and Clinical Neurophysiology, 55, 268–276. doi:10.1016/0013-4694(83)90204-3

Kileny, P. R., Edwards, B. M., Disher, M. J., & Telian, S. A. (1998). Hearing improvement after resection of cerebellopontine angle meningioma: Case study of the preoperative role of transient evoked otoacoustic emissions. Journal of the American Academy of Audiology, 9, 251–256.

Kileny, P. R., Kemink, J. L., Zimmerman-Phillips, S., & Schmaltz, S. P. (1991). Effects of preoperative electrical stimulability and historical factors on performance with multichannel cochlear implant. Annals of Otology, Rhinology & Laryngology, 100, 563–568. doi:10.1177/000348949110000708

Kileny, P. R., Niparko, J. K., Shepard, N. T., & Kemink, J. L. (1988). Neurophysiologic intraoperative monitoring: I. Auditory function. Otology & Neurotology, 9(Suppl. 1), 17–24.

Kim, A. H., Edwards, B. M., Telian, S. A., Kileny, P. R., & Arts, H. A. (2006). Transient evoked otoacoustic emissions pattern as a prognostic indicator for hearing preservation in acoustic neuroma surgery. Otology & Neurotology, 27, 372–379.

Krumm, M., Huffman, T., Dick, K., & Klich, R. (2008). Telemedicine for audiology screening of infants. Journal of Telemedicine and Telecare, 14, 102–104. doi:10.1258/jtt.2007.070612

Lancaster, P., Krumm, M., Ribera, J., & Klich, R. (2008). Remote hearing screenings via telehealth in a rural elementary school. American Journal of Audiology, 17, 114–122. doi:10.1044/1059-0889(2008/07-0008)

Laplante-Lévesque, A., Hickson, L., & Worrall, L. (2010). Factors influencing rehabilitation decisions of adults with acquired hearing impairment. International Journal of Audiology, 49, 497–507. doi:10.3109/14992021003645902

Laschinger, J. C., Owen, J., Rosenbloom, M., Cox, J. L., & Kouchoukos, N. T. (1988). Direct noninvasive monitoring of spinal cord motor function during thoracic aortic occlusion: Use of motor evoked potentials. Journal of Vascular Surgery, 7, 161–171. doi:10.1016/0741-5214(88)90389-8

Lee, J. Y., Hilibrand, A. S., Lim, M. R., Zavatsky, J., Zeiller, S., Schwartz, D. M., . . . Albert, T. J. (2006). Characterization of neurophysiologic alerts during anterior cervical spine surgery. Spine, 31, 1916–1922. doi:10.1097/01.brs.0000228724.01795.a2

Lin, F. R., Chien, W. W., Li, L., Clarrett, D. M., Niparko, J. K., & Francis, H. W. (2012). Cochlear implantation in older adults. Medicine, 91, 229–241. doi:10.1097/MD.0b013e31826b145a

Lin, F. R., Hazzard, W. R., & Blazer, D. G. (2016). Priorities for improving hearing health care for adults: A report from the National Academies of Sciences, Engineering, and Medicine. JAMA, 316, 819–820. doi:10.1001/jama.2016.7916

Luginbuhl, A., Schwartz, D. M., Sestokas, A. K., Cognetti, D., & Pribitkin, E. (2012). Detection of evolving injury to the brachial plexus during transaxillary robotic thyroidectomy. The Laryngoscope, 122, 110–115. doi:10.1002/lary.22429

Macias, A. A., Eappen, S., Malikin, I., Goldfarb, J., Kujawa, S., Konowitz, P. M., . . . Randolph, G. W. (2016). Successful intraoperative electrophysiologic monitoring of the recurrent laryngeal nerve, a multidisciplinary approach: The Massachusetts Eye and Ear Infirmary monitoring collaborative protocol with experience in over 3000 cases. Head & Neck, 38, 1487–1494. doi:10.1002/hed.24468

Maes, L., Vinck, B. M., Wuyts, F., D'haenens, W., Bockstael, A., Keppler, H., . . . Dhooge, I. (2011). Clinical usefulness of the rotatory, caloric, and vestibular evoked myogenic potential test in unilateral peripheral vestibular pathologies. International Journal of Audiology, 50, 566–576.

Malmberg, M., Lunner, T., Kähäri, K., & Andersson, G. (2017). Evaluating the short-term and long-term effects of an Internet-based aural rehabilitation programme for hearing aid users in general clinical practice: A randomised controlled trial. BMJ Open, 7(5), e013047. doi:10.1136/bmjopen-2016-013047

Manchaiah, V., Taylor, B., Dockens, A. L., Tran, N. R., Lane, K., Castle, M., & Grover, V. (2017). Applications of direct-to-consumer hearing devices for adults with hearing loss: A review. Clinical Interventions in Aging, 12, 859–871. doi:10.2147/CIA.S135390

Scope of Practice in Audiology

Megerson, S. C. (2001). Update on hearing loss recordability: OSHA call for comments. CAOHC Update, 13(2), 2, 7–8. Retrieved from http://www.caohc.org/updatearticles/summer01.pdf

Meinke, D. K. (1995). State regulation of audiometric technicians in industry. Audiology Today, 7(2), 15–17.

Melnick, W. (1984). Evaluation of industrial hearing conservation programs: A review and analysis. American Industrial Hygiene Association Journal, 45, 459–467. doi:10.1080/15298668491400106

Mishler, E. T., & Smith, P. G. (1995). Technical aspects of intraoperative monitoring of lower cranial nerve function. Skull Base Surgery, 5, 245–250.

Modi, H. N., Suh, S. W., Yang, J. H., & Yoon, J. Y. (2009). False-negative transcranial motor-evoked potentials during scoliosis surgery causing paralysis: A case report with literature review. Spine, 34, E896–E900. doi:10.1097/BRS.0b013e3181b40d4f

Morata, T., Franks, J., & Dunn, D. (1994). Unmet needs in occupational hearing conservation. The Lancet, 344, 479.

Naito, M., Owen, J. H., Bridwell, K. H., & Sugioka, Y. (1992). Effects of distraction on physiologic integrity of the spinal cord, spinal cord blood flow, and clinical status. Spine, 17, 1154–1158.

Naito, M., Owen, J. H., Schoenecker, P. L., & Sugioka, Y. (1992). Acute effect of traction, compression, and hip joint tamponade on blood flow of the femoral head: An experimental model. Journal of Orthopaedic Research, 10, 800–806. doi:10.1002/jor.1100100608

National Academies of Sciences, Engineering, and Medicine. (2016). Hearing health care for adults: Priorities for improving access and affordability. Washington, DC: The National Academies Press. Retrieved from http://nationalacademies.org/hmd/reports/2016/Hearing-Health-Care-for-Adults.aspx

Niparko, J. K., Kileny, P. R., Kemink, J. L., Lee, H. M., & Graham, M. D. (1989). Neurophysiologic intraoperative monitoring: II. Facial nerve function. American Journal of Otology, 10, 55–61.

Oliveira Beier, L., Pedroso, F., & Dornelles da Costa-Ferreira, M. I. (2015). Auditory training benefits to the hearing aid users: A systematic review. Revista CEFAC, 17(4), 1327–1332. doi:10.1590/1982-0216201517422614

Over-the-Counter Hearing Aid Act of 2017, 21U.S.C. § 360j (2017).

Owen, J. H. (1999). The application of intraoperative monitoring during surgery for spinal deformity. Spine, 24, 2649–2662.

Owen, J. H., Bridwell, K. H., & Lenke, L. G. (1993). Innervation pattern of dorsal roots and their effects on the specificity of dermatomal somatosensory evoked potentials. Spine, 18, 748–754.

Owen, J. H., Bridwell, K. H., Grubb, R., Jenny, A., Allen, B., Padberg, A. M., & Shimon, S. M. (1991). The clinical application of neurogenic motor evoked potentials to monitor spinal cord function during surgery. Spine, 16(8 Suppl.), S385-S390.

Owen, J. H., Jenny, A. B., Naito, M., Weber, K., Bridwell, K. H., & McGhee, R. (1989). Effects of spinal cord lesioning on somatosensory and neurogenic-motor evoked potentials. Spine, 14, 673–682.

Scope of Practice in Audiology

Owen, J. H., Kostuik, J. P., Gornet, M., Petr, M., Skelly, J., Smoes, C., . . . Wolfe, F. (1994). The use of mechanically elicited electromyograms to protect nerve roots during surgery for spinal degeneration. Spine, 19, 1704–1710.

Owen, J. H., Laschinger, J., Bridwell, K., Shimon, S., Nielsen, C., Dunlap, J., & Kain, C. (1988). Sensitivity and specificity of somatosensory and neurogenic-motor evoked potentials in animals and humans. Spine, 13, 1111–1118.

Owen, J. H., Naito, M., Bridwell, K. H., & Oakley, D. M. (1990). Relationship between duration of spinal cord ischemia and postoperative neurological deficits in animals. Spine, 15, 846–851.

Owen, J. H., Sponseller, P. D., Szymanski, J., & Hurdle, M. (1995). Efficacy of multimodality spinal cord monitoring during surgery for neuromuscular scoliosis. Spine, 20, 1480–1488.

Parazzini, M., Del Bo, L., Jastreboff, M., Tognola, G., & Ravazzani, P. (2011). Open ear hearing aids in tinnitus therapy: An efficacy comparison with sound generators. International Journal of Audiology, 50, 548–553. doi:10.3109/14992027.2011.572263

Parikh, S. R., Machleder, D. J., Chobot-Rodd, J., Girouard, K., Shanske, A., Stern, E., . . . Dinces, E. (2004). Building a multidisciplinary cochlear implant team. The Einstein Journal of Biology and Medicine, 21, 19–24. doi:10.23861/EJBM200421456

Park, T. S., & Owen, J. H. (1992). Surgical management of spastic diplegia in cerebral palsy. New England Journal of Medicine, 326, 745–749. doi:10.1056/NEJM199203123261106

Pearlman, R. C., & Schneider, P. L. (1994). Intraoperative neural monitoring: An introduction for perioperative nurses. AORN Journal, 59(4), 843–844, 846–849. doi:10.1016/S0001-2092(07)65342-3

Pearlman, R. C., Isley, M. R., & Ganley, J. C. (2008). Electrical artifact during intraoperative electromyographic neuromonitoring. American Journal of Electroneurodiagnostic Technology, 48, 107–118.

Pearlman, R. C., Isley, M. R., Ruben, G. D., Sandler, S. C., Weisbaum, B., Khan, M. A., . . . Shah, A. (2005). Intraoperative monitoring of the recurrent laryngeal nerve using acoustic, free-run, and evoked electromyography. Journal of Clinical Neurophysiology, 22, 148–152.

Pearlman, R. C., Naficy, M. A., Koby, M. B., & Nyanzu, M. (2012). Carotid artery compression by the hyoid bone. Vascular and Endovascular Surgery, 46, 686–687. doi:10.1177/1538574412460101

Preminger, J. E., & Yoo, J. K. (2010). Do group audiologic rehabilitation activities influence psychosocial outcomes? American Journal of Audiology, 19, 109–125. doi:10.1044/1059-0889(2010/09-0027)

Razumovsky, A. Y., Gugino, L. D., & Owen, J. H. (2006). Advanced neurologic monitoring for cardiac surgery. Current Cardiology Reports, 8(1), 17–22. doi:10.1007/s11886-006-0005-2

Rizvi, S. S., Goyal, R. N., & Calder, H. B. (1999). Hearing preservation in microvascular decompression for trigeminal neuralgia. The Laryngoscope, 109, 591–594. doi:10.1097/00005537-199904000-00013

Scope of Practice in Audiology

Rosenberg, S. I., Martin, W. H., Pratt, H., Schwegler, J. W., & Silverstein, H. (1993). Bipolar cochlear nerve recording technique: A preliminary report. Otology & Neurotology, 14, 362–368.

Schultz, T. Y. (1996, February). Alternative methods to evaluate hearing conservation program effectiveness. Paper presented at the 21st Annual Hearing Conservation Conference, National Hearing Conservation Association, San Francisco, CA.

Schwartz, D. M. (1996). Intraoperative neurophysiological monitoring during cervical spine surgery. Operative Techniques in Orthopaedics, 6(1), 6–12. doi:10.1016/S1048-6666(96)80023-1

Schwartz, D. M., & Sestokas, A. K. (2002). A systems-based algorithmic approach to intraoperative neurophysiological monitoring during spinal surgery. Seminars in Spine Surgery, 14, 136–145.

Schwartz, D. M., Auerbach, J. D., Dormans, J. P., Flynn, J., Drummond, D. S., Bowe, J. A., . . . Drummond, D.S.. J. (2007). Neurophysiological detection of impending spinal cord injury during scoliosis surgery. The Journal of Bone & Joint Surgery, 89, 2440–2449. doi:10.2106/JBJS.F.01476

Schwartz, D. M., Bloom, M. J., & Pratt, R. E. (1988). Intraoperative monitoring of the processed electroencephalogram. Seminars in Hearing, 9, 153–163.

Schwartz, D. M., Bloom, M. J., Pratt, R. E., & Costello, J. A. (1988). Anesthetic effects on neuroelectric events. Seminars in Hearing, 9, 99–111.

Schwartz, D. M., Drummond, D. S., & Ecker, M. L. (1996). Influence of rigid spinal instrumentation on the neurogenic motor evoked potential. Clinical Spine Surgery, 9, 439–445.

Schwartz, D. M., Drummond, D. S., Hahn, M., Ecker, M. L., & Dormans, J. P. (2000). Prevention of positional brachial plexopathy during surgical correction of scoliosis. Clinical Spine Surgery, 13, 178–182.

Schwartz, D. M., Schwartz, J. A., Pratt Jr, R. E., Wierzbowski, L. R., & Sestokas, A. K. (1997). Influence of nitrous oxide on posterior tibial nerve cortical somatosensory evoked potentials. Clinical Spine Surgery, 10, 80–86.

Schwartz, D. M., Sestokas, A. K., Dormans, J. P., Vaccaro, A. R., Hilibrand, A. S., Flynn, J. M., . . . Albert, T. J. (2011). Transcranial electric motor evoked potential monitoring during spine surgery: Is it safe? Spine, 36, 1046–1049. doi:10.1097/BRS.0b013e3181ecbe77

Shapiro, W. H., & Bradham, T. S. (2012). Cochlear implant programming. Otolaryngologic Clinics of North America, 45, 111–127. doi:10.1016/j.otc.2011.08.020

Shapiro, W. H., Huang, T., Shaw, T., Roland, J. T., & Lalwani, A. K. (2008). Remote intraoperative monitoring during cochlear implant surgery is feasible and efficient. Otology and Neurotology, 29, 495–498. doi:10.1097/MAO.0b013e3181692838

Shi, Y. B., Binette, M., Martin, W. H., Pearson, J. M., & Hart, R. A. (2003). Electrical stimulation for intraoperative evaluation of thoracic pedicle screw placement. Spine, 28, 595–601. doi:10.1097/01.BRS.0000049926.43292.93

Scope of Practice in Audiology

Shi, Y., Burchiel, K. J., Anderson, V. C., & Martin, W. H. (2009). Deep brain stimulation effects in patients with tinnitus. Otolaryngology—Head and Neck Surgery, 141, 285–287. doi:10.1016/j.otohns.2009.05.020

Singh, G., Pichora-Fuller, M. K., Malkowski, M., Boretzki, M., & Launer, S. (2014). A survey of the attitudes of practitioners toward teleaudiology. International Journal of Audiology, 53, 850–860. doi:10.3109/14992027.2014.921736

Smith, P. G., Backer, R. J., Kletzker, G. R., Mishler, E. T., Loosmore, J. L., Leonetti, J. P., & Bigelow, D. C. (1995). Surgical management of transcranial hypoglossal schwannomas. American Journal of Otology, 16, 451–456.

Smith, P. G., Bigelow, D. C., Kletzker, G. R., Leonetti, J. P., Pugh, B. K., & Mishler, E. T. (1993). Hearing preservation following a transtemporal resection of an acoustic schwannoma: A case report. American Journal of Otology, 14, 434–436.

Smith, S. L., Saunders, G. H., Chisolm, T. H., Frederick, M., & Bailey, B. A. (2016). Examination of individual differences in outcomes from a randomized controlled clinical trial comparing formal and informal individual auditory training programs. Journal of Speech, Language, and Hearing Research, 59, 876–886. doi:10.1044/2016_JSLHR-H-15-0162

Sommerfleck, P. A., González Macchi, M. E., Weinschelbaum, R., De Bagge, M. D., Bernáldez, P., & Carmona, S. (2016). Balance disorders in childhood: Main etiologies according to age. Usefulness of video head impulse test. International Journal of Pediatric Otorhinolaryngology, 87, 148–153. doi:10.1016/j.ijporl.2016.06.020

Spitzer, J. B., Cellum, I. P., & Bosworth, C. (2013). Stability of audiometric measures and challenges in long-term management of the elderly cochlear implant patient. Otology & Neurotology, 34, 1636–1641. doi:10.1097/MAO.0b013e31829e83c9

Stepkin R. (1993, February). Diagnostics in industry: A professional approach to loss prevention. Paper presented at the 19th Annual Hearing Conservation Conference, National Hearing Conservation Association, Albuquerque, NM.

Suter, A. H. (1978). The ability of mildly hearing-impaired individuals to discriminate speech in noise [EPA Report No. 550/9-78-100]. Washington, DC: U.S. Environmental Protection Agency.

Sutherland, C. J., Miller, D. H., & Owen, J. H. (1996). Use of spontaneous electromyography during revision and complex total hip arthroplasty. The Journal of Arthroplasty, 11, 206–209.

Swanepoel, D. W., & Hall, J. W. (2010). A systematic review of telehealth applications in audiology. Telemedicine Journal and e-Health, 16, 181–200. doi:10.1089/tmj.2009.0111

Tang, L., Thompson, C. B., Clark, J. H., Ceh, K. M., Yeagle, J. D., & Francis, H. W. (2017). Rehabilitation and psychosocial determinants of cochlear implant outcomes in older adults. Ear and Hearing, 38, 663–671. doi:10.1097/AUD.0000000000000445

Telian, S. A., Kemink, J. L., & Kileny, P. (1988). Hearing recovery following suboccipital excision of acoustic neuroma. Archives of Otolaryngology–Head & Neck Surgery, 114(1), 85-87. doi:10.1001/archotol.1988.01860130089021

Scope of Practice in Audiology

Telian, S. A., Kileny, P. R., Niparko, J. K., Kemink, J. L., & Graham, M. D. (1989). Normal auditory brainstem response in patients with acoustic neuroma. The Laryngoscope, 99, 10–14. doi:10.1288/00005537-198901000-00003

Telleria, J. J., Safran, M. R., Harris, A. H., Gardi, J. N., & Glick, J. M. (2012). Risk of sciatic nerve traction injury during hip arthroscopy—Is it the amount or duration? An intraoperative nerve monitoring study. The Journal of Bone and Joint Surgery, 94, 2025–2032. doi:10.2106/JBJS.K.01597

Terrell, J. E., Kileny, P. R., Yian, C., Esclamado, R. M., Bradford, C. R., Pillsbury, M. S., & Wolf, G. T. (1997). Clinical outcome of continuous facial nerve monitoring during primary parotidectomy. Archives of Otolaryngology–Head & Neck Surgery, 123, 1081–1087.

Tucci, D. L.., Telian, S. A., Kileny, P. R., Hoff, J. T., & Kemink, J. L. (1994). Stability of hearing preservation following acoustic neuroma surgery. The American Journal of Otology, 15, 183–188.

Tunkel, D. E., Bauer, C. A., Sun, G. H., Rosenfeld, R. M., Chandrasekhar, S. S., Cunningham, E. R., . . . Whamond, E. J. (2014). Clinical practice guideline: Tinnitus. Otolaryngology–Head and Neck Surgery, 151(2 Suppl.), S1–S40. doi:10.1177/0194599814545325

Tye-Murray, N., Spehar, B., Myerson, J., Hale, S., & Sommers, M. (2016). Lipreading and audiovisual speech recognition across the adult lifespan: Implications for audiovisual integration. Psychology and Aging, 31, 380–389. doi:10.1037/pag0000094

U.S. Department of Education. (2004). Building the legacy: IDEA 2004. Retrieved from http://idea.ed.gov/

U.S. Department of Justice. (2014). Technical assistance document on effective communication. Retrieved from https://www.ada.gov/effective-comm.pdf

U.S. Department of Justice, Civil Rights Division, & U.S. Department of Education, Office for Civil Rights, Office of Special Education and Rehabilitative Services. (2014, November). Frequently asked questions on effective communication for students with hearing, vision or speech disabilities in public elementary and secondary schools. Retrieved from https://www2.ed.gov/about/offices/list/ocr/docs/dcl-faqs-effective-communication-201411.pdf

Ueta, T., Owen, J. H., & Sugioka, Y. (1992). Effects of compression on physiologic integrity of the spinal cord, on circulation, and clinical status in four different directions of compression: posterior, anterior, circumferential, and lateral. Spine, 17(8 Suppl.), S217–S226.

Vestibular Disorders Association. (n.d.). Diagnostic tests for vestibular problems. Portland, OR: Author. Retrieved from http://vestibular.org

Warren, E., & Grassley, C. (2017). Over-the-counter hearing aids: The path forward. JAMA Internal Medicine, 177, 609–610. doi:10.1001/jamainternmed.2017.0464

Weinstein, B. E. (1996). Treatment efficacy: Hearing aids in the management of hearing loss in adults. Journal of Speech, Language, and Hearing Research, 39(Suppl.), S37–S45.

Witt, R. L., Gillis, T., & Pratt, R. (2006). Spinal accessory nerve monitoring with clinical outcome measures. Ear, Nose & Throat Journal, 85, 540–544.

Scope of Practice in Audiology

Wolfe, J., & Schafer, E. (2014). Programming cochlear implants (2nd ed.). San Diego, CA: Plural Publishing.

Xie, Y.-H., Potmesil, M., & Peters, B. (2014). Children who are deaf or hard of hearing in inclusive educational settings: A literature review on interactions with peers. Journal of Deaf Studies and Deaf Education, 19, 423–437. doi:10.1093/deafed/enu017

Yingling, C. D., & Gardi, J. N. (1992). Intraoperative monitoring of facial and cochlear nerves during acoustic neuroma surgery. Otolaryngologic Clinics of North America, 25, 413–448.

Yingling, C. D., & Gardi, J. N. (2008). Intraoperative monitoring of facial and cochlear nerves during acoustic neuroma surgery. Neurosurgery Clinics of North America, 19, 289–315. doi:10.1016/j.nec.2008.02.011

Young, W. F., Morledge, D. E., Martin, W., & Park, K. B. (1995). Intraoperative stimulation of pedicle screws: a new method for verification of screw placement. Surgical Neurology, 44, 544–547. doi:10.1016/0090-3019(95)00246-4

Yueh, B., Souza, P. E., McDowell, J. A., Collins, M. P., Loovis, C. F., Hedrick, S. C., . . . Deyo, R. A. (2001). Randomized trial of amplification strategies. Archives of Otolaryngology–Head & Neck Surgery, 127, 1197–1204. doi:10.1001/archotol.127.10.1197

RESOURCES

American Speech-Language-Hearing Association. (n.d.-a). Evidence-based practice. Retrieved from https://www.asha.org/Research/EBP

American Speech-Language-Hearing Association. (n.d.-b). Practice portal. Retrieved from https://www.asha.org/practice-portal

American Speech-Language-Hearing Association. (1991). *A model for collaborative service delivery for students with language-learning disorders in the public schools* [Relevant Paper]. Retrieved from https://www.asha.org/policy/RP1991-00123/

American Speech-Language-Hearing Association. (2003). *Evaluating and treating communication and cognitive disorders: Approaches to referral and collaboration for speech-language pathology and clinical neuropsychology* [Technical Report]. Retrieved from https://www.asha.org/policy/TR2003-00137/

Paul, D. (2013, August). A quick guide to DSM-V. *The ASHA Leader, 18,* 52–54. Retrieved from https://leader.pubs.asha.org/article.aspx?articleid=1785031

U.S. Department of Justice. (2009). *A guide to disability rights laws.* Retrieved from https://www.ada.gov/cguide.htm

Appendix I–B

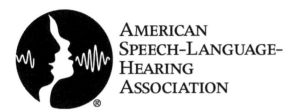
AMERICAN
SPEECH-LANGUAGE-
HEARING
ASSOCIATION

SCOPE OF PRACTICE IN SPEECH-LANGUAGE PATHOLOGY

AD HOC COMMITTEE ON THE SCOPE OF PRACTICE IN SPEECH-LANGUAGE PATHOLOGY

Reference this material as: American Speech-Language-Hearing Association. (2016). Scope of Practice in Speech-Language Pathology [Scope of Practice]. Available from www.asha.org/policy.

Scope of Practice in Speech-Language Pathology

ABOUT THIS DOCUMENT

This scope of practice document is an official policy of the American Speech-Language-Hearing Association (ASHA) defining the breadth of practice within the profession of speech-language pathology. This document was developed by the ASHA Ad Hoc Committee on the Scope of Practice in Speech- Language Pathology. Committee members were Mark DeRuiter (chair), Michael Campbell, Craig Coleman, Charlette Green, Diane Kendall, Judith Montgomery, Bernard Rousseau, Nancy Swigert, Sandra Gillam (board liaison), and Lemmietta McNeilly (ex officio). This document was approved by the ASHA Board of Directors on February 4, 2016 (BOD 01-2016). The BOD approved a revision in the prevention of hearing section of the document on May 9, 2016 (Motion 07-2016).

TABLE OF CONTENTS

- Introduction
- Statement of Purpose
- Definitions of Speech-Language Pathologist and Speech-Language Pathology
- Framework for Speech-Language Pathology Practice
- Domains of Speech-Language Pathology Service Delivery
- Speech-Language Pathology Service Delivery Areas
- Domains of Professional Practice
- References
- Resources

INTRODUCTION

The *Scope of Practice in Speech-Language Pathology* of the American Speech-Language-Hearing Association (ASHA) includes the following: a statement of purpose, definitions of *speech-language pathologist* and *speech-language pathology*, a framework for speech-language pathology practice, a description of the domains of speech-language pathology service delivery, delineation of speech-language pathology service delivery areas, domains of professional practice, references, and resources.

The *speech-language pathologist* (*SLP*) is defined as the professional who engages in professional practice in the areas of communication and swallowing across the life span. *Communication* and *swallowing* are broad terms encompassing many facets of function. *Communication* includes speech production and fluency, language, cognition, voice, resonance, and hearing. *Swallowing* includes all aspects of swallowing, including related feeding behaviors. Throughout this document, the terms *communication* and *swallowing* are used to reflect all areas. This document is a guide for SLPs across all clinical and educational settings to promote best practice. The term *individuals* is used throughout the document to refer to students, clients, and patients who are served by the SLP.

As part of the review process for updating the *Scope of Practice in Speech-Language Pathology*, the committee revised the previous scope of practice document to reflect recent advances in knowledge and research in the discipline. One of the biggest changes to the document includes the delineation of practice areas in the context of eight domains of speech-language pathology service delivery: collaboration; counseling; prevention and wellness; screening; assessment; treatment; modalities,

Scope of Practice in Speech-Language Pathology

technology, and instrumentation; and population and systems. In addition, five domains of professional practice are delineated: advocacy and outreach, supervision, education, research and administration/leadership.

Service delivery areas include all aspects of communication and swallowing and related areas that impact communication and swallowing: speech production, fluency, language, cognition, voice, resonance, feeding, swallowing, and hearing. The practice of speech-language pathology continually evolves. SLPs play critical roles in health literacy; screening, diagnosis, and treatment of autism spectrum disorder; and use of the *International Classification of Functioning, Disability and Health* (ICF; World Health Organization [WHO], 2014) to develop functional goals and collaborative practice. As technology and science advance, the areas of assessment and intervention related to communication and swallowing disorders grow accordingly. Clinicians should stay current with advances in speech-language pathology practice by regularly reviewing the research literature, consulting the Practice Management section of the ASHA website, including the Practice Portal, and regularly participating in continuing education to supplement advances in the profession and information in the scope of practice.

STATEMENT OF PURPOSE

The purpose of the *Scope of Practice in Speech-Language Pathology* is to

1. delineate areas of professional practice;
2. inform others (e.g., health care providers, educators, consumers, payers, regulators, and the general public) about professional roles and responsibilities of qualified providers;
3. support SLPs in the provision of high-quality, evidence-based services to individuals with communication, feeding, and/or swallowing concerns;
4. support SLPs in the conduct and dissemination of research; and
5. guide the educational preparation and professional development of SLPs to provide safe and effective services.

The scope of practice outlines the breadth of professional services offered within the profession of speech-language pathology. Levels of education, experience, skill, and proficiency in each practice area identified within this scope will vary among providers. An SLP typically does not practice in all areas of clinical service delivery across the life cycle. As the ASHA Code of Ethics specifies, professionals may practice only in areas in which they are competent, based on their education, training, and experience.

This scope of practice document describes evolving areas of practice. These include interdisciplinary work in both health care and educational settings, collaborative service delivery wherever appropriate, and telehealth/telepractice that are effective for the general public.

Speech-language pathology is a dynamic profession, and the overlapping of scopes of practice is a reality in rapidly changing health care, education, and other environments. Hence, SLPs in various settings work collaboratively with other school or health care professionals to make sound decisions for the benefit of individuals with communication and swallowing disorders. This *interprofessional collaborative practice* is defined as "members or students of two or more professions associated with health or social care, engaged in learning with, from and about each other" (Craddock, O'Halloran, Borthwick, & McPherson, 2006, p. 237. Similarly, "interprofessional education provides an ability to share skills and knowledge between professions and allows for a better understanding, shared values, and respect for the roles of other healthcare professionals" (Bridges et al., 2011, para. 5).

This scope of practice does not supersede existing state licensure laws or affect the interpretation or implementation of such laws. However, it may serve as a model for the development or modification of licensure laws. Finally, in addition to this scope of practice document, other ASHA professional resources outline practice areas and address issues related to public protection (e.g., A guide to disability rights law and the Practice Portal). The highest standards of integrity and ethical conduct are held paramount in this profession.

DEFINITIONS OF SPEECH-LANGUAGE PATHOLOGIST AND SPEECH-LANGUAGE PATHOLOGY

Speech-language pathologists, as defined by ASHA, are professionals who hold the ASHA Certificate of Clinical Competence in Speech-Language Pathology (CCC-SLP), which requires a master's, doctoral, or other recognized postbaccalaureate degree. ASHA-certified SLPs complete a supervised postgraduate professional experience and pass a national examination as described in the ASHA certification standards, (2014). Demonstration of continued professional development is mandated for the maintenance of the CCC-SLP. SLPs hold other required credentials where applicable (e.g., state licensure, teaching certification, specialty certification).

Each practitioner evaluates his or her own experiences with preservice education, practice, mentorship and supervision, and continuing professional development. As a whole, these experiences define the scope of competence for each individual. The SLP should engage in only those aspects of the profession that are within her or his professional competence.

SLPs are autonomous professionals who are the primary care providers of speech-language pathology services. Speech-language pathology services are not prescribed or supervised by another professional. Additional requirements may dictate that speech-language pathology services are prescribed and required to meet specific eligibility criteria in certain work settings, or as required by certain payers. SLPs use professional judgment to determine if additional requirements are indicated. Individuals with communication and/or swallowing disorders benefit from services that include collaboration by SLPs with other professionals.

The profession of speech-language pathology contains a broad area of speech-language pathology practice that includes both speech-language pathology service delivery and professional practice domains. These domains are defined in subsequent sections of this document and are represented schematically in **Figure 1**.

Scope of Practice in Speech-Language Pathology

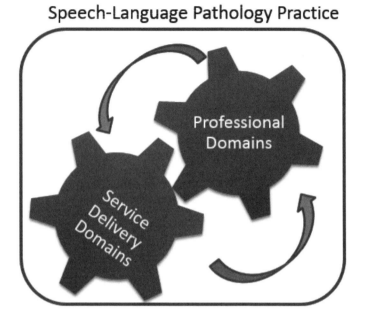

Figure 1. Schematic representation of speech-language pathology practice, including both service delivery and professional domains.

FRAMEWORK FOR SPEECH-LANGUAGE PATHOLOGY PRACTICE

The overall objective of speech-language pathology services is to optimize individuals' abilities to communicate and to swallow, thereby improving quality of life. As the population of the United States continues to become increasingly diverse, SLPs are committed to the provision of culturally and linguistically appropriate services and to the consideration of diversity in scientific investigations of human communication and swallowing.

An important characteristic of the practice of speech-language pathology is that, to the extent possible, decisions are based on best available evidence. ASHA defines evidence-based practice in speech-language pathology as an approach in which current, high-quality research evidence is integrated with practitioner expertise, along with the client's values and preferences (ASHA, 2005). A high-quality basic and applied research base in communication sciences and disorders and related disciplines is essential to providing evidence-based practice and high-quality services. Increased national and international interchange of professional knowledge, information, and education in communication sciences and disorders is a means to strengthen research collaboration and improve services. ASHA has provided a resource for evidence-based research via the Practice Portal.

The scope of practice in speech-language pathology comprises five domains of professional practice and eight domains of service delivery.

Professional practice domains:

- advocacy and outreach
- supervision

Scope of Practice in Speech-Language Pathology

- education
- administration/leadership
- research

Service delivery domains

- Collaboration
- Counseling
- Prevention and Wellness
- Screening
- Assessment
- Treatment
- Modalities, Technology, and Instrumentation
- Population and Systems

SLPs provide services to individuals with a wide variety of speech, language, and swallowing differences and disorders within the above-mentioned domains that range in function from completely intact to completely compromised. The diagnostic categories in the speech-language pathology scope of practice are consistent with relevant diagnostic categories under the WHO's (2014) *ICF*, the American Psychiatric Association's (2013) *Diagnostic and Statistical Manual of Mental Disorders*, the categories of disability under the Individuals with Disabilities Education Act of 2004 (see also U.S. Department of Education, 2004), and those defined by two semiautonomous bodies of ASHA: the Council on Academic Accreditation in Audiology and Speech-Language Pathology and the Council for Clinical Certification in Audiology and Speech-Language Pathology.

The domains of speech-language pathology service delivery complement the *ICF*, the WHO's multipurpose health classification system (WHO, 2014). The classification system provides a standard language and framework for the description of functioning and health. The ICF framework is useful in describing the breadth of the role of the SLP in the prevention, assessment, and habilitation/rehabilitation of communication and swallowing disorders and the enhancement and scientific investigation of those functions. The framework consists of two components: health conditions and contextual factors.

HEALTH CONDITIONS

Body Functions and Structures: These involve the anatomy and physiology of the human body. Relevant examples in speech-language pathology include craniofacial anomaly, vocal fold paralysis, cerebral palsy, stuttering, and language impairment.

Activity and Participation: *Activity* refers to the execution of a task or action. Participation is the involvement in a life situation. Relevant examples in speech-language pathology include difficulties with swallowing safely for independent feeding, participating actively in class, understanding a medical prescription, and accessing the general education curriculum.

CONTEXTUAL FACTORS

Environmental Factors: These make up the physical, social, and attitudinal environments in which people live and conduct their lives. Relevant examples in speech-language pathology include the role

Scope of Practice in Speech-Language Pathology

of the communication partner in augmentative and alternative communication (AAC), the influence of classroom acoustics on communication, and the impact of institutional dining environments on individuals' ability to safely maintain nutrition and hydration.

Personal Factors: These are the internal influences on an individual's functioning and disability and are not part of the health condition. Personal factors may include, but are not limited to, age, gender, ethnicity, educational level, social background, and profession. Relevant examples in speech-language pathology might include an individual's background or culture, if one or both influence his or her reaction to communication or swallowing.

The framework in speech-language pathology encompasses these health conditions and contextual factors across individuals and populations. **Figure 2** illustrates the interaction of the various components of the ICF. The health condition component is expressed on a continuum of functioning. On one end of the continuum is intact functioning; at the opposite end of the continuum is completely compromised function. The contextual factors interact with each other and with the health conditions and may serve as facilitators or barriers to functioning. SLPs influence contextual factors through education and advocacy efforts at local, state, and national levels.

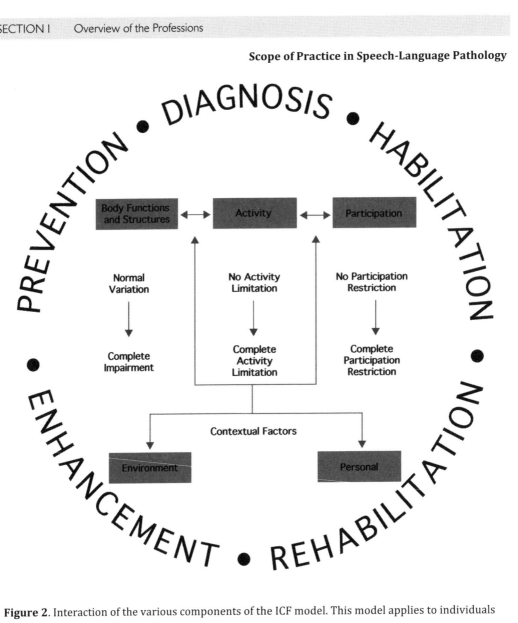

Figure 2. Interaction of the various components of the ICF model. This model applies to individuals or groups.

DOMAINS OF SPEECH-LANGUAGE PATHOLOGY SERVICE DELIVERY

The eight domains of speech-language pathology service delivery are collaboration; counseling; prevention and wellness; screening; assessment; treatment; modalities, technology, and instrumentation; and population and systems.

COLLABORATION

SLPs share responsibility with other professionals for creating a collaborative culture. Collaboration requires joint communication and shared decision making among all members of the team, including the individual and family, to accomplish improved service delivery and functional outcomes for the individuals served. When discussing specific roles of team members, professionals are ethically and legally obligated to determine whether they have the knowledge and skills necessary to perform such services. Collaboration occurs across all speech-language pathology practice domains.

As our global society is becoming more connected, integrated, and interdependent, SLPs have access to a variety of resources, information technology, diverse perspectives and influences (see, e.g., Lipinsky, Lombardo, Dominy, & Feeney, 1997). Increased national and international interchange of professional knowledge, information, and education in communication sciences and disorders is a means to strengthen research collaboration and improve services. SLPs

- educate stakeholders regarding interprofessional education (IPE) and interprofessional practice (IPP) (ASHA, 2014) principles and competencies;
- partner with other professions/organizations to enhance the value of speech-language pathology services;
- share responsibilities to achieve functional outcomes;
- consult with other professionals to meet the needs of individuals with communication and swallowing disorders;
- serve as case managers, service delivery coordinators, members of collaborative and patient care conference teams; and
- serve on early intervention and school pre-referral and intervention teams to assist with the development and implementation of individualized family service plans (IFSPs) and individualized education programs (IEPs).

COUNSELING

SLPs counsel by providing education, guidance, and support. Individuals, their families and their caregivers are counseled regarding acceptance, adaptation, and decision making about communication, feeding and swallowing, and related disorders. The role of the SLP in the counseling process includes interactions related to emotional reactions, thoughts, feelings, and behaviors that result from living with the communication disorder, feeding and swallowing disorder, or related disorders.

SLPs engage in the following activities in counseling persons with communication and feeding and swallowing disorders and their families:

- empower the individual and family to make informed decisions related to communication or feeding and swallowing issues.
- educate the individual, family, and related community members about communication or feeding and swallowing disorders.
- provide support and/or peer-to-peer groups for individuals with disorders and their families.
- provide individuals and families with skills that enable them to become self-advocates.
- discuss, evaluate, and address negative emotions and thoughts related to communication or feeding and swallowing disorders.
- refer individuals with disorders to other professionals when counseling needs fall outside of those related to (a) communication and (b) feeding and swallowing.

PREVENTION AND WELLNESS

Scope of Practice in Speech-Language Pathology

SLPs are involved in prevention and wellness activities that are geared toward reducing the incidence of a new disorder or disease, identifying disorders at an early stage, and decreasing the severity or impact of a disability associated with an existing disorder or disease. Involvement is directed toward individuals who are vulnerable or at risk for limited participation in communication, hearing, feeding and swallowing, and related abilities. Activities are directed toward enhancing or improving general well-being and quality of life. Education efforts focus on identifying and increasing awareness of risk behaviors that lead to communication disorders and feeding and swallowing problems. SLPs promote programs to increase public awareness, which are aimed at positively changing behaviors or attitudes.

Effective prevention programs are often community based and enable the SLP to help reduce the incidence of spoken and written communication and swallowing disorders as a public health and public education concern.

Examples of prevention and wellness programs include, but are not limited to, the following:

- **Language impairment:** Educate parents, teachers and other school-based professionals about the clinical markers of language impairment and the ways in which these impairments can impact a student's reading and writing skills to facilitate early referral for evaluation and assessment services.
- **Language-based literacy disorders:** Educate parents, school personnel, and health care providers about the SLP's role in addressing the semantic, syntactic, morphological, and phonological aspects of literacy disorders across the lifespan.
- **Feeding:** Educate parents of infants at risk for feeding problems about techniques to minimize long-term feeding challenges.
- **Stroke prevention:** Educate individuals about risk factors associated with stroke
- **Serve on teams:** Participate on multitiered systems of support (MTSS)/response to intervention (RTI) teams to help students successfully communicate within academic, classroom, and social settings.
- **Fluency:** Educate parents about risk factors associated with early stuttering.
- **Early childhood:** Encourage parents to participate in early screening and to collaborate with physicians, educators, child care providers, and others to recognize warning signs of developmental disorders during routine wellness checks and to promote healthy communication development practices.
- **Prenatal care:** Educate parents to decrease the incidence of speech, hearing, feeding and swallowing, and related disorders due to problems during pregnancy.
- **Genetic counseling:** Refer individuals to appropriate professionals and professional services if there is a concern or need for genetic counseling.
- **Environmental change:** Modify environments to decrease the risk of occurrence (e.g., decrease noise exposure).
- **Vocal hygiene:** Target prevention of voice disorders (e.g., encourage activities that minimize phonotrauma and the development of benign vocal fold pathology and that curb the use of smoking and smokeless tobacco products).
- **Hearing:** Educate individuals about risk factors associated with noise-induced hearing loss and preventive measures that may help to decrease the risk.
- **Concussion/traumatic brain injury awareness:** Educate parents of children involved in contact sports about the risk of concussion.

Scope of Practice in Speech-Language Pathology

- **Accent/dialect modification:** Address sound pronunciation, stress, rhythm, and intonation of speech to enhance effective communication.
- **Transgender (TG) and transsexual (TS) voice and communication:** Educate and treat individuals about appropriate verbal, nonverbal, and voice characteristics (feminization or masculinization) that are congruent with their targeted gender identity.
- **Business communication:** Educate individuals about the importance of effective business communication, including oral, written, and interpersonal communication.
- **Swallowing:** Educate individuals who are at risk for aspiration about oral hygiene techniques.

SCREENING

SLPs are experts at screening individuals for possible communication, hearing, and/or feeding and swallowing disorders. SLPs have the knowledge of—and skills to treat—these disorders; they can design and implement effective screening programs and make appropriate referrals. These screenings facilitate referral for appropriate follow-up in a timely and cost-effective manner. SLPs

- select and use appropriate screening instrumentation;
- develop screening procedures and tools based on existing evidence;
- coordinate and conduct screening programs in a wide variety of educational, community, and health care settings;
- participate in public school MTSS/RTI team meetings to review data and recommend interventions to satisfy federal and state requirements (e.g., Individuals with Disabilities Education Improvement Act of 2004 [IDEIA] and Section 504 of the Rehabilitation Act of 1973);
- review and analyze records (e.g., educational, medical);
- review, analyze, and make appropriate referrals based on results of screenings;
- consult with others about the results of screenings conducted by other professionals; and
- utilize data to inform decisions about the health of populations.

ASSESSMENT

Speech-language pathologists have expertise in the differential diagnosis of disorders of communication and swallowing. Communication, speech, language, and swallowing disorders can occur developmentally, as part of a medical condition, or in isolation, without an apparent underlying medical condition. Competent SLPs can diagnose communication and swallowing disorders but do not differentially diagnose medical conditions. The assessment process utilizes the ICF framework, which includes evaluation of body function, structure, activity and participation, within the context of environmental and personal factors. The assessment process can include, but is not limited to, culturally and linguistically appropriate behavioral observation and standardized and/or criterion-referenced tools; use of instrumentation; review of records, case history, and prior test results; and interview of the individual and/or family to guide decision making. The assessment process can be carried out in collaboration with other professionals. SLPs

- administer standardized and/or criterion-referenced tools to compare individuals with their peers;

- review medical records to determine relevant health, medical, and pharmacological information;
- interview individuals and/or family to obtain case history to determine specific concerns;
- utilize culturally and linguistically appropriate assessment protocols;
- engage in behavioral observation to determine the individual's skills in a naturalistic setting/context;
- diagnose communication and swallowing disorders;
- use endoscopy, videofluoroscopy, and other instrumentation to assess aspects of voice, resonance, velopharyngeal function and swallowing;
- document assessment and trial results for selecting AAC interventions and technology, including speech-generating devices (SGDs);
- participate in meetings adhering to required federal and state laws and regulations (e.g., IDEIA [2004] and Section 504 of the Rehabilitation Act of 1973).
- document assessment results, including discharge planning;
- formulate impressions to develop a plan of treatment and recommendations; and
- discuss eligibility and criteria for dismissal from early intervention and school-based services.

TREATMENT

Speech-language services are designed to optimize individuals' ability to communicate and swallow, thereby improving quality of life. SLPs develop and implement treatment to address the presenting symptoms or concerns of a communication or swallowing problem or related functional issue. Treatment establishes a new skill or ability or remediates or restores an impaired skill or ability. The ultimate goal of therapy is to improve an individual's functional outcomes. To this end, SLPs

- design, implement, and document delivery of service in accordance with best available practice appropriate to the practice setting;
- provide culturally and linguistically appropriate services;
- integrate the highest quality available research evidence with practitioner expertise and individual preferences and values in establishing treatment goals;
- utilize treatment data to guide decisions and determine effectiveness of services;
- integrate academic materials and goals into treatment;
- deliver the appropriate frequency and intensity of treatment utilizing best available practice;
- engage in treatment activities that are within the scope of the professional's competence;
- utilize AAC performance data to guide clinical decisions and determine the effectiveness of treatment; and
- collaborate with other professionals in the delivery of services.

MODALITIES, TECHNOLOGY, AND INSTRUMENTATION

SLPs use advanced instrumentation and technologies in the evaluation, management, and care of individuals with communication, feeding and swallowing, and related disorders. SLPs are also involved in the research and development of emerging technologies and apply their knowledge in the use of advanced instrumentation and technologies to enhance the quality of the services provided. Some examples of services that SLPs offer in this domain include, but are not limited to, the use of

Scope of Practice in Speech-Language Pathology

- the full range of AAC technologies to help individuals who have impaired ability to communicate verbally on a consistent basis—AAC devices make it possible for many individuals to successfully communicate within their environment and community;
- endoscopy, videofluoroscopy, fiber-optic evaluation of swallowing (voice, velopharyngeal function, swallowing) and other instrumentation to assess aspects of voice, resonance, and swallowing;
- telehealth/telepractice to provide individuals with access to services or to provide access to a specialist;
- ultrasound and other biofeedback systems for individuals with speech sound production, voice, or swallowing disorders; and
- other modalities (e.g., American Sign Language), where appropriate.

POPULATION AND SYSTEMS

In addition to direct care responsibilities, SLPs have a role in (a) managing populations to improve overall health and education, (b) improving the experience of the individuals served, and, in some circumstances, (c) reducing the cost of care. SLPs also have a role in improving the efficiency and effectiveness of service delivery. SLPs serve in roles designed to meet the demands and expectations of a changing work environment. SLPs

- use plain language to facilitate clear communication for improved health and educationally relevant outcomes;
- collaborate with other professionals about improving communication with individuals who have communication challenges;
- improve the experience of care by analyzing and improving communication environments;
- reduce the cost of care by designing and implementing case management strategies that focus on function and by helping individuals reach their goals through a combination of direct intervention, supervision of and collaboration with other service providers, and engagement of the individual and family in self-management strategies;
- serve in roles designed to meet the demands and expectations of a changing work environment;
- contribute to the management of specific populations by enhancing communication between professionals and individuals served;
- coach families and early intervention providers about strategies and supports for facilitating prelinguistic and linguistic communication skills of infants and toddlers; and
- support and collaborate with classroom teachers to implement strategies for supporting student access to the curriculum.

SPEECH-LANGUAGE PATHOLOGY SERVICE DELIVERY AREAS

This list of practice areas and the bulleted examples are not comprehensive. Current areas of practice, such as literacy, have continued to evolve, whereas other new areas of practice are emerging. Please refer to the ASHA Practice Portal for a more extensive list of practice areas.

1. **Fluency**
   - Stuttering
   - Cluttering

Scope of Practice in Speech-Language Pathology

2. **Speech Production**
   - Motor planning and execution
   - Articulation
   - Phonological
3. **Language**—Spoken and written language (listening, processing, speaking, reading, writing, pragmatics)
   - Phonology
   - Morphology
   - Syntax
   - Semantics
   - Pragmatics (language use and social aspects of communication)
   - Prelinguistic communication (e.g., joint attention, intentionality, communicative signaling)
   - Paralinguistic communication (e.g., gestures, signs, body language)
   - Literacy (reading, writing, spelling)
4. **Cognition**
   - Attention
   - Memory
   - Problem solving
   - Executive functioning
5. **Voice**
   - Phonation quality
   - Pitch
   - Loudness
   - Alaryngeal voice
6. **Resonance**
   - Hypernasality
   - Hyponasality
   - Cul-de-sac resonance
   - Forward focus
7. **Feeding and Swallowing**
   - Oral phase
   - Pharyngeal phase
   - Esophageal phase
   - Atypical eating (e.g., food selectivity/refusal, negative physiologic response)
8. **Auditory Habilitation/Rehabilitation**
   - Speech, language, communication, and listening skills impacted by hearing loss, deafness
   - Auditory processing

Potential etiologies of communication and swallowing disorders include

- neonatal problems (e.g., prematurity, low birth weight, substance exposure);
- developmental disabilities (e.g., specific language impairment, autism spectrum disorder, dyslexia, learning disabilities, attention-deficit disorder, intellectual disabilities, unspecified neurodevelopmental disorders);
- disorders of aerodigestive tract function (e.g., irritable larynx, chronic cough, abnormal respiratory patterns or airway protection, paradoxical vocal fold motion, tracheostomy);

Scope of Practice in Speech-Language Pathology

- oral anomalies (e.g., cleft lip/palate, dental malocclusion, macroglossia, oral motor dysfunction);
- respiratory patterns and compromise (e.g., bronchopulmonary dysplasia, chronic obstructive pulmonary disease);
- pharyngeal anomalies (e.g., upper airway obstruction, velopharyngeal insufficiency/incompetence);
- laryngeal anomalies (e.g., vocal fold pathology, tracheal stenosis);
- neurological disease/dysfunction (e.g., traumatic brain injury, cerebral palsy, cerebrovascular accident, dementia, Parkinson's disease, and amyotrophic lateral sclerosis);
- psychiatric disorder (e.g., psychosis, schizophrenia);
- genetic disorders (e.g., Down syndrome, fragile X syndrome, Rett syndrome, velocardiofacial syndrome); and
- Orofacial myofunctional disorders (e.g., habitual open-mouth posture/nasal breathing, orofacial habits, tethered oral tissues, chewing and chewing muscles, lips and tongue resting position).

This list of etiologies is not comprehensive.

Elective services include

- Transgender communication (e.g., voice, verbal and nonverbal communication);
- Preventive vocal hygiene;
- Business communication;
- Accent/dialect modification; and
- Professional voice use.

This list of elective services is not comprehensive.

DOMAINS OF PROFESSIONAL PRACTICE

This section delineates the domains of professional practice—that is, a set of skills and knowledge that goes beyond clinical practice. The domains of professional practice include advocacy and outreach, supervision, education, research, and administration and leadership.

ADVOCACY AND OUTREACH

SLPs advocate for the discipline and for individuals through a variety of mechanisms, including community awareness, prevention activities, health literacy, academic literacy, education, political action, and training programs. Advocacy promotes and facilitates access to communication, including the reduction of societal, cultural, and linguistic barriers. SLPs perform a variety of activities, including the following:

- Advise regulatory and legislative agencies about the continuum of care. Examples of service delivery options across the continuum of care include telehealth/telepractice, the use of technology, the use of support personnel, and practicing at the top of the license.
- Engage decision makers at the local, state, and national levels for improved administrative and governmental policies affecting access to services and funding for communication and swallowing issues.

- Advocate at the local, state, and national levels for funding for services, education, and research.
- Participate in associations and organizations to advance the speech-language pathology profession.
- Promote and market professional services.
- Help to recruit and retain SLPs with diverse backgrounds and interests.
- Collaborate on advocacy objectives with other professionals/colleagues regarding mutual goals.
- Serve as expert witnesses, when appropriate.
- Educate consumers about communication disorders and speech-language pathology services.
- Advocate for fair and equitable services for all individuals, especially the most vulnerable.
- Inform state education agencies and local school districts about the various roles and responsibilities of school-based SLPs, including direct service, IEP development, Medicaid billing, planning and delivery of assessment and therapy, consultation with other team members, and attendance at required meetings.

SUPERVISION

Supervision is a distinct area of practice; is the responsibility of SLPs; and crosses clinical, administrative, and technical spheres. SLPs are responsible for supervising Clinical Fellows, graduate externs, trainees, speech-language pathology assistants, and other personnel (e.g., clerical, technical, and other administrative support staff). SLPs may also supervise colleagues and peers. SLPs acknowledge that supervision is integral in the delivery of communication and swallowing services and advances the discipline. Supervision involves education, mentorship, encouragement, counseling, and support across all supervisory roles. SLPs

- possess service delivery and professional practice skills necessary to guide the supervisee;
- apply the art and science of supervision to all stakeholders (i.e., those supervising and being supervised), recognizing that supervision contributes to efficiency in the workplace;
- seek advanced knowledge in the practice of effective supervision;
- establish supervisory relationships that are collegial in nature;
- support supervisees as they learn to handle emotional reactions that may affect the therapeutic process; and
- establish a supervisory relationship that promotes growth and independence while providing support and guidance.

EDUCATION

SLPs serve as educators, teaching students in academic institutions and teaching professionals through continuing education in professional development formats. This more formal teaching is in addition to the education that SLPs provide to individuals, families, caregivers, decision makers, and policy makers, which is described in other domains. SLPs

- serve as faculty at institutions of higher education, teaching courses at the undergraduate, graduate, and postgraduate levels;
- mentor students who are completing academic programs at all levels;

Scope of Practice in Speech-Language Pathology

- provide academic training to students in related disciplines and students who are training to become speech-language pathology assistants; and
- provide continuing professional education to SLPs and to professionals in related disciplines.

RESEARCH

SLPs conduct and participate in basic and applied/translational research related to cognition, verbal and nonverbal communication, pragmatics, literacy (reading, writing and spelling), and feeding and swallowing. This research may be undertaken as a facility-specific effort or may be coordinated across multiple settings. SLPs engage in activities to ensure compliance with Institutional Review Boards and international laws pertaining to research. SLPs also collaborate with other researchers and may pursue research funding through grants.

ADMINISTRATION AND LEADERSHIP

SLPs administer programs in education, higher education, schools, health care, private practice, and other settings. In this capacity, they are responsible for making administrative decisions related to fiscal and personnel management; leadership; program design; program growth and innovation; professional development; compliance with laws and regulations; and cooperation with outside agencies in education and healthcare. Their administrative roles are not limited to speech-language pathology, as they may administer programs across departments and at different levels within an institution. In addition, SLPs promote effective and manageable workloads in school settings, provide appropriate services under IDEIA (2004), and engage in program design and development.

REFERENCES

American Psychiatric Association. (2013). *Diagnostic and statistical manual of mental disorders* (5th ed.). Washington, DC: Author.

American Speech-Language-Hearing Association. (2005). *Evidence-based practice in communication disorders* [Position statement]. Available from www.asha.org/policy.

American Speech-Language-Hearing Association. (2014). *Interprofessional education/interprofessional practice* (*IPE/IPP*). Available from www.asha.org/Practice/Interprofessional-Education-Practice/

Bridges, D. R., Davidson, R. A., Odegard, P. S., Maki, I. V., & Tomkowiak, J. (2011). Interprofessional collaboration: Three best practice models of interprofessional education. *Medical Education Online, 16.* doi:10.3402/meo.v16i0.6035. Retrieved from www.ncbi.nlm.nih.gov/pmc/articles/PMC3081249/

Craddock, D., O'Halloran, C., Borthwick, A., & McPherson, K. (2006). Interprofessional education in health and social care: Fashion or informed practice? *Learning in Health and Social Care, 5,* 220–242. Retrieved from http://onlinelibrary.wiley.com/doi/10.1111/j.1473-6861.2006.00135.x/abstract

Individuals With Disabilities Education Act of 2004, 20 U.S.C. § 1400 et seq. (2004).

Individuals with Disabilities Education Improvement Act of 2004, 20 U.S.C. § 1400 et seq. (2004).

Lipinski, C. A., Lombardo, F., Dominy, B. W., & Feeney, P. J. (1997, March 1). Experimental and computational approaches to estimate solubility and permeability in drug discovery and development settings. *Advanced Drug Delivery Reviews, 46*(1–3), 3–26. Retrieved from http://www.ncbi.nlm.nih.gov/pubmed/11259830

Rehabilitation Act of 1973, 29 U.S.C. § 701 et seq.

U.S. Department of Education. (2004). *Building the legacy: IDEA 2004.* Retrieved from http://idea.ed.gov/

World Health Organization. (2014). *International Classification of Functioning, Disability and Health.* Geneva, Switzerland: Author. Retrieved from www.who.int/classifications/icf/en/

RESOURCES

American Speech-Language-Hearing Association. (n.d.). *Introduction to evidence-based practice.* Retrieved from http://www.asha.org/Research/EBP/

American Speech-Language-Hearing Association. (n.d.). Practice Portal. Available from http://www.asha.org/practice-portal/

American Speech-Language-Hearing Association. (1991). *A model for collaborative service delivery for students with language-learning disorders in the public schools* [Paper]. Available from www.asha.org/policy

American Speech-Language-Hearing Association. (2003). *Evaluating and treating communication and cognitive disorders: Approaches to referral and collaboration for speech-language pathology and clinical neuropsychology* [Technical report]. Available from www.asha.org/policy

Paul, D. (2013, August). A quick guide to DSM-V. *The ASHA Leader, 18,* 52–54. Retrieved from http://leader.pubs.asha.org/article.aspx?articleid=1785031

U.S. Department of Justice. (2009). *A guide to disability rights laws.* Retrieved from www.ada.gov/cguide.htm

2

Professional Issues: A View from History

Judith Felson Duchan, PhD and Susan Felsenfeld, PhD

Introduction

One way to obtain a deeper perspective on the professional issues that are in this book is to step back in time. This historical view will show you that the matters covered in this book are dynamic and ever-changing. It is a mistake to think that today's professional practices arrived on the scene full-blown, with little struggle, or tweaking. Rather, our professional ancestors worked long and hard to develop today's professional practices in communication disorders. They deliberated, tried certain approaches that they then abandoned, and tried other approaches that they then changed to fit the times. A long-term view also helps one appreciate the role that social circumstances play in the formulation of professional practices. Indeed, today's professionals in the areas of speech-language pathology and audiology are still fine-tuning established practices and creating new ones to meet contemporary needs and circumstances. Professional practices within this historical perspective are rendered as processes rather than products. In this vein, our hopes for our professional progeny are that you will continue to redo, replace, or add to what we take as today's given practices.

This venture back in time tracks but a small segment of today's standard practices in communication disorders. It begins with conditions leading to the formation of the American Academy of Speech Correction in 1925. This was the organization that a half-century later, in 1978, took on the name we know today, the American Speech-Language-Hearing Association (ASHA). The chapter also describes changes in ASHA's organization over time with a particular focus on changes in its membership and certification requirements, and on changes in the scope of practices and what has influenced those changes. You will also read about the creation of the American Academy of Audiology (AAA), a second professional organization wholly devoted to professional issues in audiology. The chapter ends by identifying some trends occurring today, such as the move toward evidence-based practices that are likely to lead to significant changes that will be included in tomorrow's historical accounts.

This is not the first history to be written about the field of communication disorders and the two professional areas associated with it—speech-language pathology and audiology. One can, with some digging in obvious as well as more obscure places, find other historical renderings of various aspects of both professions. Most such depictions are short and specific, geared to a particular domain of practice, such as childhood language disorders (Aram & Nation, 1982; Leonard, 2000), phonological disorders (Bowen, 2009), voice disorders (Boone, 2010; Von Leden, 1990;); stuttering (Bobrick, 1995; Wingate, 1997), aphasia (Howard & Hatfield, 1987; Lorch, 2005; Tesak & Code, 2008), public school practices (Black, 1966; Duchan, 2009; Schoolfield, 1938), hearing aids (Deafness in Disguise, 2010), diagnostic audiology (Jerger, 2009) and aural rehabilitation (Hull, 2001; Ross, 1997). Some histories can be found tucked into larger texts or articles about a particular domain of practice. For example, a history on language disorders in children can be found in Aram and Nation (1982), Chapman (2007), and Leonard (2000); a history on aural rehabilitation is located in Hull (2001); histories on diagnostic audiology can be found in Newby (1980) and Stach (1998); and a history of phonological disorders in children is located in Bowen (2009). Many histories are recollections and memorials that provide biographical and professional information about the contributions of individuals and professional programs that have made their mark on the discipline and/or the profession (e.g., Berry, 1965; Duchan, 2011d; Jerger, 2016; Malone, 1999; Moeller, 1975).

There have been few detailed histories of professional issues such as membership and certification, professional organizations and journals, and trends in clinical practice in the United States (Jerger, 2009; Malone, 1999; Paden, 1970; Van Riper, 1981). Perhaps the best known of these is Elaine Pagel Paden's 1970 history of the American Speech and Hearing Association. In her history, Paden describes the founding of ASHA in 1925, the organization's publications over the years, the changes in membership qualifications, ethics, and relationships between ASHA and other organizations. The period covered in her book *A History of the American Speech and Hearing Association* is from 1925 to 1958.

A second history of professional issues is a 2009 publication devoted to the growth of audiology in the U.S. In it the author James Jerger describes the U.S. origins of audiology covering the years from 1922, when the first commercial audiometer appeared on the market, to 2009, when his book was published. Jerger's book begins by describing the circumstances and major players involved in the establishment of the audiology profession just after the Second World War. He then presents milestones in diagnosis and rehabilitation, with separate sections dedicated to advances in pediatric audiology, auditory processing disorders, tinnitus, and hearing conservation. Jerger's book ends with a section on professional considerations. In that section he includes the medical connection, the education requirements of audiology, the origin and nature of professional organizations devoted to different aspects of audiology, and

research support that has been available to audiologists over the years.

A third history of the profession is from Judy Duchan's website (Duchan, 2011b). Duchan shows, among other things, how the profession of speech correction grew out of the progressive movement, between 1870 and 1914—a time in which people in this country made concerted efforts to improve the lives of the disenfranchised, the impoverished, and those with disabilities.

This chapter draws from these previous histories, as well as other primary and secondary sources. The aim is to create a picture of how the professional areas of speech-language pathology and audiology in the US have developed over the years with a focus on milestones since 1925 when the group declared itself a profession in the United States. See Appendix 2–A for an outline summary of significant historical milestones.

The Profession's Organization: 1918 to Today

Just prior to the establishment of the early professional organizations made up of people interested in research and practices in speech correction, the country was experiencing social upheaval. The industrial revolution produced overcrowding and slums in the major cities. In addition, there was a large group of immigrants settling in cities, people who arrived from southern and eastern Europe following the disruptions of the First World War.

In response to these social needs, there was a movement in America called progressivism (McGerr, 2003). The aim of those involved in the movement was to create new societal structures to improve conditions for the poor, disabled, and disenfranchised. They were called "progressives" because they believed that social reforms could produce a better future. Labor unions were formed to improve wages and working conditions. Child labor laws were passed to protect children who were in the workforce. Women campaigned for the vote. Asylums for the blind, deaf, and mentally retarded were founded. Settlement houses were formed in the inner cities to provide food, clothing, education, and a sense of community to new immigrants, and compulsory education became law.

A number of professions were organized in the U.S. at this time to respond to these social needs and progressive ideals. A first agenda for these fledgling professions was to establish membership qualification requirements. Another issue that the new professions faced was creating a scope of practice for the members. One way this was done was to identify terminology and diagnostic categories for which they were responsible. College and university programs were instituted, conventions were held, and journals were created so that the newly formed profession could identify its own areas of expertise and could exclude people without the required background. In this way each profession could promulgate what it considered to be best practices for that time.

Many of the founders of the newly defined speech correction profession were members of already established professions such as medicine, education, psychiatry, psychology, and public speaking (then called elocution). Smiley Blanton, who in 1914 developed the first graduate level program in speech pathology, was strongly affiliated with the professions of psychiatry and elocution; Walter Babcock Swift, who organized a group of public school speech therapists in 1918, was a physician and public school administrator; and Carl Seashore, who promoted the founding of ASHA around 1925, was one of the first psychologists in America (see Duchan, 2011c, for biographies of these three founders).

While coming from different professional and disciplinary backgrounds, these early founders had a common interest in topics related to speech correction. They began to develop alliances with one another. Some met together in people's homes. Informal gatherings also took place at national meetings of the National Education Association (NEA) and of the National Association of Teachers of Speech (NATS). The NEA group was led by Walter Swift and consisted mostly of public school clinicians from the eastern United States. They called themselves the National Society for the Study and Correction of Speech Disorders. The second group associated with NATS was led by a small cadre of professionals whose names are among our declared founders: Lee Edward Travis, Robert West, Sara Stinchfield, and Paula Camp. This group dubbed its organization the American Academy of Speech Correction. It was the better organized of the two groups, and the one that was to eventually take hold and become the original name for the national association in 1925. That small association continued to grow into what today we call the American Speech-Language-Hearing Association (Paden, 1970).

Some 15 years later, during the Second World War, aural rehabilitation centers were established by medical departments in the armed forces to provide hearing services for military personnel (Doerfler, 1981; Jerger, 2009; Ross, 1997). The military called upon training programs in speech correction and otology to staff the centers. The personnel tested the hearing of servicemen, fitted them with hearing aids, and provided lip reading and counseling services to military personnel with hearing losses.

Following World War II these same hearing specialists returned to civilian life and lobbied for the founding

of their new area of specialty, one that they called "audiology." The field grew. Audiologists were employed by Veterans Administration Hospitals, in private practices of otolaryngologists, community hearing centers, and university speech clinics. Many of these newly minted audiologists or hearing researchers remained affiliated with the academic discipline of speech pathology, as evidenced by the 1947 renaming of the national organization to include hearing in its association title, and in 1948 with the addition of "hearing" to the name of its professional journal.

Audiologists continued to expand their services. In 1988, under the leadership of James Jerger, they formed their own organization, the American Academy of Audiology (AAA). The group held its first national convention in 1999 and in that same year began to issue the *Journal of the American Academy of Audiology* (JAAA). This publication is devoted to research and practices related to hearing and its disorders. Many audiologists belong to both AAA and ASHA and attend both national conventions. Hearing research is published in the AAA journal as well as in ASHA journals, especially the ASHA journal, begun in 1992, dedicated to audiology with an emphasis on clinical and professional issues, the *American Journal of Audiology*.

Between World War I and World War II, the fields of speech correction and audiology in the U.S. became well established. The two fields considered themselves as part of a single professional organization—the American Speech and Hearing Association or ASHA. The national organization by 1948 was working from a well-oiled constitution and set of bylaws, was meeting annually, and as of 1936, was communicating with and among its members through its own professional journal, the *Journal of Speech Disorders*. In the years that have followed, the organization and the two professional areas within it have continued to grow, creating specialty publications, increasing their membership exponentially, and expanding those domains considered to be within their scopes of practice.

Membership and Professional Qualification Requirements: 1926 to Today

In 1926, shortly after it declared itself an entity within a larger parent organization, the charter members of the American Academy of Speech Correction wrote a constitution laying out its organizational structure and its membership requirements. The constitution was approved by their host organization, the National

Association of Teachers of Speech, and was published in its journal, called the *Quarterly Journal of Speech* in 1927 (American Academy of Speech Correction, 1927, pp. 312–313). The goals laid out in the group's constitution were to provide a leadership role for stimulating interest and securing recognition of speech correction as a profession. It also aimed to raise clinical standards and encourage scholarly research (American Academy of Speech Correction, 1927, p. 312).

The bylaws of the constitution set the following criteria for membership:

i. Active present participation either in actual clinical work in speech correction or in administrative duties immediately concerned with supervision and direction of such work.

ii. Possession of an M.D., Ph.D., D.D.S., or of a master's degree, in the securing of which degree important work shall have been done in speech correction or some closely allied field such as psychology, phonetics, modern languages, mental hygiene, psychiatry, or medicine.

iii. Publication of original research in the form of a monograph, magazine article, or book.

iv. Possession of a professional reputation untainted by a past record (or present record) of unethical practices such as blatant commercialization of professional services or guaranteeing of "cures" for stated sums of money.

v. A bonafide interest in speech made manifest by continued membership in the National Association of Teachers of Speech. (American Academy of Speech Correction, 1927, p. 313).

The 1926 bylaws also stipulated that "no more than five new members can be inducted into the academy in any one year" (American Academy of Speech Correction, 1927, p. 312). The membership committee was further instructed not to elect anyone "who is not known personally to at least two members of the membership committee or to 10 members of the academy at large" (Malone, 1999, p. 75).

These restrictive criteria reveal that the Academy did not see itself as a group that represented or regulated practitioners in the field. Nor did it see itself as a group that required practitioners to pass qualification requirements in order to practice. Rather, it regarded itself as a learned or honorary society. The 25 members in 1930 were essentially the same group of people who served as charter members of the organization's formation.

In 1930, members of the Academy opened their doors to practitioners by creating a new kind of Associate membership for clinicians with a less rigorous set of

membership qualifications. Associates were required to have a bachelor's degree and three years employment in the field of speech correction. They were also required to have "adequate education in the physiology of speech and its disorders" (Paden, 1970, p. 65). In order to become an associate, one also had to be approved by a 10-member panel made up of Fellows of the organization. In 1936 the approval requirement was reduced to two members. Unlike for Fellows, members at the Associate level were not required to have a publication or outstanding achievement. Nor were they required to have an advanced degree. This group was to eventually form the bulk of the membership in the organization.

This shift in focus from a strictly academic, scholarly honorary organization to one that included practitioners is reflected in the name changes made in 1927 and 1934. In 1927 the organization changed its designation of *Academy* to *Society*, thereby changing its name from the American Academy of Speech Correction to the American Society for the Study of Disorders of Speech. In 1934 it again changed its designation, this time from *Society* to *Association*. It became known as the American Speech Correction Association. Both *Society* and *Association* have meanings that are broader and more inclusive than Academy, reflecting a change in how the leaders saw the role of the organization. Another part of the name change in 1934 was to remove the word *Study*. This, too, indicated that the organization was opening up to practitioners and shifting from a purely academic to a more clinical-based identity. Table 2–1 presents the name changes in the national organization and the years those changes took place.

A more substantive move toward a democratic organization occurred in 1942 when the organization changed its bylaws to invite practicing speech correctionists to become members of the professional organization. In keeping with this shift, three new levels of membership were established as additions to the Fellow and Associate categories (American Speech Correction Association, 1943, pp. 41–51). One new category was

Table 2–1. Name Changes of the National Association

American Academy of Speech Correction (1925)

American Society for the Study of Disorders of Speech (1927)

American Speech Correction Association (1934)

American Speech and Hearing Association (1947)

American Speech-Language-Hearing Association (1978)

for students studying to become speech pathologists. By becoming a paying member of the organization, students could receive the *Journal of Speech Disorders* at no additional cost. A second addition was an advanced level of clinical membership, called a professional member, which differentiated members with experience from those who were beginners in the profession. Professional members were required to have a master's degree.

Another level of membership was also instituted in 1942, one designed to honor outstanding members of the association. This was a precursor to today's *Honors of the Association* award that recognizes those who have made outstanding contributions to the profession. The first Honors award was given to Carl Seashore in 1944 for his contributions to the profession and to his research in the field (American Speech Correction Association, 1945, p. 1–2) See Duchan (2011d) for more on Seashore and his contributions.

As the organization approached its thirtieth birthday in the 1950s, it went through social changes that led to further revisions in its membership and credentialing policies. Elaine Paden (1970) in her history of ASHA, identified two of those social changes: (1) an increase in specialized knowledge, and (2) a growing group of non-clinical scientists seeking membership in the association. Here is Paden's description of the emerging knowledge explosion and curricular bifurcation that was going on during the 1950s.

> Increased knowledge, based both on experience and on research, spawned more course offerings, and few individuals could be expected to cover the entire span. Specialization became an accepted necessity. The most apparent partition was between the areas of speech and hearing. Although the profession had always included both aspects of communication disorders, persons were now being trained who were experts in hearing but who had only basic knowledge of the rest of the general field. Meantime, the typical speech pathologist had not had time in his academic training to become equally well prepared in the area of hearing. (Paden, 1970, p. 68)

This proliferation of information and courses in each of the two sub-areas of the profession led the 1952 executive council of the professional organization to create two separate career paths, one for speech pathology, another for audiology (American Speech and Hearing Association, 1952). This separation of certification requirements was made available at basic (clinical) and advanced (professional and fellow) levels. Some applicants received certification in both speech pathology and audiology, having fulfilled the qualification requirements in both professional tracks.

Behind the proliferation of information was a new group of research scientists in the field who did not have the clinical coursework or clinical experience required for membership. This led in 1952 to a "one-way separation" between membership and certification requirements in the organization. A researcher, or anyone with interest in the field, could become an association member without having to meet clinical requirements for certification. However, the reverse was not possible. That is, while membership without certification was permitted under these new guidelines, certification without membership was not. Those who wanted ASHA certification were required to be active association members and they had to maintain their membership throughout the time they held their certification status.

This second half of the separation between membership and certification was not to take place until 1978 following a lawsuit against ASHA by a member, Dale Bogus Lieberman, (Malone, 1999; Mylott, 2010). Lieberman's lawyers contended that ASHA was violating the Sherman Anti-Trust Act because it had a monopoly over professional certification and in that role required that those applying for certification pay their dues as members. ASHA argued that people could practice without certification, thereby showing that they were not a monopoly that was misusing its power. The case was settled out of court. Shortly thereafter ASHA separated its membership from certification, no longer requiring that professionals seeking certification be dues paying members of the organization.

In 1952, ASHA required at least 30 semester hours in the major and 275 hours of clinical practicum for basic level certification. Also required was one year of sponsored clinical experience (American Speech and Hearing Association, 1952). Neither a graduate degree nor a national examination was required for certification at this point. Advanced certification under the 1952 rules required 60 semester hours in the major, 400 hours of clinical practicum, and four years of professional experience. Those applying for advanced certification in audiology had to pass a nationally administered written and oral examination on science and practices associated with hearing and hearing loss.

Membership and certification requirements continued to change through the 1960s. In 1965 the organization returned to offering a single type of certification for both audiology and speech pathology—the Certificate for Clinical Competence (CCC), known in today's parlance as "the Cs." The new certificate merged the earlier two-tiered system of basic and advanced levels of membership into one. To qualify for certification, one had to be a graduate of a master's degree speech pathology or audiology program. The master's degree required 60 semester hours of study in specified areas and 275 hours of clinical practicum experiences. Certification in speech pathology and audiology also required nine months of supervised full-time professional employment, a letter from the candidate's academic program director, and a passing score on a national examination in their field of either speech pathology or audiology.

Over the next two decades, between 1965 and 1985, the profession continued to expand its knowledge base. Both wings of the profession felt the need to increase their professional requirements to accommodate the burgeoning scientific information. This was done by increasing the course and practicum requirements in pre-professional training programs. In 1973 the number of clinical hours required for certification increased from 275 to 300 hours, and the academic content requirements became more specific. Coursework in the professional areas increased to 75 hours (including basic sciences).

The 1993 certification and degree requirements included coursework in language disorders for the first time. For the speech-language pathology track, six hours were required in the area of language disorders and for audiologists three hours of language disorders were required. This emphasis on language disorders was reflected in yet another name change in 1978. The American Speech and Hearing Association became the American Speech-Language and Hearing Association.

Since 1993 the certification requirements in both speech-language pathology and audiology have changed several times. The number of semester hours required for undergraduate and graduate course work has varied, the composition of required courses has changed, and the clock hours required for indirect therapy observation and direct client contact has fluctuated. More recently, ASHA has changed its policy on observation hours to allow some of these to be obtained using simulated or videotaped cases (e.g., Simucase, n.d.). Still required for both sides of the profession is a passing score on the Praxis examination and a sponsored and supervised clinical fellowship following graduation.

A more recent addition for both areas of the profession is a requirement that practicing speech-language pathologists (SLPs) and audiologists engage in continuing education in order to maintain their certification. This "professional development" requirement was instituted for Speech-Language Pathologists in 1999 and for Audiologists in 2000 (American Speech-Language-Hearing Association, n.d.-a). See Chapter 3, "Establishing Competencies in Professional Education, Certification, and Licensure," for more information.

Beginning on January 1, 2020, another set of revisions to ASHA's certification standards will take effect. Rather than focusing upon curricular changes at the graduate level, many of these modifications address changes that are relevant for post-graduate students and professionals who engage in supervision activities. For example, beginning in January 2020, speech-language pathologists and audiologists who intend to supervise either graduate students or CFs must complete at least two hours of documented professional development in the area of supervision (ASHA, 2019). Beginning with the 2020–2022 certification maintenance interval, all individuals who wish to maintain their clinical certification (both CCC-SLP and CCC-A) will be required to earn at least 1.0 CMH (certification maintenance hour) in ethics. Although not yet mandated, both audiology and SLP graduate students and CFs are "encouraged to include interprofessional education and interprofessional practice into their clinical supervised experience" (ASHA, 2019). A small number of curricular changes do appear in the new standards; for example, SLP students who graduate with a master's degree in 2020 or later will need to have completed an undergraduate-level course in physics or chemistry. At present, members of the CFCC (Council for Clinical Certification in Audiology and Speech-Language Pathology) are considering whether to add a requirement for English language proficiency for both SLPs and audiologists. Because this mandate will require considerable review and discussion, if approved, it will not take effect for several years. Finally, beginning in 2020, those seeking certification must submit their application entirely online, following the respective 2020 Standards for speech (on.asha .org/2020-slp-cert) or Audiology (on.asha.org/2020-aud-cert) (Horshaw, 2019).

Leaders in ASHA have long debated about what has come to be called the entry-level degree requirement. The founders required a graduate degree for membership, a requirement that was changed when the organization opened its doors to practicing clinicians. In 1965, there were contentious debates again, but this time it was about whether to move from a bachelor's to a master's level requirement for basic membership and certification. Duane Spriestersbach, ASHA president at that time, remembers that "a lot of training programs . . . were threatened and were not at all convinced that this was necessary or appropriate" (Malone, 1999, p. 87). Both Charles Van Riper and Bryng Bryngelson argued against the upgrade for fear that current practitioners without master's degrees would be disenfranchised (Malone, 1999, p. 87). Initially, changes to what was considered the necessary entry-level degree for a practicing SLP varied as a function of work setting. The entry-level degree for clinicians working in hospitals and other non-educational agencies was changed from a bachelor's to a master's degree in 1968. For SLPs working in educational settings, primarily public and private schools, this change came much later.

In a similar vein are the recent proposals to move from a master's level to a doctoral entry-level requirement for clinical practice in speech-language pathology. Although this feels like a modern debate, discussions regarding the need for a clinical doctorate in speech pathology actually began in 1958. In that year, Virgil Anderson, a researcher in voice disorders at Stanford University and an active member of ASHA, proposed a professional doctorate in speech-language pathology, to the dismay of most of his colleagues in the organization. Here is a report from that time of how Anderson's idea was received:

> Some startled, some anxious, and some enthusiastic listeners made up the group to whom Virgil Anderson proposed a new degree, clinically oriented, at the November convention. This degree was tossed about with a great deal of speculation as to its name, its place among the time-honored MA, MS, and PhD. It was evident that its proponent was interested primarily in giving those with extensive clinical experience an opportunity to get recognition other than certification for their particular skills—especially those who might not choose to follow the path of PhD study. (Nelson, 1958, p. 81)

The idea of a doctoral-level clinical track finally took hold for audiologists some 40 years after Anderson first proposed it. In 2012, the AuD formally replaced the master's as the entry-level degree for the clinical practice of audiology (American Academy of Audiology, 2019, ASHA timeline, n.d.), although many AuD degrees were conferred prior to this date. Among other requirements, the clinical doctorate currently requires 1820 hours of supervised clinical practicum experiences and a passing score on a Praxis exam in Audiology.

Just as was the case for audiology, some professionals in speech-language pathology are now discussing whether a clinical doctoral degree in speech-language pathology is warranted (Bernthal, 2007; Lubinski, 2003). A small number of academic programs offering a clinical doctorate in speech-language pathology have been established and more are in the development stage (GRADschools.com, n.d.)

To keep pace with these developments, ASHA has published detailed programmatic guidelines for institutions that want to offer a clinical doctorate in SLP (American Speech-Language-Hearing Association, 2015). The guidelines recommend that the designator for the clinical doctoral degree be a *Doctor of Speech-Language Pathology* (*SLP-D*). These guidelines have been recog-

nized and supported by a majority of the membership of the Council of Academic Programs in Communication Sciences and Disorders (CAPCSD), who affirm the need to develop standards for program creation and accreditation (CAPSCD, 2017). Neither ASHA nor CAPCSD are suggesting that the clinical doctorate should *replace* the master's as the entry-level degree for clinical practice. Rather, the SLP-D is presently being conceived as an alternative to the research-focused Ph.D. degree, specifically designed for clinical practitioners who "want to assume advanced professional roles-such as master clinician, clinical educator, clinical administrator, or leader in a clinical setting or area of specialization-or to serve as collaborators and supporters of clinical research" (American Speech-Language-Hearing Association, 2015). Whether obtaining the SLP-D degree will result in tangible benefits, such as increases in salaries or professional advancement, remains to be seen.

For a succinct summary of the changes in ASHA certification described above, covering the years from 1925 to 2020, see the American Speech-Language-Hearing Association webpage (American Speech-Language-Hearing Association, n.d.-b).

School Certification

In the first half of the twentieth century, except in a few instances (Carrell, 1946; Gifford, 1925; Irwin, 1955), ASHA was the only organization that issued an official credential to practice as a speech-language pathologist and audiologist in any setting. In the late 1940s individual states began establishing certification requirements for public school teachers (Carrell, 1946). Speech-language pathologists working in public school settings in the decade between 1945 and 1955 were required to meet the same standards as public school teachers (Irwin, 1953, 1959), and, for some states, clinicians were required to have additional course work and experience in working with "speech handicapped school children" (Irwin, 1959). Students enrolled in curricula specializing in speech pathology needed to take additional course work in education in order to work in public schools. State departments of education later in the 1950s began to require that teachers of "speech handicapped school children" have basic speech certification from ASHA. By 1955, fifteen states required ASHA's basic certification for practicing in schools, and by 1959 the number had increased to 32 (Irwin, 1959). Today, most of the 50 state departments of education require specialized training in the field to practice in public as well as private school settings, with requirements varying from state to state (see details in American Speech Language and Hearing Association, n.d.-c).

State Licensure

In 1969 the state of Florida began a second movement at the state level to credential people. This one provided state licensure for those working in non-educational settings. Professionals working in settings that receive third-party payments such as Medicaid, insurance coverage, and Health Department monies must now have a state license to practice. Most states have established agencies (boards) in their state health departments to review and monitor practices and issue licenses in speech-language pathology and audiology (American Speech-Language-Hearing Association, n.d.-c and d).

Continuing Education

Another requirement for our professions, one involving post-graduate certification standards, has recently been put into place by ASHA. In 1999 ASHA added a continuing education requirement. To maintain their certification status, members are now mandated to pay annual membership fees and to accumulate 30 Certification Maintenance Hours of continuing education credits over a period of three years (American Speech-Language and Hearing Association, 2011). Individual states also incorporate continuing education as a requirement for state licensure as does the American Academy of Audiology. ASHA requires 30 hours of Continuing Education over a three-year period for SLPs and audiologists to maintain their clinical certification (American Speech-Language-Hearing Association, n.d.-d).

Scope of Practice and Practice Frameworks: 1926 to Today

It was not immediately clear to the founders of the speech pathology profession what services new practitioners should be providing and to whom. For example, should speech correctionists be responsible for diagnosing and treating those whose communication disorders were secondary to other disorders, such as intellectual disabilities? Should they provide services to those who wanted to improve their speech, but who had no speech problems? Should they be the ones responsible for testing and rehabilitating those with hearing losses or should they focus exclusively on the speech problems accompanying those losses? Much of the activity of the early practitioners and founders of the profession involved establishing a taxonomy and complete listing of conditions that should fall within the professed scope of practice of this new discipline.

A nomenclature committee, set up in 1927 by the American Society for the Study of Disorders of Speech, worked to provide an outline and descriptions of the various conditions that speech correctionists should know about and be responsible for. In the words of Sara Stinchfield, member and primary mover of the nomenclature committee:

> The attempt is made in this arrangement to give the student an outline of practically all of the commonly found disorders of speech, such as appear in home, school, and speech clinic, and to so group them that they may come under one of seven main headings: dysarthria, dyslalia, dyslogia, dysphasia, dysphemia, dysphonia, or dysrhythmia. . . . It was necessary for the committee on terminology to coin a number of new terms having old prefixes, frequently defining the older and better-known terms as synonymous with the coined ones. (Stinchfield, 1933, p. 29)

There was a considerable effort made by the charter members and early officers of ASHA to come up with a logical scheme and labels naming different kinds of speech disorders. An example of the exchanges on this topic is found in the following letter written in 1929 by Robert West to Elmer Kenyon, the president of the organization at that time, about what to call late developing speech:

> I rather balk at "normolalia" for infantile speech. We are not concerned with the baby talk of a baby; rather we are concerned with the baby talk of a child who has in other respects passed out of babyhood so that he has a type of speech that would be normal were he an infant. We must then choose some word that shows that it is not a normal condition. Why not then use a term translation of our phrase baby talk, such as "pedolalia"? (West, February 2, 1929) Source: From West, R. (1929, February 2). Unpublished personal letter to Elmer Kenyon. Washington, DC: American Speech-Language-Hearing Association Archives. Reprinted with permission.

While the stated purpose for the taxonomy under development was to provide students with an outline of the disorders of speech, the members of the national organization saw the classification system as a key to their newly forming professional identity.

The eventual listing of major types and subtypes of speech disorders classified by the nomenclature committee was extensive. It included over 100 different diagnostic categories with Greek and Latin names (Duchan, 2011a). The categories were grouped into six main types, some of which have withstood the tests of time (e.g., dysarthria, dysphasia, dysphonia). Our ancestors' predilection for Greek and Latin-based terminology has changed considerably over time in the U.S, being replaced by the use of accessible English terms such as *language disorders, stuttering,* or *hearing loss.* However, one can still find traces of our earlier preference for classical medical terms as evidenced by diagnostic category names that are still in use today such as *dysarthria, echolalia, aphasia, dyslexia,* and *dysphagia.*

Table 2–2 offers a comparison of some of the clinical terms used then and now. It translates the six main categories that served as a conceptual organizing structure some 80 years ago into today's parlance. It also includes the 1931 definitions, some of which contain theories about causality that have become outdated today (e.g., attributing weakened mental states or psychoses as a cause of certain communication disorders).

The scope of practice laid out by the nomenclature committee in 1931 changed dramatically following World War II. Around 1942 the term "audiology" was coined to describe the services provided to military personnel with suspected and actual hearing losses. Specialists involved in hearing testing and aural rehabilitation of military personnel during the war lobbied for the creation of a new field of audiology, one that they had been practicing in the military hospitals. Audiology was

seen then as now as a field that was separate but closely allied with speech correction. Also following the war, new attention was paid to the veterans with speech and language problems such as aphasia resulting from war-induced head injuries (Sheehan, 1948).

While services to those with aphasia and hearing impairment were provided before the war, the increase in need and funding during the war led to major upgrades in these areas of practice. Hearing loss in the Stinchfield-Robbins' 1931 taxonomy was treated as an etiology for speech problems (deaf mutism), and aphasia was seen as but a small domain that speech correctionists were trained to handle. The main emphasis of professionals in those very early years, judging from their writings and paper presentations, were in the areas of stuttering and childhood articulation disorders. However, practitioners and academics alike typically saw themselves as generalists rather than specialists. Faculty members in speech pathology typically taught courses in all areas of the field as is evidenced from the many programs that only had one faculty member specializing in speech correction.

During and following World War II, the areas of audiology and aphasia grew in importance, becoming established areas of professional specialization. This was particularly true in the newly established Veteran's Hospitals where specialized hearing and aphasia clinics and research centers were funded by the government and

Table 2–2. Comparison of Diagnostic Terminology Between 1931 and Today

Main Diagnostic Categories and Associated Definitions (Stinchfield & Robbins, 1931)	**Today's Names for 1931 Categories**
Dysarthria: Defects of articulation due to lesions of the nervous system	Dysarthria and motor speech disorders
Dyslalia: Functional and organic defects in articulation	Articulation and phonological disorders
Dyslogia: Difficulty in the expression of ideas by speech, due to psychoses	Pragmatic language disorders
Dysphasia: Impairment of language due to weakened mental imagery through disease, shock, or injury	Aphasia
Dysphemia: Variable disorders of speech due to psychoneuroses	Stuttering
Dysphonia: Defects of voice	Voice disorders
Dysrhythmia: Defects of rhythm, other than stuttering	Dysprosody; prosodic disturbances

served as a source for research studies and for experimentation and advancements in clinical methods. These Veterans' Administration (VA) clinics became epicenters of research and clinical activity in aphasia and audiology for many subsequent generations of students and professionals.

Specialty fields within any complex human service profession often begin as a research and practice subarea within a more general category of practice. This was true, for example, for autism, which was first categorized as a subtype of *emotional disturbance*. Ultimately, many clinical sub-areas were able to stand on their own, breaking off from their host categories. This happened, for example, for audiology during and after World War II and for autism spectrum disorders more recently. The degree of autonomy that any new specialty area attains depends upon factors such as the depth and scope of its research base and the success it has in creating diagnostic and therapeutic practices dedicated to that area. Typically, when a sub-specialty is gaining traction, national committees are created to carve out the details of the scope and practices. The committees specify what clinical skills are needed to serve the new population and what rules, regulations, and guidelines are needed to monitor those providing services in that area. In the last 20 years, the credibility of a new area of practice has been based largely on how well the therapy associated with that area meets the standards of evaluation associated with evidence-based practices (American Speech-Language-Hearing Association, 2006a).

Milestones for acquiring full and robust independence occur when specialty areas form their own interest groups within ASHA publish their own specialty journal, formulate their own certification standards, and develop their own evidence-based guidelines. For two relatively new specialty areas—multiculturalism and inclusive practices—the final milestone has been to infuse other areas of clinical practice with new guidelines and sensibilities specific to the sub-specialty.

Table 2–3 shows the origins and early developmental progression of seven specialty areas that have evolved in the last 50 years. Included in the table are indicators of the primary forces that drove the expansion of the area, some of the earliest and most seminal published work in the area, references to key federal laws governing practice in the area, ASHA guidelines and position statements about the area, whether and when members in that area became a special interest group (SIG) within ASHA, and the emergence of a professional journal dedicated to that practice domain.

The specialty areas listed in Table 2–3 established themselves in the profession in a variety of ways. As can be seen from the Table, different specialty areas came about as a result of different driving forces. Notable

among these driving forces were social reform movements, technological and internet advances, and changing conceptual frameworks.

Specialties Arising from Social Reform Movements

Reverberations from the civil rights movements in the 1960s were deeply felt in speech-language pathology. The first wave of changes was to remove clinical practice biases toward those who spoke in dialects other than Standard American English. African Americans in the profession, such as Orlando Taylor, Ron Williams, and Vicki Deal-Williams, lobbied for clinicians to treat dialect differences as legitimate and normal departures from Standard English and to differentiate them from errors arising from language disorders (Deal-Williams, 2009; Moore, 2009; Taylor, 1969; Williams, 1975).

The civil rights movement in the profession has grown steadily over the last 50 years, leading to new ASHA mandates and guidelines for best practices, ASHA's Office of Multicultural Affairs (est. 1969), and one of ASHA's 18 special interest divisions entitled Communication Disorders and Sciences in Culturally and Linguistically Diverse (CLD) Populations.

A second wave of social changes came from the disability rights movement in the 1970s. New legislation growing out of the movement included Public Law 94-142 in 1975, its reenactment as the Individuals with Disabilities Education Act (IDEA) in 1990, and the American Disabilities Act of (1990). These have all strongly affected professional practices. The inclusion movement in public education, for example, is based on the concepts arising in the disability movement that children with severe communication needs have the right to regular education. The service emphasis within this view is to find ways to support children so they can access and participate in regular classroom activities (American Speech-Language and Hearing Association, 1996b). Similarly, the focus on altering environments to include adults with disabilities has led to new interventions and clinical responsibilities that promote participation and engagement in everyday life activities (for example, Life participation approach to aphasia [LPAA] Project Group, 2011).

The disability rights movement required that clinicians reframe their services by shifting from a traditional medically based model, with its focus on remediation of individual disabilities, to a socially based one that works to reduce barriers and promote communication access (Duchan, 2001; LPAA Project Group, 2011; Lubinski, 2008; Simmons-Mackie, 2000). The model is variously referred to as the social model (Byng & Duchan, 2005; Simmons-Mackie, 2000), life participation model

Table 2–3. Seven Specialty Areas that Emerged Between 1960 and 2019

Specialty Area	Impetus for the Area's Emergence	Early Literature	Federal Legislation	ASHA Activities	ASHA Special Interest Group (SIG)	Specialty Journal(s)
(Central) auditory processing disorders (CAPD)	Information processing theories	Myklebust, 1954; Katz, 1968; Keith, 1977		ASHA 1993 Task Force on CAPD; ASHA 2002 working group on APD		
Augmentative and alternative communication (AAC)	Advances in technology	McDonald & Schultz, 1973; Vanderheiden, 1976; Vanderheiden et al., 1976.	US Technology Related Assistance Act, 1988; US Title 1 Programs for individuals with developmental disabilities, 2000.	ASHA 1981 Ad hoc committee on AAC; ASHA 1981 Position statement on AAC	SIG 12 Augmentative and Alternative Communication	*Augmentative and Alternative Communication,* established in 1984
Autism spectrum disorders	Shift from psychodynamic to learning theory and cognitive/ linguistic explanations	Kanner, 1943; Rutter, 1966; Lovaas, 1987	US Education for All Handicapped Children Act, 1975	ASHA 2003, Ad hoc committee on autism spectrum disorders; ASHA 2006, Position statement on autism spectrum disorders.		*Journal of Autism and Developmental Disorders,* established in 1970
Dysphagia	Advances in technology	Larsen, 1972; Logemann, 1983		ASHA 1987 Ad hoc committee on dysphagia, ASHA 1987 Technical report on dysphagia, ASHA 2004, Guidelines	SIG 13 Swallowing and Swallowing Disorders	*Dysphagia,* established in 1985
Language/learning disabilities	Information processing theories	Strauss & Lehtinen, 1947; Kirk & McCarthy, 1961	National Joint Committee on Learning Disabilities, 1975 (see Abrams, 1987)	ASHA 1976 ASHA 1982, Position Statement on Language/ Learning disabilities	SIG 1 Language Learning and Education	*Topics in Learning Disabilities,* established in 1967; *Topics in Language Disorders,* established in 1980

continues

Table 2–3. *continued*

Specialty Area	Impetus for the Area's Emergence	Early Literature	Federal Legislation	ASHA Activities	ASHA Special Interest Group (SIG)	Specialty Journal(s)
Inclusive practices	Social reform/ disability movement	Wilcox, Kouri, & Caswell, 1991; Duchan, 2001; LPAA Project Group, 2011	US Rehabilitation Act of 1973; US Education for all Handicapped Children Act, 1975; US Americans with Disabilities Act, 1990a; US IDEA, 1990	ASHA 1996b, Position statement on inclusive practices.		
Multiculturalism	Social reform/civil rights movement	Baratz, 1969; Taylor, 1969; Williams, 1975		ASHA 1969, Office of Multicultural Affairs established; ASHA 1983, Position statement on multiculturalism	SIG 14 Cultural and Linguistic Diversity SIG 17 Global Issues in Communication Sciences and Related Disorders	

(LPAA Project Group, 2011), communication access model (Byng & Duchan, 2004), or the environmental approach (Lubinski, 2008).

Social model practices have had a strong impact on scope of practices for children as well as adults. Interventions were created for supporting children's communication, including training in conversational skills for family members of children with communication disabilities (Hanen, 1975), developing competence-based approaches for school service personnel (Jorgensen, McSheehan, & Sonnenmeier, 2009), and adapting the curriculum and delivery systems to accommodate children in regular classrooms (Erickson, Koppenhaver, Yoder, & Nance, 1997). Conversational partner training was also developed to support adults with communication difficulties (Kagan, Black, Duchan, Simmons-Mackie, & Square, 2001; McVicker, Parr, Pound, & Duchan, 2009). Principles of universal design were applied to create communicatively accessible environments in public institutions (American Speech-Language-Hearing Association, n.d.-e; Lubinski, 2008; Parr, Pound, & Hewitt, 2006; Pound, Duchan, Penman, Hewitt, & Parr, 2007).

The Influence of Technologies on the Growth and Shaping of Specialties

Technological changes have had a strong influence on clinical practices in speech-language pathology and audiology since the earliest years of the professions' formation. One way our early disciplines endeavored to establish themselves as respectable professions was to become more "scientific." To that end, efforts were made to develop measuring devices for understanding mechanisms underlying speech production and perception (Scripture, 1899) and for evaluating clinical performance (Travis, 1957).

Carl Seashore exemplifies the group of founders who were also inventors. He invented several instruments for measuring aspects of sound, voice, and music during his time at the University at Iowa. In 1902, he developed the Voice Tonoscope, to record, measure, and display (via waveforms) various aspects of the human voice (Malin, 2011). Seashore's Tonoscope provided an early model for modern voice instrumentation such as the Visipitch.

Another of Seashore's inventions was an early version of an audiometer. This machine, called the Iowa Pitch Range Audiometer, presented a series of clicks of increasing intensity through a telephone receiver held up to the test-taker's ear. After several unsuccessful iterations, Seashore finally came up with a prototype audiometer that could measure hearing thresholds—not only at a range of sound intensities but also at various frequencies—and could deliver the auditory stimuli under headphones. Lee Edward Travis, also from the University of Iowa, shared Seashore's interest in developing ways to measure speech and hearing behaviors. Travis was one of the first researchers in America to use electrophysiological methods (EMG and EEG) to measure motor movements and brain activity (Lindsley, 1976) and he became one of our field's most prolific and adventurous scientists in the early years of the profession.

Research laboratories early in our professions' history also served as incubators for technological advances in speech and hearing instrumentation. In 1922, inventors at Bell Telephone Labs developed the first hearing aid, weighing in at 200 pounds; in 1929 they developed the first prototype of an artificial larynx; in 1937 they invented a speech synthesizer; and in 1941, they produced the first speech spectrograph (Engineering & Technology History Wiki, Bell Labs n.d.). All of these inventions led to transformational changes in research and practice in both speech pathology and audiology.

Technological advances in the speech and hearing science did not, however, always translate to similar advances in clinical practice. Charles Van Riper (1986), another early pioneer in our field, writes about his experiences as a new faculty member and speech clinician at Western Michigan University in 1936:

> I had no equipment at all in that first speech clinic except three tuning forks that I used to test hearing. . . . There were no audiometers back then. I also bought a throat mirror and some tongue depressors, made models of the larynx out of clay, drew charts showing the various speech organs, and contrived a skeleton out of paper mache [sic], coat hangers [sic] and tape. . . . Oh yes, I also had a toothbrush which I used to cure lisping. I'd brush it along the midline of the tongue, tell the kid to close his teeth and blow along the place that tingled. Damned if it didn't work on a lot of them. (Van Riper, 1986, p. 91)

Van Riper's observations reflected the experiences of many speech-language pathologists well into the 1980s, many of whom had little more than a cassette tape recorder and Language Master[1] at their disposal. This experience is changing in many work settings, although clinicians "in the trenches" still rely upon ingenuity and creativity to measure and motivate clients when technology is not available.

---

[1]A Language Master was a portable recording machine that used magnetized cards that could record a few seconds of (clinician) speech. A parallel track could be recorded over by the client. The tracks could be played back over and over again for comparison. This was a very popular "electronic" therapy aid throughout the 1970s and into the 1980s.

Technology's Spawning of New Areas of Clinical Practice. Technological advances have not only revolutionized how we carry out our research and clinical practice but have given birth to new areas of clinical practice. For example, the development of high-tech communication devices for clients with multiple disabilities has led to the emergence of a specialty area called Augmentative/Alternative Communication (AAC). Practices and research in AAC began in the 1980s with increasing demand for speech-language services for non-speaking populations. Devices were invented that were both "low" and "high" tech. The high-tech devices allowed for the storage and retrieval of electronic messages and many could also produce synthesized speech. The first known AAC device was developed in 1969 by an undergraduate engineering student (Barry Romich) and his friend (Ed Prentke) from a discarded teletype machine (Prentke-Romich Company, n.d.-a). These two entrepreneurs would soon form the Prentke Romich Company, now one of the largest and most successful developers of speech generating devices in the nation. A relatively recent trend in the AAC field has been to use tablets as AAC devices for clinical practice and communication (Leibs, 2018).

Another significant technological advance in recent times has been the introduction of cochlear implants. This breakthrough has allowed persons who have never had functional hearing to perceive sound and speech, often for the first time. This surgical implant, which externally resembles a hearing aid, works (generally speaking) by producing an electrical current that stimulates surviving regions of the auditory nerve. Surprisingly, the possibility that electrical currents might be used to stimulate audition was reportedly first suggested by Alessandro Volta in 1800 (Traynor, 2016; Volta, 1800). An empirical test of this theory, however, could not be done safely until much later. Exploratory surgical studies on a small number of adults with profound deafness were performed in 1961 (House & Berliner, 1991) and in 1964 (Simmons et al, 1965). These pioneering studies paved the way for the aggressive development of this technology. According to ASHA, the first single channel cochlear implant was introduced in 1972 (American Speech-Language-Hearing Association, 2004b). From that date until the mid-1980s, approximately 1000 children and adults received cochlear implants. In 1984, the first multi-channel cochlear implant system was placed on the market. Since then, manufacturers of cochlear implants have continued to improve the technology.

In 2017, the National Institutes on Deafness and Other Communication Disorders estimated that 324,200 people worldwide had cochlear implants, with approximately 96,000 of these residing in the United States (National Institute on Deafness and Other Communication Disorders, 2017). Audiologists have the primary responsibility for teaching recipients how to use their implant successfully and for monitoring the effectiveness of the device. Recently, the American Board of Audiology established clinical practice guidelines for audiologists who manage implant patients. This organization also offers specialty certification to audiologists who provide cochlear implant services (American Board of Audiology, 2011).

Another area of clinical practice, swallowing disorders, can serve as a case study for how technology has expanded research and scope of practice in speech-language pathology. Students who received a master's degree in Communication Sciences and Disorders in the 1970s and early 1980s had no coursework in dysphagia (i.e., swallowing disorders). Today, virtually every accredited master's program in the country has a required course devoted solely to this topic.

Rigorous dysphagia assessment by SLPs cannot be performed in modern times without technology. Diagnosing swallowing disorders typically involves real-time swallow studies that are minimally invasive, efficient, and cost-effective. They include videofluoroscopy (also known as the modified barium swallow) and fiberoptic laryngoscopy (also known as FEES).

Although fiberoptic laryngoscopy technologies have existed since the mid-1960s their routine use in the assessment of dysphagia, often in combination with videofluoroscopy, did not become standard practice until the 1980s (Langmore, 2017). Initially, physicians (typically laryngologists) were the medical practitioners who performed and interpreted these procedures.

In 1983, Dr. Jeri Logemann published a seminal book on the evaluation and treatment of swallowing disorders (Logemann, 1983), arguing that SLPs had the appropriate background to work with the dysphagia population. She went on to promote immediate speech-language pathology curricular changes that would ensure that future graduates would have technical skills for providing swallowing assessment and interventions (Logemann, 2006).

Other advocates for broadening the SLP scope of practice to include dysphagia management soon emerged. Today, a Special Interest Group (SIG 13) on Swallowing and Swallowing Disorders (Dysphagia) has been created by ASHA, as well as a Specialty Board Certification (BCS-S) in swallowing (American Speech-Language-Hearing Association, 2006b).

The Impact of Computers and the Internet. In the last 20 years, with the introduction and increased availability of computers, software, and the internet, basic practices have changed significantly in almost every health-related discipline. Today's clinicians in every work environment use computers and the internet as routine parts of their clinical practice. Specialized software aids practitioners in report writing, billing, and client scheduling. Several standardized speech and language tests now include an optional computer-based scoring system. Therapy sessions incorporate games and apps. Computer-based intervention programs are used to treat specific disorders, such as deficits in auditory processing.

The way in which both researchers and clinicians obtain information has also changed significantly. Paper journals have all but disappeared. When clinicians or scientists need to find information about a particular topic, they will almost invariably begin that search using Google Scholar and the more specialized search engines maintained online by ASHA such as the Practice Portal (American Speech-Language-Hearing Association, n.d.-f) and the online repository for all ASHA journals, known as ASHAWire (American Speech-Language-Hearing Association, n.d.-g). When clinicians want to find creative games or projects to use in therapy, they may turn to commercial sites such as Speech Therapy Ideas (Speech Therapy Ideas, n.d.).

The Influence of Conceptual Frameworks on Specialties

The last 50 years of our history have seen a number of changes in practices that have come about as a result of new ways of looking at disabilities and their etiologies. The area of autism offers a sterling example of how shifts in conceptual frameworks have altered our scope of practice. Leo Kanner first portrayed autism in 1943 as a kind of emotional disorder (Kanner, 1943). The disorder, in his view as a psychoanalyst, was caused by lack of maternal affection. Following Kanner the entire medical establishment in the U.S. considered the communication difficulties of those with autism as being secondary to their emotional disability. Therapies began with work on the emotional problem, in hopes that the communication disabilities would then take care of themselves. The most blatant version of this view was that of Bruno Bettelheim, who advocated removing children from their homes to give them the love that they were deprived of by their "refrigerator mothers" (Bettelheim, 1950). Physicians and psychologists, not communication specialists, were the professionals seen as having the needed expertise in emotional rehabilitation.

Another prevailing framework that kept SLPs out of the clinical loop when providing services to those with autism was information processing theory. These so-called box-and-arrow models adopted by the field offered no place for emotional content in communication process (Baker, Croot, McLeod, & Paul, 2001; Duchan, 2011e). Since autism was seen as an emotionally based problem, SLPs were given no role in diagnosis or rehabilitation of this population.

But this all changed with the 1987 work of Ivar Lovaas, a behavioral psychologist, who published a study showing that nonverbal children with autism could learn to speak (Lovaas, 1987). Thus began a shift in thinking about the disorder. Once it became general consensus that autism was a social-communicative disability, SLPs played a major role in research and practice in the area. Clinicians and researchers focused on intentionality, social skill building, and providing augmentative and alternative communication opportunities to children with autism, thereby creating what is now an important area in our scope of practice.

The linguistic revolution of the 1970s created an even broader tectonic shift in scope of clinical and research practices for the field of speech pathology. It was a time when a new discipline was emerging in the social sciences, one grounded in theories and research in the fields of psychology and linguistics. The combined discipline came to be called psycholinguistics.

One such framework that became popular was based upon psycholinguistic models of language processing that differentiated perceptual-motor-based problems from higher order cognitive-linguistic ones (Kirk & McCarthy, 1961; Myklebust, 1954; Wepman, Jones, Bock, & Van Pelt, 1960). Tests such as the *Illinois Test of Psycholinguistic Ability*, or *ITPA* (McCarthy & Kirk, 1961), became widely used and therapy programs for children with language disorders quickly emerged that were based upon this modular conceptualization of the language processing system (e.g., Kirk & Kirk, 1971). Seemingly diverse disorders such as hearing loss and aphasia that had been treated as separate areas of practice became conceptually associated within these psycholinguistic processing models. The effort for diagnosticians, then, was not only to identify and differentiate disorders from one another, but also to determine how each disorder impacted other areas in the psycholinguistic processing system. Conceptual models such as these helped lead to the growth in the 1960s of new areas of specialization, considerably expanding professional practice areas. Thus, while each new specialty area clearly had its own historical origins and milestones, some general growth trends became apparent when examining them together.

The psycholinguistic framework that focused on language structure and processing shifted the thinking and practice in areas such as delayed speech, articulation problems, and aphasia. The shifts led to name changes of the well-worn categories, with delayed speech becoming childhood language disorders and articulation problems changing to phonological disorders. Linguistic analyses became substituted for or added to diagnostic testing methods and newly devised language therapies targeted linguistic rules or psychological processes such as memory and attention (Duchan, 2011c).

In the 1970s, the psycholinguistic model provided clinicians with a framework for the construction of yet another diagnostic group, children with language-learning disabilities (LLD). The psycholinguistic focus on researching, identifying, and treating LLD children was so influential that leaders in the profession, such as Kay Butler, started a movement to have the term *language* added to ASHA's title and to change the professionals name from *speech pathologist* to *speech-language pathologist*. These changes were acted upon in 1978 when the field and professionals added language to their titles.

This emphasis on language learning and processing positioned clinicians in public schools to play a key role in identifying and providing services to children with language-learning problems. Fred Spahr, the managing director for ASHA from 1980 to 2003, commented on the impact of adding language and LLD to ASHA's scope of practices in schools:

> There have been big changes also in speech-language pathology in the schools. When I first began at ASHA almost 90% of the caseloads of school-based clinicians were made up of children with articulation disorders. Today 90% of their caseloads are children with language-based disorders. This change is owing to the foresight of leaders in the late 1970s and early 1980s who recognized that the education and training of speech pathologists (as they were known then) would allow us to deal with issues related to language and language training in children. And today this training has allowed clinicians to enter the important area of literacy. (Uffen, 2003)

In audiology, one can also see the influence of an elaborately detailed information-processing conceptual framework. Audiologists who had previously focused on peripheral aspects of hearing began to emphasize stages of processing of auditory information including what came to be called central auditory processing. Tests measuring different kinds of processing have evolved, research has been conducted to locate the source of the auditory processes in the neurological system, and therapies have been devised to remediate central auditory processing disorders (American Speech-Language-Hearing Association, 1996a; Keith, 1977; Masters, Stecker, & Katz, 1992). Audiologists have also expanded their diagnostic and intervention services to include tinnitus, vestibular disorders, and cochlear implants. Developments in hearing aid technology and the license to dispense hearing aids greatly enhanced audiologists' scope of practice.

Recent Trends

The new millennium brings its own set of professional issues, adding to and continuing with those that came before. These involve upheavals in population demographics, the economy, educational and medical practices, information technology, and globalization. In order to accommodate this changing world, SLPs and audiologists are changing how they go about their business.

For example, two new special interest groups have been created in ASHA. Special Interest Group 17 is dedicated to dispensing information and dealing with issues related to Globalization and Special Interest Group 18, is dedicated to dealing with the impact of the newest technology on professional practices, or what the founders of the division have called Telepractice. The most recent Special Interest Group 19, developed in 2015, is one that focuses on areas of Speech Science (American Speech-Language-Hearing Association, n.d.-h).

Among the most robust and far-reaching changes affecting professional practices are those coming from the evidence-based practice movement. This movement entered our field in the late 1990s following the lead of medical researchers in Canada and England (Dollaghan, 2007; Sackett, Straus, Richardson, Rosenberg, & Haynes, 2000). An important catalyst for the movement was the writings of David Sackett and his colleagues in the *British Journal of Medicine*. While the movement as such is a twentieth and twenty-first century one, Sackett and others have traced its philosophical origins to the late nineteenth century (Sackett, Rosenberg, Gray, Haynes, & Richardson, 1996, p. 71). It was then, in France, that positivism first took root (Comte, 1907). The positivist view of the world and of how science is best carried out favors sense experience over subjective experience and positive, measurable data over derived or inferential (deep structure) information. Positivism has led to other movements in the profession, including the standardized testing movement beginning in the 1970s, and the profession's effort to obtain measurable outcomes for therapy practices that took hold in 1990s (Fratalli, 1998). Evidence-based practice in our profession builds upon these earlier movements by favoring standardized and well-controlled data collection to evaluate therapy efficacy and efficiency (American Speech-Language-Hearing Association, 2005).

This positivist bias of the evidence-based movement is reflected in its focus on large research studies, especially those using randomized, experimentally controlled trials. The studies tend to be about the usefulness of a particular kind of treatment within a particular domain of practice. Evidence-based studies have been done to evaluate the effectiveness or efficacy of many areas of practice, such as augmentative communication intervention (Schlosser, 2000) and auditory processing disorder therapies (Fey, Richard, Geffner, Kamhi, Medwetsky, Paul, Ross-Swain, Wallach, & Frymark, 2010). Areas that have received particular attention in the evidence-based literature are those whose practices have been controversial (e.g., Lof & Watson, 2008 on nonspeech oral motor exercises).

Besides focusing primarily on randomized controlled studies, the evidence-based practice movement has given rise to a healthy literature comparing the findings from different studies. These research studies involving what has been called meta-analyses have been done in different areas of practice, including, for example, treatments for developmental speech and language delay and aphasia (Law, Garrett, & Nye, 2004; Robey, 1998).

The emphasis on empirical, measurable research outcomes from controlled studies has tended to result in inattention to significant and helpful areas of evidence, such as the voice of the client (Kovarsky, 2008; Kovarsky & Curran, 2007) the degree of client engagement in the therapeutic activity (Simmons-Mackie & Kovarsky, 2009) and the quality of the relationship between those involved in the clinical interaction (Duchan, 2011e; Fourie, 2011). Some have argued that the experiment itself can bias the results being obtained (Duchan, 1993, 1995). Indeed, the major figures in the evidence-based practices field, including Sackett et al. (1996) and Dollaghan (2007), have bemoaned the narrow, positivist view that has come to dominate the evidence-based literature. These authors have argued for enriching and expanding on the definition of evidence in typical evidence-based discussions to include phenomenological or subjective evidence as well as results of qualitative research. Those promoting a broader view of evidence have also argued that clinicians should base their decision making not only on research evidence, but also on evidence gathered from their own clinical experience and from their clients' values, goals, and preferences (Dollaghan, 2007; Sackett et al, 2000). Sackett and his colleagues have observed that:

> Without clinical expertise, practice risks becoming tyrannized by evidence, for even excellent external evidence may be inapplicable or inappropriate for an individual patient. Without current best evidence, practice risks becoming rapidly out of date, to the detriment of patients. (Sackett et al., 1996, p. 72)

See Chapter 8, "Applying Evidence to Clinical Practice," for more information.

Summary

In this short history of the profession of communication disorders we have tried to show how professional practices in both speech-language pathology and audiology have changed considerably over the years and how they continue to change. Our aim has been to capture the dynamics and direction of growth by focusing on the founding of the organization, changes in membership and certification requirements, and the factors influencing growth and specialization in the field.

In the early days of the professional organization, leaders worked to establish an honorary academy, to create by-laws that included goals and membership requirements, and to carve out a scope of practice. Later the organization opened its doors to clinicians. Still later, it began credentialing its members creating criteria for providing services in speech pathology and audiology. ASHA increased its training and credentialing requirements to keep up with burgeoning information associated with different areas of practice. In its latest stages, the organization began to expand into new areas of specialty. These new specialty areas have their own histories, with different driving forces, modes of independence, and growth patterns. The areas that were most successful in establishing professional autonomy within the organization were ones that were associated with social changes taking place in society (multicultural and inclusionary practices following a social model), ones that changed with technology (e.g., stuttering, AAC, cochlear implants, dysphagia) and ones that were consistent with newly emerging conceptual frameworks (autism, language and learning disabilities, and auditory processing disorders.) Together, these shifts in practices illustrate the complexity and dynamic nature of professional issues in the field. The historical events described in this chapter have been offered as a context for understanding how some of today's practices came about, as well as a context for understanding that today's practices are about to become tomorrow's history.

Critical Thinking

1. Can you give several examples of how professional issues of today are a continuation of those of the past?

2. How have the histories of audiology and speech-pathology differed over the years?

3. How have social attitudes and changes in the society affected professional practices of the past?

4. What are some other societal trends, besides ones mentioned in this chapter, that have had an impact on professional practices?

5. How has technology influenced clinical practice? What technological advances may be on the horizon that will promote future changes?

6. What are the pros and cons of evidence-based practices?

7. What aspects of today's professions need changing and why do you think they should be changed?

8. What avenues are available to you to bring about changes in the profession?

9. How might a view from history aid in the understanding and enactment of current professional practices?

References

Abrams, J. (1987). National Joint Committee on Learning Disabilities: History, mission, process. *Journal of Learning Disabilities, 20*(2), 102–106.

Academy of the Doctors of Audiology. (n.d.). *AuD timeline.* Retrieved from https://www.audiologist.org/history/aud-timeline/

American Academy of Audiology. (2019). *AuD facts.* Retrieved from https://www.audiology.org/education-research/education/students/aud-facts/

American Academy of Speech Correction. (1927). Association News. *Quarterly Journal of Speech, 12,* 311–317.

American Board of Audiology. (2011). *Cochlear implant specialty certification.* Retrieved from http://www.boardofaudiology.org/cochlear-implant-specialty-certification/

American Speech Correction Association. (1943). Membership regulation. *Journal of Speech Disorders, 8*(1), 41–51.

American Speech Correction Association. (1945). The American Speech Correction Association presents the honors of the association to Carl Emil Seashore. *Journal of Speech Disorders, 10,* 1–2.

American Speech and Hearing Association. (1952). Clinical certification requirements of the American Speech and Hearing Association. *Journal of Speech and Hearing Disorders, 17,* 249–254.

American Speech and Hearing Association. (1969). *Office of Multicultural Affairs.* Retrieved from http://www.asha.org/practice/multicultural/about.htm

American Speech and Hearing Association. (1976). Learning disabilities. *ASHA, 18,* 282–290.

American Speech-Language-Hearing Association (1981). Report of ad hoc committee on communication processes and nonspeaking persons. Position statement on nonspeech communication. *ASHA, 23*(8), 577–581.

American Speech-Language-Hearing Association. (1982). Position statement on language learning disorders. *ASHA, 11,* 937–944.

American Speech-Language-Hearing Association. (1983). Social dialects and implications of the positions on social dialects [Position paper], *ASHA, 25*(9), 23–27.

American Speech-Language-Hearing Association. (1987). Dysphasia. *ASHA, 29,* 57–58.

American Speech-Language-Hearing Association. (1996a). Central auditory processing: Current status of research and implications for clinical practice. *American Journal of Audiology, 5,* 41–54.

American Speech-Language-Hearing Association. (1996b). *Inclusive practices for children and youths with communication disorders* [Position statement]. Retrieved from https://www.asha.org/policy/PS1996-00223/

American Speech-Language-Hearing Association. (2003). *Cochlear implants.* Retrieved from https://www.asha.org/policy/tr2004-00041/#sec1.2

American Speech-Language-Hearing Association. (2004a, updated 2017). *Guidelines for speech-language pathologists performing videofluoroscopic swallowing studies* [Guidelines]. Retrieved from https://www.asha.org/policy/GL2004-00050.htm

American Speech-Language-Hearing Association. (2004b). *Technical report: Cochlear implants.* Retrieved on from https://www.asha.org/policy/TR2004-00041/

American Speech-Language-Hearing Association. (2005). *Evidence based practices in communication disorders.* Retrieved from https://www.asha.org/policy/PS2005-00221/

American Speech-Language-Hearing Association. (2006a). *Roles and responsibilities of speech-language pathologists in diagnosis, assessment, and treatment* of autism spectrum disorders across the life span [Position statement]. Retrieved from https://www.asha.org/policy/ps2006-00105/

American Speech-Language-Hearing Association. (2006b). *Speech-Language Pathologists (SLPs) as the preferred providers for dysphagia services.* Retrieved from https://www.asha.org/uploaded Files/slp/clinical/dysphagia/TalkingPointsprefer provider.pdf

American Speech-Language-Hearing Association. (2011). *A chronology of changes in ASHA's certification standards.* Retrieved from http://www.asha.org/Certification/CCC_history.htm

American Speech-Language-Hearing Association. (2015). *Guidelines for the clinical doctorate in speech-language pathology.* Retrieved from https://www.asha.org/policy/GL2015-00341/

American Speech-Language-Hearing Association. (2019). *Certification standards to change in 2020.* Retrieved from https://www.asha.org/Certification/Certification-Standards-Change-in-2020/

American Speech-Language-Hearing Association. (n.d.-a). *Maintaining your certification.*

American Speech-Language-Hearing Association. (n.d.-b). *A chronology of changes in ASHA's certification standards.* Retrieved from http://www.asha.org/certification/CCC_history.htm

American Speech-Language-Hearing Association. (n.d.-c). *State teacher credentialing requirements.* Retrieved from https://www.asha.org/advocacy/state/StateTeacherCredentialingRequirements/

American Speech-Language-Hearing Association. (n.d.-d). *ASHA state by state.* Retrieved from https://www.asha.org/advocacy/state/

American Speech-Language-Hearing Association. (n.d.-e). *Universal design for learning.* Retrieved from https://www.asha.org/SLP/schools/Universal-Design-for-Learning/

American Speech-Language-Hearing Association. (n.d.-f). *The practice portal.* Retrieved from https://www.asha.org/practice-portal/

American Speech-Language-Hearing Association. (n.d.-g). *ASHAwire.* Retrieved from https://pubs.asha.org/

American Speech-Language-Hearing Association. (n.d.-h). *About Special Interest Group 19: Speech science.* Retrieved from https://www.asha.org/SIG/19/About-SIG-19/

Aram, D., & Nation, J. (1982). Historical heritage of child language disorders. In D. Aram & J. Nation (Eds.), *Child language disorders* (pp. 7–31). St. Louis, MO: C.V. Mosby.

Baker, E., Croot, K., McLeod, S., & Paul, R. (2001). Psycholinguistic models of speech development and their application to clinical practice. *Journal of Speech-Language and Hearing Research, 44,* 685–702.

Baratz, J. (1969) Language and cognitive assessments of Negro children: Assumptions and research needs. *ASHA, 11,* 87–91.

Bernthal, J. (2007, May 29). Looking back and to the future of professional education in speech-language pathology. *The ASHA Leader.* Retrieved from https://leader.pubs.asha.org/doi/10.1044/leader.AN.12072007.14

Berry, M. (1965). Historical vignettes of leadership in speech and hearing: III Stuttering. *ASHA, 7,* 78–79.

Bettelheim, B. (1950) *Love is not enough: The treatment of emotionally disturbed children.* Glencoe, IL: Free Press.

Black, M. (1966). The origins and status of speech therapy in the schools. *ASHA, 8,* 419–425.

Bobrick, B, (1995). *Knotted tongues: Stuttering in history and a quest for a cure.* New York, NY: Simon & Schuster.

Boone, D. (2010). A historical perspective of voice management: 1940–1970. *Perspectives on Voice and Voice Disorders, 20,* 47–55.

Bowen, C. (2009). *Children's speech sound disorders.* New York, NY: Wiley.

Byng, S., & Duchan, J. (2004) Challenging aphasia therapies. In J. Duchan & S. Byng (Eds.), *Challenging aphasia therapies* (pp. 8–18). London, UK: Psychology Press.

Byng, S., & Duchan, J. (2005). Social model philosophies and principles: Their applications to therapies for aphasia. *Aphasiology, 19,* 906–922.

Carrell, J. (1946). State certification of speech correctionists. *Journal of Speech Disorders, 11*(2), 91–95.

Chapman, R. (2007). Children's language learning: An interactionist perspective. In R. Paul (Ed.), *Language disorders from a developmental perspective.* (pp. 3–53). Mahwah, NJ: Lawrence Erlbaum.

Comte, A. (1907). *A general view of positivism.* London, UK: Routledge and Sons.

Council of Academic Programs in Communication Sciences and Disorders. (2017). *Resolution: Clinical doctorate in speech-language pathology.* Retrieved from http://www.capcsd.org/wp-content/uploads/2017/10/Clinical-Doctorate-in-SLP-Proposed-Resolution-Passed-August-15-2017.pdf

Deafness in Disguise. (2010). *Concealed hearing devices of the 19th century.* St. Louis, MO: Washington University School of Medicine. Retrieved from http://beckerexhibits.wustl.edu/did/19thcent/index.htm

Deal-Williams, V. (2009). The roots of our experience: Trials and triumphs. *The ASHA Leader.* Retrieved from https://leader.pubs.asha.org/doi/10.1044/leader.AN2.14042009.20

Doerfler, L. (1981). A short history of audiology and aural rehabilitation. *ASHA, 23,* 858.

Dollaghan, C. (2007). *The handbook for evidence-based practice in communication disorders.* Baltimore, MD: Paul H. Brookes.

Duchan, J. (1993). Issues raised by facilitated communication for theorizing and research on autism, *Journal of Speech and Hearing Research, 36,* 1108–1119.

Duchan, J. (1995). The role of experimental research in validating facilitated communication. *Journal of Speech and Hearing Research, 38,* 207–210.

Duchan, J. (2001). Impairment and social views of speech-language pathology: Clinical practices re-examined. *Advances in Speech-Language Pathology, 3*(1), 37–45.

Duchan, J. (2009). The early years of speech-language and hearing services in US schools. *Language, Speech, and Hearing Services in Schools.* Retrieved from http://lshss.asha.org/cgi/content/abstract/41/2/152

Duchan, J. (2011a). *Diagnostic taxonomy of Stinchfield and Robbins.* Retrieved from http://www.acsu.buffalo.edu/~duchan/history_subpages/stinchfieldtaxonomy.html

Duchan, J. (2011b). *Emergence of professionalism in late 19th and early 20th century America.* Retrieved from http://www.acsu.buffalo.edu/~duchan/new_history/hist19c/professionalism.html

Duchan, J. (2011c). *The linguistic era, 1965–1975. In getting here: A short history of speech-language pathology in America.* Retrieved from http://www.acsu.buffalo.edu/~duchan/1965-1975.html

Duchan, J. (2011d). *Pioneers of speech-language pathology and audiology.* Retrieved from http://www.acsu.buffalo.edu/~duchan/biographies.html

Duchan, J. (2011e). How conceptual frameworks influence discovery and depictions of emotions in clinical relationships. *Topics in Language Disorders, 31*(4), 300–309.

Engineering & Technology History Wiki: Bell Labs. (n.d.). Retrieved on April 11, 2019 from https://ethw.org/Bell_Labs

Erickson, K., Koppenhaver, D. Yoder, D., & Nance, J. (1997). Integrated communication and literacy instruction for a child with multiple disabilities. *Focus on Autism and Other Developmental Disabilities, 12*(3), 142–150.

Fey, M., Richard, G., Geffner, G., Kamhi, A., Medwetsky, L., Paul, D., . . . Frymark, T. (2010) Auditory processing disorders and auditory/language interventions: An evidence-based systematic review. *Language, Speech, and Hearing Services in Schools.* Retrieved from https://pubs.asha.org/doi/10.1044/0161-1461(2010/10-0013)

Fourie, R. (Ed.). (2011). *Therapeutic processes for communication disorders.* New York, NY: Psychology Press.

Frattali, C. (1998). Outcomes measurement: definitions, dimensions and perspectives. In C. Frattali (Ed.) *Measuring outcomes in speech-language pathology* (pp. 1–27). New York, NY: Thieme.

Gifford, (1925). Speech correction work in the San Francisco Public Schools. *Quarterly Journal of Speech Education, 11,* 277–381.

GRADschools.com. (n.d.). *Find Doctor of Clinical Science (CScD) and Speech Pathology Doctorate degrees.* Retrieved from https://www.gradschools.com/doctorate/communication-science-disorders/speech-pathology

Hanen, A. (1975). *It takes two to talk.* Toronto, CA: Hanen Centre.

Horshaw, G. E. (2019). Know when to apply for your CCCs. *ASHA Leader, 24*(8), 44–45.

House, W., & Berliner, K. (1991). Cochlear implants: From idea to clinical practice. In H. Cooper (Ed.). *Cochlear implants: A practical guide* (pp. 9–33). San Diego, CA: Singular Publishing.

Howard, D., & Hatfield F. (1987). *Aphasia therapy: Historical and contemporary issues.* London, UK: Erlbaum.

Hull, R. (Ed.) (2001). *Aural rehabilitation: Serving children and adults* (4th ed.). San Diego: Singular Publishing.

Irwin, R. (1953). State certification in speech and hearing therapy. *The Speech Teacher*, 2, 124–128.

Irwin, R. (1955). State programs in speech and hearing therapy. Part II: Certification. *The Speech Teacher*, 4, 253–258.

Irwin, R. (1959). Speech therapy in the public schools: State Legislation and Certification. *Journal of Speech and Hearing Disorders*, 24, 2, 127–143.

Jerger, J. (2009). *Audiology in the USA*. San Diego, CA: Plural Publishing.

Jerger, J. (2016). *A life in audiology*. San Diego, CA: Plural Publishing.

Jorgensen, C., McSheehan, M., & Sonnenmeier, R. (2009). *The Beyond Access Model: Promoting membership, participation and learning for students with disabilities in the general education classroom.* Baltimore, MD: Paul H. Brookes.

Kagan, A., Black, S., Duchan, J., Simmons-Mackie, N., & Square, P. (2001). Training volunteers as conversation partners using "Supported Conversation for Adults with Aphasia" (SCA): A controlled trial, *Journal of Speech, Language, and Hearing Research*, 44(3), 610–623.

Kanner, L. (1943). Autistic disturbances of affective contact. *Nervous Child*, 2, 217–250.

Katz, J. (1968). The SSW Test: An interim report. *Journal of Speech and Hearing Disorders*, 33, 132–146.

Keith, R. (Ed.). (1977). *Central auditory dysfunction.* New York. NY: Grune & Stratton.

Kirk, S., & Kirk, W. (1971). *Psycholinguistic learning disabilities: Diagnosis and remediation.* Urbana, IL: University of Illinois Press.

Kirk, S., & McCarthy, J. (1961). *Illinois Test of Psycholinguistic Abilities.* Urbana, IL: The University of Illinois Press.

Kovarsky, D. (2008). Representing voices from the life-world in evidence-based practice. *International Journal of Language and Communication Disorders*, 43(Suppl. 1), 47–57.

Kovarsky, D., & Curran, M. (2007). The missing voice in the discourse of evidence-based practice. *Topics in Language Disorders*, 27(1), 50–61.

Langmore, S. (2017). History of fiberoptic endoscopic evaluation of swallowing for evaluation and management of pharyngeal dysphagia: Changes over the years. *Dysphagia*, 32(1), 27–38.

Larsen, G. (1972). Rehabilitation for dysphagia paralytica, *Journal of Speech and Hearing Disorders*, 37, 187–194.

Law, J., Garrett, Z., & Nye, C. (2004). The efficacy of treatment for children with developmental speech and language delay/disorder: A meta-analysis. *Journal of Speech-Language-Hearing Research*, 47, 924–943.

Leibs, A. (2018). Top alternative and augmentative communication (AAC) apps for iPad. *Lifewire.* Retrieved from https://www.lifewire.com/top-alter native-and-augmentative-communication-198828

Leonard, L. (2000). *Children with specific language impairment.* Boston, MA: The MIT Press.

Lindsley, D. B. (1976). The first half of a remarkable life and career: The Nebraska and Iowa years. In D. Tweedie & P. Clement (Eds.). *Psychologist Pro Tem: In honor of the 80th birthday of Lee Edward Travis.* Los Angeles, CA: University of Southern California Press.

Lof, G., & Watson, M. (2008). A nationwide survey of nonspeech oral motor exercise use: Implications for evidence-based practice. *Language, Speech, and Hearing Services in Schools*, 39, 392–407.

Logemann, J. (1983) *Evaluation and treatment of swallowing disorders.* San Diego, CA: College-Hill Press.

Logemann, J. (2006). Preparation of speech-language pathologists in the United States: Master's Degree. *Folia Phoniatrica and Logopaedica*, 58(1), 55–58.

Lorch, M. (2005). Guest editor, special issue. The history of aphasiology. Special issue, *Journal of Neurolinguistics*. 18, 4.

Lovaas, O. (1987). Behavioral treatment and normal educational and intellectual functioning in young autistic children. *Journal of Consulting and Clinical Psychology*, 55, 3–9.

LPAA Project Group. (2011). *Life participation approach to aphasia.* Retrieved from https://www .asha.org/public/speech/disorders/LPAA.htm

Lubinski, R. (2003). Revisiting the Professional doctorate in medical speech-language pathology. *Journal of Medical Speech-Language Pathology*, 11, lix-lxii.

Lubinski, R. (2008). Environmental approach to adult aphasia. In R. Chapey (Ed.), *Language intervention strategies in aphasia and related neurogenic communication disorders* (5th ed.). Baltimore, MD: Williams and Wilkins.

Lubinski, R., & Higginbotham, J. (Eds.). (1997). *Communication technologies for the elderly: Vision, hearing, and speech.* San Diego, CA: Singular Publishing.

Malin, C. (2011). Not just your average beauty: Carl Seashore and the history of communication research in the United States. *Communication Theory, 21,* 3. Retrieved from https://academic .oup.com/ct/article-abstract/21/3/299/4085680

Malone, R. (1999). *The first 75 years: American Speech-Language-Hearing Association.* Rockville, MD: American Speech-Language and Hearing Association.

Masters, M., Stecker, N., & Katz, J. (1992). *Central auditory processing disorders: Mostly management.* New York, NY: Allyn & Bacon.

McCarthy, J., & Kirk, W. (1961). *Illinois Test of Psycholinguistic Abilities (Experimental edition).* Champaign, IL: University of Illinois.

McDonald, E., & Schultz, A. (1973) Communication boards for cerebral palsied children. *Journal of Speech Hearing Disorders, 38,* 72–88.

McGerr, M. (2003). *A fierce discontent: The rise and fall of the progressive movement in America, 1870–1920.* New York, NY: Free Press.

McVicker, S., Parr, S., Pound, C., & Duchan, J. (2009). The Communication Partner Scheme: A project to develop long-term, low-cost access to conversation for people living with aphasia. *Aphasiology, 23*(1), 52–71.

Moeller, D. (1975). *Speech pathology and audiology: Iowa origins of a discipline.* Iowa City, IA: The University of Iowa.

Moore, M. (2009, March 4). 1968: Orlando Taylor looks back. *ASHA Leader.* Retrieved from https://leader.pubs.asha.org/doi/10.1044/leader .AN3.14042009.21

Mullennix, J., & Stern, S. (Eds.) (2010). *Computer synthesized speech technologies: Tools for aiding impairment.* Hershey, PA: Medical Information Science Reference.

Myklebust, H. (1954). *Auditory disorders in children.* New York, NY: Grune and Stratton.

Mylott, K. (2010). *1978: SLP sues ASHA; Case raised issue—Did ASHA act like a monopoly?* Retrieved from http://ashawatch.blogspot.com/2010/08/ 1974-asha-member-sues-asha-case-raised.html

National Institute on Deafness and Other Communication Disorders. (2017). *Cochlear implants.* Retrieved from https://www.nidcd.nih.gov/health/ cochlear-implants

Nelson, S. (1958). News and announcements. *Journal of Speech and Hearing Disorders, 23*(1), 81–92.

Newby, H. (1980). *Audiology.* New York, NY: Appleton-Century-Crofts.

Paden, E. (1970). *A history of the American Speech and Hearing Association.* Washington, DC: American Speech and Hearing Association.

Parr, S., Pound, C., & Hewitt, A. (2006). Communication access to health and social services. *Topics in Language Disorders, 26*(3), 189–198.

Pound, C., Duchan, J., Penman, T., Hewitt, A., & Parr, S. (2007). Communication access to organisations. *Aphasiology, 21,* 23–38.

Prentke-Romich Company. (n.d.-a). *History.* Retrieved from https://www.prentrom.com/50/

Robey, R. (1998). A meta-analysis of clinical outcomes in the treatment of aphasia. *Journal of Speech, Language, and Hearing Research, 41,* 172-187.

Ross, M. (1997) A retrospective look at the future of aural rehabilitation. *Journal of the Academy of Rehabilitative Audiology, 30,* 11–20. Retrieved from http://www.hearingresearch.org/ross/aural_ rehabilitation/a_retrospective_look_at_the_future_ of_aural_rehabilitation.php

Rutter, M. (1966). Behavioral and cognitive characteristics. In J. K. Wing (Ed.), *Early childhood autism: Clinical, educational and social aspects.* London, UK: Pergamon Press.

Sackett, D., Rosenberg, W., Gray, J., Haynes, R., & Richardson. W. (1996). Evidence-based medicine. What it is and what it isn't. *British Medical Journal, 312,* 71–72.

Sackett, D., Straus, S., Richardson, W., Rosenberg, W., & Haynes, R. (2000). *Evidence-based medicine: How to practice and teach EBM.* Edinburgh, Scotland: Churchill Livingstone.

Schlosser, R. W. (2000). *The efficacy of augmentative and alternative communication intervention: Toward evidence-based practice.* San Diego, CA: Academic Press.

Schoolfield, L. (1938). The development of speech correction in America in the 19th century. *Quarterly Journal of Speech, 24,* 101–116.

Scripture, E. W. (1899). *Researches in experimental phonetics. Observations on rhythmic action.* Studies from the Yale Psychological Laboratory, VII. New Haven CT: Yale University.

Sheehan, V. (1948). Techniques in the management of aphasia. *Journal of Speech and Hearing Disorders, 13,* 241–246.

Simmons, F., Epley, J., Lummis, R., Guttmann, N., Frishkopf, L., Harmon, L., & Swicker, E. (1965). Auditory nerve: Electrical stimulation in man. *Science, 148*(3666), 104–106.

Simmons-Mackie, N. (2000). Social approaches to the management of aphasia. In L. Worrell & C. Fratalli (Eds.), *Neurogenic communication disorders: A functional approach* (pp. 162–168). New York: NY: Thieme.

Simmons-Mackie, N., & Kovarsky, D. (Eds.). (2009). Engagement in clinical interaction. *Seminars in Speech and Language, 30*(1), 5–10.

Simucase. (n.d.). *Explore Simucase: See how Simucase helps SLP students and professionals learn in a virtual environment.* Retrieved from https://www.simucase.com/explore

Speech Therapy Ideas. (n.d.). *Speech therapy ideas.* Retrieved from https://www.speechtherapyideas.com/

Stach, B. (1998). *Clinical audiology: An introduction.* San Diego, CA: Singular Publishing.

Stinchfield, S. (1933). *Speech disorders.* New York, NY: Harcourt Brace.

Stinchfield, S., & Robbins, S. (1931). *A dictionary of terms dealing with disorders of speech.* Boston, MA: Expression Company.

Strauss, A., & Lehtinen, L. (1947). *Psychopathology and the education of the brain-injured child.* New York, NY: Grune and Stratton.

Taylor, O. (1969). Social and political involvement of the American Speech and Hearing Association. *ASHA, 11,* 216–218.

Tesak, J., & Code, C. (2008). *Milestones in the history of aphasia: Theories and protagonists.* New York, NY: Psychology Press.

Travis, L. E. (1957). *Handbook of speech pathology and audiology.* New York, NY: Appleton Century Crofts.

Traynor, R. (2016). Electrical stimulation of hearing. *Hearing: Health and Technology Matters.* Retrievedfrom https://hearinghealthmatters.org/hearinginternational/2016/cochlear-implants/

Uffen, E. (2003, October 7). Goodbye Fred. *ASHA Leader.* https://doi.org/10.1044/leader.FTR1.08182003.4

United States Congress. (1973). Rehabilitation Act. Retrieved from https://www.access-board.gov/the-board/laws/rehabilitation-act-of-1973

United States Congress. (1975). Education for All Handicapped Children Act (PL 94-142). Retrieved from https://www.govinfo.gov/content/pkg/STATUTE-89/pdf/STATUTE-89-Pg773.pdf

Unites States Congress. (1988). Technology-Related Assistance for Individuals with Disabilities Act of 1988, P.L. 100-407, Title I (U.S.C. 2201-2217). Retrieved from https://www2.ed.gov/pubs/Biennial/336.html

United States Congress. (1990a). Individuals with Disabilities Education Act (IDEA). Reauthorized in 2004. Retrieved from https://sites.ed.gov/idea/

United States Congress. (1990b). Americans with Disabilities Act. Retrieved from http://www.ada.gov.

United State Congress. (2000). Title 1: Program for individuals with developmental disabilities, Public Law 106–402. Retrieved from https://www.congress.gov/106/plaws/publ402/PLAW-106publ402.pdf

Vanderheiden, G. (1976). Providing a child with a means to indicate. In G. Vanderheiden, K. Grilley, & K. McDonald (Eds.), *Non-vocal communication techniques and aids for the severely physically handicapped.* Baltimore, MD: University Park Press.

Vanderheiden, G. (2002). A journey through early augmentative communication and computer access. *Journal of Rehabilitation Research and Development, 39*(6 Suppl.), 39–53. Retrieved from http://www.rehab.research.va.gov/jour/02/39/6/sup/vanderheiden.html

Vanderheiden, G., Grilley, K., & McDonald, K. (Eds.) (1976). *Non-vocal communication techniques and aids for the severely physically handicapped.* Baltimore, MD: University Park Press.

Van Riper, C. (1981). An early history of ASHA. *ASHA, 23*, 855–858.

Van Riper, C. (1986). *Charles Gage Van Riper: An autobiography*. Unpublished manuscript.

Volta A. (1800). On the electricity excited by the mere contact of conducting substances of different kinds. *Philosophical Trans*, 90, 403–431.

Von Leden, H. (1990). Pioneers in the evolution of voice care and voice science in the United States of America. *Journal of Voice, 4*, 99–106.

Wepman, J., Jones, L., Bock, D., & Van Pelt, D. (1960). Studies in aphasia: Background and theoretical formulations. *Journal of Speech and Hearing Disorders, 25*, 323–332.

Wilcox, M. J., Kouri, T. A., & Caswell, S. B. (1991). Early language intervention: A comparison of classroom and individual treatment. *American Journal of Speech Language Pathology, 1*(1), 49–62.

Williams, R. (1975). *Ebonics: The true language of black folks*. St. Louis, MO: Institute of Black Studies.

Wingate, M. (1997). *Stuttering: A short history of a curious disorder*. Westport, CT: Bergin & Garvey.

Worrall, C., & Frattali (Eds.) *Neurogenic communication disorders: A functional approach* (pp. 162–168). NY: Thieme.

Appendix 2–A

◇◇

A Few Milestones in the History of Speech-Language Pathology and Audiology in the United States

- **1870–1914** Period of progressive movement in the United States, one that promoted values that provided a context for development of the helping professions.

- **1914** Establishment of the first graduate-level program in speech pathology, organized by Smiley Blanton at the University of Wisconsin.

- **1918** Walter Babcock Swift organized public school clinicians in the Northeast. Their group, affiliated with the National Education Association, was called the National Society for the Study and Correction of Speech Disorders.

- **1922** First commercial audiometer made available.

- **1925** Formation of the American Academy of Speech Correction.

- **1926–1927** Formation and approval of the constitution of the American Academy of Speech Correction, including bylaws.

- **1927** American Academy of Speech Correction renamed American Society for the Study of Disorders of Speech

- **1930** American Academy of Speech Correction created an associate level of membership, allowing practitioners to become members.

- **1934** American Society for the Study of Disorders of Speech renamed the American Speech Correction Association.

- **1945** Establishment of audiology as a profession following World War II.

- **1947** American Speech Correction Association renamed the American Speech and Hearing Association.

- **1952** Two sets of membership requirements were created by the American Speech and Hearing Association, one for speech pathology and one for audiology.

- **1965** Certificate of Clinical Competence was established for both speech pathologists and audiologists.

- **1968** Master's-level degree was required for speech-pathologists to practice in hospitals and agencies.

- **1969** State of Florida began a movement for state certification of professionals in speech pathology to work in non-educational settings.

- **1970** American Speech and Hearing Association published Elaine Pagel Paden's book tracing its history from its 1925 origins.

- **1978** American Speech and Hearing Association was renamed the American Speech-Language-Hearing Association.

- **1978** Certification and membership requirements were separated. One could become certified without being a member of the association.

- **1988** Formation of the American Academy of Audiology (AAA).

- **1990** Special Interest Divisions program was created by the American Speech-Language-Hearing Association to have members affiliate by individual specialties.

- **1993** Language requirements were instituted for certification.

- **1997** The professional doctorate in audiology was established. It became the entry level degree in audiology in 2012.

- **1999** First national convention of AAA was held.

- **1999** First issue of the *Journal of the American Academy of Audiology* was published.

- **2009** James Jerger published his book on the *History of Audiology.*

- **2012** ASHA Special Interest Divisions restructured into ASHA Special Interest Groups with a strong focus on continuing education.

- **2013** ASHAWire, an online compendium of ASHA journal articles became available.

- **2019** Establishment of a new peer-reviewed scholarly journal *Perspectives of the ASHA Special Interest Groups*

3

Establishing Competencies in Professional Education, Certification, and Licensure

Lissa Power-deFur, PhD

Introduction

We tend to look for initials after a person's name when selecting a professional to work for us—from automotive to financial, from medical to recreational; we like to look for letters: ASE, CMT, CFP, CFA, RDN.[1] Why? We like to know that the person we have selected to work for us is competent in his or her field. Table 3–1 indicates the initials, often reflecting the credentials, of a variety of the professionals with whom speech-language pathologists (SLPs) and audiologists (AUDs) might work.

These initials indicate that the professional has met the standards for practice in that profession. The credentials reflect certifications or registrations that demonstrate the individual has met the national expectations for the field. Persons who have achieved credentials have voluntarily met professional standards designed to ensure high quality. They have demonstrated the knowledge, skills, and expertise established by their academic and clinical preparation and, in general, successfully passed a national examination.

This chapter will explore the competencies required for certification, licensure, and professional education for SLPs and AUDs. As these standards intersect with the ethical standards of professional organizations, telepractice, and international practice, readers will want to connect the information in this chapter with the information in Chapters 5 ("Professional Ethics") 7 ("International Alliances"), and 27 ("Technology for Student Training, Professional Practice, and Service Delivery").

It is best to begin by reviewing some terminology: accreditation, credentialing, credential, certification, and license. The lay public often uses these terms interchangeably. However, there are distinctive differences in meaning, as shown in Table 3–2.

Credentialing requirements are not static, as credentialing agencies periodically update requirements to reflect changes in practice patterns, consumer protection approaches, and legislative intent.

---

[1]ASE = National Association of Automotive Service Excellence, CMT = Certified Massage Therapist, CFP = Certified Financial Planner, RDN = Registered Dietitian.

Table 3–1. Credentials of Professionals With Whom Speech-Language Pathologists and Audiologists May Work

CDAL	Certified Director of Assisted Living
CGC	Certified Genetic Counselor
DDS	Doctor of Dental Surgery
DMD	Doctor of Dental Medicine
DO	Doctor of Osteopathic Medicine
DPH	Doctor of Public Health
FAAP	Fellow of the American Academy of Pediatrics
JD	Juris Doctor
LCSW	Licensed Clinical Social Worker
LPC	Licensed Professional Counselor
MD	Medical Doctor
MPH	Master of Public Health
OTR	Registered Occupational Therapist
PA	Physician Assistant
PsyD	Doctor of Psychology
PT	Physical Therapist
RDN	Registered Dietitian Nutritionist
RN	Registered Nurse
RRT	Registered Respiratory Therapist

Table 3–2. Various Terms Associated With Credentialing

Accreditation	A process of evaluating an education or credentialing program based on specific standards
Certification	A process whereby an individual earns a certificate after having met academic and professional standards
Credential	A designation of a qualification or achievement
Credentialing	The process of evaluating an individual's or organization's qualifications in comparison with established standards
License	An official permit to do something (e.g., drive a car or practice as a speech-language pathologist or audiologist)
Licensure	Regulation of a license, typically by a state agency

Agencies and organizations make such changes based upon new research that informs evidence-based practice. Legislative and regulatory requirements are generally more responsive to public issues and concerns. A fundamental value of credentialing programs is that whenever changes are proposed, credentialing agencies inform licensees and certified professionals (the persons who may be impacted by those changes) of the opportunity for comment on proposed changes. This chapter will provide an overview of requirements but will refrain from addressing specific requirements, as these are not static. Rather than providing specifics that may have changed by the time the reader reviews the information herein, this chapter will provide links and resources for professionals and aspiring professionals to meet their obligations to understand and adhere to current requirements.

How Do You Know You Are Competent?

Aspiring SLPs and AUDs want to present themselves to the public and their peers as competent professionals. Professionals demonstrate this through attainment of credentials; in our professions, this is professional certification. In addition to demonstrating professional credibility and achieving public recognition, attainment of a profession-specific credential is generally needed for employment and reimbursement for clinical services provided (ASHA, n.d.-d).

The Institute for Credentialing Excellence (ICE) is an organization that accredits credentialing programs. ICE identifies an assessment-based certificate program as one that (a) provides instruction to enable acquisition of specified learning outcomes in terms of knowledge, skills, and abilities; (b) evaluates participants' attainment of these outcomes; and (c) awards certificates to those participants who meet the standards for assessment (Institute for Credentialing Excellence, 2010). ICE points out that a certificate of attendance (or participation) signifies presence or participation in a program or event only, but when there is no required demonstration, it does not establish that the individual met the learning outcomes.

ICE further identifies the characteristics of professional certification—that it is a process in which persons elect to be evaluated by a credentialing organization to determine if they have met standards for knowledge, skills, and competencies set by that certifying entity (Institute for Credentialing Excellence, 2010). The national credential that SLPs and AUDs acquire is a certification credential. This reflects an independent assessment of individuals' competencies as required for

performance in speech-language pathology and audiology. The intention is to demonstrate that individuals have met the work-related knowledge, skills, and competencies of the profession and have met the requirements of the certification program (e.g., academic preparation, years of professional experience). Certification also measures continued competence through recertification and renewal programs (Institute for Credentialing Excellence, 2010).

American Speech-Language-Hearing Association (ASHA)

ASHA established its program for certifying SLPs and AUDs in 1952 (American Speech-Language-Hearing Association, n.d.-a). Since that time, the number of certified SLPs has reached 175,025 per year-end 2018 statistics. The number of certified AUDs has reached 13,407, with 813 individuals dually certified in audiology and speech-language pathology (American Speech-Language-Hearing Association, n.d.-h). The first certification program did not require a graduate degree or national examination. This was replaced in 1965 with the Certificate of Clinical Competence (CCC), which required a master's degree or equivalent, supervised full-time employment, and a passing score on the National Examination in Speech Pathology and/or Audiology (NESPA). Over the years, the semester hours of graduate coursework, practicum, clinical fellowship, and exam requirements have evolved. The most recent update applies to persons applying for certification after January 1, 2020. The ASHA website (https://www.asha.org/certification/) includes the current standards in both speech-language pathology and audiology (American Speech-Language-Hearing Association, n.d.-g).

The National Commission for Certifying Agencies (NCCA), an independent organization that accredits over 300 personnel certification programs, accredits ASHA's certification program (Institute for Credentialing Excellence, n.d.-b). ASHA's program is governed by the Council for Clinical Certification, a group of SLPs, AUDs, and members of the public (American Speech-Language-Hearing Association, n.d.-j). The purpose of this external accreditation is to have a third-party evaluation of the certification program, for ensuring the health, welfare, and safety of the public (Institute for Credentialing Excellence, n.d.-a, n.d.-c). Like our own individual professional certification as an audiologist and/or speech-language pathologist, this accreditation reflects excellence on the part of the certification agency.

As is common with credentialing programs, the CCC requires certain basic elements: (a) academic preparation, (b) clinical experience, and (c) demonstration of knowledge through a national examination.

The academic preparation is completion of a master's (SLP) or doctoral (Audiology) degree (or equivalent) from an institution accredited by the Council on Academic Accreditation in Audiology and Speech-Language Pathology (CAA). The clinical experience begins during the graduate program with students required to amass hours in a variety of discipline-specific areas (American Speech-Language-Hearing Association, n.d.-m).

The CCC in Speech-Language Pathology includes a Clinical Fellowship period following graduation, in which the graduate (a "Clinical Fellow") receives mentoring/supervision. This mentor must be an individual holding the CCC in speech-language pathology (American Speech-Language-Hearing Association, n.d.-m). Students and graduates may hear the outdated term "Clinical Fellowship Year" to refer to this period after graduation. The term "Clinical Fellowship" is now used, dropping "Year," as the period of fellowship does not necessarily equate to a calendar year. The Clinical Fellowship (CF) is a transition period after completion of a speech-language pathology master's degree (or equivalent) and the period when the SLP provides clinical services independently. The CF is a minimum 36-week full-time (or equivalent part-time experience) mentored professional experience. As noted above, the mentor must hold ASHA certification in speech-language pathology. (*Note*: Individuals can verify current ASHA certification status using the ASHA Certification Verification System at https://www.asha.org/Certification/cert-verify/). The purpose of this transition period is to integrate and apply information from the graduate program, evaluate strengths and limitations, refine clinical skills, and move to independent practitioner (American Speech-Language-Hearing Association, n.d.-m).

As graduates move into their CF experience, they will want to be sure this experience meets the requirements. These include opportunities for evaluation and treatment, with 80% of the time spent on clinical activities. Failure to ensure that the CF experience meets these requirements may have devastating consequences for the new graduate, as the new SLP may be required to repeat some or all of the CF experience prior to earning the Certificate of Clinical Competence. ASHA offers suggestions to graduates to ask when considering a CF placement that new graduates will want to review as they pursue their first professional positions (American Speech-Language-Hearing Association, n.d.-m). See Chapter 26, "Supervision and Mentoring," for more information on the CF experience.

Credentialing generally involves achieving a passing score on an exam to demonstrate one's acquisition of the requisite knowledge to enter the profession. In our fields, the Educational Testing Service (ETS) currently administers the national examination in speech-language pathology and audiology, the Praxis examination (American Speech-Language-Hearing Association, n.d.-j). (Students will remember ETS from their completion of the SAT and GRE exams!) ETS develops test questions through a rigorous process, designed to meet high standards for assessments. Professionals and discipline specific specialists meet with ETS and their experts to ensure the assessments reflect the skills being assessed (Educational Testing Service, n.d.-b). The certification agency sets the passing score, for example, the Council for Clinical Certification at ASHA sets the passing score, which is 162 in speech-language pathology and 170 in audiology at the time of this writing (American Speech-Language-Hearing Association, n.d.-k). ETS provides reasonable accommodations for test takers with disabilities or health-related needs. Test takers must submit requests and ETS must approve accommodations prior to scheduling tests (Educational Testing Service, n.d.-a).

The American Academy of Audiology (AAA)

The American Academy of Audiology operates a credentialing program for AUDs, enabling them to become Board Certified in Audiology (American Board of Audiology, 2016, n.d.-a, n.d.-b, n.d.-c). AAA's purpose for board certification is comparable to the industry standard—demonstration that the individual meets professional standards. Board certification is based on education (doctoral degree in audiology from a regionally accredited institution), state licensure (which may be submitted within one year if eligible for a license, but does not hold at the time of application), professional experience (minimum of 2000 hours), and information on employment history (American Board of Audiology, 2016). AAA identifies that Board Certified in Audiology allows for expedited licensure in a number of states (American Board of Audiology, 2016).

Professional Development and Certification Maintenance

Achievement of certification does not end an individual's commitment to being a qualified professional. Certification and licensing entities, especially those certifying SLPs and AUDs, expect practitioners to maintain their competency through ongoing professional development (American Speech-Language-Hearing Association, n.d.-i). This requirement, generally termed certification maintenance, covers a set period (e.g., 2 years, 3 years). For example, state licensure boards establish a timeframe during which the licensed practitioner must complete a specified amount of professional development hours.

(A professional development hour is considered 60 minutes of professional development.) Following specific timeframes, set by the credentialing agencies, professionals must attest that they have completed the needed professional development for certification maintenance.

Licensure boards often audit professional development, so individuals must ensure they have the records to support such attestation. ASHA and AAA operate continuing education registries (American Academy of Audiology, 2016; American Speech-Language-Hearing Association, n.d.-n) that facilitate tracking of continuing education units (CEUs). These registries are comparable to a college registrar, maintaining a cumulative record of courses and CEUs. Like registrars, transcripts can be issued, which demonstrate that an individual has met CE requirements for licensure when needed. State licensure agencies do not necessarily require specific providers of CEUs, but the use of ASHA and AAA CEUs and their registries greatly facilitates maintenance of continuing education requirements as mandated by state licensure boards.

The credentialing organization (e.g., ASHA or the state licensure board) may have specific professional development topic requirements and it is incumbent upon the credentialed professional to be aware of and meet these requirements. For example, ASHA certification requirements and many states' licensure requirements specify completion of professional development in ethics as a requirement for continuing certification or licensure.

ASHA offers Continuing Education (CE) units, with a host of ASHA approved CE providers (American Speech-Language-Hearing Association, n.d.-c). ASHA's Continuing Education Board (CEB), a board of AUDs and SLPs, establish standards for offering continuing education, which CE providers must meet. CE providers plan, offer, and assess their CE courses, ensuring that they meet the high standards set by the CEB. CEB designed these standards to conform to industry standards, as identified by the International Association for Continuing Education and training (IACET) (American Speech-Language-Hearing Association, n.d.-n).

When pursuing professional development, professionals will want to assure themselves that the CE provider is offering a program of quality. Some hints for selecting and evaluating CE courses include:

- Review promotional materials to ensure they include learning outcomes, faculty qualifications, availability of CEUs, refund/cancellation policies, and instructional methods.

- Ensure that CE instructors disclose any relevant financial or non-financial relationships they have with the course content. Most CE organizations expect such disclosure to ensure balance, independence, objectivity, and scientific rigor in the educational events. In other words, the instructor should present without bias, conflicts of interest, or personal gain.

- Ensure that the CE reflects evidence-based practice by looking for citations on slides or handouts and on a reference list (American Speech-Language-Hearing Association, n.d.-n).

How Can You Demonstrate Your Excellence in a Particular Area of Practice?

ASHA certification and AAA board certification demonstrate entry-level credentials to work as SLPs or AUDs. Many professionals develop expertise in certain areas of the profession and wish to demonstrate that specialized knowledge and skill to the public. Professionals who hold the credential to practice in their field (i.e., the Certificate of Clinical Competence or Board Certification in Audiology) seek formal recognition of their advanced knowledge and skills. ASHA, AAA, and others have created credentials to recognize specialized areas of practice. These recognitions have various terms but are all designed to demonstrate to consumers, colleagues, employers, and payers that the individual has expertise beyond that required for general certification. As stated by Brian Shulman, "[S]pecialty recognition advances the professions. With the continued changes and challenges impacting healthcare and educational systems, specialists are integral members of the service delivery team" (American Speech-Language-Hearing Association, n.d.-o). These voluntary programs enable consumers to identify professionals with recognized specialties. Such recognition promotes practitioners' advanced practice areas, validates their expertise, and may support professional advancement. Professionals aspiring for such special recognition find that the professional development required to attain the recognition is enriching. A variety of organizations offers such specializations, as shown in Table 3–3. Professionals desiring to attain such specialization will be mindful to review the requirements to plan their acquisition of professional development and clinical experiences to align with the specialization standards. It is likely that continued specializations will emerge; for example, a specialization in Autism is in development at ASHA at the time of this writing. Professionals desiring specialization will want to monitor the ASHA and AAA websites to keep track of such developments. Information on how to apply for clinical specialty certification is available through ASHA (American Speech-Language-Hearing Association, n.d.-b).

Table 3–3. Advanced Certification in Speech-Language Pathology and Audiology

Granting Organization	Specialization	For More Information
Academy of Neurologic Communication Disorders and Sciences (Academy of Neurologic Communication Disorders and Sciences, n.d.)	ANCDS Board Certification	https://www.ancds.org/ancds-board-certification
Alexander Graham Bell Association for the Deaf and Hard of Hearing (Alexander Graham Bell Association for the Deaf, n.d.)	Listening and Spoken Language Certification	https://www.agbell.org/Professionals/Professional-Development
American Academy of Audiology (American Academy of Audiology, n.d.-d)	■ Cochlear Implant Specialty Certification ■ Pediatric Audiology Specialty Certification	https://www.boardofaudiology/org/board-certified-in-audiology
American Board of Child Language and Language Disorders (American Speech-Language-Hearing Association, n.d.-e)	Child language and language disorders	https://www.asha.org/certification/specialty
American Board of Fluency and Fluency Disorders (American Speech-Language-Hearing Association, n.d.-e)	Fluency and fluency disorders	https://www.asha.org/certification/specialty
American Board of Swallowing and swallowing disorders (American Speech-Language-Hearing Association, n.d.-e)	Swallowing and swallowing disorders	https://www.asha.org/certification/specialty
American Audiology Board of Intraoperative Monitoring (American Speech-Language-Hearing Association, n.d.-e)	Intraoperative monitoring	https://www.asha.org/certification/specialty

The National Board for Professional Teaching Standards (NBPTS) established standards for teachers to demonstrate that that they have the knowledge and expertise to have a positive impact on student learning in 1989 (National Board for Professional Teaching Standards, n.d.). Teachers achieving "national board certification" generally receive a pay increase and other recognition of their expertise. As many SLPs work in school settings, ASHA has provided a comparison between the NBPTS and the ASHA Certification in Speech-Language Pathology and in Audiology (American Speech-Language-Hearing Association, n.d.-f). This provides professionals with information to advocate

that the CCC is a specialization comparable to that of NBPTS. As local school districts have the authority to make decisions regarding recognition of board certified teachers, this information gives SLPs and AUDs the tools to advocate inclusion in any such recognition program.

State Licensure

In order to provide services to consumers, professionals must hold a license to practice in the state in which they provide services. All 50 states require licensure to work as a SLP or audiologist (National Council of State Boards of Examiners, n.d.-b). State licensure requirements generally track the ASHA certification requirements, but it is common for states to include state-specific requirements. As a result, applicants for licensure will want to review carefully the licensure requirements in the state in which they plan to practice. In general, it is in the professionals' best interest to retain ASHA certification, as this facilitates licensure across the country. Professionals must remember that the ASHA certification is voluntary, but licensure as SLPs or AUDs in the state in which they are practicing is mandatory. Failure to meet licensure requirements (including maintenance requirements) can result in fines or withholding or removal of licensure. SLPs and AUDs may not practice (i.e., serve clients) without a current license from the state where they serve the client. In our mobile and tech-savvy culture, it may be common for an SLP or AUD to practice in another state, either face-to-face or through telepractice. If this is the case, the professional must hold licensure in the state where the client is located. Individuals pursuing telepractice will want to carefully review Chapter 27, "Technology for Student Training, Professional Practice and Service Delivery," and comply with the licensure requirements for each state in which they will be practicing.

In some states, an individual holds a single license issued by one entity, a board of audiology and speech-language pathology, to work in both education and health care settings. This is termed "universal licensure"—in which one license (credential) serves all settings. Many states, however, require separate credentialing to work in public education settings. In these states, the state boards of education set these standards for school-based personnel, which may be unrelated to the requirements of the state licensure board for work in other settings. (Interestingly, the requirement for a credential to work in public schools preceded the establishment of requirements for working in all other settings. When states began passing licensure for SLPs and AUDs, this resulted in dual credentials in many states. The move toward "universal licensure" is relatively recent.) An SLP employed by public education agencies may hold a credential from that state's department of education with an endorsement in speech-language services. (This credential is termed a license in some states and certification in other states. The endorsement in speech-language will have different terms across the country, but "speech-language" is generally a component of the term.) Those individuals must also hold a license from the state's board of audiology and speech-language pathology if they choose to work for any other employer (e.g., health care, contract agency, private practice). ASHA maintains a website of state requirements for licensure, tracking information regarding whether a separate credential is required to work in the schools (http://www.asha.org/advocacy/state). This site also includes information on licensure requirements related to support personnel, dispensing hearing aids, and continuing education requirements.

The National Council on State Licensure Boards (NCSB) is an organization that represents state licensure boards in audiology and speech-language pathology. Their role is to engage licensure boards in discussion of regulatory and policy issues related to licensure in our fields (National Council on State Boards of Examiners, n.d.-a, n.d.-e, n.d.-d, n.d.-e). Their website includes links to state licensure agencies and summarizes current licensure requirements in such areas as continuing education, hearing aid dispensing with an audiology license, support personnel requirements (e.g., speech-language pathology assistants), and telepractice (http://www.ncsb.org). Individuals are encouraged to access the website of the state's licensure board (or department of education if a separate license is required). This will enable the professional to verify the information on both the NCSB and ASHA sites. Although both NCSB and ASHA strive to keep their sites up-to-date, states may update information at any time and professionals will want to verify they have the most current information to obtain and maintain a license to practice in the state where they are serving clients.

Individuals who provide telepractice services in multiple states, who live at the juncture of two or more states and service clients in both states, or who travel to serve clients in more than one state often find it challenging to secure and maintain licensure in all states. Professionals must pay license fees and meet the requirements for continuing education in each state in which they practice. Responding to this challenge, the NCSB and ASHA are currently working on a draft licensure compact for audiology and speech-language pathology (National Council of State Boards of Examiners, n.d.). On September 27, 2018, NCSB reported that it was working collaboratively with the NCSB Advisory Committee and the Draft Team to develop a "Licensure Compact for Audiology and Speech-Language Pathology" (Phillips, 2018).

Occasionally, professionals will practice in other countries. A few countries have credentialing requirements, but most do not. Individuals must review the requirements to practice abroad prior to initiating services. This includes individuals on short-term mission or professional trips to other countries. It is common for agencies supporting such trips to require persons to demonstrate their license to practice in order to be granted permission to practice in another country. For more information on international practice of speech-language pathology, please consult Chapter 7, "International Alliances."

How Do You Know Your University Graduate Program Will Ensure You Become Competent?

Students desiring to become SLPs and AUDs will want to make sure that their graduate education program is qualified to provide them with the necessary training and clinical experience to enter the profession. Accreditation is the credentialing vehicle for colleges and universities (frequently termed institutions of higher education, IHEs). The purpose of this accreditation is to evaluate a program in comparison with standards specified by an external, third party. Accreditation enables the university to inform the public about the external evaluator that reviewed the program. (Institute for Credentialing Excellence, n.d.-c). The Council of Higher Education Accreditation (CHEA) establishes standards for accrediting organizations to ensure academic quality, improvement, and accountability (CHEA, n.d.). CHEA recognizes various regional accreditation agencies for accreditation of IHEs, as shown in Table 3–4.

CHEA also recognizes accreditation organizations, to ensure that these organizations ensure the quality and accountability of the higher education programs in those particular professions. The Council on Academic Accreditation in Audiology and Speech-Language Pathology (CAA) is the CHEA approved entity that accredits graduate programs in our fields. CAA comprises professionals in the field from both university and clinical settings as well as a public member (Council on Academic Accreditation, 2010). The CAA first established standards in the 1960s, with the first accreditation of speech-language pathology and audiology programs awarded in 1965 (CAA, n.d.-b). Earlier iterations of CAA had different names, first the American Board of Examiners for Speech Pathology and Audiology (ABESPA), then the Educational Testing Board (ETB), followed by the Educational Standards Board (ESB), and finally CAA as of 1996 (CAA, n.d.-b).

The accrediting agency for our graduate education programs has a long history of recognition, first recognized in 1964 by the Council on Postsecondary Accreditation (now CHEA) and, shortly after, in 1967, by the U.S. Secretary of Education (now referred to as the U.S.

Table 3–4. Regional Organizations That Accredit Institutions of Higher Education That Are Recognized by the Council of Higher Education

Regional Accrediting Organization	Scope of Accreditation
Higher Education Learning Commission (HLC)	Degree granting institutions (associate, baccalaureate, master's or doctoral degrees) Arizona, Arkansas, Colorado, Illinois, Indiana, Iowa, Kansas, Michigan, Minnesota, Missouri, Nebraska, New Mexico, North Dakota, Ohio, Oklahoma, South Dakota, West Virginia, Wisconsin, Wyoming
Middle States Commission on Higher Education (MSCHE)	Degree granting institutions offering one or more postsecondary education programs in Delaware, the District of Columbia, Maryland, New Jersey, New York, Pennsylvania, Puerto Rico, and the Virgin Islands
New England Commission of Higher Education (NECHE)	Institutes that award bachelor's, master's, and doctoral degrees and certain associate degree-granting institutes in Connecticut, Maine, Massachusetts, New Hampshire, Rhode Island, Vermont, and internationally
Southern Association of Colleges and Schools Commission on Colleges (SACSCOC)	Degree granting institutions of higher education in Alabama, Florida, Georgia, Kentucky, Louisiana, Mississippi, North Carolina, South Carolina, Tennessee, Texas, Virginia, Latin America, and certain international sites
WASC Senior College and University Commission (WSCUC)	Baccalaureate degree or higher institutions in California, Hawaii, and the Pacific Basin

Source: Based on information from CHEA, n.d.

Department of Education [USDE] recognition) (Council on Academic Accreditation in Audiology and Speech-Language Pathology, n.d.-b). These recognitions are the "Good Housekeeping Seal of Approval" for the accreditation standards set for our professions—that they have high expectations for academic quality and accountability. In addition, USDE recognition is critical for eligibility to participate in federal student aid and other federal programs (Council on Academic Accreditation in Audiology and Speech-Language Pathology, n.d.-b).

CAA is responsible for formulating standards for graduate programs that provide entry-level preparation in audiology or speech-language pathology (Council on Academic Accreditation in Audiology and Speech-Language Pathology, n.d.-a). These standards are designed to ensure that students entering the field have been appropriately prepared to serve the public. Entry-level preparation is at the masters' level in speech-language pathology and the clinical doctoral level in audiology. As a result, CAA standards only address these degree programs. They do not address bachelor level programs in Communication Sciences and Disorders nor do they address research doctorates (e.g., Ph.D.) in either field or clinical doctorates in speech-language pathology. In addition to creating standards, CAA evaluates programs that apply for accreditation on a voluntary basis. Evaluation includes review of university programs' self-studies and on-site visits. Accredited programs are recognized and lists of such programs are available to the public and key agencies.

As is typical of standards, the CAA has reviewed and revised the standards numerous times over the years. Perhaps one of the more significant revisions was the move in accreditation of audiology graduate programs from the masters to the doctoral level. Revisions have also created standards for program improvement. Higher education programs are expected to institute ongoing review of their current programs to keep up with the dynamic changes that occur in evidence-based practices, technology, shifts in policy, insurability, law, and general political and social movements that affect our services and scope of practice. In light of this, higher education programs need to ensure that their curriculum anticipates, captures, and/or adjusts course content to meet the needs of the marketplace through continual reflection and improvement. These standards promote excellence in the preparation of future SLPs and AUDs. The CAA publishes the current standards for accreditation of graduate programs at https://caa.asha.org/reporting/standards/

Financial Aid and Scholarships

The cost of getting a graduate degree in speech-language pathology and audiology is significant. Students may wish to review the resources found in Table 3–5 for links to information about financial aid and scholarships. The list includes those that are specific to Communication Sciences and Disorders and some that are generic.

As many universities have scholarships, fellowships, and graduate assistants available, students will want to contact the financial aid office, graduate school, and speech-language pathology and audiology program at their university for more information. An additional resource is https://www.speechpathologygraduateprograms.org/slp-scholarship-guide/ and search by state.

What Are Some Pointers for Maintaining My Credentials?

Congratulations! You are well on your way to demonstrating your qualifications now that you have (or are on your way to have):

- graduated from a regionally accredited university that holds CAA accreditation in audiology and/or speech-language pathology, gathering the required knowledge and skills needed for entrance into the professions;

- passed the national certification exam; and

- completed needed clinical experience with required supervision and mentoring.

Entering the field, you may be considering attaining recognition of specialization, with plans to achieve a credential documenting your expertise.

However, this chapter would be incomplete if it did not remind credentialed professionals of the following:

- Read the requirements for the state(s) where you have chosen to practice. Identify whether your state required a separate credential to work for public education agencies (i.e., school districts) and for all other settings or if a single license from the state's board of audiology and speech-language pathology is sufficient.

- Attend to the requirements for licensure (or certification) in the state where you provide clinical services. Be sure to note the dates for license renewal and completion of continuing education requirements. Identify if there are required professional development topics and the number of continuing education units required for renewal. Failure to hold a current license to practice can result in fines and other consequences.

- Retain your national certification. Most states' licensure requirements build upon national certification requirements, so retaining this

Table 3–5. Financial Aid and Scholarship Information

Financial Aid:

Free Application for Federal Student Aid (FAFSA)
  - https://studentaid.ed.gov/sa/fafsa
    ☐ Subsidized and unsubsidized loans and federal grants (PELL)

State Government Financial Aid Information
  - https://www2.ed.gov/about/contacts/state/index.html

Direct PLUS Loan (for graduate or professional students OR parents of undergraduate students)
  - https://studentaid.ed.gov/sa/types/loans/plus

Federal Supplemental Educational Opportunity Grant (undergraduates with high financial need)
  - https://studentaid.ed.gov/sa/types/grants-scholarships/fseog

Scholarships and Awards—CSD Program Specific

American Speech-Language-Hearing Association: Minority Student Leadership Program
  - https://www.asha.org/Students/MSLP-Award/

American Speech-Language-Hearing Association: Student Ethics Essay Award
  - https://www.asha.org/practice/ethics/essay_award/

American Speech-Language-Hearing Association: Students Preparing for Academic-Research Careers Award
  - https://www.asha.org/Students/SPARC-Award/

American Speech-Language-Hearing Foundation Graduate Student Scholarship
  - https://www.ashfoundation.org/Apply/Graduate-Student-Scholarship/

Council of Academic Programs in Communication Sciences and Disorders: Frances J. Laven Scholarship
  - http://www.capcsd.org/funding-opportunities/scholarships/frances-j-laven-scholarship-2/

EBS Healthcare Scholarship
  - http://www.ebshealthcare.com/school-based-scholarships
    ☐ Scholarship for school-based pediatric clinicians.

National Student Speech Language Hearing Association Scholarship
  - https://www.nsslha.org/Programs/Scholarships/
    ☐ Scholarship application opens October 2019 and is due December 4, 2019

National Black Association for Speech-Language and Hearing: Supporting Career Growth through Mentoring Scholarship
  - https://www.nbaslh.org/scholarships

Sertoma Communicative Disorders Scholarship Program
  - https://sertoma.org/what-we-do/scholarships/

Scholarships and Awards—General Application (Non-CSD Specific)

American Business Clubs (AMBUCS) Scholarship
  - https://ambucs.org/therapists/scholarship-program/
    ☐ Scholarship for physical therapy, occupational therapy, speech-language pathology, and hearing/audiology.

Jacob K. Javits Fellowship Program
  - https://www2.ed.gov/programs/jacobjavits/index.html

National Achievement Scholarship Program
  - https://www.nationalmerit.org/s/1758/interior.aspx?sid=1758&gid=2&pgid=433

National Association of Junior Auxiliaries
  - http://www.najanet.org/naja-scholarship/

National Merit Scholarship Program
  - https://www.nationalmerit.org/s/1758/interior.aspx?sid=1758&gid=2&pgid=424

certification facilitates attainment of licensure when moving to another state. If an individual drops certification, for whatever reason, the professional must meet the current requirements (rather than the requirements when originally certified). For example, the applicant must meet current requirements for coursework and clinical experience, which may have changed since the applicant was originally credentialed. Professionals should be certain to check certification requirements and timelines when considering applying for recertification.

■ Continuing education is crucial. Maintain an accurate record of your continuing education and ensure that you pursue continuing education from recognized continuing education providers.

With these caveats, you can be sure that you will have the opportunity to enjoy practicing in your profession for decades!

Summary

SLPs and AUDs have the honor of serving persons with speech, language, hearing, and swallowing difficulties, opening avenues for communication and swallowing. The clients we serve deserve to have the very best services from highly qualified personnel. Our professions of speech-language pathology and audiology meet the public's desire for competent professionals by achieving the credentials that demonstrate our knowledge, skills, and expertise. By attaining national certification, SLPs and AUDs demonstrate that they have met the high standards for serving the public. Some professionals pursue additional credentials to demonstrate their expertise in a particular area of practice, achieving these specializations from any of a variety of professional organizations. In addition, professionals ensure they acquire and maintain their license to practice in the state where they provide services, as this licensure is the standard required to demonstrate state specific competencies. Licensure and certification are essential to demonstrate that our professions have high regard for the client's welfare, as they demonstrate that the professionals have met the standards for knowledge, skills, and abilities.

Critical Thinking

1. Review the licensure requirements for the state where you plan to practice. Are there any differences between those requirements and those for the Certificate of Clinical Competence?

2. Review the requirements to provide services in the public schools. Does your state require a single credential or is a second credential from the Board of Education required? If a second credential is required, how is it different from the state licensure requirements?

3. An employer offers a new graduate employment to begin the week after graduation. Can the graduate accept this offer? If not, what should the graduate say to the employer?

4. What is the benefit to the consumer to receive services from a licensed SLP or AUD? What is the benefit to receive services from an ASHA-certified SLP or AUD?

5. The lobbyist for your state speech-language-hearing association has informed the board that there is a movement to "sunset" (i.e., eliminate) licensure requirements for many professions, including speech-language pathology and audiology. What should be the association's response?

6. What is the benefit to the consumer to receive services from a SLP or AUD who has achieved specialty certification?

7. A SLP accepts employment in the state where he resides and is licensed. The employer directs him begin providing telepractice services to individuals in three other states. Can the SLP do this? If not, what should he say to his employer?

8. Why is continuing education a critical component of serving as a professional? (Review Chapter 5, "Professional Ethics," when considering this question.)

References

Academy of Neurologic Communication Disorders and Sciences. (n.d.). *ANCDS board certification*. Retrieved from https://www.ancds.org/ancds-board-certification

Alexander Graham Bell Association for the Deaf and Hard of Hearing. (n.d.). *The LSLS certification*. Retrieved from https://www.agbell.org/Professionals/Professional-Development

American Academy of Audiology. (n.d.). *CEU reporting*. Retrieved from http://www.audiology.org/ceu-reporting

American Board of Audiology. (2016). *Candidate handbook and application for certification* [PDF file]. Retrieved from http://www.boardofaudiology.org/board-certified-in-audiology/

American Board of Audiology. (n.d.-a). *Board certified in audiology.* Retrieved from http://www.boardofaudiology.org/board-certified-in-audiology/

American Board of Audiology. (n.d.-b). *Certificate programs.* Retrieved from http://www.boardofaudiology.org/certificate-programs.shtml

American Board of Audiology. (n.d.-c). *Cochlear implant specialty certification.* Retrieved from http://www.boardofaudiology.org/cochlear-implant-specialty-certification/

American Board of Audiology. (n.d.-d). *Pediatric audiology specialty certification (PASC).* Retrieved from http://www.boardofaudiology.org/pediatric-audiology-specialty-certification/

American Speech-Language-Hearing Association. (n.d.-a). *A chronology of changes in ASHA's certification standards.* Retrieved from https://www.asha.org/certification/CCC_history/

American Speech-Language-Hearing Association. (n.d.-b). *Apply for clinical specialty certification.* Retrieved from https://www.asha.org/Certification/specialty/Apply-for-Clinical-Specialty-Certification/

American Speech-Language-Hearing Association. (n.d.-c). *ASHA continuing education approved continuing education provider status.* Retrieved from https://www.asha.org/ce/for-providers/

American Speech-Language-Hearing Association. (n.d.-d). *Benefits of ASHA certification.* Retrieved from https://www.asha.org/certification/cert_benefits/

American Speech-Language-Hearing Association. (n.d.-e). *Clinical specialty certification.* Retrieved from https://www.asha.org/certification/specialty/

American Speech-Language-Hearing Association. (n.d.-f). *Comparison requirement with NBPTS.* Retrieved from https://www.asha.org/uploaded Files/ComparisonReqwithNBPTS(1).pdf

American Speech-Language-Hearing Association. (n.d.-g). *General information about ASHA certification.* Retrieved from https://www.asha.org/certification/aboutcertificationgeninfo/

American Speech-Language-Hearing Association. (n.d.-h). *Highlights and trends: Member and affiliate counts, year-end 2018.* Retrieved from https://www.asha.org/uploadedFiles/2018-Member-Counts.pdf

American Speech-Language-Hearing Association. (n.d.-i). *Maintaining your certification.* Retrieved from https://www.asha.org/certification/maintain-ccc/

American Speech-Language-Hearing Association. (n.d.-j). *Praxis examination in audiology and speech-language pathology.* Retrieved from https://www.asha.org/certification/praxis/

American Speech-Language-Hearing Association. (n.d.-k). *Praxis score and score reports.* Retrieved from https://www.asha.org/certification/praxis/praxis_scores/

American Speech-Language-Hearing Association. (n.d.-l). *Selecting a clinical fellowship (CF) setting.* Retrieved from https://www.asha.org/certification/SelectingCFSetting/

American Speech-Language-Hearing Association. (n.d.-m). *Speech-language pathology clinical fellowship.* Retrieved from https://www.asha.org/certification/clinical-fellowship/

American Speech-Language-Hearing Association. (n.d.-n). *The ASHA CE Registry: Convenient, accessible, secure.* Retrieved from https://www.asha.org/CE/CEUs/default/

American Speech-Language-Hearing Association. (n.d.-o). *Value of clinical specialty certification.* Retrieved from https://www.asha.org/Certification/specialty/Value-of-Clinical-Specialty-Certification/

Council on Academic Accreditation in Audiology and Speech-Language Pathology. (2010). *Accreditation handbook.* Rockville, MD: American Speech-Language-Hearing Association.

Council on Academic Accreditation in Audiology and Speech-Language Pathology. (n.d.-a.). *About.* Retrieved from https://caa.asha.org/about/

Council on Academic Accreditation in Audiology and Speech-Language Pathology. (n.d.-b.). *Accreditation milestones.* Retrieved from https://caa.asha.org/about/accreditation-milestones/

Council for Higher Education Accreditation. (n.d.). *Regional accrediting organizations.* Retrieved from https://www.chea.org/regional-accrediting-organizations

Educational Testing Services. (n.d.-a.). *Accommodations for test takers with disabilities or health related needs.*

Retrieved from https://ets.org/gre/revised_general/register/disabilities?WT.ac+rx28

Educational Testing Services. (n.d.-b.). *The Praxis study companion: Speech-language pathology.* Retrieved from http://www.ets.org/praxis

Institute for Credentialing Excellence. (n.d.-a.). *Accreditation.* Retrieved from https://www.credentialingexcellence.org/accreditation

Institute for Credentialing Excellence. (n.d.-b.). *NCAA accreditation.* Retrieved from https://www.credentialingexcellence.org/page/ncca-mission-and-vision

Institute for Credentialing Excellence. (n.d.-c.). *2017–2018 ICE annual report* [PDF file]. Retrieved from https://www.credentialingexcellence.org/p/cm/ld/fid=271

Institute for Credentialing Excellence. (2010). *Defining features of quality certification and assessment-based certificate programs* [PDF file]. Retrieved from https://www.credentialingexcellence.org/page/assessment-based-certificate-programs-524

National Board for Professional Teaching Standards. (n.d.). *National board standards.* Retrieved from https://www.nbpts.org/standards-five-core-propositions/

National Council of State Boards of Examiners. (n.d.-a.). *Continuing education requirements.* Retrieved from http://www.ncsb.info/continuing

National Council of State Board Examiners. (n.d.-b.). *History of legislation.* Retrieved from http://www.ncsb.info/history-by-state

National Council of State Boards of Examiners. (n.d.-c.). *States permitting hearing aid dispensing with audiology license.* Retrieved from http://www.ncsb.info/dispensing

National Council of State Boards of Examiners. (n.d.-d.). *States with regulation of support personnel.* Retrieved from http://www.ncsb.info/support

National Council of State Board Examiners. (n.d.-e.). *States that regulate audiology and speech-language pathology.* Retrieved from http://www.ncsb.info/regulate

Phillips, K. (2018). *Draft licensure compact for audiology and speech-language pathology.* Retrieved from http://www.ncsb.info/newsletters/6695708

4

Professional Organizations

Sue T. Hale, MCD and Fred H. Bess, PhD

Introduction

This chapter introduces you to opportunities for affiliating with professional organizations. The benefits of membership are highlighted, but the more important objective is to help you discover the service, leadership, and learning opportunities these organizations present. Scenarios in the opening section set the stage for what associations can do for their members. A brief review of the construct of professional organizations is provided. The American Speech-Language-Hearing Association (ASHA) and the American Academy of Audiology (AAA) are highlighted as the two primary organizations for our professions. Related professional organizations, state associations, and student organizations are also described.

Practical Dilemmas and Affiliation

Consider the following:

- The only speech-language pathologist working in a rural school district has concerns about the size of the caseload the school district requires to be served. Unlike the predecessor in this position, this clinician serves a number of children who exhibit multiple and severe handicaps. How does the speech-language pathologist demonstrate that the current caseload/workload with fewer children is equivalent in effort to that of the previous clinician who saw greater numbers of children with less severe disorders?

- An audiologist is approached by a hearing aid manufacturer who offers an all-expense-paid educational opportunity regarding a new product line the manufacturer sells. The conference will take place for two hours a day during a five-day stay at an exclusive ski resort. The company representative also encourages the audiologist to invite a family member or spouse to come along. How should the audiologist respond?

- A speech-language pathologist in a medical setting is assigned to provide intervention for patients who require systems for alternative/augmentative communication, an area of practice with which the clinician has had little experience or education. How can the clinician locate relevant educational events and materials to assist in developing the necessary skills and knowledge to provide services in this area?

- An audiologist wants to communicate with other audiologists who are researching hearing aid products and cochlear implants. Where can the audiologist locate colleagues with similar interests?

- A speech-language pathologist is concerned about reimbursement levels for services provided to hospital outpatients. How can the speech-language pathologist maximize the value of advocacy efforts for legislation of this nature?

In each instance, affiliation with a professional association and taking advantage of the member benefits of that association will assist the professionals facing these practical dilemmas. Professional associations available to speech-language pathologists and audiologists support members in dealing with all of the instances listed previously: clarifying caseload versus workload issues to employers, handling ethical dilemmas in the workplace, accessing continuing education opportunities, affiliating with other professionals who have similar interests, and participating in grassroots and coordinated advocacy efforts. These are just a few of the benefits available to speech-language pathologists and audiologists who are members of professional associations.

Students in training who affiliate with organizations targeted to their interests and needs gain firsthand knowledge of the structure and benefits of these associations prior to entering the workforce. Student organizations provide opportunities for leadership development and volunteer service as well as educational materials and scholarly and professional publications. These organizations facilitate the transition of students to the workplace in regard to standards and credentialing, ethics, and networking. Two organizations available to students in communication sciences and disorders are the National Student Speech Language Hearing Association (NSSLHA), which is affiliated with ASHA, and the Student Academy of Audiology (SAA), which is affiliated with AAA. These organizations will be described in more detail later in the chapter.

How Do Professional Organizations Work?

Professional associations offer an array of services and benefits to members as well as provide support and advocate on behalf of consumers served by those members.

Professional associations have a targeted scope of activity, typically related to a particular discipline. Individuals who wish to affiliate with the association often have to meet requirements that relate to degrees held and other educational and professional qualifications.

Professional associations have a number of common characteristics. These organizations often take responsibility for providing members with educational programs and materials, scientific and professional publications, targeted legislative advocacy activities, standards and scopes of practice, marketing resources, and public information. An important characteristic of most professional organizations is a requirement that members agree to abide by a Code of Ethics, a set of standards for professional conduct that delineate responsibilities of the members to consumers, colleagues, and the profession. Professional associations are usually nonprofit organizations governed by a Board of Directors and operated with publicly accessible bylaws. The bylaws, which contain the organization's mission and goals, also describe the governance structure and how the work of the association is conducted. Most professional organizations operate with a combination of volunteer leaders, who often assume positions on the Board of Directors or other policy-making groups, and paid staff members who engage in day-to-day operations and support member services.

Professional organizations derive a large portion of the operating budget from member dues, but additional fiscal resources are often generated by conventions and continuing education activities, publications and product sales, affiliations with commercial entities (affinity credit cards, professional and casualty insurers, convention exhibitors), corporate sponsors, and investments. These sources of income support the member benefits and consumer advocacy goals of the organization.

ASHA and AAA are two national organizations with members from the professions of speech-language pathology and audiology. ASHA has members from both professions, while AAA has members from the profession of audiology.

ASHA: A National Professional Organization for Speech-Language Pathologists and Audiologists

The American Speech-Language-Hearing Association is the largest and oldest scientific and professional organization representing the professions of speech-language pathology and audiology. ASHA began with a meeting in May 1925 in the home of Lee Edward Travis. There were fewer than 25 individuals at that first meeting, and they came together because they all held an interest in speech and its disorders. It was more than a decade before the number of members reached 60, and the organization began publishing its first scholarly journal. In 1947, the organization embraced the profession of audiology and was named the American Speech and Hearing Association. In the 1960s, the association established national standards for accrediting graduate training program and credentialing service providers. In 1978, the organization changed its name once again to reflect the component of language in its research and clinical pursuits and became the American Speech-Language-Hearing Association. Throughout its history, the association has been characterized by enormous growth in membership and a corresponding need for greater staff support. In 2007 the association moved to its current headquarters in Rockville, Maryland, a 140,000-square-foot facility holding Gold Leadership in Energy and Environmental Design (LEED) certification due to its environmentally focused construction and usage. About 300 staff members work in the ASHA National Office. See Chapter 2 for more on the founding of the professions.

Purpose

Bylaws address the purposes of an association. The purposes of ASHA, as stated in its bylaws (ASHA, 2017), are as follows:

1. To encourage basic scientific study of the processes of individual human communication with special reference to speech, language, hearing, and related disorders;

2. To promote high standards and ethics for the academic and clinical preparation of individuals entering the discipline of human communication sciences and disorders;

3. To promote the acquisition of new knowledge and skills for those within the discipline;

4. To promote investigation, prevention, and the diagnosis and treatment of disorders of human communication and related disorders;

5. To foster improvement of clinical services and intervention procedures concerning such disorders;

6. To stimulate exchange of information among persons and organizations, and to disseminate such information;

7. To inform the public about communication sciences and disorders, related disorders, and the professionals who provide services;

8. To advocate on behalf of persons with communication and related disorders;

9. To promote the individual and collective professional interests of the members of the Association.

Source: Reprinted with permission from American Speech-Language-Hearing Association. (2017). American Speech-Language-Hearing Association. (2017). *Bylaws of the american speech-language-hearing association* [Bylaws]. Available from http://www.asha.org/policy © Copyright 2017 American Speech-Language-Hearing Association. All rights reserved.

The ASHA bylaws address many other issues and serve to provide information about all aspects of the operation and mission of the association, including governance, standards, the Code of Ethics, publications, and other key organizational components.

Membership

At the end of 2018, ASHA currently had more than 200,000 individuals associated with the organization. This number reflects certified members, noncertified members, nonmember certificate holders, and international affiliates, who are audiologists; speech-language pathologists; and speech, language, or hearing scientists. The number also includes members of the National Student Speech-Language-Hearing Association at undergraduate and graduate levels of training in the discipline as well as support personnel in audiology and speech-language pathology. At the end of 2018, ASHA affiliates included more than 170,000 certified members who are speech-language pathologists and approximately 12,500 certified member audiologists. Approximately 800 individuals were certified in both speech-language pathology and audiology (ASHA, 2019a). At the end of 2018, ASHA membership was 95.4% female, a continuation of a trend that has seen a gradual reduction in the percentage of males in the association. Also at the end of 2018, racial/ethnic minority-group members were 8.2% of those affiliated with the association, and 22.1% of members were 55 years of age or older (ASHA, 2019a). Two of these demographic factors are concerning to the association.

Efforts have been initiated to recruit and retain males in the professions, but the numbers indicate that these efforts have not met with great success. The association has also worked to increase the number of professionals from racial and ethnic minorities, but the overall percentage in relation to the total membership has increased only slightly since 2003. Success in the recruitment and retention of males and minority professionals is essential for a diverse workforce to be available to address the communication needs of all citizens. The relatively large number of older members with retirement on the horizon has been a concern for the association for a number of years. However, the distribution of members by age suggests that younger members are increasing and equalizing the age distribution of the workforce. While members up to the age of 45 now make up approximately 57% of the total membership, a critical concern remains regarding the number of younger members who will obtain research and teaching degrees to address future educational needs and contribute to the knowledge base. ASHA in partnership with the Council of Academic Programs in Communication Sciences and Disorders is devoting large amounts of energy and resources to address the doctoral shortage. See Chapter 8 for further discussion of demographics of the profession.

It should be mentioned that the number of audiologists who are members of ASHA and hold the Certificate of Clinical Competence (CCC) has held steady in recent years. While negligible changes in the total number of audiologists affiliated with ASHA have been observed and retention of audiology members/affiliates/certificate holders has held annually above 96%, the number of speech-language pathologists continues to increase annually. The result is that the percentage of audiology members in relation to the total ASHA membership has declined. These demographic trends will continue to engage the interest and attention of ASHA organizers for the foreseeable future (ASHA, 2019a).

Standards

A key component of the American Speech-Language-Hearing Association is its standards program, which addresses issues of credentialing of individual service providers as well as accreditation of academic training. ASHA has offered the CCC in audiology and speech-language pathology for more than 50 years. These certificates have become nationally recognized credentials by governmental and educational agencies. The CCC standards have served as the model for the state licensure requirements in many states. Additionally, ASHA supports the accreditation of graduate programs in communication sciences and disorders through the Council on Academic Accreditation in Audiology and Speech-Language Pathology (CAA), an accreditor recognized by the Secretary of the U.S. Department of Education and the Council for Higher Education Accreditation of the U.S. Department of Education. Students who wish to receive the ASHA CCC must complete the requisite academic and clinical training in a CAA-accredited graduate training program. The newest CAA standards for graduate education and ASHA standards for professional credentialing in both audiology and speech-language

pathology emphasize the attainment of knowledge and skills to address speech, language, and hearing needs across the life span and with a variety of disorders. See Chapter 3 for an in-depth discussion of CAA accreditation and ASHA certification and see the list of resources at the end of this chapter for web addresses of ASHA certification and accreditation programs.

Governance

The governance structure of an association describes how policies are made, states who is responsible for certain work in the organization, and serves to guide a consumer or member in determining where to go for assistance with a certain problem or question. The governance structure of ASHA is described in detail in Article IV of the bylaws (ASHA, 2017, Article IV, 4.1–4.2). A visual display of the structure is presented in Figure 4–1 (ASHA, 2018).

For ASHA, the work of governance is conducted by the Board of Directors (BOD), which holds the duties for policy making and fiscal responsibility. The BOD consists of 16 ASHA members and the ASHA CEO. The President Elect (who then serves as president and past president) and 10 Vice Presidents who serve 3-year terms are elected by the membership in an electronic vote. The President Elect, Vice President for Planning, Vice President for Government Relations and Public Policy, Vice President for Science and Research, and Vice President for Finance may be audiologists or speech-language pathologists. Audiologists are represented on the BOD by the Vice President for Academic Affairs in Audiology, Vice President for Standards and Ethics in Audiology, and Vice President for Audiology Practice. Three similar vice-presidential positions exist for speech-language pathology. The vice presidents who hold the positions associated with a specific profession are elected by a vote of ASHA members in that profession. The other members of BOD are the Chief Executive Officer of the association, who is a nonvoting member, the Chairs of two advisory bodies, the Audiology Advisory Council, and the Speech-Language Pathology Advisory Council, who are elected by the respective councils. The National Advisor of the National Student Speech-Language-Hearing Association is also a member of the BOD chosen by the student association.

The Advisory Councils (ACs) are two bodies composed of ASHA members from each of the 50 states and the District of Columbia and representatives from the National Student Speech Language Hearing Association and ASHA's International Affiliates. The states and the two representative groups elect one speech-language pathologist and one audiologist to serve in each of the ACs and to consider matters of importance to the association.

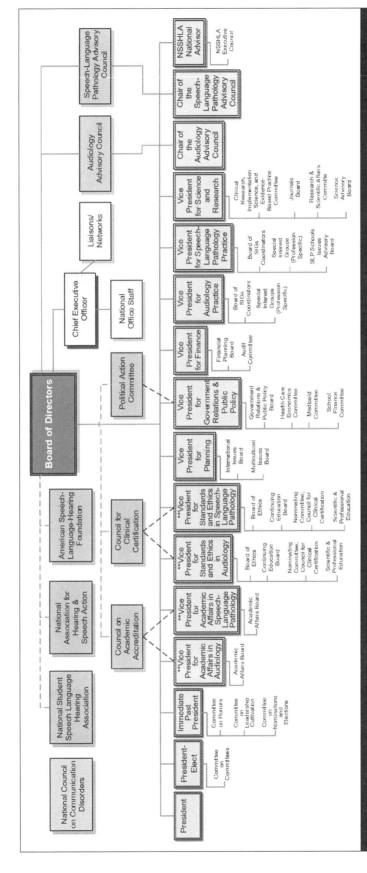

Figure 4–1. ASHA Governance Structure. *Source:* Reprinted with permission from ASHA Governance Structure. https://www.asha.org/uploadedFiles/ASHA-Governance-Structure.pdf Copyright 2018 by American Speech-Language-Hearing Association. All rights reserved.

Through electronic discussions and face-to-face meetings, the ACs provide guidance and input to the BOD. The Chair of each AC is elected by that body and serves on the BOD as a full voting member (ASHA, 2017).

ASHA has recently conducted a study of its governance structure, and changes to the composition of the board may result from that work.

The National Office

In addition to the volunteer leadership of the association, a national office staff of approximately 300 members works in the day-to-day operation of the Association. The Chief Executive Officer works closely with Chief Operating Officers in speech-language pathology, audiology, science and research, multicultural affairs, communications, and operations to conduct the work of the National Office. These executives, referred to as the Facilitating Team, guide the work clusters in the National Office. The work clusters include academic affairs, certification, ethics; audiology practices; speech-language pathology practices; multicultural affairs; governmental relations and public policy; governance and operations; professional education; marketing and sales; public relations; publishing; NSSLHA, the Action Center; the National Center for Evidence-Based Practice; and other administrative and operational groups.

The administrators and staff in the National Office work to accomplish association purposes, develop and implement work plans to achieve association objectives, and monitor long-term operations. The National Office relates to members directly through the Action Center call line and other forms of person-to-person communication. ASHA participates in a variety of social media platforms to enhance member outreach efforts, including Facebook, Twitter, Instagram, LinkedIn, Pinterest, YouTube, and the ASHAsphere Blog. Additionally, staff within the office maintain and update the website to maximize its benefit to members, students, and consumers. ASHA now distributes all of its journals to members electronically and through its website, and all articles in ASHA journals are archived on the site and available to members. Working with the volunteer leadership, the national office staff members are often the most direct link between the association and the members, and the work of the national office is essential to the association.

The Future

ASHA's future is dependent on many issues, many of which are tied to the ability to remain responsive and effective in a world where information must be gained and shared instantaneously and across national borders. Members will value services that meet their expectations for immediacy, accuracy, and currency. The ASHA website provides information regarding web-based seminars and dialogues and telecommunications of all types, which are association activities that address those expectations.

In addition, ASHA has developed a strategic plan to address concerns and issues that are considered central to the continuing mission of the association and its service to consumers and members. The Strategic Pathway to Excellence suggests a means for addressing key issues for the future. The vision of the Association is "making effective communication, a human right, accessible and achievable for all" (ASHA, 2019b). This vision rests on the mission of empowering the members and the professions to advocate on behalf of people with communication and related disorders, advance the science of the discipline, and promote effective human communication. Through the Strategic Pathway to Excellence, ASHA continues its commitment to the global professional community while maintaining a focus on the research, educational, legislative, and practice needs of its current members.

Special Interest Groups

Special Interest Groups were established within ASHA to promote knowledge and skills in specialized areas. ASHA members may join one or more of the Special Interest Groups and have access to educational programs, research, publications, and dialogue with members with similar interests. The Groups, which are closely aligned with the ASHA structure, have their own coordinating committees and have the opportunity to determine what programs and issues are most germane to the members of the group at any given time. This model provides members with an opportunity to gain leadership experience and influence practice patterns within an area of specialization.

Eighteen Special Interest Groups address the diverse areas of language learning, neurogenic disorders, voice disorders, fluency disorders, orofacial disorders, hearing research and diagnostics, aural rehabilitation, hearing conservation, hearing disorders in childhood, issues in higher education, administration and supervision, augmentative and alternative communication, swallowing and swallowing disorders, communication issues in culturally and linguistically diverse populations, gerontology, school-based issues, global issues, telepractice, and speech science (ASHA, 2019c).

AAA: A National Professional Organization for Audiologists

The American Academy of Audiology (AAA) is the world's largest professional organization of, by, and for audiologists. The impetus for AAA dates back to the 1987 ASHA convention in New Orleans when a mini-seminar was presented on "The Future of Audiology." Richard Talbott chaired the session and recruited five well-known audiologists to discuss such critical issues as future needs and potential employment of audiologists, the knowledge base required to meet the future needs, the level of academic training needed to achieve the knowledge base, and the university faculty/supervisory personnel needs for training audiologists. One of the panel members, James Jerger, concluded his presentation by noting that it was now time for a new professional organization of, by, and for audiologists. Jerger's comments were met with an enthusiastic response. As a follow-up to the ASHA session, 32 audiology leaders met in Houston, Texas, in early 1988 at the invitation of James Jerger (Baylor College of Medicine). The purpose of the study group was to establish an independent, freestanding, national organization for audiologists. The group voted unanimously to develop a new organization for audiologists, to be called the American College of Audiology, and the first National Office was established at Baylor College of Medicine. In addition, an ad hoc steering committee was appointed to develop bylaws. Finally, before leaving the Houston meeting, each member of the founders group contributed $20 to establish the organization's first budget (Stach, 1998).

In the few short months to follow, remarkable progress was made. The newly developed bylaws for the organization were approved, the organization was renamed the American Academy of Audiology, the Academy was incorporated under the laws of the state of Tennessee, an organizational structure was established and officers elected, dues were established, committee assignments were made, dates for the first annual meeting were determined, and a major membership drive was launched. In 1989, the first AAA convention was held at Kiawah Island, South Carolina, and the response exceeded all expectations: Close to 600 participants, including 45 "charter" exhibitors, attended the meeting and literally overflowed the conference facilities.

Since 1989, the AAA has undergone significant growth in membership and development. By 1993, the AAA reached a point in membership size and fiscal responsibilities that it became necessary to move the National Office to Washington, DC, and contract staff to assist in the organization's management. Today, the AAA National Office is located in Reston, Virginia.

Purpose

According to the AAA bylaws (American Academy of Audiology, 2017), the Academy is a professional organization of individuals dedicated to providing quality

hearing and balance care by advancing the profession of audiology through leadership, advocacy, education, public awareness, and support of research. The focus is to enhance the ability of AAA members to achieve career and practice objectives through professional development, education, research, and increased public awareness of hearing disorders and audiologic services.

Membership

AAA currently has more than 12,000 members, an impressive number given the relatively short time the organization has been in existence. Moreover, the number of new members added each year is growing substantially. The demographic breakdown of the AAA membership is similar to that of ASHA—approximately 79% of the membership of AAA is female, and 64% hold doctoral degrees (this number will grow significantly now that the doctor of audiology degree is required to practice in the profession). Fifty-five percent of those with doctorates earned the AuD degree. Finally, ~12% of audiologists are over age 55.

Both ASHA and AAA have been concerned about the inability to attract additional males and minorities into the profession despite the development of special recruitment initiatives. Equally disturbing is the number of professionals who are 55 years or older, most of whom will be retiring within the next 10 years. These demographic concerns have been discussed earlier in the membership section related to ASHA.

Standards

Similar to ASHA, the AAA has developed a standards program for certifying audiologists. The program, offered by the American Board of Audiology (ABA), certifies audiologists whose knowledge base and clinical skills are consistent with professionally established standards and who continue to add to their knowledge through various forms of continuing education. The ABA is working toward having states and government agencies recognize ABA certification. A goal of AAA has always been to serve as the professional home for all audiologists, including those from other countries. Accordingly, the ABA Board developed a policy for certification of international audiologists. Eligibility requirements for international certification through AAA appear on the ABA website.

The ABA has begun to develop specialty certifications such as the Pediatric Audiology Specialty Certification (PASC) and the Cochlear Implant Specialty Certification (CISC), both of which are voluntary certification programs. To achieve specialty certification, specific requirements unique to a given specialty area must be met—details of the specialty certification programs offered by the ABA can also be found on the AAA website. See the Resources section for web addresses of organizations. Finally, the ABA administers assessment-based certificate programs in specialty areas of practice or a set of specific skills. Examples of specialty certificate programs include Audiology Preceptor (CH-AP) and Tinnitus Management (CH-TM).

The AAA has also developed an accreditation process for universities offering AuD graduate training. Beginning in 2003, the Accreditation Commission for Audiology Education (ACAE) began developing education standards for AuD training programs. The ACAE is an independent 501(c)(3) non-profit organization established by representative members of the AAA and the Academy of Doctors of Audiology. The purpose of ACAE accreditation is to recognize, reinforce, and promote high-quality performance in AuD educational programs through a rigorous verification process—a process designed to ensure that AuD programs prepare graduates who meet high standards and who demonstrate competencies considered essential for practice at the doctoral level. The ACAE adopted the recently revised standards (March 2016) following a rigorous peer review process. The standards can be found online at ACAE's website (http://www.acaeaccred.org/standards). In addition to ACAE, a technology company has been contracted for the development of a web-based accreditation system. The Computerized Accreditation Program (CAP) is an innovative online accreditation system combining high-quality standards with state-of-the art technology. The result is accreditation *plus* an interactive, web-based process designed to facilitate ease in management and provide valuable information to program directors, faculty, students, and communities of interest. Some of the proposed features of the system include online participation, an interactive self-study process, and the ability to retrieve national trends and analyses from a data warehouse.

Governance and the National Office

The governance structure of AAA is described in Article III of the bylaws (AAA, 2017). The structure is purposely designed to be streamlined so that the leadership can respond in a timely manner to its membership as well as to topical issues on the national front that arise from time to time throughout the year. To this end, the Academy is governed by a Board of Directors composed of 12 Fellows, including the President, President-Elect, Immediate Past President, and nine Members-At-Large. Each member of the board is elected by the membership at large and possesses the power to vote on issues before the board. In addition to other

duties, the Board of Directors is expected to (1) grant membership to those applicants whose qualifications, in the board's judgment, meet the requirements set forth by the bylaws; (2) establish boards, committees, and task forces, as necessary, to guide and assist the Academy in its mission, and appoint the Chair of such groups; and (3) transact all such other business in the interest of the membership.

The national office is composed of an Executive Director and an office staff who work closely with the President, other board members, and volunteers from the membership to facilitate operational activities of the Academy. Examples of such activities include government relations, credentialing, public relations, marketing, publications, continuing education, and professional education.

The Future

The AAA has experienced extraordinary growth and success during the first three decades of its existence. The future of AAA, however, will depend on the ability of the Academy leadership to continue to meet the ever-changing needs of audiologists and the profession as well as to develop effective tools to measure progress. Indeed, those organizations that fail to define their goals and critical success factors for the future and to communicate the goals to their members will not be successful. To this end, AAA leadership has developed a comprehensive strategic plan that sets the course for the future of the profession. Goals, strategies, and action plans have been developed to help ensure that the Academy will achieve its vision of advancing the science and practice of audiology and achieving public recognition of audiologists as experts in hearing and balance. Some of the objectives in the AAA strategic plan (2018–2019) include the following: (1) provide innovative educational resources to support quality audiology services; (2) promote high-quality standardized education; (3) increase effectiveness of communications and technology; (4) deliver tangible personal benefits to the membership; (5) create strategic partnerships to achieve more together; (6) help shape federal and state policy; and (7) increase initiatives directly linked to recognition of audiologists and the audiology enterprise.

Related Professional Organizations

Related professional organizations are available to individuals with research, clinical, or educational interests that may not be fully addressed within the scope of

ASHA or AAA. Examples of these organizations are the Academy of Neurologic Communication Disorders and Sciences (ANCDS), an organization with professional, clinical, educational, scientific, and charitable interests directed toward the quality of life for adults and children with neurologic communication disorders; the Acoustical Society of America, an organization involved in the scientific pursuit of acoustics information, which includes members from diverse scientific professions, including physics, engineering, biology, psychology, and speech and hearing; and the Council for Exceptional Children (CEC), an organization dedicated to improving educational outcomes for students with exceptionalities such as developmental disabilities, learning disabilities, and communicative disabilities and deafness.

These are just a few of the many examples of related professional organizations that may engage the student or professional with special interests in a focused educational, clinical, or research area. A listing of some relevant related professional organizations is provided in the Resources section at the end of the chapter.

State Organizations

State organizations in speech-language pathology and audiology are often affiliated with a larger national organization and have similar purposes and structure when this is the case. For example, many state speech-language hearing associations are recognized affiliates of ASHA. As such, they have access to ASHA's state-national relations resources, which provide informational and sometimes financial assistance with legislation, licensure, and other state-focused issues. The Council of State Association Presidents meets twice annually, once in the spring in conjunction with the ASHA State Policy Workshop and on the day prior to the annual ASHA convention. Contact information for state associations and other information pertinent to state licensing and teacher certification is found in the "ASHA State by State" section of the ASHA website.

Similar to ASHA, AAA members are usually associated with state organizations which exist in all 50 states and the U.S. Territory of Puerto Rico. These state audiology associations work in concert with AAA on state-related issues—and they have access to the many benefits and resources provided by the Academy. For example, state affiliates often work with AAA to prepare educational materials to assist members to understand licensure and certification issues and support individual audiologists in resolving specific licensure concerns.

State organizations have an opportunity to influence practice issues, regulations, funding decisions, and other aspects of the day-to-day practice of the profes-sions within a locale. As such, these organizations offer students and professionals the opportunity to become engaged in activities of vital importance to their current or future livelihood.

Students are often provided reduced fees or even free memberships and convention registration if they assist with state activities. Assisting at the state association level is an excellent means to enter the volunteer workforce that is so essential to the viability of professional organizations. Students who affiliate with state associations while they are in their training programs have an opportunity to network with individuals who may ultimately be future employers or mentors when the students graduate.

Student Organizations

Training programs in communication sciences and disorders typically have local chapters of the National Student Speech Language Hearing Association (NSSLHA) and the Student Academy of Audiology (SAA). Like the earlier model, NSSLHA, which is recognized and affiliated with ASHA, includes student members who are preparing for careers in audiology or in speech-language pathology. SAA, which is affiliated with AAA, includes student members preparing for careers in audiology—it is the official national student organization of the AAA that serves as a collective voice for students and advances the rights, interests, and welfare of students pursuing careers in audiology.

NSSLHA

As the only student association formally recognized by ASHA, NSSLHA has representatives on the Audiology Advisory Council and the Speech-Language Pathology Advisory Council, and its National Advisor is a member of the ASHA Board of Directors. Additionally, NSSLHA has student representatives on a number of the ASHA councils and boards. The requirements for membership in NSSLHA are that an undergraduate or graduate student has an interest in the study of normal and disordered human communication behavior and is enrolled either part or full time in a training program in communication sciences. Local chapters in university settings allow students opportunities for leadership development, volunteerism, philanthropic work, professional networking, educational events, reduced ASHA convention registration, and a reduction in ASHA certification fees if membership is maintained throughout the graduate training program. The website for the NSSLHA organization is provided in Resources at the end of the chapter.

SAA

The SAA essentially replaced a former student organization, the National Association of Future Doctors of Audiology (NAFDA). Founded in 1998 by an AuD doctoral student, NAFDA provided a number of benefits to students such as a student newsletter, an academic journal, and an online forum and chatroom. For a brief period, both SAA and NAFDA existed as separate organizations but with similar objectives—SAA was the official student organization associated with AAA, and NAFDA was a student organization independent of AAA. In 2008, NAFDA and the AAA announced an agreement to merge NAFDA into AAA's SAA. The unified SAA created new bylaws and now conducts the business of fine-tuning the student organization for the profession of audiology. Some of the benefits of SAA include elected representatives with ties to AAA, educational opportunities, student publications/newsletters, student-related sessions at the AAA annual meeting, and importantly, the opportunity for mentored leadership.

International Professional Organizations

For those who have an interest in international professional issues in speech-language pathology and audiology, affiliation with a number of professional organizations may be useful. For example, the International Society of Audiology and the International Association of Logopedics and Phoniatrics (IALP) provide membership and educational opportunities. In addition, you will read about professional organizations in other countries in Chapter 7, "International Alliances." There you will read about associations in other English-speaking countries, including Australia, Canada, New Zealand, South Africa, and the United Kingdom.

Summary

Students are encouraged to affiliate with national professional organizations as well as state organizations, special interest groups, and related professional organizations. Early involvement in these associations provides opportunities for volunteering, networking, advocacy, and learning. An excellent training ground for these experiences is active participation in a student organization affiliated with a national association, such as the National Student Speech Language Hearing Association or the Student Academy of Audiology. Being a member of a larger group makes it more likely that problems can be solved and answers to questions can be obtained in a coordinated, consistent, and effective manner. Being

aware of the history and governance of associations will also help students as they choose to affiliate with those associations that will continue to be the most effective in representing member interests and in relating to the larger global community.

Critical Thinking

1. What are the advantages of membership in a national professional organization?

2. Refer to the opening scenarios. What specific kinds of assistance could these individuals expect to get from their national professional organization(s)?

3. Create scenarios specific to your own area of interest or a problem you might encounter as a professional and discuss resources your professional organization might provide to address the issue.

4. What valuable experiences are likely to be gained from affiliation with a state organization, a special interest group, or a related professional organization?

5. Should a graduate student in audiology affiliate with NSSLHA, SAA, or both? Should a practicing audiologist hold membership in AAA, ASHA, or both?

6. After you graduate and hold a professional degree, you may be advised by a colleague that there is more value to belonging to a state organization and that using your limited resources to join a national professional organization is unwise. On what basis would your colleague make that argument? What support could you provide for joining a national organization?

7. Leadership in a student organization is often viewed as a resumé builder. In what way could you relate leadership experiences to a prospective employer so that the employer would value the experience and expect resulting transferable skills?

8. Professional organizations rely heavily on volunteer leadership, notably in committee service and board positions. What are the expected consequences, both positive and negative, if you volunteer as a leader for a professional organization?

9. When you graduate, you will join one or more professional organizations. Create a plan for 10 years postgraduation that will allow you to become a leader in one of those organizations.

10. Interview several audiologists about what they think about having two major professional organizations devoted to hearing and its disorders (ASHA and AAA). What are the advantages and disadvantages of having these two professional organizations for practicing clinicians? With which organization(s) do you see yourself affiliating and why?

References

Accreditation Commission for Audiology Education (ACAE). (2016). *Accreditation Standards for the Doctor of Audiology (Au.D.) Program.* Retrieved from http://www.acaeaccred.org/standards

American Academy of Audiology. (2017). *Bylaws of the American Academy of Audiology.* Retrieved from http://www.audiology.org/

American Speech-Language-Hearing Association. (2017). *Bylaws of the American Speech-Language-Hearing Association* [Bylaws]. Retrieved from http://www.asha.org/policy.

American Speech-Language-Hearing Association. (2018). *ASHA governance structure.* Rockville, MD: Author. Retrieved from http://www.asha.org/uploadedfilesabout/governance/ASHAGovStructure.pdf

American Speech-Language-Hearing Association. (2019a). *ASHA summary membership and affiliation counts, year-end 2018.* Retrieved from http://www.asha.org

American Speech-Language-Hearing Association. (2019b). *Strategic pathway to excellence.* Rockville, MD: Author. Retrieved from https://www.asha.org/uploadedFiles/Strategic-Pathway-to-Excellence-Map.pdf

American Speech-Language-Hearing Association. (2019c). *Special interest groups.* Rockville, MD: Author. Retrieved from https://www.asha.org/SIG/About-Special-Interest-Groups/

Stach, B. (1998). In the beginning—1987–1988. *Audiology Today,* 6–11.

Resources

National Professional Organizations

Accreditation Commission for Audiology Education (ACAE)
11480 Commerce Park Drive, Suite 220
Reston, VA 20191

Phone: 202-986-9500
Website: http://www.acaeaccred.org

American Academy of Audiology
11480 Commerce Park Drive, Suite 220
Reston, VA 20191
Phone: 703-790-8631
Website: http://www.audiology.org
American Board of Audiology
http://www.audiology.org/development/boardcertification

American Speech-Language-Hearing Association
10801 Rockville Pike
Rockville, MD 20852
Phone: 301-897-5700
Website: http://www.asha.org
Council for Clinical Certification
http://www.asha.org/certification/
Council on Academic Accreditation
https://caa.asha.org/

National Student Speech Language Hearing Association
10801 Rockville Pike
Rockville, MD 20852
Phone: 301-471-0481
Website: http://www.nsslha.org

Student Academy of Audiology
11480 Commerce Park Drive, Suite 220
Reston, VA 20191
Phone: 703-790-8631
Website: http://www.audiology.org/education/students/SAA

State Professional Organizations

For a complete list of state professional associations affiliated with ASHA,
http://www.asha.org/advocacy/state/

Related Professional Organizations

Academy of Doctors of Audiology (ADA)
http://www.audiologist.org

Academy of Federal Audiologists and Speech-Language Pathologists (AFASLP)
http://afaslp.org/

Academy of Neurologic Communication Disorders and Sciences (ANCDS)
http://www.ancds.org

Academy of Rehabilitative Audiology (ARA)
http://www.audrehab.org

Acoustical Society of America (ASA)
http://www.acousticalsociety.org

Alexander Graham Bell Association for the Deaf and Hard of Hearing
http://www.agbell.org

American Academy of Private Practice in Speech Pathology & Audiology (AAPPSPA)
http://www.aappspa.org

American Auditory Society (AAS)
http://www.amauditorysoc.org

American Cleft Palate-Craniofacial Association (ACPA)
http://www.acpa-cpf.org

American Society for Deaf Children (ASDC)
http://www.deafchildren.org

American Tinnitus Association (ATA)
http://www.ata.org

Better Hearing Institute (BHI)
http://www.betterhearing.org

Brain Injury Association of America
http://www.biausa.org

Canadian Association of Speech-Language Pathologists and Audiologists (CASLPA)
http://www.caslpa.ca

Council for Exceptional Children (CEC)
http://www.cec.sped.org

Council of Academic Programs in Communication Sciences and Disorders (CAPCSD)
http://www.capcsd.org

Educational Audiology Association (EAA)
http://www.edaud.org

Hearing Loss Association of America (HLAA)
http://hearingloss.org/

International Association of Logopedics and Phoniatrics (IALP)
http://www.ialp.info/

International Association of Orofacial Myology (IAOM)
http://www.iaom.com

The International Dyslexia Association (IDA) (formerly Orton Dyslexia Society)
http://www.interdys.org

International Society for Augmentative and Alternative Communication (ISAAC)
http://www.isaac-online.org

International Society of Audiology (ISA)
http://www.isa-audiology.org

Linguistic Society of America (LSA)
http://www.lsadc.org

National Aphasia Association (NAA)
http://www.aphasia.org

National Black Association for Speech-Language and Hearing (NBASLH)
http://www.nbaslh.org

National Institute on Deafness and Other Communication Disorders (NIDCD)
http://www.nidcd.nih.gov

National Rehabilitation Association (NRA)
http://www.nationalrehab.org

National Stuttering Association (NSA)
http://www.nsastutter.org

Stuttering Foundation of America
http://www.stutteringhelp.org

5

Professional Ethics

◇◇◇

Jaynee A. Handelsman, PhD

Introduction

Ethical behavior is the cornerstone of professionalism and is essential to maintaining the highest standards of practice. This chapter will explore various topics related to professional ethics in speech-language pathology and audiology including standards of professional conduct, conflicts of interest, the role of professional associations, ethical issues in practice management, ethical issues in supervision and academia, how to manage ethical dilemmas, and unethical behavior complaint processes for the American Speech-Language-Hearing Association (ASHA) and the American Academy of Audiology (AAA). The importance of ethics education will be discussed, including some specific examples of education provided by our professional associations. Finally, some critical thinking questions will be listed to help readers think about how these issues might apply to their specific professional contexts.

Standards of Professional Conduct

Standards of professional conduct for audiologists and speech-language pathologists (SLPs) are established by various entities including professional associations, places of employment, and legal regulatory agencies such as state licensure boards. There are some important distinctions between professional associations and legal regulatory bodies that SLPs and audiologists need to appreciate. For example, the purpose of professional associations is to bring together individuals that have a common professional purpose and agree to uphold specific high standards of practice. On the other hand, the purpose of state regulatory bodies is to determine the legal requirements for licensure to practice and to regulate licensed professionals (Frazek, 2003). Codes of Conduct or Standard Practice Guidelines are often developed and published by institutions to document behavioral expectations of all employees and employees may be required to attest to having read and agreed to complying with the policies. ASHA members, certificate holders, and those in the application process are obligated the follow the ASHA Code of Ethics (Code) and the ASHA Board of Ethics (BOE) has jurisdiction over these individuals to adjudicate complaints of unethical behavior (ASHA, 2016a). They are also required to adhere to licensure laws and other applicable standards of practice.

It is important for SLPs and audiologists to understand the ethical codes of the professional associations to which they belong as well as the licensure regulations of the state(s) in which they practice (Frazek, 2003). When working internationally, they are also bound by the standards and laws of the country in which they are working. In some states the standards for professional conduct are quite similar between professional associations' Codes of Ethics and the requirements for licensure. In other states there are important differences. For example, in some states speech-language pathologists are able to legally practice in a school setting without ASHA certification. However, if the SLP is a member of ASHA, they would also need to hold the CCC in order to ethically practice. Specifically, Principle of Ethics II, Rule B states that "members who do not hold the Certificate of Clinical Competence may not engage in the provision of clinical services" (ASHA, 2016a, p. 6). Similarly, audiologists working in many settings are not required to hold the Certificate of Clinical Competence in Audiology (CCC-A) in order to practice legally. However, in order to be a member of ASHA, they would need to hold the CCC-A in order to ethically practice.

Audiologists and speech-language pathologists should also be aware of the standard practice guidelines of their place of employment. There may be circumstances in which those guidelines exceed the requirements imposed by the professional associations as well as licensure boards. Failure to adhere to the standard practice guidelines of a place of employment could put the individual's job in jeopardy.

Conflicts of Interest

Conflicts of interest occur when there are competing priorities affecting the decisions we make. For example, a speech-language pathologist may have authored and published an assessment tool for literacy that is very popular among professionals. A conflict is present if that speech-language pathologist is in a position of making purchasing decisions about clinic materials in her clinic. In that case, the conflict is real because the author of the tool stands to benefit financially from the purchase by way of royalties. A second example is a hearing scientist who has developed a technology to mitigate tinnitus while working at a university using grant funds and then subsequently creates a start-up company with the intent of ultimately patenting and selling it. The conflict occurs when the faculty member has a financial interest in the company and still wants to serve as the primary investigator on a project to assess its effectiveness with patients and to enroll patients.

Perceived conflicts of interest occur when there is no real opportunity for the individual to benefit personally, financially, or professionally from a particular circumstance. However, consumers or other individuals may have concerns about bias entering the decision making. An example of a perceived conflict of interest can occur when the Council on Academic Accreditation (CAA) is evaluating educational programs for the purpose of determining if that program meets accreditation standards. In order to avoid perceived conflicts based on potential bias, council members are recused from participating in the evaluation of programs within their state. While a particular council member may not have any relationship with the other academic programs in his or her state, there may be a perception of bias should that member be involved in the program evaluation.

We are all faced with making decisions in our personal and professional lives that impact and ultimately determine our behavior, the people we interact with as friends and colleagues, where we spend time, and the relative value we place on how those things shape our lives. In making each choice, we consider various options and determine which variables are most important to us. There are consequences for each choice we make (Handelsman, 2006).

The ASHA Code has for many years included a statement that conflicts of interest are unethical. The specific language occurs in Principle of Ethics III, Rule B, which states that "individuals shall avoid engaging in conflicts of interest whereby personal, financial, or other considerations have the potential to influence or compromise professional judgment and objectivity" (ASHA, 2016a, p. 7). The American Academy of Audiology (AAA) Code of Ethics specifies in Principle 4, Rule 4c that "individuals shall not participate in activities that constitute a conflict of professional interest" (AAA, 2018, p. 1).

One of the challenges for audiologists and speech-language pathologists has to do with implied expectations or "strings." Something as simple as accepting lunch from a manufacturer's representative might carry with it an expectation of bias to use that company's products. Another example of a possible "string" involves a physician who refers patients to an individual speech-language pathologist or audiologist expecting the professional in our discipline to reciprocate by referring patients for surgical management. In the same way, a colleague you know from a professional association volunteer experience might expect you to recommend her graduate program to students you know. In all three examples, the key to knowing whether there are expectations of reciprocity is clear and honest communication (Handelsman, 2006). Audiologists and speech-language pathologists must be aware of both real conflicts of interest and those that are perceived in order to avoid both.

The Role of Professional Associations

In establishing their codes of conduct, many professional associations have moral principles that underlie their guidelines (Kitchner, 1984). For most groups, these principles include freedom of action and choice, justice and fairness, doing good for others, preventing or avoiding harm, and fidelity and loyalty (Bupp, 2012). The core principles of the ASHA Code focus on honoring professional boundaries and responsibilities to individuals served, colleagues, students, support personnel, and the public (ASHA, 2016a). These principles include: responsibilities to individuals served; responsibilities for one's own professional competence; responsibilities to the public; and responsibilities to inter- and intraprofessional relationships (ASHA, 2016a).

The ASHA Board of Ethics (BOE) is a semiautonomous body of ASHA that is charged by the ASHA Bylaws with four important functions including: (1) creating, publishing, and, as needed, amending a Code of Ethics (hereinafter the "Code") that specifies the professional ethical responsibilities of members and certificate holders; (2) developing ethics educational materials for distribution; (3) adjudicating complaints of unethical behavior by individuals who are bound by the Code; and (4) making decisions as specified in the semi-autonomous bodies agreement (ASHA, 2018). BOE members are appointed by the Committee on Committees of the ASHA Board of Directors (BOD) at their third meeting of the year. The ASHA Board of Directors is responsible for approving all modifications to the Code as well as the policies and procedures proposed by the BOE relative to adjudicating complaints of Code violations (ASHA, 2018). Sanctions for violations are determined by the BOE and will be outlined in another section of this chapter.

ASHA has been committed to providing a framework for ethical behavior from the beginning. The first Code was published in 1952 and it has been modified over the years as the professions and society overall have changed (ASHA, 2016a). The Code was most recently revised in 2016 to include: an updated preamble; a new technology section; 15 new Rules of Ethics; and revisions to two Principles of Ethics. The revised code is intended to provide greater clarity about the Code and how a specific rule might apply to members faced with an ethical dilemma (Bupp, 2016). Changes to the Code were made based upon themes from previously adjudicated cases, from input from ASHA staff, and from peer review. For a list of themes that are addressed in the 2016 Code, please refer to the Code of Ethics Revision Summary that is available on the ASHA website (ASHA, 2016b).

The purpose of the Code is to protect consumers of our services as well as to protect the integrity of the discipline including audiologists, speech language pathologists, and speech-language-hearing scientists in their roles as educators, supervisors, mentors, clinical service providers, researchers, and administrators. As previously mentioned, individuals bound by the Code include ASHA members holding the Certificate of Clinical Competence (CCC), members not holding the CCC, nonmember certificate holders, and those in the application process (ASHA, 2016a).

The Code includes four Principles of Ethics, which form the underlying philosophical basis of the Code, as well as the Rules of Ethics that are specific statements about acceptable and unacceptable behavior. The Principles "are reflected in the following areas: (I) responsibility to persons served professionally and to research participants, both human and animal; (II) responsibility for one's professional competence; (III) responsibility to the public; and (IV) responsibility for professional relationships" (ASHA, 2016a, p. 2). Principle I is supported by 20 Rules that specify expected behaviors as well as those that are prohibited. Principle II is supported by 8 Rules, Principle III is supported by 7 Rules, and Principle IV is supported by 20 statements of appropriate and inappropriate behavior (ASHA, 2016a). Overall, the Code is intended to provide guidance to members, certificate holders, and applicants for membership and certification as they make decisions about professional behavior. The intention is not to outline specific circumstances that professionals may encounter (ASHA, 2018). The 2016 Code is appended to this chapter and is available from http://www.asha.org/policy

It is important to note that an effective Code requires fairness in the administration and enforcement of all of its elements as well as complete compliance by members and certificate holders. Decisions by the BOE are made on a case-by-case basis taking into account the merits of each (ASHA, 2018). The policies and procedures that are used by the BOE in adjudicating cases will be reviewed in a later section of this chapter.

The American Academy of Audiology (AAA) also has a Code of Ethics that specifies standards of professional behavior for audiologists who are members of AAA, including student members. It is divided into two parts: (Part I) Statement of Principles and Rules; and (Part II) Procedures for the Management of Alleged Noncompliance (AAA, 2018). There is considerable overlap between the information that is included in the AAA Principles and Rules and the ASHA Code, although the formatting is quite different. For example, the AAA Code includes eight Principles as opposed to four in the ASHA Code, and each Principle is supported by between 1 and 5 Rules as opposed to between 7 and 20 Rules. Although the structure of the AAA Code is different from the ASHA Code, it too specifies standards of conduct that protect the integrity of the profession while also protecting the welfare of individuals served (AAA, 2018). The procedures for addressing potential noncompliance with the AAA code will also be discussed in a later section of this chapter.

Ethical Issues in Practice Management

While there are ethical issues that cross all professional domains in which speech-language pathologists, audiologists, and speech and hearing scientists work, there are some issues that primarily affect clinical practice and practice management. The following sections address some of the ethical issues related to clinical practice, including relationships with vendors, professional communication, and other miscellaneous topics such as confidentiality, billing practices, and documentation.

Relationships with Vendors

The importance of avoiding or managing conflicts of interest was discussed in an earlier section of this chapter. Audiologists and speech-language pathologists who are in practice often have the need to have professional relationships with vendors, including making decisions about equipment purchases as well as recommending particular products for patients or clients to improve their ability to communicate. For example, a pediatric audiologist working with a child with newly diagnosed hearing loss typically makes recommendations to the family regarding the most appropriate amplification options given the degree and configuration of the hearing loss in addition to other factors. Similarly, a speech-language pathologist working with a patient with neurodevelopmental disabilities that prevent him from using speech to communicate may recommend the most appropriate augmentative and alternative communication (AAC) device given his abilities and communication needs. An audiology and speech pathology clinic manager who has the responsibility to purchase equipment and materials for use in the clinic should make those decisions based on what is best given the population being served and the needs of the professionals serving the individuals coming to the clinic.

In all three examples listed above, there is a potential risk of conflict based on relationships with vendors, particularly when there are incentives for purchasing a particular product. For example, audiologists attending professional meetings are frequently invited to private dinners paid for by individual hearing aid manufacturers or equipment vendors in appreciation for the use of their products. Similarly, a clinic manager may be compelled by a colleague to purchase a product created by her. Another example of a possible conflict is that some hearing aid manufacturers offer summer "camps" over several days for audiology doctoral students free of charge. While the educational opportunity is excellent, the conflict occurs because the hearing aid company is completely underwriting the cost of attending, often including travel. As mentioned earlier, decisions should be made based on what is best for the patient or clinic rather on the basis of personal or professional gain. The AAA Code compels members to "provide only services and products that are in the best interest of those served" (AAA, 2018, p. 1). Principle of Ethics I of the ASHA Code has to do with professionals honoring their responsibility to persons served and to participants in research and scholarly activities. Rule K specifically addresses evaluating the effectiveness of technology employed and products dispensed, and making decisions about both based on their potential benefit to individuals served (ASHA, 2016a).

Professional Communications

There are important ethical issues related to professional communication, including with individuals served, colleagues within the discipline, and professionals outside the discipline with whom they collaborate. Some areas for consideration include offering second opinions regarding hearing status or communication options, dismissing patients when the speech-language pathologist or audiologist believes it is in the best interest of the individual served, and transparency related to the relative costs of services and devices (bundling versus unbundling) (Metz, 2006). This section of the chapter explores two topics that are relevant to both audiologists and speech-language pathologists. Specifically, issues related to providing second opinions and dismissal of patients are highlighted.

Speech-language pathologists and audiologists are often asked to provide second opinions. It is important that the clinician demonstrates sensitivity when providing that opinion. As professionals, we need to be aware of and sensitive to all of the individuals involved with a case including the patient/family as well as the other professionals who have been involved in the case. We need to recognize that we are now part of a team that is larger than our immediate colleagues. If parents request second opinion about their child's hearing status from a pediatric audiology clinic due to concerns about speech and language development, it is important that the audiologist providing a second opinion report the results to the parents and offer them a variety of options for follow-up. If the child has documented hearing loss, the audiologist must provide information about management options in an unbiased manner. Similarly, if an individual who is an actor asks for a second opinion from a professional voice clinic about healthy voice use, the speech-language pathologist also must provide recommendations in an unbiased fashion. The audiologist or speech-language pathologist needs to be aware of the need to communicate recommendations with referral sources, with patient/clients and their families when appropriate, and with other health care or educational personnel as needed. They also need to be transparent about management options including returning to the provider of the first opinion (Metz, 2006).

Another issue related to professional communication has to do with dismissing patients when the speech-language pathologist or audiologist believes it is in the best interest of the individual served, or when the professional determines that there are client variables that are negatively impacting progress. Consider an audiologist who has been working with an adult with hearing loss in an effort to fit and program hearing aids that will help to improve her ability to hear in a variety of contexts. The audiologist has tried many hearing aid fitting strategies and hearing aids from multiple manufacturers, yet the individual continues to struggle and is not satisfied. In that case, it may be in the best interest of the patient to try a different audiologist for hearing loss management strategies. It may also be the case that the individual served was only trying hearing aids because her family pressed her to do so, yet her lack of interest in hearing aids prevents her from succeeding. A clinician can ethically dismiss a patient if notification is provided in writing, including the reason for dismissal, and then offers to provide copies of patient records when a release of information is provided (Metz, 2006).

Consider the speech-language pathologist who has been involved in the diagnosis of a three-year old child that is not talking and has normal hearing. The child demonstrates characteristics of autism spectrum disorder (ASD) so the SLP recommends referral to an interdisciplinary autism clinic for evaluation. The parents are not yet ready to accept the possibility that their child may have autism and refuse to follow-up on the recommendation. While the SLP is able to provide therapy to improve communication options, progress may be negatively impacted by the child's behavior and the parents' unwillingness to pursue an autism evaluation. If the

SLP believes it is in the best interest of the child to refer to a different provider, it may be ethically appropriate to do so.

Clearly, SLPs and audiologists must attend to how decisions they make relative to professional communication apply to the ethical practice requirements imposed by our professional associations' Codes. Principle of Ethics I Rule B in the ASHA Code specifies the requirement that audiologists and speech-language pathologists utilize all resources, including referral, to ensure that the needs of individuals are met (ASHA, 2016a). The AAA Code compels members to use all available resources, including referrals to other professionals when appropriate (AAA, 2018).

Other Issues Related to Clinical Practice Management

There are several additional ethical issues related to audiology and speech-language practice that warrant consideration including the importance of maintaining confidentiality, the appropriate use of informed consent for clinical procedures, documentation, marketing, and impaired practitioners. The ASHA website has valuable information about how to navigate in an ethical manner around these issues and others we have already mentioned. Denton (2009) provided advice about potential ethical traps in private practice, although the topics are relevant to practice in all environments. Please refer to his article as well as relevant Issues in Ethics Statements for helpful information about these ethical issues (ASHA, 2019). Chapters 6 and 20 also provide a more in-depth discussion on some of these issues.

Ethical Issues in Supervision

There are a number of ethical issues related to supervision and delegation of service provision to students and clinical fellows, including conflicts of interest, licensure, being sure to identify student status in clinical interactions, balancing the needs of student experience against the need for clinical experience, and being sure to model professional behavior to learners in the clinical setting. While specific examples of the application of the ASHA Code and the AAA Code to supervision exceed the limits of this chapter, excellent guidance is provided in the ASHA Issues in Ethics Statements related to supervision as well as on the ASHA practice portal section on clinical education and supervision (ASHA, 2019a, b). See Chapter 26 for further discussion on supervision. It is important for audiologists and speech-language pathologists to be aware of their responsibilities to uphold the responsibility to persons served by delegating tasks related to the provision of professional services only to those having appropriate knowledge and skills and necessary supervision to ensure the welfare of individuals served (ASHA, 2016a).

Ethical Issues in Academia

As is the case with ethical issues in supervision, there are issues that specifically relate to academia including academic integrity, research responsibilities, and student/faculty relationships. The ASHA Code provides guidance for each of these topics. For example, Principle of Ethics I, Rule I addresses ethical practice surrounding participation in research or teaching demonstrations and Principle of Ethics II, Rule P addresses the confidentiality of participants in research (ASHA, 2016a). Principle of Ethics II, Rule C addresses the responsibility of those members who are engaged in research to comply with all institutional, state, and federal regulations.

Chabon, Hale, and Wark (2008) discussed the complexities of relationships in the student-supervision-client paradigm that frequently occur in academia. For example, clients have the right to know that a student is involved in providing care and it is the student's responsibility to inform them of their student status. Patients have a right, once informed, to refuse services provided by a student. Patients should also feel confident that their best interests are held paramount. Given the timing of clinical rotations in academia, clinical supervisors are ultimately responsible for ensuring appropriate continuity of care (Chabon et al., 2008).

Ethical Dilemmas

Audiologists and SLPs are inevitably faced with ethical dilemmas due to pressures applied by employers regarding caseload or schedules, billing practices of their places of employment, the requirements for supervision of students and clinical fellows, or academic expectations for teaching and participation in research. It is important for professionals in the discipline to have a strategy for maintaining their ethical standards of conduct in the face of ethical dilemmas.

Ethical Dilemma Examples

Bupp (2012) outlined several examples of ethical dilemmas based on inquiries to the ASHA office and complaints filed about potential violations of the ASHA Code. A brief summary of some of the topics outlined is provided here. For a complete description of the nine dilemmas covered, please refer to Bupp (2012).

One of the topics included has to do with documentation of clinical encounters. An example is when a supervisor asks an SLP to "sign off" on paperwork for individuals the SLP did not evaluate or treat, including services provided by students or assistants the SLP did not adequately supervise. Another example is when ASHA members are asked to alter or supplement evaluation or treatment paperwork in order to increase reimbursements (Bupp, 2012). Audiologists and SLPs must adhere to their ethical responsibilities as outlined by our professional associations' codes of ethics related to documentation.

A related situation in which audiologists and speech-language pathologists are faced with an ethical dilemma has to do with employer demands relative to caseloads, time limits, and productivity quotas. Employer expectations can place the professional in an untenable situation of having to choose between ethical behavior and meeting the demands of the employer. When the expectations of ethical behavior and employer demands are diametrically opposed, the ASHA Ethics Office staff are available to provide assistance (Bupp, 2012).

A third type of ethical dilemma has to do with impaired practitioners. While recognizing and dealing with impaired professionals and clinical fellows is complex, it is important and may have both legal and ethical ramifications (Bupp, 2012). National mental health statistics and surveys of ASHA members suggest that a subset of speech-language pathologists and audiologists may be affected by mental health conditions, substance abuse, or both (Bupp, 2012). Because impaired professionals pose a liability to patients and colleagues, having a plan to deal with this ethical dilemma that involves appropriate personnel is important (Bupp, 2012).

Unethical Practice Complaint Process

In the next sections of the chapter, the policies and procedures for filing an unethical practice complaint for ASHA and AAA will be discussed as well as the procedures employed to adjudicate complaints for each association. In addition, various types of complaints, possible sanctions, and the appeals process are summarized.

ASHA

As was mentioned earlier in this chapter, the Board of Ethics is charged with maintaining and administering the Code as well as providing education in order to ensure that individuals understand its significance (ASHA, 2017b). The jurisdiction of the BOE is limited to member and certificate holders and they are only able to adjudicate cases that are brought to them. Complaints of unethical behavior can be filed by individuals who are affiliated with ASHA as well as others, including patients, consumers, licensure boards, students, and employers (ASHA, 2016a).

Unlike licensure boards, the BOE does not have investigative powers, nor are they able to compel witnesses to testify or produce documents as evidence of wrongdoing. However, since members and certificate holders are obligated by the Code to self-disclose their own unethical behavior and to report unethical behavior of others, they assist the BOE in enforcing the Code (ASHA, 2016a).

An important concept in ethical practice has to do with "willful blindness," which has to do with the members' responsibility to address unethical conduct on the part of others, even when it seems awkward or difficult. The ASHA Code Principle IV, Rules M and N specify that ASHA members who are aware of areas of noncompliance are expected to work collaboratively with colleagues to resolve the situation where possible or to inform the Board of Ethics through its established procedures. Rule N specifies that ASHA members recognize their responsibility to report individuals from other professions to the appropriate regulatory bodies when they are aware of unethical behavior.

ASHA has established a complaint process that is intended to allow for due process and ensure fairness. Information about the process is easily accessible on the ASHA website or by contacting the national office staff for assistance. ASHA will not accept anonymous complaints or agree to keep confidential the identity of the person filing the complaint (complainant) from the person about whom the complaint is rendered (respondent). Part of the reason for this policy is to enable the respondent to present and support a claim of bias when appropriate. Also, individuals are less likely to file malicious or frivolous complaints if the respondent is aware of their identity. Finally, transparency regarding the identity of the complainant helps the BOE determine the credibility of the evidence submitted (ASHA, 2012).

In its deliberations, the BOE will only consider evidence that is provided by the complainant and the respondent. When a complaint is filed, the respondent is given a copy of the complaint and the opportunity to submit a written response to the BOE. The adjudication process is confidential. If the BOE determines that there is not sufficient evidence to support a claim of wrongdoing, both the complainant and the respondent are notified of the decision and the case is considered closed. If the BOE finds there is sufficient evidence of a Code violation, both parties will be notified about the specific Rules of Ethics that were violated and the BOE will determine a sanction (ASHA, 2018).

AAA

The Ethical Practices Committee (EPC) is responsible for responding to inquiries submitted about ethical behavior and adjudicating allegations of Code violations by members of AAA. Allegations of suspected Code violations can be made to the EPC by AAA members or consumers of members' services. Complaints must be made in writing including documentation to support the claim. The complainant will be asked to sign a Waiver of Confidentiality permitting the EPC to disclose his/her name and the complaint details should that be necessary during the investigation. However, a signed waiver is not required in order to move forward with deliberations. In the case of the EPC learning from a state licensure board that a member's license has been suspended or revoked, the EPC will proceed with its investigation without having a complainant. The Chair of the EPC is permitted to communicate with other agencies or individuals in order to gather additional information that may be needed at any time during the deliberations (AAA, 2018).

Following receipt of a complaint, the EPC will convene to discuss the merits of the alleged violation of the Code. If the allegations include behaviors that have a high likelihood of being illegal, the case may be referred to the appropriate agency and the EPC will suspend its investigation until the legal process is complete (AAA, 2018).

If the EPC finds sufficient preliminary evidence that a violation of the Code has occurred, the member will be notified in writing about the complaint including a description of the circumstances of the alleged behavior and which ethical principle(s) and/ or rules are implicated in the complaint. The member will be asked to provide a written response to the allegation and supporting documents within 30 days (AAA, 2018).

Following receipt of a response from the member, the EPC will convene in person or via teleconference to consider all of the evidence. If no response is received from the respondent, the EPC will still convene to review the existing evidence. If the EPC finds sufficient evidence of a Code violation, the member will be notified of his/her right to a hearing in person or by teleconference, the ethical noncompliance being cited, possible sanctions, and the right to defend the charges. This is the final opportunity for the respondent to provide additional information to the EPC. If the EPC finds that there is insufficient evidence of a Code violation, all parties will be notified and the case closed. If the ruling is that sufficient evidence exists, the Principle(s)/ Rule(s) will be cited and sanction(s) will be specified (AAA, 2018).

There are some important differences between the procedures of the EPC and the ASHA BOE. First, while ASHA will not allow anonymous complaints, the EPC will convene to discuss a case even when the complainant refuses to sign a waiver that would allow the EPC to share his or her identity with the respondent. A second difference has to do with the timing of the respondent knowing about the complaint and having a chance to provide evidence of compliance with the Code. Specifically, in the ASHA BOE procedures, the respondent is notified immediately of the complaint. The respondent is also given a copy of the complaint so an appropriate response can be submitted to the BOE. The BOE does not meet until the response has been received and deliberations occur only in person. In addition, the ASHA BOE does not have investigative ability and will only consider the evidence provided by the complainant and the respondent, whereas the EPC procedures allow the Chair to seek information from individuals and/or agencies to obtain information about the case beyond that is beyond what is including by the complainant or respondent. Differences in possible sanctions are discussed in another section of this chapter.

Types of Complaints

The most common types of ethics complaints are reflected in the topics included in the ASHA Issues in Ethics Statements (ASHA, 2019a). The BOE creates these documents in order to address specific issues of ethical conduct. They are intended to provide guidance in ethical decision making. The topics included reflect issues that have been referred to the ASHA BOE. For a complete list of Issues in Ethics statements and the advice presented, please refer to ASHA (2019a).

Sanctions

Possible sanctions for violation of the ASHA Code are either private or public. Public sanctions provide evidence to other ASHA members that the Code is important and ASHA is willing to enforce its standards. Additionally, public sanctions may serve as education for the respondent as well as all members of the Association. Sanctions include: reprimand (private); censure (public reprimand); or withholding, suspension, or revocation of membership and/or certification for a specified time period, including up to life. Public sanctions resulting from a violation of the ASHA Code are published in the *ASHA Leader* including the name of the respondent and the specific Rules of Ethics that were violated. This information is also forwarded to the appropriate state licensure body (ASHA, 2018).

Possible sanctions for violations of the AAA Code include: an educative letter; cease and desist order; reprimand; mandatory continuing education; probation of suspension; suspension of membership; or revocation of membership. Sanctions are imposed by a simple majority vote of the EPC with the exception of revocation of membership, which requires a two-thirds majority vote of the EPC. In order to educate the membership, the circumstances and nature of all cases are published in *Audiology Today* and on the AAA website, although the members' names are not revealed (AAA, 2018).

Disclosure

The 2016 ASHA Code provides greater clarity about professional self-disclosure than did previous versions. The Code provides guidance for members and certificate holders about ethical reporting including the need to report one's own violation of the Code. Examples of violations of the Code that must be self-disclosed include misdemeanors, felonies, public sanctions, and denials of licenses or other credentials (ASHA, 2016a).

During the process of applying for ASHA membership and/or certification, applicants are required to answer three questions related to previous behavior that resulted in criminal conviction or formal professional discipline. Applicants must answer the questions honestly as well as supply documentation related to the conviction or discipline when asked to do so. The obligation to self-disclose continues following the application process through Principle IV, Rules R, S, and T of the Code (ASHA, 2016a).

Honesty and transparency in reporting information are foundational to proper, professional, and ethical conduct. While various work environments can create a tension between the obligation to choose ethical behavior versus personal preference and the opportunity for personal gain, audiologists and speech-language pathologists are expected to remain ethically compliant with the Code, including accurate self-disclosure (ASHA, 2016a). There is no clear statement regarding self-disclosure in the AAA Code.

Appeals

Both AAA and ASHA have appeals processes for individuals found to be in violation of their respective Codes. The AAA member may appeal the final decision of the EPC to the Academy Board of Directors (BOD). Requests for appeal must be made within 30 days of notification of the final decision, stating the basis for the appeal. No new information can be provided during that time period. The AAA BOD will review all of the evidence and deliberate the case at the earliest possible BOD meeting. The decision by the BOD is considered final (AAA, 2018).

The policies and procedures of the ASHA BOE include two levels of appeal following the initial determination. Specifically, when a Code violation has been determined and a sanction imposed, the respondent may request Further Consideration by the BOE within 30 days of the initial determination. The respondent is permitted to submit a written defense prior to the hearing and the complainant is also able to provide additional information. Further Consideration hearings are held before the adjudicating body of the BOE. The respondent may appear in person and may be accompanied by counsel. The respondent must be available for questioning by the BOE at the time of the hearing and must not permit counsel to answer questions. Following the Further Consideration hearing, the BOE shall render a decision and notify the respondent (ASHA, 2017b).

The respondent may appeal the Board of Ethics Decision After Further Consideration to the ASHA Ethics Appeal Panel in writing within 30 days after the decision was mailed to the respondent. The only basis for appeal is if the BOE did not follow its own procedures and/or the decision was arbitrary and capricious and without evidentiary basis. The three members on the appeal panel will not consider any evidence other than that included in the record of the Further Consideration Hearing and their decision is final (ASHA, 2017b).

Ethics Education

Our professional associations provide ample opportunities for ethics education for speech-language pathologists and audiologists, much of which is accessible from the associations' websites and at both state and national conferences For example, the AAA website has a section called "Ethics News" that includes articles from *Audiology Today* related to ethical issues audiology practice (AAA, 2019b). There is also an *Ethics in Audiology* (Second Edition) CEU Program that is available from eAudiology, which is intended to provide in-depth information on ethical conduct in various clinical, educational, and research settings (AAA, 2019a).

The ASHA website has an entire section on ethics under the Practice Management area, which is intended to promote standards of ethical conduct and integrity in the work of speech-language pathologists, audiologists, and speech and hearing scientists. Active links are provided to the Code, processes and procedures related to ethics complaint adjudication, ethics guidance, hot topics related to ethics, sanctions and violations history, student ethics essay awards, and ethics education (ASHA, 2019c). While there is a specific area for ethics education, one could argue that all of the content on this page is educational. In addition, there are typically multiple offerings at the yearly ASHA convention on the topic of ethics. Readers should note that beginning in 2020, ASHA certificate holders are required to earn 1 of their 30 required certification maintenance hours in Ethics. Many states also require continuing education in Ethics for license holders in both audiology and speech-language pathology, and that information is available from https://www.asha.org/advocacy/state/. Finally, those who hold the American Board of Audiology certification also have an ethics requirement in their recertification of the credential (http://www.boardof audiology.org).

Recent Changes and Future Directions

There have been substantial changes in health care in the last decade that have impacted the professions of speech-language pathology and audiology, including the move toward electronic medical records, increased inclusion of technicians and assistants in the provision of care, and the onset of telepractice in both professions. These changes have been in response to the need for seamless communication and patient/family centered care, increased efficiency, and the desire to make care accessible in areas of the country in which qualified professionals do not practice. These trends will undoubtedly continue in the coming years as we move toward the provision of exceptional services for all individuals needing our care in spite of dwindling resources. It is important that as the professions move in the directions mentioned above, we continue to uphold our responsibility to ensure the welfare of individuals served and to protect the reputation and integrity of the discipline (ASHA, 2016a).

Summary

This chapter has provided a summary of various topics related to professional ethics in speech-language pathology, audiology, and speech and hearing science, including standards of professional conduct, conflicts of interest, the role of professional associations, ethical issues in practice management, ethical issues in supervision and academia, how to manage ethical dilemmas, and unethical behavior complaint processes for the American Speech-Language-Hearing Association (ASHA) and the American Academy of Audiology (AAA). The importance of ethics education and some specific examples of education provided by our professional associations were highlighted. Critical thinking questions are listed in the next session to help readers think about how these issues might apply to their specific professional contexts.

Critical Thinking

1. Your supervisor has asked you to bill for therapy services provided by a speech-language pathology assistant that you did not supervise. Review the ASHA Code and determine which Principle(s) and Rule(s) are relevant to the situation. How would you respond to your supervisor in order to avoid violating your ethical responsibilities?

2. You are supervising a student in a clinical externship whose performance is below expectations and who is not responsive to your attempts to improve her performance. You are concerned that the quality of the services provided may be compromised because of the student's placement, yet you are being pressured by her university to let her continue in the clinical placement. Describe the ethical dilemma facing you and what actions are most appropriate for you to take.

3. You have been invited by a vendor to attend a workshop about its products at a resort in the Rocky Mountains. The vendor has offered to pay for all of your expenses during the workshop as well as the cost of travel. Consider the information provided in this chapter about relationships with vendors and conflicts of professional interest. How might you deal with the invitation in a way that does not cause you to compromise your ethical obligations?

4. You are a research assistant in a hearing science laboratory working on a project supported by your mentor. You are being pressured by another senior faculty member to change directions with your research. You are enthusiastic about your project and want to bring it to conclusion. How would you resolve the conflict between your goals and those of the other faculty member?

5. You have had an assistant assigned to help you with your growing caseload. As a supervisor, what are some of the ethical considerations you need to address as you assume this responsibility?

6. Telepractice and the use of technology in the supervision of students and clinical fellows have improved our ability to expand our reach to remote areas of the country. What are some of the issues related to maintaining ethical standards of care while not being physically present with patients, students, or clinical fellows?

7. You are a preceptor for an audiology student completing his final full-time externship. Please review the ASHA and AAA Codes to consider how each Code addresses students providing clinical services. What is the student's responsibility in terms of disclosing his role to patients/clients? What title is appropriate for him to use when signing documents? What is your ethical responsibility to the student and to the patients/clients being served under your direction?

8. You are aware that one of your speech-language-pathology colleagues has been drinking alcohol in the parking lot before reporting to work as well as on her lunch break and you notice that she is clearly unable to perform her duties in a responsible manner during the day. Consider the ASHA Code of Ethics. What is your ethical responsibility to remain compliant with the Code? What is your colleague's responsibility? What Principles and Rules are relevant to this issue, and where might you find additional guidance from the BOE?

References

American Academy of Audiology. (2018). *Code of Ethics.* Retrieved from https://www.audiology.org/publications-resources/document-library/code-ethics Republished with permission from the American Academy of Audiology. http://www.audiology.org

American Academy of Audiology. (2019a). *Ethics in audiology (second edition) CEU program.* Retrieved from https://www.audiology.org/professional-development/eaudiology/ethics-audiology-second-edition-ceu-program

American Academy of Audiology. (2019b). Ethics News. Available from https://www.audiology.org/about-us/membership/ethics/ethics-news

American Speech-Language-Hearing Association. (2012). *Why ASHA does not accept anonymous ethics complaints* [From the Director of Ethics]. Retrieved from http:/www.asha.org/practice/ethics/anonymous/

American Speech-Language-Hearing Association. (2016a). *Code of Ethics* [Ethics]. Retrieved from http://www.asha.org/policy Republished with permission.

American Speech-Language-Hearing Association. (2016b). *Code of Ethics (2016) revision summary.* Retrieved from https://www.asha.org/Practice/ethics/Code-of-Ethics-2016-Revision-Summary/

American Speech-Language-Hearing Association. (2017a). *Bylaws of the American Speech-Language-Hearing Association* [Bylaws]. Retrieved from http://www.asha.org/policy

American Speech-Language-Hearing Association. (2017b). *Practices and procedures for appeals of board of ethics decisions* [Ethics]. Retrieved from http://www.asha.org/policy

American Speech-Language-Hearing Association. (2018). *Practices and procedures of the Board of Ethics* [Ethics]. Retrieved from http://www.asha.org/policy

American Speech-Language-Hearing Association. (2019a). *Issues in ethics statements.* Retrieved from https://www.asha.org/Practice/ethics/ethics_issues_index/

American Speech-Language-Hearing Association. (2019b). *Clinical education and supervision.* Retrieved from https://www.asha.org/PRPSpecificTopic.aspx?folderid=8589942113&section=Overview

American Speech-Language-Hearing Association. (2019c). *Ethics resources.* Retrieved from https://www.asha.org/practice/ethics/

Bupp, H. (2012). 9 upsetting dilemmas. *The ASHA Leader, 17*(14), 10–13. https://doi.org/10.1044/leader.FTR1.17142012.10

Bupp, H. (2016). What's new in the 2016 Ethics Code. *The ASHA Leader, 21*(7), 58–59. https://doi.org/10.1044/leader.AN1.21072016.58

Chabon, S. S., Hale, S. T., & Wark, D. J. (2008). Triangulated ethics: the patient-student-supervisor relationship. *The ASHA Leader, 13*(2), 26–27. https://doi.org/10.1044/leader.FTR6.13022008.26

Denton, D. (2009). Watch out for these ethical traps in private practice. *The ASHA Leader, 14*(10), 47. https://doi.org/10.1044/leader.IPP2.14102009.47

Frazek, M. (2003, February). Ethics vs. legal jurisdiction. *The ASHA Leader.* Retrieved from http://www.asha.org/practice/ethics/ethics-juridiction/

Handelsman, J. (2006). Recognizing when strings are attached. *The ASHA Leader, 11*(1), 18. https://doi.org/10.1044/leader.MIW.11012006.18

Kitchner, K. S. (1984). Intuition, critical evaluation and ethical principles. The foundation for ethical decisions in counselling psychology. *Counselling Psychologist, 12*, 43–55.

Metz, M. J. (2006). Ethics of professional communication. In T. Hamill (Ed.), *Guidelines for ethical conduct in clinical, educational, and research settings* (pp. 37–47). Reston, VA: American Academy of Audiology.

Resources

American Academy of Audiology
https://www.audiology.org/about-us/membership/ethics

American Speech-Language-Hearing Association
https://www.asha.org/practice/ethics

Appendix 5–A

◇◇◇

American Academy of Audiology Code of Ethics

Preamble

The Code of Ethics of the American Academy of Audiology specifies professional standards that allow for the proper discharge of audiologists' responsibilities to those served, and that protect the integrity of the profession. The Code of Ethics consists of two parts. The first part, the Statement of Principles and Rules, presents precepts that members (all categories of members including Student Members) effective January 1, 2009 of the Academy agree to uphold. The second part, the Procedures, provides the process that enables enforcement of the Principles and Rules.

Part I. Statement of Principles and Rules

PRINCIPLE 1: Members shall provide professional services and conduct research with honesty and compassion, and shall respect the dignity, worth, and rights of those served.

> **Rule 1a:** Individuals shall not limit the delivery of professional services on any basis that is unjustifiable or irrelevant to the need for the potential benefit from such services.

> **Rule 1b:** Individuals shall not provide services except in a professional relationship and shall not discriminate in the provision of services to individuals on the basis of sex, race, religion, national origin, sexual orientation, or general health.

PRINCIPLE 2: Members shall maintain the highest standards of professional competence in rendering services.

> **Rule 2a:** Members shall provide only those professional services for which they are qualified by education and experience.

> **Rule 2b:** Individuals shall use available resources, including referrals to other specialists, and shall not give or accept benefits or items of value for receiving or making referrals.

> **Rule 2c:** Individuals shall exercise all reasonable precautions to avoid injury to persons in the delivery of professional services or execution of research.

> **Rule 2d:** Individuals shall provide appropriate supervision and assume full responsibility for services delegated to supportive personnel. Individuals shall not delegate any service requiring professional competence to unqualified persons.

> **Rule 2e:** Individuals shall not knowingly permit personnel under their direct or indirect supervision to engage in any practice that is not in compliance with the Code of Ethics.

> **Rule 2f:** Individuals shall maintain professional competence, including participation in continuing education.

PRINCIPLE 3: Members shall maintain the confidentiality of the information and records of those receiving services or involved in research.

> **Rule 3a:** Individuals shall not reveal to unauthorized persons any professional or personal information obtained from the person served professionally, unless required by law.

PRINCIPLE 4: Members shall provide only services and products that are in the best interest of those served.

> **Rule 4a:** Individuals shall not exploit persons in the delivery of professional services.

> **Rule 4b:** Individuals shall not charge for services not rendered.

> **Rule 4c:** Individuals shall not participate in activities that constitute a conflict of professional interest.

> **Rule 4d:** Individuals using investigational procedures with human participants or prospectively collecting research data from human participants shall obtain full informed consent from the participants or legal representatives. Members conducting research with human participants or animals shall follow accepted standards, such as those promulgated in the current Responsible Conduct of Research by the U.S. Office of Research Integrity.

PRINCIPLE 5: Members shall provide accurate information about the nature and management of communicative disorders and about the services and products offered.

Rule 5a: Individuals shall provide persons served with the information a reasonable person would want to know about the nature and possible effects of services rendered or products provided or research being conducted.

Rule 5b: Individuals may make a statement of prognosis, but shall not guarantee results, mislead, or misinform persons served or studied.

Rule 5c: Individuals shall conduct and report product-related research only according to accepted standards of research practice.

Rule 5d: Individuals shall not carry out teaching or research activities in a manner that constitutes an invasion of privacy or that fails to inform persons fully about the nature and possible effects of these activities, affording all persons informed free choice of participation.

Rule 5e: Individuals shall maintain accurate documentation of services rendered according to accepted medical, legal and professional standards and requirements.

PRINCIPLE 6: Members shall comply with the ethical standards of the Academy with regard to public statements or publication.

Rule 6a: Individuals shall not misrepresent their educational degrees, training, credentials, or competence. Only degrees earned from regionally accredited institutions in which training was obtained in audiology, or a directly related discipline, may be used in public statements concerning professional services.

Rule 6b: Individuals' public statements about professional services, products or research results shall not contain representations or claims that are false, misleading, or deceptive.

PRINCIPLE 7: Members shall honor their responsibilities to the public and to professional colleagues.

Rule 7a: Individuals shall not use professional or commercial affiliations in any way that would limit services to or mislead patients or colleagues.

Rule 7b: Individuals shall inform colleagues and the public in an objective manner consistent with professional standards about products and services they have developed or research they have conducted.

PRINCIPLE 8: Members shall uphold the dignity of the profession and freely accept the Academy's self-imposed standards.

Rule 8a: Individuals shall not violate these Principles and Rules nor attempt to circumvent them.

Rule 8b: Individuals shall not engage in dishonesty or illegal conduct that adversely reflects on the profession.

Rule 8c: Individuals shall inform the Ethical Practices Committee when there are reasons to believe that a member of the Academy may have been in noncompliance with the Code of Ethics.

Rule 8d: Individuals shall fully cooperate with reviews being conducted by the Ethical Practices Committee in any matter related to the Code of Ethics.

Part II. Procedures for the Management of Alleged Noncompliance

Members of the American Academy of Audiology are obligated to uphold the Code of Ethics of the Academy in their personal conduct and in the performance of their professional duties. To this end, it is the responsibility of each Academy member to inform the Ethical Practice Committee of possible noncompliance with the Ethics Code. The processing of alleged noncompliance with the Code of Ethics will follow the procedures specified below in an expeditious manner to ensure that behaviors of noncompliant ethical conduct by members of the Academy are halted in the shortest time possible.

Procedures

1. Suspected noncompliance with the Code of Ethics shall be reported in letter format, giving documentation sufficient to support the alleged noncompliance. Letters must be addressed to:

2. American Academy of Audiology Chair, Ethical Practices Committee 11480 Commerce Park Dr. Suite 220 Reston, VA 20191. Following receipt of a report of suspected noncompliance, at the discretion of the Chair, the Ethical Practices Committee will request a signed Waiver of Confidentiality from the complainant indicating that the complainant will allow the Ethical Practice Board to disclose his/her name and complaint details should this become necessary during investigation of the allegation.

   a. The Committee may, under special circumstances, act in the absence of a signed Waiver of Confidentiality. For example, in cases where the Ethical Practice Committee has received information from a state licensure board of a member having his or her license suspended or revoked, then the Ethical Practice Committee will proceed without a complainant.

b. The Chair may communicate with other individuals, agencies, and/or programs for additional information as may be required for Committee review at any time during the deliberation.

3. The Ethical Practice Committee will convene to review the merit of the alleged noncompliance as it relates to the Code of Ethics

a. The Ethical Practice Committee shall meet to discuss the case, either in person, by electronic means, or by teleconference. The meeting will occur within 60 days of receipt of the Waiver of Confidentiality, or of notification by the complainant of refusal to sign the waiver. In cases where another form of notification brings the complaint to the attention of the Ethical Practice Committee, the Committee will convene within 60 days of notification.

b. If the alleged noncompliance has a high probability of being legally actionable, the case may be referred to the appropriate agency. The Ethical Practice Committee will postpone member notification and further deliberation until the legal process has been completed.

4. If there is sufficient evidence that indicates noncompliance with the Code of Ethics has occurred, upon majority vote, the member will be forwarded a Notification of Potential Ethics Concern.

a. The circumstances of the alleged noncompliance will be described.

b. The member will be informed of the specific Code of Ethics principle(s) and/or rule(s) that may conflict with member behavior.

c. Supporting AAA documents that may serve to further educate the member about the ethical implications will be included, as appropriate.

d. The member will be asked to respond fully to the allegation and submit all supporting evidence within 30 calendar days.

5. The Ethical Practices Committee will meet either in person or by teleconference:

a. within 60 calendar days of receiving a response from the member to the Notification of Potential Ethics Concern to review the response and all information pertaining to the alleged noncompliance, or

b. within sixty (60) calendar days of notification to member if no response is received from the member to review the information received from the complainant.

6. If the Ethical Practice Committee determines that the evidence supports the allegation of noncompliance, the member will be provided written notice containing the following information:

a. The right to a hearing in person or by teleconference before the Ethical Practice Committee;

b. The date, time, and place of the hearing;

c. The ethical noncompliance being charged and the potential sanction

d. The right to present a defense to the charges.

At this time the member should provide any additional relevant information. As this is the final opportunity for a member to provide new information, the member should carefully prepare all documentation.

7. Potential Rulings.

a. When the Ethical Practices Committee determines there is insufficient evidence of ethical noncompliance, the parties to the complaint will be notified that the case will be closed.

b. If the evidence supports the allegation of Code noncompliance, the Code(s)/Rule(s) will be cited and the sanction(s) will be specified.

8. The Committee shall sanction members based on the severity of the noncompliance and history of prior ethical noncompliance. A simple majority of voting members is required to institute a sanction unless otherwise noted. Sanctions may include one or more of the following:

a. Educative Letter. This sanction alone is appropriate when:

1) The ethics noncompliance appears to have been inadvertent.

2) The member's response to Notification of Potential Ethics Concern indicates a new awareness of the problem and the member resolves to refrain from future ethical noncompliance.

b. Cease and Desist Order. The member signs a consent agreement to immediately halt the practice(s) that were found to be in noncompliance with the Code of Ethics

c. Reprimand. The member will be formally reprimanded for the noncompliance with of the Code of Ethics.

d. Mandatory continuing education

1) The EPC will determine the type of education needed to reduce chances of recurrence of noncompliance.

2) The member will be responsible for submitting documentation of continuing education within the period of time designated by the Ethical Practices Committee.

3) All costs associated with compliance will be borne by the member.

e. Probation of Suspension. The member signs a consent agreement in acknowledgement of the Ethical Practice Committee decision and is allowed to retain membership benefits during a defined probationary period.

1) The duration of probation and the terms for avoiding suspension will be determined by the Ethical Practice Committee.

2) Failure of the member to meet the terms for probation will result in the suspension of membership.

f. Suspension of Membership.

1) The duration of suspension will be determined by the Ethical Practice Committee.

2) The member may not receive membership benefits during the period of suspension.

3) Members suspended are not entitled to a refund of dues or fees.

g. Revocation of Membership. Revocation of membership is considered the maximum consequence for noncompliance with the Code of Ethics.

1) Revocation requires a two-thirds majority of the voting members of the EPC.

2) Individuals whose memberships are revoked are not entitled to a refund of dues or fees.

3) One year following the date of membership revocation the individual may reapply for, but is not guaranteed, membership through normal channels, and must meet the membership qualifications in effect at the time of reapplication.

9. The member may appeal the Final Finding and Decision of the Ethical Practice Committee to the Academy Board of Directors. The route of Appeal is by letter format through the Ethical Practice Committee to the Board of Directors of the Academy. Requests for Appeal must:

a. be received by the Chair of the Ethical Practice Committee within 30 days of the Ethical

Practice Committee notification of the Final Finding and Decision,

b. state the basis for the appeal and the reason(s) that the Final Finding and Decision of the Ethical Practice Committee should be changed,

c. not offer new documentation.

The EPC chair will communicate with the Executive Director of the Academy to schedule the appeal at the earliest feasible Board of Director's meeting.

The Board of Directors will review the documents and written summaries and deliberate the case.

The decision of the Board of Directors regarding the member's appeal shall be final.

10. In order to educate the membership, upon majority vote of the Ethical Practice Committee, the circumstances and nature of cases shall be presented in Audiology Today and in the Professional Resource area of the AAA website. The member's identity will not be made public.

11. No Ethical Practice Committee member shall give access to records, act or speak independently, or on behalf of the Ethical Practice Committee, without the expressed permission of the members then active. No member may impose the sanction of the Ethical Practice Committee or interpret the findings of the EPC in any manner that may place members of the Ethical Practice Committee or Board of Directors, collectively or singly, at financial, professional, or personal risk

12. The Ethical Practice Committee Chair and Staff Liaison shall maintain electronic records that shall form the basis for future findings of the Committee.

Confidentiality and Records

Confidentiality shall be maintained in all Ethical Practice Committee discussion, correspondence, communication, deliberation, and records pertaining to members reviewed by the Ethical Practice Committee.

1. Complaints and suspected noncompliance with the Code of Ethics are assigned a case number.

2. Identity of members involved in complaints and suspected noncompliance cases and access to EPC files is restricted to the following:

a. EPC members

b. Executive Director

c. Agent/s of the Executive Director

d. Other/s, following majority vote of EPC

3. Original records shall be maintained at the Central Records Repository at the Academy office in a locked cabinet.

a. One copy will be sent to the Ethical Practice Committee Chair or member designated by the Chair.

b. Redacted copies will be sent to members.

4. Communications shall be sent to the members involved in complaints by the Academy office via certified or registered mail, after review by Legal Counsel, as needed.

5. When a case is closed,

a. The Chair will forward all documentation to the Staff Liaison to be maintained at the Academy Central Records Repository.

b. Members shall destroy all material pertaining to the case.

6. Complete records generally shall be maintained at the Academy Central Records Repository for a period of 5 years.

a. Records will be destroyed five years after a member receives a sanction less than suspension, or five years after the end of a suspension, or after membership is reinstated.

b. Records of membership revocations for persons who have not returned to membership status will be maintained indefinitely.

Source: American Academy of Audiology Code of Ethics. (2018). Code of Ethics. Available from https://www.audiology.org/publications-resources/document-library/code-ethics. Reprinted with permission from the American Academy of Audiology. http://www.audiology.org

Appendix 5–B

◇◇

American Speech-Language-Hearing Association Code of Ethics

Preamble

The American Speech-Language-Hearing Association (ASHA; hereafter, also known as "The Association") has been committed to a framework of common principles and standards of practice since ASHA's inception in 1925. This commitment was formalized in 1952 as the Association's first Code of Ethics. This Code has been modified and adapted as society and the professions have changed. The Code of Ethics reflects what we value as professionals and establishes expectations for our scientific and clinical practice based on principles of duty, accountability, fairness, and responsibility. The ASHA Code of Ethics is intended to ensure the welfare of the consumer and to protect the reputation and integrity of the professions.

The ASHA Code of Ethics is a framework and focused guide for professionals in support of day-to-day decision making related to professional conduct. The Code is partly obligatory and disciplinary and partly aspirational and descriptive in that it defines the professional's role. The Code educates professionals in the discipline, as well as students, other professionals, and the public, regarding ethical principles and standards that direct professional conduct.

The preservation of the highest standards of integrity and ethical principles is vital to the responsible discharge of obligations by audiologists, speech-language pathologists, and speech, language, and hearing scientists who serve as clinicians, educators, mentors, researchers, supervisors, and administrators. This Code of Ethics sets forth the fundamental principles and rules considered essential to this purpose and is applicable to the following individuals:

- a member of the American Speech-Language-Hearing Association holding the Certificate of Clinical Competence (CCC)

- a member of the Association not holding the Certificate of Clinical Competence (CCC)

- a nonmember of the Association holding the Certificate of Clinical Competence (CCC)

- an applicant for certification, or for membership and certification

By holding ASHA certification or membership, or through application for such, all individuals are automatically subject to the jurisdiction of the Board of Ethics for ethics complaint adjudication. Individuals who provide clinical services and who also desire membership in the Association must hold the CCC.

The fundamentals of ethical conduct are described by Principles of Ethics and by Rules of Ethics. The four Principles of Ethics form the underlying philosophical basis for the Code of Ethics and are reflected in the following areas: (I) responsibility to persons served professionally and to research participants, both human and animal; (II) responsibility for one's professional competence; (III) responsibility to the public; and (IV) responsibility for professional relationships. Individuals shall honor and abide by these Principles as affirmative obligations under all conditions of applicable professional activity. Rules of Ethics are specific statements of minimally acceptable as well as unacceptable professional conduct.

The Code is designed to provide guidance to members, applicants, and certified individuals as they make professional decisions. Because the Code is not intended to address specific situations and is not inclusive of all possible ethical dilemmas, professionals are expected to follow the written provisions and to uphold the spirit and purpose of the Code. Adherence to the Code of Ethics and its enforcement results in respect for the professions and positive outcomes for individuals who benefit from the work of audiologists, speech-language pathologists, and speech, language, and hearing scientists.

Terminology

ASHA Standards and Ethics—The mailing address for self-reporting in writing is American Speech-Language-Hearing Association, Standards and Ethics, 2200 Research Blvd., #313, Rockville, MD 20850.

■ **advertising**—Any form of communication with the public about services, therapies, products, or publications.

■ **conflict of interest**—An opposition between the private interests and the official or professional responsibilities of a person in a position of trust, power, and/or authority.

■ **crime**—Any felony; or any misdemeanor involving dishonesty, physical harm to the person or property of another, or a threat of physical harm to the person or property of another. For more details, see the "Disclosure Information" section of applications for ASHA certification found on www.asha.org/certification/AudCertification/and www.asha.org/certification/SLPCertification/.

■ **diminished decision-making ability**—Any condition that renders a person unable to form the specific intent necessary to determine a reasonable course of action.

■ **fraud**—Any act, expression, omission, or concealment—the intent of which is either actual or constructive—calculated to deceive others to their disadvantage.

■ **impaired practitioner**—An individual whose professional practice is adversely affected by addiction, substance abuse, or health-related and/or mental health–related conditions.

■ **individuals**—Members and/or certificate holders, including applicants for certification.

■ **informed consent**—May be verbal, unless written consent is required; constitutes consent by persons served, research participants engaged, or parents and/or guardians of persons served to a proposed course of action after the communication of adequate information regarding expected outcomes and potential risks.

■ **jurisdiction**—The "personal jurisdiction" and authority of the ASHA Board of Ethics over an individual holding ASHA certification and/or membership, regardless of the individual's geographic location.

■ **know, known, or knowingly**—Having or reflecting knowledge.

■ **may vs. shall**—*May* denotes an allowance for discretion; *shall* denotes no discretion.

■ **misrepresentation**—Any statement by words or other conduct that, under the circumstances, amounts to an assertion that is false or erroneous (i.e., not in accordance with the facts); any statement made with conscious ignorance or a reckless disregard for the truth.

■ **negligence**—Breaching of a duty owed to another, which occurs because of a failure to conform to a requirement, and this failure has caused harm to another individual, which led to damages to this person(s); failure to exercise the care toward others that a reasonable or prudent person would take in the circumstances, or taking actions that such a reasonable person would not.

■ **nolo contendere**—No contest.

■ **plagiarism**—False representation of another person's idea, research, presentation, result, or product as one's own through irresponsible citation, attribution, or paraphrasing; ethical misconduct does not include honest error or differences of opinion.

■ **publicly sanctioned**—A formal disciplinary action of public record, excluding actions due to insufficient continuing education, checks returned for insufficient funds, or late payment of fees not resulting in unlicensed practice.

■ **reasonable or reasonably**—Supported or justified by fact or circumstance and being in accordance with reason, fairness, duty, or prudence.

■ **self-report**—A professional obligation of self-disclosure that requires (a) notifying ASHA Standards and Ethics and (b) mailing a hard copy of a certified document to ASHA Standards and Ethics (see term above). All self-reports are subject to a separate ASHA Certification review process, which, depending on the seriousness of the self-reported information, takes additional processing time.

■ **shall vs. may**—*Shall* denotes no discretion; *may* denotes an allowance for discretion.

■ **support personnel**—Those providing support to audiologists, speech-language pathologists, or speech, language, and hearing scientists (e.g., technician, paraprofessional, aide, or assistant in audiology, speech-language pathology, or communication sciences and disorders). For more information, read the Issues in Ethics Statements on Audiology Assistants and/or Speech-Language Pathology Assistants.

- **telepractice, teletherapy**—Application of telecommunications technology to the delivery of audiology and speech-language pathology professional services at a distance by linking clinician to client/patient or clinician to clinician for assessment, intervention, and/or consultation. The quality of the service should be equivalent to in-person service. For more information, see the telepractice section on the ASHA Practice Portal.

- **written**—Encompasses both electronic and hard-copy writings or communications.

Principle of Ethics I

Individuals shall honor their responsibility to hold paramount the welfare of persons they serve professionally or who are participants in research and scholarly activities, and they shall treat animals involved in research in a humane manner.

Rules of Ethics

A. Individuals shall provide all clinical services and scientific activities competently.

B. Individuals shall use every resource, including referral and/or interprofessional collaboration when appropriate, to ensure that quality service is provided.

C. Individuals shall not discriminate in the delivery of professional services or in the conduct of research and scholarly activities on the basis of race, ethnicity, sex, gender identity/gender expression, sexual orientation, age, religion, national origin, disability, culture, language, or dialect.

D. Individuals shall not misrepresent the credentials of aides, assistants, technicians, support personnel, students, research interns, Clinical Fellows, or any others under their supervision, and they shall inform those they serve professionally of the name, role, and professional credentials of persons providing services.

E. Individuals who hold the Certificate of Clinical Competence may delegate tasks related to the provision of clinical services to aides, assistants, technicians, support personnel, or any other persons only if those persons are adequately prepared and are appropriately supervised. The responsibility for the welfare of those being served remains with the certified individual.

F. Individuals who hold the Certificate of Clinical Competence shall not delegate tasks that require the unique skills, knowledge, judgment, or credentials that are within the scope of their profession to aides, assistants, technicians, support personnel, or any nonprofessionals over whom they have supervisory responsibility.

G. Individuals who hold the Certificate of Clinical Competence may delegate to students tasks related to the provision of clinical services that require the unique skills, knowledge, and judgment that are within the scope of practice of their profession only if those students are adequately prepared and are appropriately supervised. The responsibility for the welfare of those being served remains with the certified individual.

H. Individuals shall obtain informed consent from the persons they serve about the nature and possible risks and effects of services provided, technology employed, and products dispensed. This obligation also includes informing persons served about possible effects of not engaging in treatment or not following clinical recommendations. If diminished decision-making ability of persons served is suspected, individuals should seek appropriate authorization for services, such as authorization from a spouse, other family member, or legally authorized/appointed representative.

I. Individuals shall enroll and include persons as participants in research or teaching demonstrations only if participation is voluntary, without coercion, and with informed consent.

J. Individuals shall accurately represent the intended purpose of a service, product, or research endeavor and shall abide by established guidelines for clinical practice and the responsible conduct of research.

K. Individuals who hold the Certificate of Clinical Competence shall evaluate the effectiveness of services provided, technology employed, and products dispensed, and they shall provide services or dispense products only when benefit can reasonably be expected.

L. Individuals may make a reasonable statement of prognosis, but they shall not guarantee—directly or by implication—the results of any treatment or procedure.

M. Individuals who hold the Certificate of Clinical Competence shall use independent and evidence-based clinical judgment, keeping paramount the best interests of those being served.

N. Individuals who hold the Certificate of Clinical Competence shall not provide clinical services solely by correspondence, but may provide services via telepractice consistent with professional standards and state and federal regulations.

O. Individuals shall protect the confidentiality and security of records of professional services provided, research and scholarly activities conducted, and products dispensed. Access to these records shall be allowed only when doing so is necessary to protect the welfare of the person or of the community, is legally authorized, or is otherwise required by law.

P. Individuals shall protect the confidentiality of any professional or personal information about persons served professionally or participants involved in research and scholarly activities and may disclose confidential information only when doing so is necessary to protect the welfare of the person or of the community, is legally authorized, or is otherwise required by law.

Q. Individuals shall maintain timely records and accurately record and bill for services provided and products dispensed and shall not misrepresent services provided, products dispensed, or research and scholarly activities conducted.

R. Individuals whose professional practice is adversely affected by substance abuse, addiction, or other health-related conditions are impaired practitioners and shall seek professional assistance and, where appropriate, withdraw from the affected areas of practice.

S. Individuals who have knowledge that a colleague is unable to provide professional services with reasonable skill and safety shall report this information to the appropriate authority, internally if a mechanism exists and, otherwise, externally.

T. Individuals shall provide reasonable notice and information about alternatives for obtaining care in the event that they can no longer provide professional services.

Principle of Ethics II

Individuals shall honor their responsibility to achieve and maintain the highest level of professional competence and performance.

Rules of Ethics

A. Individuals who hold the Certificate of Clinical Competence shall engage in only those aspects of the professions that are within the scope of their professional practice and competence, considering their certification status, education, training, and experience.

B. Members who do not hold the Certificate of Clinical Competence may not engage in the provision of clinical services; however, individuals who are in the certification application process may engage in the provision of clinical services consistent with current local and state laws and regulations and with ASHA certification requirements.

C. Individuals who engage in research shall comply with all institutional, state, and federal regulations that address any aspects of research, including those that involve human participants and animals.

D. Individuals shall enhance and refine their professional competence and expertise through engagement in lifelong learning applicable to their professional activities and skills.

E. Individuals in administrative or supervisory roles shall not require or permit their professional staff to provide services or conduct research activities that exceed the staff member's certification status, competence, education, training, and experience.

F. Individuals in administrative or supervisory roles shall not require or permit their professional staff to provide services or conduct clinical activities that compromise the staff member's independent and objective professional judgment.

G. Individuals shall make use of technology and instrumentation consistent with accepted professional guidelines in their areas of practice. When such technology is not available, an appropriate referral may be made.

H. Individuals shall ensure that all technology and instrumentation used to provide services or to conduct research and scholarly activities are in proper working order and are properly calibrated.

Principle of Ethics III

Individuals shall honor their responsibility to the public when advocating for the unmet communication and swallowing needs of the public and shall provide accurate information involving any aspect of the professions.

Rules of Ethics

A. Individuals shall not misrepresent their credentials, competence, education, training, experience, and scholarly contributions.

B. Individuals shall avoid engaging in conflicts of interest whereby personal, financial, or other considerations have the potential to influence or compromise professional judgment and objectivity.

C. Individuals shall not misrepresent research and scholarly activities, diagnostic information, services provided, results of services provided, products dispensed, or the effects of products dispensed.

D. Individuals shall not defraud through intent, ignorance, or negligence or engage in any scheme to defraud in connection with obtaining payment, reimbursement, or grants and contracts for services provided, research conducted, or products dispensed.

E. Individuals' statements to the public shall provide accurate and complete information about the nature and management of communication disorders, about the professions, about professional services, about products for sale, and about research and scholarly activities.

F. Individuals' statements to the public shall adhere to prevailing professional norms and shall not contain misrepresentations when advertising, announcing, and promoting their professional services and products and when reporting research results.

G. Individuals shall not knowingly make false financial or nonfinancial statements and shall complete all materials honestly and without omission.

Principle of Ethics IV

Individuals shall uphold the dignity and autonomy of the professions, maintain collaborative and harmonious interprofessional and intraprofessional relationships, and accept the professions' self-imposed standards.

Rules of Ethics

A. Individuals shall work collaboratively, when appropriate, with members of one's own profession and/or members of other professions to deliver the highest quality of care.

B. Individuals shall exercise independent professional judgment in recommending and providing profes-sional services when an administrative mandate, referral source, or prescription prevents keeping the welfare of persons served paramount.

C. Individuals' statements to colleagues about professional services, research results, and products shall adhere to prevailing professional standards and shall contain no misrepresentations.

D. Individuals shall not engage in any form of conduct that adversely reflects on the professions or on the individual's fitness to serve persons professionally.

E. Individuals shall not engage in dishonesty, negligence, fraud, deceit, or misrepresentation.

F. Applicants for certification or membership, and individuals making disclosures, shall not knowingly make false statements and shall complete all application and disclosure materials honestly and without omission.

G. Individuals shall not engage in any form of harassment, power abuse, or sexual harassment.

H. Individuals shall not engage in sexual activities with individuals (other than a spouse or other individual with whom a prior consensual relationship exists) over whom they exercise professional authority or power, including persons receiving services, assistants, students, or research participants.

I. Individuals shall not knowingly allow anyone under their supervision to engage in any practice that violates the Code of Ethics.

J. Individuals shall assign credit only to those who have contributed to a publication, presentation, process, or product. Credit shall be assigned in proportion to the contribution and only with the contributor's consent.

K. Individuals shall reference the source when using other persons' ideas, research, presentations, results, or products in written, oral, or any other media presentation or summary. To do otherwise constitutes plagiarism.

L. Individuals shall not discriminate in their relationships with colleagues, assistants, students, support personnel, and members of other professions and disciplines on the basis of race, ethnicity, sex, gender identity/gender expression, sexual orientation, age, religion, national origin, disability, culture, language, dialect, or socioeconomic status.

M. Individuals with evidence that the Code of Ethics may have been violated have the responsibility to work collaboratively to resolve the situation where possible or to inform the Board of Ethics through its established procedures.

N. Individuals shall report members of other professions who they know have violated standards of care to the appropriate professional licensing authority or board, other professional regulatory body, or professional association when such violation compromises the welfare of persons served and/or research participants.

O. Individuals shall not file or encourage others to file complaints that disregard or ignore facts that would disprove the allegation; the Code of Ethics shall not be used for personal reprisal, as a means of addressing personal animosity, or as a vehicle for retaliation.

P. Individuals making and responding to complaints shall comply fully with the policies of the Board of Ethics in its consideration, adjudication, and resolution of complaints of alleged violations of the Code of Ethics.

Q. Individuals involved in ethics complaints shall not knowingly make false statements of fact or withhold relevant facts necessary to fairly adjudicate the complaints.

R. Individuals shall comply with local, state, and federal laws and regulations applicable to professional practice, research ethics, and the responsible conduct of research.

S. Individuals who have been convicted; been found guilty; or entered a plea of guilty or nolo contendere to (1) any misdemeanor involving dishonesty, physical harm—or the threat of physical harm—to the person or property of another, or (2) any felony, shall self-report by notifying ASHA Standards and Ethics (see Terminology for mailing address) in writing within 30 days of the conviction, plea, or finding of guilt. Individuals shall also provide a certified copy of the conviction, plea, nolo contendere record, or docket entry to ASHA Standards and Ethics within 30 days of self-reporting.

T. Individuals who have been publicly sanctioned or denied a license or a professional credential by any professional association, professional licensing authority or board, or other professional regulatory body shall self-report by notifying ASHA Standards and Ethics (see Terminology for mailing address) in writing within 30 days of the final action or disposition. Individuals shall also provide a certified copy of the final action, sanction, or disposition to ASHA Standards and Ethics within 30 days of self-reporting.

Source: American Speech-Language-Hearing Association. (2016). Code of Ethics [Ethics]. Available from www.asha.org/policy Reprinted with permission from the American Speech-Language-Hearing Association.

6

Professional Accountability

◇◇

Shelly S. Chabon, PhD and Becky Sutherland Cornett, PhD

Introduction

Although neither of us is a quilter, we have decided to use the quilt as a metaphor for discussing accountability in delivering high value care. Like a quilt, our clinical services, or "product" are put together bit by bit, using materials and resources that represent individual preferences, abilities, outlooks and interests, evidence, knowledge, ethical and regulatory guidelines, and, organizational parameters. Like a quilt, each of these pieces may be important, but the whole is greater than the sum of its parts. In the end, a quilt, like clinical outcomes, tells a story, about our values, how we conducted our work, how we reconciled choices between service levels and service quality, between policies and practices, between what the patient desires and what the organization offers, between what we know and what we have yet to discover. The quilter and the clinician share an interpretative role in the art and science of professional accountability.

Speech-language pathologists and audiologists bear the responsibility for binding together these multiple remnants into a fabric of personal, public, and professional legitimacy. Our patients trust us to listen, to understand, and to do what is right, fair, and just. We are held to account for what we do or do not do and are therefore ethically obliged to anticipate and evaluate the impact of our words and actions. The true and enduring testament of accountability is to support our patients' needs in a way that clearly appreciates their expectations and values.

Cornett and Chabon (1988) described three attitudes central to providing high-quality, accountable services:

- A *therapeutic attitude* refers to interpersonal skills that create an atmosphere in which change can occur.

- A *professional attitude* encompasses expertise (knowledge and skill sets), professional norms (e.g., certification, codes of conduct, quality measures), professional identity (memberships, collegiality), legal identity (licensure), business acumen, and personal traits.

- A *scientific attitude* represents theoretical knowledge and the ever-increasing scientific data base that informs our evolving understanding of human communication and communication disorders.

131

We are duty-bound to consider the attitudes, knowledge, and skills we bring to our work and to examine the myriad patterns of influence and infrastructure on our patients' outcomes.

In this chapter, we ask you to redefine or reimagine researcher and clinician roles, and to recognize their bidirectionality. We ask for a balance, not a trade-off, between efficiency and equity in treatment, between what the clinician perceives to be priorities and what patients value most. We ask for individual and collective accountability for the inputs, outcomes, and impacts of our clinical work.

Professional accountability requires knowledge of our ethical commitments to enable outcomes that support the patient's participation in daily life. "Effectiveness" in the pursuit and accomplishment of discrete goals of little practical application to our patients' everyday lives compromises our professionalism.

Navran (2013) reminds us that "we are accountable for the effectiveness, the timeliness and the quality of what we do even if we were not responsible for the decision that it be done or the decision that it be done by us. And, of course, we are accountable for the means by which we accomplish the task." Claiming or "owning" our actions and decisions is at the core of accountable care. It would not be acceptable to assert a lack of responsibility for workplace policies, just for the duty to execute them. This is an artificial separation, because as professionals we are accountable for the standards we follow as well as how we choose to implement them.

Clarity of professional guidelines is not always available. These documents tend to be intentionally general so that they may be interpreted across varied and diverse situations and individuals. The effective and efficient use of policy statements coheres around the obligation to preserve the adequacy of resources to support the integration and stabilization of clinician and patient shared decision making. It is only through the application of diverse perspectives that we can find true accountability as a standard of thoroughness and thoughtfulness.

Accountable Care

"Accountable care" refers broadly to organizing and delivering health care services that are focused on effectiveness and efficiency—achieving superior results while demonstrating a high degree of stewardship of financial, human, and material resources.

The quest for accountability within the health care community is long-standing, multi-faceted, and continues to evolve as health care practitioners and organizations are challenged to provide care that is highly reliable and valuable to all stakeholders. The key ques-

tion has not changed for habilitation and rehabilitation professionals: How do we know, and how can we show that what we do in therapy makes a difference? (Douglass, 1983, p. 117). Robert Douglass, founder of the communication disorders program at California State University, delineated the following precepts of clinical accountability:

- The welfare of the patient is paramount.

- A regimen of treatment is followed that consists of systematically applied procedures.

- The ability of a professional, as demonstrated in knowledge and skills, is directly related to the capacity to be helpful to a client.

- Members of a profession are answerable for their actions on behalf of their clients.

- The clinical activities of members of a profession must be accounted for or explained in some formal manner (pp. 107–108).

Concluding the article "A Principal Calling: Professionalism and Health Care Services," Cornett (2006) said:

The work we do as health care professionals carries special obligations because we influence people's lives in such basic ways. Our "product" is clinical service to individuals who are vulnerable. Our duty to that "product" requires nothing less than the highest degree of involvement in examining our attitudes toward our professional duties, and in building a solid infrastructure of knowledge, skills, standards and principles to which we can be held accountable. Health care professionals are not expected to have all the answers—but we are expected to keep seeking them. Inquiry, introspection, and integrity are the keys to professionalism. (p. 308)

Although health professionals have long been subject to requirements and standards, calls for heightened accountability arose when the Institute of Medicine (now Health and Medicine Division of the National Academy of Medicine) published *To Err Is Human: Building a Safer Health Care System* (2000), which found that the health care industry was at least a decade behind other high-risk industries in ensuring basic safety. *Crossing the Quality Chasm: A New Health System for the 21st Century* (2001) called for new rules for the twenty-first century health care system with safety as a system priority; care is based on continuous healing relationships instead of number of visits; decision making is evidence based; the patient is the source of control; knowledge is shared and information flows freely; waste is continuously decreased; and cooperation among clinicians is a priority.

Subsequently, the Institute for Healthcare Improvement (IHI) promoted the Triple Aim framework, seeking to optimize health system performance by redesigning care to:

- Improve the patient experience of care (including quality and satisfaction)
- Improve the health of populations
- Reduce the per capita cost of health care.

We are still struggling to achieve these goals well into the twenty-first century.

Managing Risks and "Risk Intelligence" for Accountable Clinicians and Organizations

The health care industry is highly regulated because our business involves caring for human lives with all associated risks. Moreover, misalignment of incentives among the players—individual and institutional providers and suppliers, life science and medical device companies, government and commercial payers, employers, and patients—also fuels the perceived need for a myriad of laws, regulations, rules, and guidance. Additional pressure results from years of reports of low-value care (offering few or no benefits) and waste in the system, amounting to approximately 30% of all health expenditures (O'Neill & Scheinker, 2018). Waste is categorized as: failures of care delivery, failures of care coordination, over-treatment, administrative complexity, pricing failures, and fraud and abuse.

Under the fee-for-service (FFS) system, payers and policymakers often assumed that providers are incentivized to maximize visits, sessions, tests, procedures, surgeries, and high cost care venues. Consequently, regulatory compliance requirements for payment have focused on rules for documenting assessment and treatment and for coding and billing of services according to type of practitioner and place of service. Detailed rules are also described for patient safety and privacy of health information as the result of numerous failures in these areas in the health care industry. These requirements, forming important basic infrastructure for accountability, will not be discussed here. Readers are referred to ASHA's Practice Portal and Chapter 14, "Health Care Legislation, Regulation, and Financing," for updated trends, issues, and requirements associated with laws and regulations, which will change as the system moves from FFS to other forms of payment in which providers assume increasing risk for improving the health and well-being of a patient population for a pre-determined payment.

Understanding and participating in ongoing risk management activities for organizations (and individuals) is also a basic component of professional accountability. The National Institutes of Health (NIH) succinctly describes *risk management* as a continuous process designed to proactively identify and mitigate risks to help promote the achievement of an organization's objectives, strategy, and mission. Risk management drives accountability by assigning responsibility to personnel for considering risk as part of their daily jobs.

According to Doherty and Carino (2018), current critical risks facing the health care industry include:

- Professional liability: 4 in 10 Americans experienced a medical error in 2017; the top errors are: misdiagnosis, delayed diagnosis, medication error, and inaccurate medical advice.

- Opioid litigation against providers: litigation has focused previously on pharmaceutical companies manufacturing opioids and distributors.

- Health care infections: health care acquired infections (HAI) cost the U.S. health system billions of dollars a year and lead to the loss of thousands of lives.

- Clinical alarm fatigue: Although clinical alarms associated with heart monitors, ventilators, infusion pumps, compression devices, beds, chairs, and other equipment are designed to draw attention to a potential problem with a patient, overwhelmed health professionals may become desensitized to them and then fail to respond or delay responding, resulting in patient harm or death.

- Workplace violence and disruptive behavior: 75% of workplace violence occurs in health care and social service settings.

- Cyber risk: Electronic health records have created new patient privacy exposures. Data breaches and network disruptions can jeopardize an organization's financial stability, security and reputation. Forty-seven percent of providers reported data-security violations in 2017.

- Emergency preparedness: Centers for Medicare and Medicaid Services conditions of participation require specific elements of compliance pertaining to natural and man-made disasters and other life-safety issues.

Management consultant Frederick (Rick) Funston created the concept of "risk intelligence" in 2001. He described "risk intelligence" as understanding the risks of action and inaction. A risk intelligent enterprise (or professional) integrates people, processes, and tools to facilitate decision making to create value and to preserve value.

Deloitte's report *Cultivating a Risk Intelligent Culture: Understand, Measure, Strengthen and Report* (2012) presented key characteristics of a risk intelligent culture:

- Individuals demonstrate a commonality of purpose, values, and ethics.

- Risk is considered in all activities—from strategic planning to daily operations.

- The ability of the organization to manage risk is continuously improving.

- Everyone encourages timely, transparent, and open communication.

- People understand the value that risk management brings to the organization.

- People take personal responsibility for the management of risk and proactively seek to involve others as applicable.

- People are comfortable challenging others, including authority figures. The people who are being challenged respond positively (p. 2).

Maintaining a risk intelligent culture is essential to professional accountability and organizational viability.

Raising the Bar on Accountability: The Value Equation

The publication of the landmark article "What Is Value in Health Care?" (Porter, 2010) was a tipping point in the long journey of health care reform. Porter's definition of value provided the shared goal he envisioned to refocus the industry on changing the nature of accountability among all stakeholders. That definition has frequently been portrayed as an equation:

$$\text{VALUE} = \frac{\text{health outcomes achieved}}{\text{per dollar spent}}$$

Porter contended that achieving high value for patients must become the overarching goal, focusing on "what matters for patients and unites all actors in the system" (p. 2477).

Purchasers and payers have sought to hold providers increasingly accountable for performance on measures of safety, clinical care processes, efficiency and cost reduction, and patient and caregiver experience of care through pay-for-performance and value-based purchasing initiatives for over a decade. Provider enrollment in Medicare and commercial payer accountable care organizations (ACOs) has increased slowly, because health care institutions and individual providers have been reluctant to assume performance risk and financial risk for specified populations of covered lives. Their reluctance is largely based on the disconnects between legacy models of patient care and payment that rely upon volumes of tests, procedures, visits, sessions, and surgeries and new payment models that require providers to rethink volume in favor of services that measurably improve the overall health and quality of life of the populations served at reduced cost (value).

Although no universal set of value-based health measures have been implemented, policymakers and advisory groups continue to work on developing these measures. It is useful to present the Institute for Healthcare Improvement's Triple Aim Measures (http://www.ihi.org) to illustrate the challenge. The measures are categorized according to IHI's Triple Aims, shown in Table 6–1.

In the past few years, provider associations, foundations, and not-for-profit institutes and organizations have led the way in identifying "low-value" care. Although definitions vary, low-value care generally includes tests, procedures, and services that should not be performed given their potential for harm or the existence of comparably effective and often less expensive alternatives (Schpero, 2014). Chief among these efforts is the Choosing Wisely® campaign, an initiative of the American Board of Internal Medicine (ABIM). This effort seeks to advance a national dialogue on avoiding unnecessary medical tests, treatments, and procedures. Materials have been developed for patient use and practitioner use. Recommendations are included for occupational therapy, physical therapy, and hearing problems.

Initiatives to identify and promote health benefits plans that "get more health out of every dollar spent" are anchored at the University of Michigan's Center for Value-Based Insurance Design (VBID). According to the center, plans that incorporate VBID principles increase access to necessary treatments, improve adherence to medication and treatment plans, engage patients, and ensure the best clinical outcomes for employees and enrollees, ultimately decreasing long-term health care costs and increasing patient quality of life and productivity. The premise of VBID Health is to align patients' out-of-pocket costs, such as copayments and deductibles, with the value of health services. By reducing barriers to high-value treatments (through lower costs to patients) and discouraging low-value treatments (through higher costs to patients), plans can improve

Table 6–1. IHI Triple Aim Measures

Dimension	Measure
Population Health	1. Health/Functional Status: single-question (e.g., from CDC HRQOL-4) or multi-domain (e.g., SF-12, EuroQoL)
	2. Risk Status: composite health risk appraisal (HRA) score
	3. Disease Burden: Incidence (yearly rate of onset, avg. age of onset) and/or prevalence of major chronic conditions; summary of predictive model scores
	4. Mortality: life expectancy; years of potential life lost; standardized mortality rates. *Note: Healthy Life Expectancy (HLE) combines life expectancy and health status into a single measure, reflecting remaining years of life in good health. See http://reves.site.ined.fr/en/DFLE/definition/*
Patient Experience	1. Standard questions from patient surveys, for example: ■ Global questions from US CAHPS or How's Your Health surveys ■ Experience questions from NHS World Class Commissioning or CareQuality Commission ■ Likelihood to recommend
	2. Set of measures based on key dimensions (e.g., US IOM Quality Chasm aims: Safe, Effective, Timely, Efficient, Equitable and Patient-centered)
Per Capita Cost	1. Total cost per member of the population per month
	2. Hospital and ED utilization rate

Source: Reprinted from Stiefel, M., & Nolan, K. *A Guide to Measuring the Triple Aim: Population Health, Experience of Care, and Per Capita Cost.* IHI Innovation Series white paper. (Available on http://www.IHI.org) ©2018 Reprinted with permission of the Institute for Health Care Improvement.

health outcomes. VBID is used in a growing number of Medicare Advantage plans and managed Medicaid plans and by many commercial insurers. Resources at vbid.org include: the MedInsight Health Waste Calculator and Low-Value Care Reduction Toolkits for providers, employers, and payers.

The health care community is also engaging in better defining, describing, and practicing high-value care. Examples include the American College of Physicians (ACP) High Value Care (HVC) Initiative, offering resources for clinicians (e.g., a high value care coordination toolkit and video learning modules) and medical educators (curricula for medical residents and fellows and toolkits for faculty). (See acponline.org.) Ninety partner institutions are involved in the High Value Academic Practice Alliance, responding to the concern that the cost of health care is the biggest financial concern facing American families. Alliance members are identifying opportunities and implementing initiatives that improve patient care quality and safety while reducing costs by consulting an architecture of high-value health care. The pillars are:

■ diagnostic and therapeutic efficiency (precision practice);

■ quality-driven care pathways (evidence shows that pathways improve outcomes and reduce length of stay);

■ care transitions including hospital discharge (decreasing preventable readmissions);

■ optimized patient care setting (avoid unnecessary use of inpatient care and emergency departments); and

■ preventive medicine and healthy lifestyle (promote a healthy lifestyle to reduce risk of disease and chronic conditions; use of evidence-based screening tests for early diagnosis; adhere to preventive care guidelines).
(More information is found at hvpaa.org.)

Rehabilitation professionals are also under pressure to better define high-value care. The Improving Medicare Post-Acute Care Transformation (IMPACT) Act of 2014, implemented beginning in FY2019 standardizes assessments across the spectrum of post-acute care (PAC) providers, establishes public reporting of quality measures across settings, provides quality measures to consumers upon care transition, and requires the Department of Health and Human Services (DHHS) and the Medicare Payment Advisory Commission (MedPAC) to conduct studies and reports to link payment to quality. HHS and MedPAC must develop a plan to link post-acute payment to quality of care, review current risk adjustment methodologies, and study the effect of socioeconomic status on quality, resource use, and other measures. In FY2022, MedPAC is to report to Congress on establishing prospective payment for post-acute care. Moreover, a study published in *JAMA Internal Medicine* (McWilliams et al., 2017) reported: "post-acute care is thought to be a major source of wasteful spending. The extent to which accountable care organizations (ACOs) can limit post-acute care spending has implications for the importance and design of other payment models that include post-acute care" (p. 518). The study concluded that provider participation in the Medicare Shared Savings Program (MSSP) was associated with significant reductions in post-acute spending without deterioration of quality of care.

Achieving the Triple Aim for rehabilitation professionals will require individual and collective effort to determine which interventions reflect best practices to achieve maximum efficiency and will link treatment to results that describe our impact on individual's everyday lives. Two efforts may be keys to success: a "build-out" of the Rehabilitation Treatment Taxonomy (RTT) and reporting of *participation outcomes.*

Leaders in the medical rehabilitation field have recognized the need for a common framework to define and describe rehabilitation treatments. A classification system or taxonomy allows comparisons between and among treatment methods and materials to identify clinical best practices. Proponents observed that treatments are often named by the type of professional who delivers the services (e.g., OT, PT, SLP), or the problem treated (e.g., "gait training," "spoken language comprehension") rather than by specific approach, procedure, environmental modification, medication, device, or other service. Although patient deficits have been well delineated and status at discharge documented and measured, interventions have not been delineated well.

A grant by the National Institute on Disability and Rehabilitation Research (NIDRR, now National Institute on Disability, Independent Living and Rehabilitation) in 2008 funded the development of the conceptual framework to specify treatments by rehabilitation professionals in all areas of rehabilitation in terms of "active ingredients." This work was reported in a special supplement of *Archives of Physical Medicine and Rehabilitation* (Dijkers, 2014). Subsequently, a 2018 Patient-Centered Outcomes Research Institute (PCORI) grant was issued to Albert Einstein Health Network to develop a manual to help rehabilitation providers use standard ways to define treatments. The 2019 publication describes targets (the specific functional problem presented) and "ingredients" (the types of interventions offered). Three types of treatments are addressed:

- Body functions treatments make a body part work better.

- Skills and habits treatments help people get better at doing something that needs practice, such as walking.

- Representations focus on thoughts, feelings, and knowledge.

Turkstra and colleagues (2016) stressed the importance of adopting the taxonomy to speech-language pathology practice, research and knowledge translation in the article "Knowing What We're Doing: Why Specification of Treatment Methods Is Critical for Evidence-Based Practice in Speech-Language Pathology." We will also be aided in the future to specify inputs, outputs, and impact by software that extracts data from unstructured text, analyses of massive integrated databases, and software and analytic methods that are not yet applied or created in a rapidly evolving technology environment.

A focus on participation outcomes is also recommended as a key to success for practitioners and patients as part of a value-oriented health system. The World Health Organization (WHO) defines participation as taking part in life situations (2001). According to Baum (2011) "people receive services to live their lives" (p. 171). Baum's Coulter Memorial Lecture "Fulfilling the Promise: Supporting Participation in Daily Life" presented a model of rehabilitation service that focused on participation. She contended "disability is not a problem originating with a person; it exists when there is a poor person-environment fit." In Baum's view, rehabilitation should focus not on disability or deficits, but on enablement and participation. Focusing on participation helps fill the gap between biomedical science and population science and the gap between the biomedical system in which people receive health care and the broader sociocultural system in which people live. Rehabilitation services today seem primarily to be focused on intermediate measures (percent correct on tests, scale scores, or achieving levels on discrete measures of function). These measures are important to improve, test, and review inputs, but the final measure should be that the person is able to participate in activities that will provide quality to his or her life. Baum concluded by stating that rehabilitation professionals must "fulfill the promise that our science and professions offer: we will be known for our efforts to help people participate in their daily lives" (p. 174).

In the field of communication disorders, Baylor and colleagues have contributed significantly to our understanding of the role of participation-focused treatment in delivering high-value care. Communicative participation is "taking part in life situations in which information or ideas are exchanged between people" (Eadie et al., 2006). These professionals teach us that participation is influenced by speech-language symptoms (communication effort), health status, physical environment, personal outlook (resilience), situations encountered, and social environment (support system). Successful intervention requires a holistic, cross-cutting approach.

The University of Washington researchers developed the Communication Participation Item Bank (CPIB) (Baylor et al., 2013) an instrument designed for community-dwelling adults across different communication disorders and life situations. The items ask about the extent to which the respondent's condition interferes with participation in a wide range of speaking situations such as talking to people you do not know, talking on the telephone to get information, ordering a meal in a restaurant, and talking in groups of people. According to the authors, having a unidimensional patient-reported outcome (PRO) instrument dedicated to the construct of communicative participation will facilitate advancement of both clinical and scholarly work in the area of communicative participation. Optimizing participation might be regarded as the ultimate outcome of intervention in that patients or clients are able to do the things they want and need to do in their daily lives.

A Key Opportunity to Shape the Future of Accountability: Learning Health Systems

Don't be a know-it-all, be a learn-it-all—Satya Nadella, describing his leadership vision at Microsoft Corporation, based on the book *Mindset* by Carol Dweck (2016)

The Learning Health System (LHS) approach to professional accountability and engagement illustrates Nadella's vision well. The LHS was conceived by the Committee on the Learning Health Care System in America at the Institute of Medicine (IOM) and described in the landmark report *Best Care at Lower Cost: The Path to Continuously Learning Health Care in America* (2012). The committee contended that the entrenched challenges of the U.S. health care system demanded a transformed approach to improving outcomes of care at lower cost for all stakeholders: "left unchanged, health care will continue to underperform; cause unnecessary harm; and strain national, state, and family budgets. The actions required to reverse this trend will be notable, substantial, and sometimes disruptive—and absolutely necessary" (p. 4). The transformation recommended is a system that learns—in real time and with new tools, including the increasing power of technology—to manage problems presented by patients in new and better ways, continuously updated as knowledge evolves.

According to the committee, characteristics of a continuously learning health care system include:

■ Real-time access to knowledge—reliably capture, curate, and deliver the best available evidence to improve clinical decision making.

■ Digital capture of the care experience—use digital platforms for real-time generation and application of knowledge.

■ Engaged, empowered patients—promote the inclusion of patients and families as vital members of the continuously learning health care team.

■ Incentives aligned for value—incentives are actively aligned to encourage continuous improvement, identify and reduce waste, and reward high-value care.

■ Full transparency—systematically monitor the safety, quality, processes, prices, costs, and outcomes of care; make information available for care improvement and informed choices.

■ Leadership-instilled culture of learning—leaders are committed to a culture of teamwork, collaboration, and adaptability in support of continuous learning.

■ Supportive system competencies—complex care operations are constantly refined through skill-building, systems analysis, and information development, with feedback loops for continuous learning and systems improvement.

Embi and Payne (2013) described an approach to implement a learning health system in their article: "Evidence-generating medicine: Redefining the research-practice relationship to complete the evidence cycle."

They argued that the success of improving health care value lies in leveraging point-of-care activities, data, and resources to generate evidence through routine practice. A paradigm shift is needed to redefine the relationship between research and practice as bidirectional rather than unidirectional (which depends on research findings from historical data analysis). The evidence-generating approach creates a virtuous cycle in which clinical practice is not distinct from research. Evidence-generating health care does not supplant clinical trials; it allows clinicians to chart a course of systematic use of external and internal data sources to optimize care and use of resources.

Nationwide Children's Hospital in Columbus, Ohio formed a local learning health system—the Learn from Every Patient™ program—to simultaneously provide clinical care while systematically collecting data for quality improvement and research projects on all patients (Lowes et al., 2017; Noritz, Boggs, Lowes, & Smoyer, 2018). Clinicians create data collection tools in the electronic health record to discretely capture data for clinical, quality, and research use. Results include reducing the need for inpatient admissions, reducing lengths of stay, improving workflow efficiency, and reducing costs—while focusing on offering an excellent patient experience.

Accountable clinicians in a learning health system develop and advance knowledge and skill sets such as data analytics, adaptive learning, systems science, team science, implementation science, and performance management that expand and evolve. The Michigan Medicine Department of Learning Health Sciences is the nation's first basic science department focused on the sciences related to learning across multiple levels of scale. Faculty members and students work to improve health in systemic ways by advancing the sciences that make learning effective, routine, and efficient. Learning is viewed as a continuous process of discovery and implementation, leading to innovation. The department offers research, educational, and service programs designed to facilitate the application of learning and to transform health care organizations into learning health systems. *Learning Health Systems* is an international, peer-reviewed open access online journal, published in collaboration with the University of Michigan, that advances learning health systems. Readers are encouraged to review the special issue Learning Health Systems: Connecting Research to Practice Worldwide (January 2019).

Professional accountability in the twenty-first century and beyond requires what Daugherty and Wilson (2018) call *relentless reimagining*—the rigorous discipline of creating new processes and business models from scratch, rather than simply automating (or tweaking) old processes. Their book is about reimagining work in the age of artificial intelligence (AI)—how AI can help people transform work, organizational processes, business models, and entire industries. The capability to reimagine enables individuals to more easily adapt to —and thrive in—a different everyday world, one that embraces using advanced technology as a tool and that requires continuous learning and striving to achieve better results—relentlessly.

Conclusion

We return to the quilt metaphor as we imagine the future place of accountability within the professions. As noted earlier, each quilt is made of unique pieces bound together to create a glorious work of art, comforting to body and soul. Over time, some pieces may unravel or become frayed or new color choices sought to replace the originals. Similarly, within our own professions, new tools will emerge, some old concepts will be discarded in favor of new ones, some methods will become obsolete, and our knowledge and skills will evolve in response to scientific, technological, and social changes. Clinicians must piece together qualitative and quantitative data, clinical evidence, and patients' hopes and goals. This intertwining of multiple bits of information and perspectives will lead to functional, personalized, and powerful outcomes.

Expectations for accountability in health care will no doubt advance in the years to come and we are individually and collectively, through our professional organization, responsible for scrutinizing and assuming responsibility for the new patterns that emerge. It is our ethical and professional imperative to seek common threads of understanding among those with different views of health, illness, and ability. Professional accountability, like quilting, reflects our heritage and our future.

Summary

In this chapter we have attempted to stitch together the components of professional accountability in ways that are both theoretical and practical—providing a foundation for conducting clinical practice, teaching, research, or business management in speech-language pathology and audiology. We described "accountable care" and presented current barriers that challenge our ability to be accountable in a fragmented health care system; discussed aspects of risk management, emphasizing the importance of developing and maintaining a "risk intelligent" culture; and urged all readers to engage in continuous learning and relentless reimagining to fulfill Carolyn Baum's wish that we will be known for our efforts to help people participate in their daily lives.

Critical Thinking

1. A "risk intelligent" culture in health care addresses both *performance risk* and *financial risk*. Given the emphasis on *value* (results achieved per dollar spent) instead of *volume* of procedures and services/visits, how should rehabilitation professionals conduct daily practice activities to respond to these challenges?

2. What information would be needed to write participation outcomes for a 29-year-old male with traumatic brain injury following a motor vehicle accident?

3. What did Dr. Carolyn Baum mean when she said: "disability is not a problem originating with a person; it exists when there is a poor person-environment fit"? What are the implications of her statement for designing clinical practice strategies in a learning health system?

4. Using Choosing Wisely™ as a guide, give an example of a high-value intervention and a low-value intervention, including the basis for your classification, for a child for whom English is not the first language.

5. How is "evidence-based" health care different from "evidence-generating" care?

6. What components are essential in a high-value care curriculum for speech-language pathologists and audiologists?

References

Baum, C. (2011). Fulfilling the promise: Supporting participation in daily life. *Archives of Physical Medicine and Rehabilitation*, 92(2), 169–175.

Baylor, C., Yorkston, K., Eadie, T., Kim, J., Chung, H., & Amtmann, D. (2013). The communicative participation item bank (CPIB): Item bank calibration and development of a disorder-generic short form. *Journal of Speech-Language-Hearing Research*, 56(4), 1190–1208.

Committee on the Learning Health Care System in America, Institute of Medicine of the National Academies. (2012). *Best care at lower cost: The path to continuously learning health care in America. Report Brief*. Washington, DC: National Academies Press.

Committee on Quality of Health Care in America, Institute of Medicine of the National Academies.

(2000). *To err is human: Building a safer health system*. Washington DC: National Academies Press.

Committee on Quality of Health Care in America, Institute of Medicine of the National Academies. (2001). *Crossing the quality chasm: A new health system for the 21st century*. Washington DC: National Academies Press.

Cornett, B. S. (2006). A principal calling: Professionalism and health care services. *Journal of Communication Disorders*, 39(4), 301–309.

Cornett, B. S., & Chabon, S. (1988). *The clinical practice of speech-language pathology*. Columbus, OH: Merrill.

Daugherty, P., & Wilson, H. J. (2018). *Human + machine: Reimagining work in the age of A.I.* Cambridge, MA: Harvard Business Review Press.

Deloitte LLC (2012). *Cultivating a risk intelligent culture: Understand, measure, strengthen and report*. Chicago, IL: Deloitte Development LLC.

Dijkers, M. (Ed.) (2014). Toward a taxonomy of rehabilitation treatments. *Archives of Physical Medicine and Rehabilitation*, 95(1 Suppl.), S1–S94.

Doherty, D., & Carino, R. (2018). *Critical risks facing the health care industry*. Retrieved from https://www.chubb.com/microsites/_assets/doc/healthcare-risk-collateral/chubb-healthcare-critical-risk-whitepaper.pdf.

Douglass, R. (1983). Defining and describing clinical accountability. *Seminars in Speech and Language*, 4(2), 107–108.

Dweck, C. (2016). *Mindset: The new psychology of success*. New York, NY: Ballantine.

Eadie, T., Yorkston, K., Klasner, E., Dudgeon, B., Deitz, J., Baylor, C., Miller, R., & Amtmann, D. (2006). Measuring communicative participation: A review of self-report instruments in speech-language pathology. *American Journal of Speech-Language Pathology*, 15(4), 307–320.

Embi, P., & Payne, P. (2013). Evidence-generating medicine: Redefining the research-practice relationship to complete the evidence cycle. *Medical Care*, 51(Suppl. 8), S81–S87.

Lowes, L., Noritz, G., Newmeyer, A. Embi, P., Yin, H., & Smoyer, W. (2017). Learn from every patient: Implementation and early results of a learning health system. *Developmental Medicine & Child Neurology*, 59(2), 183–191.

McWilliams, J., Gilstrap, L., Stevenson, D., Chernew, M., Huskamp, H., & Grabowski, D. (2017). Changes in postacute care in the Medicare shared savings program. *JAMA Internal Medicine*, *1777*(4), 518–526.

Navran, F. (2013). *Ethics thoughtpieces: Accountability.* Retrieved from https://www.tei.org.za/index.php/resources/articles/business-ethics/6832-accountability.

Noritz, G., Boggs, A., Lowes, L., & Smoyer, W. (2018). Evidence that local learning health systems can systematically learn and improve patient care: A report from the 'learn from every patient' program. *Pediatric Quality & Safety*, *3*(5), e100.

O'Neill, D., & Scheinker, D. (2018, May 31). Wasted health spending: Who's picking up the tab? *Health Affairs* blog. Retrieved from https://www.healthaffairs.org/do/10.1377/hblog20180530.245587/full/

Porter, M. (2010). What is value in health care? *New England Journal of Medicine*, *363*, 2477–2481.

Schpero, W. (2014). Limiting low-value care by 'choosing wisely.' *Virtual Mentor*, *16*(2), 131–134.

Turkstra, L., Norman, R., Whyte, J., Dijkers, M., & Hart, T. (2016). Knowing what we're doing: Why specification of treatment methods is critical for evidence-based practice in speech-language pathology. *American Journal of Speech-Language Pathology*, *25*(2), 164–171.

World Health Organization. (2001). *International classification of functioning, disability, and health.* Geneva, Switzerland: Author.

7

International Alliances

Robert M. Augustine, PhD, Tina K. Veale, PhD, and Kelly M. Holland, MEd

Introduction

International alliances provide experiences to promote global competencies for audiologists and speech-language pathologists. Disciplinary societies, such as the American Speech-Language-Hearing Association (ASHA), create international alliances to foster the exchange of global practices, research, and knowledge essential for advancing the discipline and the professions. For pre-service students, an international alliance develops global competencies for meeting standards of practice required to assess and treat multicultural patients and to collaborate with multicultural professionals on interprofessional teams, both domestically and abroad. Universities that invest in international alliances for their students and faculty create distinctive and diverse communities attractive to multicultural recruitment and career success. For in-service practitioners who seek global careers, the alliances create pathways to access the expertise, professional networks, and international credentialing required for practice in English-speaking and non-English speaking countries. Service-learning alliances create the potential for access to sustainable services and cohorts of practitioners who hone culturally appropriate skills and knowledge for underresourced countries. Service-learning alliances also provide opportunities to share best practices for the advancement of effective treatment outcomes on a global scale. For researchers, international alliances connect the science and evidence behind diagnostic and intervention tools to foster cross-cultural applications. This chapter will explore a variety of international alliances designed to guide achievement of the competencies associated with global career paths and characteristics that define a quality experience.

Definition of an International Alliance

The American Council on Education Center for Internationalization and Global Engagement defines an international alliance as a collaboration with international partners. The purpose of the alliance is to prepare those who participate with competencies, sometimes referred to as *knowledge and skills*, needed to achieve career success in the global community that represents today's workforce (Helms, 2015).

Competencies and Outcomes Associated with an International Alliance

Graduate degrees from accredited programs in audiology and speech-language pathology that lead to clinical practice require demonstration of a wide range of competencies that are specified by discipline certification standards and state licensing requirements. While employers expect knowledge and skills competency in disciplinary practice areas for employees holding the master's degree and the professional doctorate, the qualities they most desire for entry-level professionals include a range of transferrable professional competencies (Council of Graduate Schools, 2007; Gallagher, 2014, 2015). These skills are embedded within graduate training programs in audiology and speech-language pathology, and students are expected to demonstrate competencies in these skills in addition to clinical practice skills.

Transferrable professional competencies include leadership, communication, critical thinking and problem solving, collaborative teaming, and access to a network of new professionals who contribute additional expertise to the employer's network. Employers most value employees who have developed transferrable professional competencies within the context of integrated professional experiences (Gallagher, 2014, 2015). When leadership, communication, critical thinking, problem solving, and collaboration are practiced simultaneously with disciplinary competencies, the skills translate more readily to the workplace than when they are acquired in discrete experiences through workshops or seminars. Sekuler (2011) found that the global diversity of today's workforce requires transferrable professional knowledge and skills, such as leadership, entrepreneurship, and knowledge transfer as pathways to valuable career opportunities for those with global competencies. Further supporting the Council of Graduate Schools (2007), Gallagher (2014, 2015), and Sekuler (2011), the National Association of Colleges and Employers (NACE) identifies eight transferrable competencies essential for "career readiness" of college graduates (NACE, 2019). "Global/intercultural fluency," defined as understanding and valuing multicultural differences, is included among the transferrable competencies essential for career readiness identified by NACE (2019). For professionals who seek to practice clinically, foster research, or advance to leadership roles within the global workplace, transferrable global knowledge and skills are essential.

Hyter, Roman, Staley, and McPherson (2017) completed a comprehensive literature review to achieve two important aims related to understanding the competencies, or knowledge and skills associated with global careers in audiology and speech-language pathology. The first was to explain the role of globalization's impact on the professions. The second was to develop an initial model of global knowledge and skills important for practice in the professions of audiology and speech-language pathology. Hyter et al. (2017) shared that professionals gain global competence from the experience of living and working with people from multiple cultures. They stated that study abroad experiences, in conjunction with coursework and practicum, lead to those competencies. Based on their analysis, Hyter et al. (2017) established the "Framework for Global Engagement Competencies." This framework expands the global competencies in audiology and speech-language pathology to include "dispositions" and "attitudes" in addition to "knowledge" and "skills" identified by Helms (2015) and Sekuler (2011). The model offers a rubric for defining and evaluating competencies organized into categories. For example, the authors note that humility, self-reflection, empathy, inquisitiveness, and promotion of social justice are behaviors that exemplify competencies associated with a person's "dispositions." Understanding one's own culture and that of others, the impact of economic privilege, and the political and cultural elements of the country are among the competencies associated with "knowledge." Evidence of competencies associated with "skills" includes experience with diverse cultures and the ability to create an environment that is culturally/globally responsive; while evidence of the competencies associated with "attitudes" includes reciprocity of knowledge and beliefs associated with communication as a human right. Appendix 7–A includes the framework created by Hyter et al. (2017) to guide professionals in self-analysis of current global competence. It can also serve as a tool to guide development of the kind of international alliance that can foster development of global competencies that are important for global practice or research.

Harten, Franca, Boyer, and Pegoraro-Krook (2018) affirm the workforce demand for global competencies, such as those developed through international alliances. They recommend that universities develop international alliances to address the growing need for globally prepared practitioners and researchers, as outlined by ASHA (2018c). International alliances add global cultural competencies to the knowledge, skills, and related competencies associated with multicultural domestic competence that are essential for practitioners and researchers in the global community. The knowledge and skills acquired within international alliances establish interprofessional collaborations required for culturally informed and appropriate practices. When the international alliances follow best practice guidelines, the alliances also create sustainable services in countries where audiology and speech-language pathology services may not exist or are limited. International alliances that seek to establish sustainable services within an underresourced country support the advocacy roles of professionals in training and those who are credentialed. Sustainable services have the potential to foster international alliances focusing on research that can further inform global practice. These alliances reflect the level of cultural awareness and diverse perspectives that build on the global knowledge competencies described by Hyter et al. (2017) and impact practice as envisioned by Franca, Flowers, Smith, and Pitt (2007).

Aligned with perspectives on the importance of international alliances promoting global competencies, Randazzo and Garcia (2018) amplify the importance of globally prepared professionals. For practitioners who aim to offer culturally relevant services in under-resourced environments, specific knowledge and expertise are required. The authors connect their work to the World Health Organization *World Report on Disability* (WHO, 2011). Based on an international service delivery model in Cambodia, Randazzo and Garcia (2018) identified guidelines for effective global service delivery models in underresourced countries. The guidelines are based on "biopsychosocial" clinical practices. Biopsychosocial clinical practices use culturally appropriate training to engage members of the family and community as intervention partners so that services will continue after the professionals depart. This approach is in contrast to the traditional model of training a clinical service provider for that role. Randazzo and Garcia (2018) identified culturally relevant, holistic, accessible, and sustainable clinical competencies as those aligned with biopsychosocial practices. They suggested that international alliances that provide voluntary short-term access to services in underresourced countries should be coordinated with local health care programs to promote sustainability of services through the transfer of expertise to providers who reside locally.

International alliances create experiences for professionals in training, credentialed professionals, and researchers that are essential for developing the knowledge, skills, dispositions, and attitudes required for career success in today's global community. Global competencies integrated with disciplinary competencies lead to acquisition of the transferrable professional knowledge, skills, and professional networks essential for today's global clinical and research communities.

International Alliances Promoting Global Competencies Grounded in Standards of Practice

As our global society evolves, it is increasingly important that educators and health care providers, such as speech-language pathologists (SLPs) and audiologists, are prepared to deliver services that are relevant in a multicultural context. The International Issues Board of the American Speech-Language-Hearing Association (ASHA, 2019a) monitors global issues that impact science and our professions, and emphasizes the multicultural impact that professionals trained in communication sciences and disorders can exact.

ASHA Standards of Practice Aligned with Global Competencies

The Scope of Practice in Speech-Language-Pathology (CFCC/SLP, 2018a) specifies that SLPs must be skilled in providing services that are culturally and linguistically appropriate for their clients. The Council for Clinical Certification in Audiology and Speech-Language Pathology (CFCC/SLP, 2018a) requires that candidates for the Certificate of Clinical Competence (CCC/SLP) understand the cultural correlates associated with their clinical practices. Similarly, the Scope of Practice in Audiology (ASHA, 2018a) acknowledges that audiologists provide "person-centered care" that includes competence in considering the psychological, social, cultural, and environmental factors that influence treatment; and the Council for Clinical Certification in Audiology (CFCC/A, 2018b) includes competencies for applying cultural correlates to assessment and treatment in audiology practice.

ASHA Standards of Practice Aligned with the World Health Organization's International Classification of Functioning

The CFCC's diagnostic categories are aligned with the World Health Organization's (WHO, 2001) *International Classification of Functioning, Disability, and Health* (ICF). The ICF framework for management of health (WHO, 2001) is utilized in many countries as a collaborative approach for evaluating health and disability status (McNeilly, 2018). It focuses on the contexts that may impact an individual's life, including family, work, government agencies, laws, and cultural beliefs that can positively or negatively influence health conditions and outcomes. The Scope of Practice in Audiology (ASHA, 2018a) and Speech-Language Pathology (ASHA, 2016), Certificate of Clinical Competence in speech-language pathology (CCC/SLP; CFCC/SLP, 2018a), Certificate of Clinical Competence in audiology (CFCC/A, 2018b), and ICF framework (WHO, 2001) each identify the critical role of cultural competence.

ASHA Standards of Practice Aligned with Interprofessional Practice

In addition to alignment with WHO standards, ASHA (2016, 2018a, 2018b) and McNeilly (2018) acknowledge the integration of interprofessional practice competencies within the scopes of practice in audiology and speech-language pathology. The Interprofessional Education Collaborative (2016) specifies among its core competencies for interprofessional collaborative practice that members of collaborative teams embrace and mutually respect the cultural diversity and unique cultural values of patients and of the members of the health professions who may represent many domestic and global cultures. Building on a shared vision, interprofessional practice fosters the community-building essential for sustainable practice. Such effective approaches to clinical management require an understanding of the cultural issues that influence health care and education.

ASHA's Strategic Pathways Aligned with Global Competencies

Further supporting the standards of global competence associated with international alliances that foster global competencies, the American Speech-Language-Hearing Association's *Strategic Pathway to Excellence* (ASHA, 2018c) specifically identifies enhancing international engagement and increasing the cultural competence of ASHA members as strategic objectives. *ASHA's Envisioned Future: 2025* verifies the goal of collaborating with speech-language, hearing, and health organizations worldwide to strengthen the exchange of knowledge.

Another of ASHA's strategic pathways to excellence is "practicing at the top of the license." McNeilly (2018) states that practice at the top of the license means providing services that meet standards of inclusivity and evidence, while also addressing the needs of the client and family members who are impacted by the communication disorder. Inclusive competencies for speech-language pathologists and audiologists, such as those outlined above that embrace and mutually respect cultural diversity, lead to enhanced service delivery for clients while simultaneously helping service providers to practice at the top of their license (McNeilly, 2018).

Role of International Alliances Meeting Global Competencies Aligned with Standards of Practice

An international alliance creates a broad multicultural knowledge base and offers strategies for engaging with families to enhance clinical outcomes. An international professional network provides access to resources for clinical decision making and practice resources important for serving the broad demographic of a multicultural society. The opportunity to complete a clinical practicum experience at an international location, or to study and observe clinical practice internationally, creates a foundational understanding of the global community (Helms, 2015).

International alliances are designed to provide pre-professionals, certified practitioners, and researchers with a wide range of options (initial exposure, courses, clinical practicum, research engagement) needed to meet the demands for career success in a global community. The alliance may provide a pathway to credentialed clinical practice in English-speaking countries, including Canada, the United Kingdom, and Australia. The experience may include practice in non-English speaking countries for practitioners fluent in multiple languages. The alliance may serve as a pathway to promote and advocate for sustainable services in underresourced countries where speech-language pathology and audiology services are limited or unavailable. The alliance can create international research partnerships to promote global investigation of dynamic research questions. Presenting new knowledge in international forums provides a context for broadening the impact of research and fosters important professional partnerships (Watters et al., 2010).

Types of International Alliances that Promote Global Competence

International alliances are developed and offered by a variety of organizations, including professional societies, colleges and universities, service-learning programs, and research and scholarship programs.

Augustine (2012) outlined practices that promote global collaborations at colleges and universities where challenges, such as funding and curricular expansion, can be barriers to establishing international alliances. For professional programs where the academic offerings must meet accreditation standards in order for graduates to be eligible for clinical practice, domestic and international disciplinary societies can eliminate barriers by establishing collaborative standards of accreditation and practice that promote global exchange of professionals. This approach, sometimes called "globalization of the profession," has been more widely adopted in business and engineering. ASHA's International Issues Board (IIB) (ASHA, 2019a) currently provides leadership to facilitate global relationships that advance the science and research of the professions. Examples from ASHA's IIB and from other organizations are outlined in more detail in the section that follows.

Programs that seek to globalize their curriculum through international alliances can create a *global mentor or supervisors' network* to connect students and practitioners with certified personnel abroad. This ensures that their global clinical experiences will meet certification standards. Another important practice includes hosting a *global ambassadors program* that connects those who are ready to launch global careers with international opportunities for employment.

Colleges and universities offer alliances to achieve important mission-focused goals. One goal is to promote global competencies for both degree-seeking and non-degree seeking students or program alumni. Universities also create alliances to promote international scholarship and facilitate scholarly exchanges, each of which is important to the institution's commitment to knowledge creation.

Disciplinary and health organizations create international alliances to achieve the international goals established by their governing boards often through service-learning models. Service-learning programs foster alliances to strengthen access to services in underserved areas and create international learning experiences for practitioners, university faculty, and practicum students. The societies also collaborate with universities to strengthen opportunities for international exchange of knowledge and to create new educational programs at international locations.

Research alliances are available through several key programs that are designed to foster global exchanges of knowledge and scholarship. Research alliances strengthen research evidence for practice and add new knowledge about the cultural elements of practice important for achieving treatment outcomes.

International Alliances Promoting Global Competencies Through the American Speech-Language-Hearing Association and Other National Organizations

In service to achieving the strategic goals of promoting international engagement and practicing at the top of the license and with an aim to globalize professional knowledge, skills, and research, ASHA and other national organizations have established several important international alliances. Those previewed here represent examples of high-impact alliances with potential for replication by other organizations.

Mutual Recognition of Professional Credentials

Among ASHA's international alliances is the *2017 Agreement for Mutual Recognition of Professional Association Credentials* (ASHA, 2017). This powerful international alliance creates a pathway for mutual recognition of the requirements for certification or membership of speech-language pathologists. Such organizations in English-speaking countries include the American Speech-Language-Hearing Association, the Speech-Language and Audiology Association of Canada, the Irish Association of Speech-Language Therapists, the New Zealand Speech-Language Therapists' Association, the Royal College of Speech and Language Therapists, and the Speech Language Association of Australia Limited.

The *Agreement for Mutual Recognition of Professional Association Credentials* advanced by ASHA's Special Interest Group 17 Global Issues in Communication Sciences and Related Disorders (SIG 17) (ASHA, 2019b) creates an efficient process for earning mutual certification in participating countries. Once certification in the home country is achieved, professionals are recognized as having the qualifications required for credentialing needed to practice within these English-speaking countries. The agreement alerts those who earn mutual certification that other legal or immigration standards emerging from national, state, or provincial laws may need to be considered. This agreement was designed to promote global exchange. Details for earning mutual recognition credentials, including any additional requirements related to examinations, internships, or certification, are available at: https://www.asha.org/uploadedFiles/Cred RecognitionAgreement.pdf (ASHA 2017).

The ASHA-PAHO Collaboration

Adding to the opportunities that foster achievement of the standards of practice associated with international alliances, ASHA serves as a non-state actor (NSA) in an alliance with the Pan American Health Organization (PAHO). Through the ASHA-PAHO Collaboration, ad hoc committees created educational programs in Honduras and Guyana, along with educational resources and opportunities to foster sustainable services (Waterson, Duttine, Roman, & Caesar, 2018).

ASHA's Special Interest Group 17

The mission of ASHA's Special Interest Group 17 Global Issues in Communication Sciences and Related Disorders

(ASHA, 2019b) focuses on programs to advance research, clinical practice, and related experiences that promote globalization of the professions. In addition to the alliances described, SIG 17 publishes Perspectives of the ASHA Special Interest Group 17, offers webinars, discussions, courses, and conference and convention sessions on globalization and global careers. The group hosts an online community to discuss international issues along with an annual meeting at the ASHA Convention each November. Details on all of the resources available through SIG 17 are available at https://www.asha.org/SIG/17/About-SIG-17/

Europe's International Alliances Promoting Global Competencies

Beyond the United States, speech-language pathology has been acknowledged as a global autonomous profession practiced across many countries. To create standards for competent speech-language therapists (SLTs) to practice across cultures in Europe, the *Network for Tuning Standards and Quality of Education Programs in Speech and Language Therapy/Logopedics across Europe* (NetQues) was initiated. This multi-nation collaboration created benchmarks for educational and clinical competencies of SLTs in participating countries in Europe and has developed a model of cross-borders collaboration in education and research to improve clinical practice (Patterson, Hansson, Lowit, Stansfield, & Trinite, 2015). The principles of practice emerging from this alliance have amplified competencies in diversity and multiculturalism to form benchmarks for clinical practice across many countries and cultures in Europe.

International Alliances Promoting Global Competencies Through Colleges and Universities

Colleges and universities are an essential resource for access to international alliances that provide a pathway to global competencies. Some alliances offer an experience limited to learning about how audiology and speech-language pathology are practiced at an international location and the requirements for practice. Short-term alliances also focus on fostering interest in returning for a more long-term program designed to acquire multicultural, interprofessional, and global competencies. Other alliances offer experiences to achieve standards of academic and cultural competence for careers in global markets. Selecting the most suitable alliance requires

an understanding of the characteristics that define their quality.

Characteristics of High-Quality Alliances

The American Council on Education Center for Internationalization and Global Engagement (2015) offers a summary of the essential elements for prospective students or practitioners to consider when seeking a successful international alliance to promote global career options. International alliances vary in scope and mission. To evaluate such programs and their value to individuals seeking global competence, the American Council on Education (ACE) developed parameters for assessing international alliances. The assessment parameters include transparency, engagement, and quality assurance. Understanding these criteria can guide development or selection of an international alliance (ACE, 2015).

Transparency. ACE (2015) identified transparency as a critical element to assess when considering international alliances. The Organisation for Economic Co-operation and Development (OECD) defines transparency as a complete description of the "knowledge, understanding and skills that a successful student should acquire" through this alliance (OECD, 2005). When developing an international alliance experience, it is critical to articulate a well-defined list of competencies that will be developed and methods for assessing their acquisition upon completion of the experience. The competencies should be clearly specified in published materials, along with credit or non-credit policies and support services that strengthen success. Cost and financial aid relative to the experience should also be clearly stated (New England Association of Schools and Colleges, 2003). In fields such as communication sciences and disorders that require program accreditation, public information should specify how the experience facilitates professional development of students or faculty in support of the program's stated mission and its accreditation standards.

Some alliances are designed to develop broad cultural competencies and networking important for future research and practice. These alliances may focus on visiting research laboratories and/or clinical facilities to observe research or practice. Some may focus on service delivery and provide appropriately credentialed alumni with opportunities to engage in community service abroad. Other alliances may be specifically designed to meet learning outcomes that demonstrate alignment with clinical certification and/or program accreditation standards. When alliance experiences are an integral part of a degree program, whether elective or required, the program should specify learning objectives, associated educational activities that will be assessed to show knowledge and skill acquisition, and the certification standards to which these are mapped. As in other courses, how learning will be assessed and the standards for doing so should be explicit. These elements are typically presented as part of a course syllabus similar to those of other courses in the approved program of study. The alliance experience may also be an integral program element that is used as evidence of meeting accreditation standards. Materials promoting the alliance must state that the program meets standards for regional and discipline accreditation, name the accrediting bodies, and specify how the experience helps the program to demonstrate accreditation standards. Examples of how an international alliance can support program accreditation include, but are not limited to, development of faculty sufficiency through interprofessional research and teaching collaborations; development of student competencies through culturally relevant instruction, research, or clinical practice opportunities; and/or demonstration of curriculum sufficiency through development of coursework that develops international professional competencies not otherwise available within the degree program.

Engagement. Another factor for evaluating an international alliance is the engagement of the program faculty and the alliance institution (ACE, 2015). It is important that faculty have decision-making responsibilities associated with the alliance as their engagement shapes the nature and quality of the experience. Faculty engagement may range from a single faculty member with an international network who initiates alliances and serves as a champion to foster additional faculty and student engagement, to faculty who teach and lead programs as program directors. When deciding whether to participate in an international experience, students should understand the level of faculty engagement. This factor is an essential element for participants to examine to be sure the program will meet their needs and help them achieve their individual objectives. The university should also have the infrastructure to support faculty alliances. For example, universities typically designate a study abroad administrative unit that systematically reviews its programs and can provide information about the value of the program to anyone interested in the program.

Quality Assurance. Programs ensure quality using a variety of standards that often focus on three key areas of measurement: accreditation, assessment of student learning outcomes, and risk assessment. Quality assurance may begin with the regional and academic accreditation of the program. The accreditation should

be public, and students completing the degrees should know prior to initiating the program that their degree will meet required standards of practice. They should be able to determine the stated goals for an international experience and see how the experience will fulfill those goals. If a stated goal is earning one or more degrees through a joint or dual degree alliance, the student should understand the specific role of the international alliance experience in attaining their degree(s). Accrediting bodies require this kind of information to be publicized to students in a transparent manner, and the university to deliver the experience as stated publicly.

In addition to accreditation, all programs that offer international experiences should have published assessment data relative to the student learning outcomes of each experience. These data should verify that students who participated in the program achieved the desired learning outcomes and stated objectives of each experience. Assessment data showing student learning outcomes should be publicized and made readily available, either online or upon request.

Finally, programs should provide information about potential risks of international alliance experiences. The Forum on Education Abroad (2011) established that all participants in an international alliance should be informed about the potential risks of participation and how to manage those risks. Common risk factors when traveling abroad include economic, health, and safety concerns. These issues are often manageable, but participants should be informed of the risks, suggested strategies for dealing with them, and the university and program supports that will be available to assist in risk management during the experience.

College and University Alliances for Students and Alumni

College and university alliances range from faculty-led programs abroad and international exchanges to dual and joint degree programs. A variety of offerings allows students to assess which type of program may be best suited to their interests, their degree, and their future employment. In the fields of audiology and speech-language pathology, some faculty-led programs and exchanges are offered on a recurring basis so that multiple cohorts of students have access to the experience. Dual and joint degree programs are less common offerings for students. Faculty members leading degree programs may hold joint appointments in both a U.S. institution and an international university and may hold credentials to practice and supervise at an international location. Faculty-led international programs may be taught at one or more partner university or clinical facility abroad and may include a third-party organization responsible for the structure of the experience. International alliance experiences may be open to alumni as well as enrolled students. Alumni can enhance the international experience for student participants while simultaneously expanding their own cultural competence.

Faculty-Led Study Abroad Programs. Universities often offer opportunities for informal international alliance experiences that incorporate study at one or more international locations. These experiences are led or taught by domestic program faculty members alone or in collaboration with international faculty members on site. They are informal in the sense that they are not necessary to degree completion, may not be offered for academic credit, and may be offered infrequently depending on demand and faculty availability.

Important considerations for informal faculty-led alliances include student status and transcript-approved credit. In terms of student status to participate in an international alliance experience, requirements often vary. Programs may be offered to students currently enrolled in a degree program, students enrolled at the university but not in the program that developed the experience, or to credentialed practitioners who return as non-degree-seeking students who may or may not be affiliated with the institution. Programs often include an opportunity to network with clinical service providers and administrators to foster interest in international clinical practice. Designed to be experiential in nature, the programs may help participants understand the steps needed to be eligible to practice internationally. Faculty-led programs may be offered during scheduled university breaks when students are not enrolled in other classes, during breaks between academic terms, or at times when practicing professionals can participate. Faculty-led programs often offer opportunities to observe clinical practice, sometimes across multiple international locations. This allows participants to broaden their perspective on practice standards and methods and helps them understand international similarities and differences in the practice of audiology and speech-language pathology.

Faculty-led programs may vary in terms of the academic credit associated with the experience. Some programs are offered for academic credit, while others may be offered for optional or no academic credit. Credit-bearing seminars compliment the international experience by increasing content knowledge, providing clinical practice experience, and/or allowing for evidence-based research in an international forum. Non-credit opportunities are equally valuable experiences and may include acknowledgment of the experience on the participant's academic transcript upon successful completion of the program.

Availability of programs in an abbreviated format, offered during one- or two-week breaks in the traditional academic schedule, and led by program faculty familiar to participants, make these informal alliances ideal as an initial global immersion experience. Their structure increases opportunities for participation by both degree and non-degree-seeking practicing professionals.

The program in Communication Sciences and Disorders (CSD) at Illinois State University (ISU) (Illinois State University, 2019) offers graduate and undergraduate students an experience that meets the characteristics of a high-quality international alliance. Led by the program's faculty and clinical educators, the international program features a one- to two-week experience over an institutional break that is designed to foster knowledge of the cultural and historical context of the professions and health care in the countries visited. The three-hour credit-bearing program focuses on competencies related to service delivery and clinical practice models employed within the countries visited. The course of study specifies learning outcomes and how these are assessed. This international experience connects students to an international network of practicing professionals and has been identified as a distinction that is attractive to potential program applicants. Dr. Ann Beck, Chair, stated, "The faculty value the cultural knowledge and skills that CSD students at ISU gain and equally value achievement of the institution's commitment to promoting cultural knowledge through international experiences" (A. Beck, personal communication, March 4, 2019).

De Diego-Lazaro (2018) provided an example of a study abroad program designed to foster cultural competence for students in training and to establish sustainable practices after the program concludes. The collaborators include Arizona State University, a nonprofit organization, and a facility in Jinotega, Nicaragua that provides education for individuals with hearing impairment. Practices from this program include an offer of academic credit, comprehensive predeparture training, immersion during a scheduled university break, opportunities to develop or further develop a second language, and transparent and clearly defined goals leading to cultural competencies. Students and supervisors collaborate with teachers and families to develop intervention strategies for clients that are sustainable upon their departure. An important contribution from this project was the application of the Cultural Awareness and Competence Scales (CACS) (De Diego-Lazaro, 2016) to assess outcomes in a pre- and post-study abroad design. While the number of students assessed using CACS was too small to apply statistical analysis, a descriptive qualitative analysis of data before and after study abroad experiences suggested increases in cultural competencies, but less impact on cultural awareness and self-efficacy. The authors suggested that a longer experience may be essential for advancing competencies in these areas.

Exchange Programs. One type of inter-institutional collaboration with an international partner, typically a university, is an international exchange program. The collaborating or "exchange" universities develop a formal legal agreement often called a "Memorandum of Understanding" or "Memorandum of Agreement" (MOU/MOA). The MOU establishes guiding principles of the alliance. The Council of Graduate Schools (2010) identified 10 principles of effective graduate-level collaborations during the 2009 Strategic Leaders Global Summit on Graduate Education. Denecke and Kent (2010) created an MOU Checklist to guide development of international collaborations; and Klomparens (2008) developed best practice guidelines on inter-institutional agreements. Best practice principles for MOUs and inter-institutional agreements should include clearly established benefits for all stakeholders, including the students, faculty, institutions, and countries. Another important standard includes identification of the learning outcomes and ways they will be measured. A third standard requires identification of support mechanisms to foster the success of those who participate. Appendix 7–B includes the *MOU Checklist for International Collaborations* created by Denecke and Kent (2010) to guide best practices for development of MOUs/MOAs.

Based on the MOU, exchange programs may be designed as a one- or two-way exchange. A one-way alliance may present a student from an institution in the United States with a cultural immersion opportunity abroad for a term of study or a longer period. At some universities, a one-way alliance may be referred to as "direct enrollment with the international institution." A one-way alliance does not require that students from the United States "exchange" with an equal number of students from an international partner institution. This type of agreement allows students from the United States to experience cultural immersion abroad. Alternatively, other one-way agreements that do not require an exchange create access to multicultural students who can be recruited from the collaborating international institution in order to systematically introduce domestic students to multicultural perspectives.

For students from the United States going abroad through a one-way exchange, the program must demonstrate that the curriculum at the international location meets regional and professional accreditation requirements, that the international partner has the faculty and clinical supervisors who meet required standards, and that there are appropriate housing and support services for domestic students who participate. To allow for the transfer of academic credit, courses and practicum expe-

riences must meet university and program requirements, as governed by clinical certification and program accreditation standards. Program faculty serve in an advisory capacity and support participation in the program. A site visit by a department or program representative to the international location prior to enrollment of students ensures that all of the curricular, facilities, and housing arrangements are in place to support the students who participate in the program.

One-way programs are also valued as an opportunity for students in the United States to study with well-regarded international faculty members. The study may include courses that offer advanced coursework in a specialized area of the curriculum, provide access to content knowledge that may not be available at the U.S. university, and allow comparative study of educational systems in the host country. In some cases, areas of specialization in the curriculum may be linked to a student's research interests. The alliance is often accompanied by opportunities to observe and network with professionals who are practicing in a variety of clinical locations. Some one-way programs are specifically developed to provide advanced clinical training and intra-professional practice. Another important goal of a one-way international program is for students in the United States to learn about international disciplinary organizations that influence practice abroad. Knowledge of the requirements for clinical practice beyond those expected for practice in the United States helps participants plan for future international employment, if that is their goal.

Students from the United States enrolled in a one-way study abroad program at an international location must work with their academic advisor to confirm that the specialized course of study meets requirements for transfer of academic credit upon return from the international experience. Based on a student's intended career pathway, the focus of the program may be on coursework, research, supervised clinical practicum in a multicultural environment, or a combination of these activities. The program may require certain courses for all participants, such as an introductory course to the culture. Some programs may allow a student and faculty advisor to develop coursework that is highly specific to the student's interests.

Exchange programs, sometimes referenced as "reciprocating exchanges" (Harten, Franca, Boyer, & Pegoraro-Krook, 2018) require that domestic students exchange with international students from a partnering institution, and that a balance of exchanges is achieved over a specified period of time. During an exchange, the international partner selects candidates to study in the United States, and the domestic university selects candidates to study at the international partner university. The MOU outlines the process used to maintain an equal balance of exchange students. Each institution benefits from the disciplinary and cultural knowledge shared by engagement with students who participate in the exchange.

Students considering participation in an exchange program value strategies that help to manage program costs. The MOU between the collaborating institutions typically specifies that exchange students are assessed costs associated with enrolling in the home institution. The programs often offer comparable living accommodations at the exchange institution, as well. Given the familiar parameters of the cost structure of their home university, and the assurance of housing at the partner institution, students may feel more comfortable enrolling in an international exchange experience.

Another valuable function of an exchange alliance is to offer a predetermined curriculum that is completed by all students selected for the exchange. Exchange programs may be part of an undergraduate curriculum or a graduate curriculum. The curriculum is delivered in English and transfers back to the student's home institution at the conclusion of the exchange. The curriculum is developed in conjunction with university constituents for study abroad experiences (i.e., study abroad office; registrar; student health services) to ensure that it meets required regional and disciplinary clinical certification and accreditation standards, as appropriate. The curriculum may include didactic courses or clinical practicum experiences. Program faculty and advisors are tasked with confirming that the experiences meet clinical certification and/or program accreditation standards so that the courses taken abroad apply to the student's degree program. A member of the program faculty provides advisement to exchange students and maintains contact with exchange students during the experience.

Exchanges often include opportunities for the students to present and share information about the discipline and their culture to a broad range of constituents, including current students, program alumni, practitioners, and faculty. The value of the exchange to students is the opportunity to learn about the discipline from local practitioners and faculty, and to master transferrable competencies associated with multicultural awareness via engagement with them and other students at the site. The opportunity for a full-term or longer period of study establishes a long-term impact for the participant and fellow participants, creating an international network of colleagues for years to come. The networks foster additional interest in both practice at an international location and practice in the United States and help create pipelines of potential professionals who have developed the transferrable international competencies important to preparing for an international career.

Exchange programs following an MOU that adhere to principles of best practices also include a comprehensive orientation or predeparture program. This ensures that those selected for the program have the required travel documents and guidance on travel practices prior to initiating the program. This predeparture program is often delivered by the university study abroad or international office prior to departure, and additional support is available during the term abroad. When exchange students return to the home department following an exchange, they are often invited to share their experience with the larger program community. An established study abroad exchange often advances an alliance toward a "transformational" high-impact learning experience that strengthens a student's disciplinary, research, and professional competencies and career pathways (American Council on Education, 2015, p. 36). In 2007, the National Survey of Student Engagement (NSSE) stated the following based on survey results: "Students who took part in one or more 'high-impact' practice such as a learning community, research with faculty, study abroad, and culminating senior experience reported greater levels of deep learning and greater gains in learning and personal development" (National Survey of Student Engagement, 2007, p. 13).

Dr. Yvette D. Hyter, Professor and Graduate Coordinator of the Speech, Language and Hearing Sciences (SLHS) Program at Western Michigan University (WMU), shared the evolution of the WMU SLHS summer study abroad program in Senegal, Africa. The program also reflects the standards of best practice described previously. The Cultural Connections Senegal Summer Program (Western Michigan University, 2019) evolved from a collaboration with a visiting scholar with ties to the country. The program then advanced with two grants from the Fulbright-Hays Program that funded the travel critical for strengthening the network of relationships needed in order to create the current faculty-led study abroad experience. Faculty from multiple colleges and disciplines, including speech-language and hearing sciences, special education, education, political science, health administration, and others contribute to the program's interdisciplinary and interprofessional experiences. The program's learning outcomes promote understanding of cultural differences in order to think critically about culturally responsive practices across the multiple disciplines participating in the program. A comprehensive predeparture program includes the cultural history of Senegal. While on-site, the participants visit surrounding communities to learn about the culture and history of the country, and to gain insights about how communities have addressed the effects of globalization with limited resources. The program supports undergraduates, graduates, and practicing professionals who may enroll as non-degree or temporary students. Three hours of credit are earned, and participants are required to complete a capstone project. Dr. Hyter shared the following observation about the program in Senegal: "The most important goal for this program is to develop reciprocal and sustainable practices. Our intent is to walk side-by-side with our collaborators and learn how to contribute through their knowledge of the culture." Dr. Hyter noted that reciprocity to advance to an exchange program is a future goal (Y. Hyter, personal communication, March 11, 2019).

Dual Degree and Joint Degree Programs. Dual international degrees offer a course of study, usually between one domestic university and one international university, that earns two diplomas, including one from each institution upon completion of the degree requirements. In contrast, a joint international degree provides a curriculum of study, typically at one domestic and one international university, that leads to a single diploma upon completion of the work at the participating institutions. The single diploma, issued by the domestic institution, should either include the seals and signatures of officials from both institutions or be accompanied by documents such as transcripts or certificates that verify the international elements of the program.

Joint and dual degree programs are international alliances that often evolve over a period of time in which the partner institutions have benefited from an informal alliance and determined that strengthening the alliance by creating a degree program would be mutually beneficial. Joint and dual degrees are sometimes initiated through faculty who are alumni of an international university and have maintained an ongoing strategic research or professional relationship with the institution. An alumnus faculty connection is important for program success and sustainability because such individuals are stakeholders in both university partners and often committed to the long-term success of the degree program that is created. Dual and joint degree programs may also emerge from networking with faculty at international universities via research, service, or professional outreach at international conferences and meetings. Based on the informal alliances, programs can establish an equal and vested interest in a formal strategic international alliance. Factors that motivate shifting from an informal or "ad hoc" alliance to a formal strategic long-term arrangement are connected to a commitment to meeting academic program or institutional goals to foster tangible benefits. Such benefits include attracting international students to the program to bolster program quality through the multicultural competencies in research and practice that these degrees create (Denecke & Kent, 2010).

Denecke and Kent (2010) further described other features of dual and joint degrees that should be considered as universities evaluate their potential for achieving program and institutional goals. Joint and dual degrees are more prevalent at the master's level in comparison to doctoral study. Dual and joint degrees have been most frequently developed in the disciplines of business and engineering, fields that also require attention not only to regional accreditation and state oversight, but also academic accreditation. These disciplines are often used as templates for considering development of dual or joint programs. Non-financial factors to consider for strategic long-term international alliances include negotiating the memorandum of understanding, ensuring sustainability, and recruiting students. Financial factors focus on the funding needed to develop the programs and the fee structures important to their success. Resolution of academic credit issues can present challenges; however, many institutions have established "double counting" and thesis/dissertation credit policies that can be attractive to applicants.

Among available degree options, dual degrees are the most prevalent, but are rare in professional fields leading to clinical practice. The challenges associated with meeting disciplinary program accreditation standards, as well as credentialing standards required for practice, can present barriers for degree programs in clinical practice disciplines. Joint and dual degree programs typically require that faculty travel between alliance locations, often requiring institutional or external funds to support their travel requirements. These degree programs may be offered for a specific period of time, and decisions regarding their continuance may depend upon student, faculty, and university assessment of their effectiveness in meeting expected outcomes.

College and University Offices and Agencies that Guide Access to International Alliances

Academic programs in communication sciences and disorders are the initial starting point for seeking an international experience while studying or after degree completion. An academic advisor or faculty mentor can provide guidance and assistance in finding a program that best suits an individual student's degree progress and interests.

The university's study abroad office is another resource for students, or practitioners returning for professional development, who seek a study abroad experience when a program or department currently does not offer a program. The study abroad office may have information on international experiences offered through partner universities or through other programs that may be valuable to those in the speech-language pathology and audiology disciplines.

The university's office of international students and scholars, or international services office, can provide information about multicultural experiences offered on the campus. Engaging with the local international community, composed of international students, faculty, and staff, may help begin a network important for access to a future international experience.

Individuals may seek to research programs on their own, without the assistance of a university. In the field of international education there are private companies, non-profit and for-profit organizations that offer a wide variety of programs including study, internship, research, volunteer, and work abroad opportunities. It is imperative prior to committing to a program that an individual is able to verify the operating status of the company, partners with whom they work, professional associations that they belong to, and alumni who have successfully completed the program. A thorough investigation of participant support services is recommended, ranging from housing to visa application assistance to professional liability insurance for experiences in clinical settings.

Many university study abroad offices are open to assisting in the research of a unique program. They may allow a student to petition for an independent study opportunity not already vetted and approved by the institution. A petition may consist of a written proposal, estimated budget, and faculty letters of support. A committee composed of faculty and staff review the petition and determine if the program is suitable for an academic credit-bearing experience. If the program is not associated with university credit, the institution may not engage in a petition process with the student but will instead point to outside vetting resources to ensure the program is safe and well executed.

International Immersion Experiences

Some international alliances are developed as guided immersion experiences that afford participants the chance to advance their bilingual competencies while collaborating with local practitioners in service delivery. EBS United, a non-profit division of EBS Healthcare, provides a bilingual immersion program that is designed to help clinical professionals as they seek to advance their skills in listening, speaking, reading, and writing in Spanish during coordinated volunteer experiences (EBS United, 2019). According to Jose Galarza who coordinates this program for EBS Healthcare, there has been a significant increase in interest among SLPs and other clinicians who seek short-term experiences to increase their cultural awareness and improve their second language proficiency (J. Galarza, personal communication,

February 10, 2019). The EBS Bilingual Immersion Program has been previously hosted in Mexico, Ecuador, and Costa Rica; and new sites continue to be developed. It is a three-week experience that pairs participants with a host family for the duration of their stay. This provides opportunities for contextualized language practice and cultural experiences in home and community settings. Participants also attend "language school" daily where they experience intensive, formalized instruction in the Spanish language. They work toward improved language comprehension, speaking, reading, and writing, as these skills are all critical for the bilingual practitioner. Lastly, participants are placed in a community agency that delivers services to individuals with communication disorders. While program participants do not assume primary responsibility for assessment or treatment during this experience, they collaborate with providers on site who do so. This part of the experience is much like a practicum experience in graduate school or a professional apprenticeship.

There are very few master's-prepared SLPs in Latin American countries. Rather, individuals with a variety of types and degrees of preparation identify themselves as speech-language therapists and provide communication services. There is a great need for more practicing professionals. In order to provide effective services in a Latin American country, practitioners must be able to speak Spanish fluently, both in conversation and in the professional discourse of the discipline. Because there are few available assessment or treatment materials, they must be able to create their own culturally appropriate tests and therapy tools. They should understand the infrastructure of the country in which they choose to practice, as the ways in which clients are referred for services vary significantly. There are few positions advertised for SLPs or other therapists even though there is a great need for service delivery. As such, a practitioner who would like to work in a Latin American country may need to do his/her own investigation of job possibilities and create the opportunity through his/her personal connections. Pay structures are often considerably lower for therapists who work abroad, so advanced financial planning for people considering this path is also important. Maintaining professional credentials earned in the United States, such as ASHA certification and state practice licensure for SLPs, is highly recommended (J. Galarza, personal communication, February 10, 2019).

The best pathway toward successful international employment, if desired, may be a step-wise approach that begins with an immersion experience and extends to a bilingual practitioner position in the United States. As the clinician develops the necessary cultural competencies and professional or personal connections in a target region abroad, plans can be made to transition to work in that country in the future.

International Alliances Through Service-Learning for Practitioners and Students

Service-learning experiences involve the provision of volunteer service to underserved countries that have little to no access to audiology and speech-language pathology services. Such international alliances create cultural competencies for the volunteers, including student clinicians and their faculty supervisors and collaborators, and also provide access to services for communities that are underserved. Such alliances should be guided by principles of best practice for each discipline delivering services and should incorporate clinical methods that are relevant to and appropriate for other cultures (Karle, Christensen, Gordon, & Nystrup, 2008). Service-learning opportunities are most often non-credit bearing experiences, and can be arranged by a number of organizations, groups, or individuals.

Alliances Promoting Sustainable Practices

Gill, Bharadwaj, Chance, Quick, and Wainscott (2016a) identified recent global developments that positively influence the potential for expansion of speech-language pathology services in underserved countries. Global efforts to educate more countries about health-related services and strengthen access offer new opportunities for collaborative international alliances. Universities may partner with international universities and local agencies to create long-term volunteer international immersion opportunities that lead to critically needed sustainable services and training programs within underserved host countries. Gill, Bharadwaj, Quick, Wainscott, and Chance (2016b) offer an exemplary international alliance model of long-term volunteering to establish sustainable services where access is limited or not available. The long-term volunteer program included a partnership between a charitable organization, the Connective Link Among Special Needs Programs International, the University of Zambia, Texas Woman's University, George Washington University, and Texas Tech University. The partnership was supported by university professors, lecturers, students, and practicing SLPs who volunteered to create an SLP training program that would provide long-term access to service after the volunteers were gone. Gill et al. (2016b) stated that the alliance was guided by principles of community-based participatory research developed by Israel, Schulz, Parker, and Becker (1998). These principles were designed to foster cultural relevance and sustainability of volunteer programs, and equally important, to avoid the failures associated with methods of practice that are not relevant to other cul

tures, as described by Karle, Christensen, Gordon, and Nystrup (2008). Guided by these principles, the university-agency volunteer service alliance resulted in a cohort of new master's-prepared practitioners and opportunities for their employment. Factors contributing to the program's success were building on existing strengths, creating culturally sensitive materials, achieving mutual benefits for all partners, recognizing and facilitating community involvement promoting co-learning, and cultivating a long-term solution.

Alliances Promoting Exchange of Best Practices

Ross-Swain, Fogel, and Schneider (2017) offered an alliance to promote international interprofessional collaboration. This alliance focused on the exchange of professional views on practice and the sharing of best practices globally. The collaborators in the exchange were 12 SLP members of the California Speech-Language-Hearing Association representing multiple work settings and representatives of the Finnish National Board of Education. The collaborating team met in Finland to review practices, including an emphasis on early intervention and implementation of interprofessional collaborations among many professions. These practices, along with other investments in education, have reduced the impact of speech-language delays on educational and social achievement and earned Finland "high global status" (Ross-Swain et al., 2017). An important practice for maximizing treatment outcomes emerged from this exchange. Participants conducted a systematic review of Finland's interprofessional collaborative practices that employ a cross-training of professionals model, consisting of multidisciplinary teams that include physicians, social workers, SLPs, and psychologists, to provide services to families. The intervention approaches used in Finland offer models for interprofessional collaborations that integrate international-level expertise into clinical practice.

International Alliances Promoting Global Research for Scholars

Universities and academic programs frequently promote development of transferrable global competencies using an international faculty model. Visiting international scholars may offer courses, practicum, and research that contribute to students' degrees. Programs may use a faculty exchange model, similar to the student exchange model, but faculty members execute the exchange. As with student exchanges, faculty exchanges and visiting international scholar programs typically require a Memorandum of Understanding, agreed to by both institutions, that specifies details about the experience including support from the home institution and support from the exchange institution. Typical arrangements require that the home institution handle compensation and travel for the faculty member; while appropriate housing will be provided by the exchange institution, along with access to office, laboratory, library, internet, and related university facilities.

Faculty exchange programs often promote joint research in areas of specialization and provide graduate students with access to an international research mentor. For example, there may be subsequent opportunity to continue the experience through a student exchange or one-way program of study at the international faculty member's institution. Another important outcome may include presenting research at the international university or at an international research conference. Networking with other international scholars and opportunities to publish in international journals are additional outcomes that enhance the value of faculty exchanges. Similarly, faculty in the program who exchange with the international partners may form research alliances with faculty and graduate students at the international location who may, in turn, be invited to the United States to discuss their projects and network with domestic students and faculty.

Visiting international scholars are often invited to teach courses or to engage in clinical supervision to foster mastery of internationally focused content and practice strategies. Visiting scholars may focus on case studies in rare disorder areas or offer new insights on treatment emerging from internationally focused evidence. Program alumni and practitioners are often invited to seminars to learn more about requirements for practice at the international location and to foster an interest in preparing for an international career pathway. Visiting scholars may also be invited to campus via faculty who have earned a Fulbright Award, as described below.

Research Alliances Through the Fulbright Program

The Fulbright Program (United States Bureau of Education and Cultural Affairs Exchange Programs, 2019) is a prestigious international exchange program that supports both faculty and student exchanges with the goal of fostering knowledge that transcends borders. The Fulbright Program was one of the earliest forms of funding committed to establishing international alliances through multiple forms of engagement for university faculty and students. Fulbright is sponsored by the United States government and funded by the Bureau of Educational and Cultural Affairs of the Department of State.

The Fulbright Scholars Program for U.S. Scholars offers faculty who hold terminal degrees and academic appointments, university administrators, and professionals across many disciplines competitive grant-funded support to pursue multiple projects. For example, Fulbright Scholars may propose a teaching award designed to advance the academic mission of both the home and the host institution, while also reflecting the culture of the host country. Teaching awards often create long-term curricular alliances that infuse transferrable multicultural competencies across both institutions. Research awards create opportunities to understand research questions from multicultural perspectives and address critical gaps in our understanding of human communication and evidence-based practice. Scholar awards may also consider joint teaching/research projects that connect the teaching and research missions of both universities. An essential element of all of the programs for scholars includes establishing a long-term alliance to broaden the impact of the project beyond the universities. A very important program for early career scholars is the Fulbright Postdoctoral and Early Career Awards. These awards provide an early career international alliance and network to scholars from across the globe. Creating an early career alliance and network fosters the long-term potential for high-impact international collaborations important for both research and professional practice. The Fulbright Student Program is specifically designed to provide graduate students with research and teaching opportunities abroad.

In addition to creating alliances abroad, Fulbright provides resources to promote access to visiting international scholars in multiple ways. The Visiting Scholars program offers access for international scholars to conduct research and/or lecture in the United States. The Scholar-in-Residence program creates access to international scholars for institutions that lack a strong international component or that are minority serving. The Outreach Lecturing Fund (OLF) creates access to visiting scholars who are already in the United States and are interested in establishing liaisons with other institutions. There are a wide range of options for the Scholars and Students Programs that can be reviewed at the Fulbright website, Fulbright Scholar Program (2019) https://www.cies.org/about-us

Molrine and Drayton (2013) provided an example of research conducted in part through a Fulbright Exchange Scholars grant. The project focused on competencies associated with culturally sensitive speech-language pathology service delivery in the English-speaking twin island Republic of Trinidad and Tobago. The cohort of eight SLPs, six trained in accredited programs in the

United States and two trained in the United Kingdom, and each of whom were currently practicing in Trinidad and Tobago, identified modifications needed in a graduate program aligned with speech-language pathology certification standards (ASHA, 2014) that were designed to lead to cultural competence. Their research revealed that understanding cultural, ethnic, and language use differences, understanding the need for intense client/family education, and collaborating with social and health systems were among the components needed to achieve cultural competence.

Research Alliances Through the Fogarty International Center

The Fogarty International Center also provides funding for scholars to advance the mission of the National Institutes of Health (NIH) and the National Institute on Deafness and Other Communication Disorders (NIDCD) through funding to facilitate research collaborations between U.S. and international scholars. Research on deafness and communication disorders are among the research topics where funding is available. Training awards often focus on low-resource locations that advance scientific knowledge for development of the best tools and practices for diagnosis and treatment. Funding support through the Fogarty Program (NIH, 2019) may be accessed at https://www.fic.nih.gov/Funding/Pages/Fogarty-Funding-Opps.aspx

Research Alliances Through Partnerships With Health/Medical Organizations

Legg and Penn (2014) developed a model for conducting research abroad that was partially funded by a partnership with the Medical Research Council of South Africa. Their anthropological research in an underresourced area of South Africa focused on addressing gaps in our understanding of culturally sensitive approaches to aphasia. Legg and Penn (2014) found that treatment outcomes rely on building culturally relevant spaces of support within the community. Their work again amplified the importance of evaluating cultural and social factors that support clinical treatment. Culturally relevant clinical practices are essential for creating the family and community networks that ensure sustained clinical improvements in patients, such as their clients with aphasia.

Research Alliances Through Other Research Partnerships

ASHA provides additional resources for research funding leading to international research alliances. ASHA members can access resources such as modules to guide development of interdisciplinary collaborations and Clinicians and Researchers Collaborating, (CLARC) among other resources at this link: https://www.asha.org/research/

Summary

International alliances produce benefits that extend well beyond the experience itself. For credentialed professionals, acquiring cultural competence through an international alliance provides a pathway to career success in today's global workforce. For students, an international experience expands their knowledge of clinical practice standards and methods in another country, enhances their bilingual competence, and encourages them to envision creative solutions for improving access to speech-language pathology and audiology services in underserved global communities. For faculty, international alliances extend their knowledge of pedagogy and forge new research alliances. For individuals with communication and hearing disorders, international alliances not only provide necessary services for the duration of the program, but may indeed be the impetus for creating sustainable services for their community for years into the future.

The combined impact of an international alliance is difficult to estimate, but hard to overstate. While speech-language pathologists and audiologists have not traditionally relocated outside the United States for employment, more are embracing bilingual practice and looking for opportunities to make a difference for underserved populations. Universities in partnership with one another, combined with faculty committed to developing global competencies for future speech-language pathologists and audiologists, will continue to advance these professions as they meet the challenge of increasing the cultural relevance of clinical practice for clients around the world through international alliances.

Critical Thinking

1. Multicultural competence and global competence are sometimes used interchangeably to label the knowledge and skills required to assess and treat individuals with speech-language-hearing disorders from diverse cultures. What distinguishes global competence from multicultural competence?

2. What professional advantages can audiologists and speech-language pathologists in training or in early clinical practice gain from participating in

international learning/clinical experiences? How can their expertise be distinguished from other practitioners who have not engaged in international learning/clinical experiences?

3. What can an experienced/mid-career audiologist or speech-language pathologist gain from participation in a service-learning international alliance? How does this experience lead to "practicing at the top of the license" and/or "biopsychosocial clinical practice"?

4. Speech-language-hearing science research associated with an international alliance may allow for a stronger research design. Give one example and state how the validity of research findings may be enhanced.

5. Speech-language-hearing science research associated with an international alliance also presents inherent challenges. Give an example of a common challenge associated with clinical research in another country, and state how validity of the research findings may be compromised by this design factor.

6. International alliances that create sustainable access to audiology and speech-language pathology services in underresourced countries are high-impact projects. What parameters are important to an alliance in order to ensure its long-term/sustainable impact?

7. Advancing a global career requires learning, clinical, disciplinary, and related experiences that build global competencies. Identify four actions that an audiologist or speech-language pathologist can take to establish a global career pathway.

8. What domestic alliances can campus-based professionals create in an effort to facilitate future international opportunities? Identify three colleagues or departments that may provide a starting point.

References

American Council on Education. (2015). *International higher education partnerships: A global review of standards and practices.* Washington, DC: American Council on Education Center for Internationalization and Global Engagement Insights. Retrieved from https://www.acenet.edu/news-room/Documents/CIGE-Insights-Intl-Higher-Ed-Partnerships.pdf

American Speech-Language-Hearing Association. (2014). *2014 Standards for clinical certification in speech-language pathology.* Rockville, MD: Author. Retrieved from https://www.asha.org/uploadedFiles/2014-SLP-CCC-Application-Standards.pdf

American Speech-Language-Hearing Association. (2016). *ASHA scope of practice in speech-language pathology.* Rockville, MD: Ad Hoc Committee on Scope of Practice in Audiology. Retrieved from https://www.asha.org/policy/sp2016-00343/

American Speech-Language-Hearing Association. (2017). *Agreement for the mutual recognition of professional association credentials 2017.* Rockville, MD: Author. Retrieved from https://www.asha.org/uploadedFiles/CredRecognitionAgreement.pdf

American Speech-Language-Hearing Association. (2018a). *ASHA scope of practice in audiology.* Rockville, MD: Ad Hoc Committee on Scope of Practice in Audiology. Retrieved from https://www.asha.org/policy/sp2018-00353/

American Speech-Language-Hearing Association. (2018b). ASHA renews status with World Health Organization. *ASHA Leader, 10*(10), 63. Retrieved from https://leader.pubs.asha.org/toc/leader/23/10

American Speech-Language-Hearing Association. (2018c). *Strategic pathway to excellence.* Rockville, MD: Author. Retrieved from https://www.asha.org/uploadedFiles/ASHA-Strategic-Pathway-to-Excellence.pdf

American Speech-Language-Hearing Association. (2019a). *International Issues Board.* Rockville, MD: Author. Retrieved from https://www.asha.org/about/governance/committees/ committeesmart forms/international-issues-board/

American Speech-Language-Hearing Association. (2019b). *Special Interest Group 17, Global issues in communication sciences and related disorders.* Rockville, MD: Author. Retrieved from https://www.asha.org/SIG/17/

Augustine, R. (2012). Career expectations of students and faculty. *Proceedings from the Sixth Annual Strategic Leaders Global Summit: From Brain Drain to Brain Circulation: Graduate Education for Global Career Pathways, September 4–6, 2012 Bavaria, Germany.* Washington, DC: Council of Graduate Schools.

Council for Clinical Certification in Audiology and Speech-Language Pathology of the American

Speech-Language-Hearing Association. (2018a). *2020 Standards for the certificate of clinical competence in speech-language pathology*. Rockville, MD: American Speech-Language-Hearing Association. Retrieved from https://www.asha.org/certification/2020-slp-certification-standards/

Council for Clinical Certification in Audiology and Speech-Language Pathology of the American Speech-Language-Hearing Association. (2018b). *2020 Standards for the certificate of clinical competence in audiology*. Rockville, MD: American Speech-Language-Hearing Association. Retrieved from https://www.asha.org/certification/2020-audiology-certification-standards/

Council of Graduate Schools. (2007). *Task Force Report on the Professional Doctorate*. Washington, DC: Council of Graduate Schools. Retrieved from https://cgsnet.org/task-force-report-professional-doctorate

Council of Graduate Schools. (2010). Principles and Practices of Effective Collaborations. *Global Perspectives on Graduate International Collaborations: Proceedings of the 2009 Strategic Leadership Global Summit on Graduate Education*. Washington, DC: Council of Graduate Schools.

De Diego-Lazaro, B. (2016). *Cultural Awareness and Competence Scales*. Unpublished scale. Arizona State University.

De Diego-Lazaro, B. (2018). A study abroad to Nicaragua: Measuring cultural competence in speech and language pathology students. *Perspectives of the ASHA Special Interest Group 17, 3*(Part 1), 38–48. Retrieved from https://pubs.asha.org/doi/full/10.1044/persp3.SIG17.38

Denecke, D., & Kent, J. (2010). *Joint degrees, dual degrees, and international research collaborations: A report on the CGS Graduate International Collaborations Project*. Washington, DC: Council of Graduate Schools. Retrieved from https://cgsnet.org/joint-degrees-dual-degrees-and-international-research-collaborations-0

EBS United. (2019). *Bilingual immersion programs*. West Chester, PA: EBS United. Retrieved from http://ebsunited.com/bilingual-immersion-programs

Forum on Education Abroad. (2011). *Standards of good practice for education abroad*. Carlisle, PA: Author. Retrieved from http://www.forumea.org/wp-content/uploads/2014/10/ForumEA-StandardsGoodPractice2011-4thEdition.pdf

Franca, M., Flowers, C., Smith, L., & Pitt, J. (2007). The impact of multiculturalism in rehabilitation education. *Rehabilitation Counselors and Educators Journal, 1*(1), 51–59.

Gallagher, S. (2014). *Major employers' hiring practices and the evolving function of the professional master's degree* (Doctoral dissertation). College of Professional Studies, Northeastern University, Boston, Massachusetts.

Gallagher, S. (2015). *Yes, master's: A graduate degree's moment in the age of higher education innovation*. Retrieved from http://www.nebhe.org/thejournal/yes-masters-a-graduate-degrees-moment-in-the-age-of-higher-education-innovation/

Gill, C., Bharadwaj, S., Chance, P., Quick, N., & Wainscott, S. (2016a). Impetus for change: Speech-language pathology around the globe. *Perspectives of the ASHA Special Interest Group 17, 1*(Part 1), 3–6. Retrieved from https://pubs.asha org/doi/pdf/10.1044/persp1.SIG17.3

Gill, C., Bharadwaj, S., Quick, N., Wainscott, S., & Chance, P. (2016b). From volunteering to academic programming: A case example. *Perspectives of the ASHA Special Interest Group 17, 1*(Part 1), 7–11. Retrieved from https://pubs.asha. org/doi/pdf/10.1044/persp1.SIG17.7

Harten, A., Franca, M., Boyer, V., & Pegoraro-Krook, M. (2018). Across the universe of speech-language-pathology: Developing international alliances. *Perspectives of the ASHA Special Interest Group 17, 3*(Part 1), 49–58. Retrieved from https://pubs.asha.org/doi/ full/10.1044/persp3.SIG17.49

Helms, R. M. (2015). *International higher education partnerships: A global review of standards and practices*. Washington, DC: American Council on Education. Retrieved from https://www.acenet.edu/news-room/Documents/CIGE-Insights-Intl-Higher-Ed-Partnerships.pdf

Hyter, Y., Roman, T., Staley, B., & McPherson, B. (2017). Competencies for effective global engagement: A proposal for communication sciences and disorders. *Perspectives of the ASHA Special Interest Group 17, 2*(Part 1), 9–20. Retrieved from https://pubs.asha.org/doi/full/ 10.1044/persp2.SIG17.9

Illinois State University. (2019). *Communication Sciences and Disorders Study Abroad and Travel Experiences*. Normal, IL: Illinois State University. Retrieved from https://csd.illinoisstate.edu/getInvolved/studyAbroad/

Interprofessional Education Collaborative. (2016). *Core competencies for interprofessional collaborative practice: Report of the Expert Panel.* Washington, DC. Retrieved from https://ipecollaborative.org/uploads/IPEC-Core-Competencies.pdf

Israel, B., Schulz, A., Parker, E., & Becker, A. (1998). Review of community-based research: Assessing partnership approaches to improve public health. *Annual Review Public Health, 19,* 173–202.

Karle, H., Christensen, L., Gordon, D., & Nystrup, J. (2008). Neo-colonialism versus sound globalization policy in medical education. *Medical Education, 10,* 954–958. Retrieved from https://www.ncbi.nlm.nih.gov/pubmed/18823513

Klomparens, K. (2008). Inter-institutional agreements. *Global Perspectives on Graduate Education: Proceedings of the Strategic Leaders Global Summit on Graduate Education.* Washington, DC: Council of Graduate Schools.

Legg, C., & Penn, C. (2014). The relevance of context in understanding the lived experience of aphasia: Lessons from South Africa. *Perspectives of the ASHA Special Interest Group 17, 4*(Part 1), 4–11. Retrieved from https://pubs.asha.org/toc/ashagics/4/1

McNeilly, L. (2018). Requisite knowledge for teaching graduate students to utilize the International Classification of Functioning, Disability and Health Framework. *Perspectives of the ASHA Special Interest Group 17, 3*(Part 2), 14–21. Retrieved from https://pubs.asha.org/doi/full/10.1044/persp3.SIG17.78

Molrine, C., & Drayton, K. (2013). International clinical standards and cultural practices in speech-language pathology graduate education: A model from Trinidad and Tobago. *Perspectives of the ASHA Special Interest Group 17, 3*(Part 1), 14–21. Retrieved from https://pubs.asha.org/doi/pdf/10.1044/gics3.1.14

National Association of Colleges and Employers. (2019). *Career readiness for new college graduates: A definition of competencies.* Bethlehem, PA: National Association of Colleges and Employers. Retrieved from https://www.naceweb.org/uploadedfiles/pages/knowledge/articles/career-readiness-fact-sheet-jan-2019.pdf

National Institutes of Health. (2019). *Fogarty International Center.* Bethesda, MD: Fogarty International Center. Retrieved from https://www.fic.nih.gov/Funding/Pages/Fogarty-Funding-Opps.aspx

National Survey of Student Engagement. (2007). *Experiences that Matter: Enhancing Student Learning and Success Annual Report 2007.* Bloomington, IN:

Indiana University Center for Postsecondary Research. Retrieved from http://nsse.indiana.edu/NSSE_2007_Annual_Report/docs/withhold/NSSE_2007_Annual_Report.pdf#page=12

New England Association of Schools and Colleges. (2003). *Principles of Good Practice in Over-seas International Education Programs for Non-U.S. Nationals.* Burlington, MA: New England Association of Schools and Colleges. Retrieved from https://cihe.neasc.org//sites/cihe.neasc.org/downloads/POLICIES/Pp47_Overseas_progams_for_non-US_Nationals.pdf

Organisation for Economic Co-operation and Development. (2005*). Guidelines for quality provision in cross-border higher education.* Paris, France: OECD. Retrieved from http://www.oecd.org/edu/skills-beyond-school/35779480.pdf

Patterson, A., Hansson, K., Lowit, A., Stansfield, J., & Trinite, B. (2015). EU collaboration in speech and language therapy education: The NetQues Project. *Perspectives of the ASHA Special Interest Group 17, 5,* 21–31. Retrieved from https://pubs.asha.org/doi/pdf/10.1044/gics5.1.21

Randzaao, M., & Garcia, F. (2018). An international service delivery model for sustainable practices: Insights from Cambodia. *Perspectives of the ASHA Special Interest Group 17, 3*(Part 1), 4–13. Retrieved from https://pubs.asha.org/ doi/full/10.1044/persp3.SIG17.4

Ross-Swain, D., Fogel, B., & Schneider, E. (2017). International interprofessional collaboration: The benefits of global networking. *Perspectives of the ASHA Special Interest Group 17, 2*(Part 2), 73–81. Retrieved from https://pubs.asha.org/doi/pdf/10.1044/persp2.SIG17.73

Sekuler, A. (2011). Ecosystems for developing transferrable skills. Washington, DC: Council of Graduate Schools. *Proceedings from the 2011 Strategic Global Summit on Graduate Education: Global Perspectives on Career Outcomes for Graduate Students.*

United States Bureau of Education and Cultural Affairs Exchange Programs. (2019). *Fulbright Scholar Program.* Retrieved from https://www.cies.org/about-us

Waterson, L., Duttine, A., Roman, T. R., & Caesar, L. (2018). The American Speech-Language-Hearing Association–Pan American Health Organization Partnership: Progress, future plans and connecting to World Health Organization Rehabilitation 2030. *Perspectives of the ASHA Special Interest Group 17, 3*(Part 1), 60–68.

Retrieved from https://pubs.asha.org/doi/pdf/10.1044/2018_PERS-SIG17-2018-0000

Watters, C., King, M., Min, K., Chambaz, J., Jablonski, C., & DePauw, K. (2010). National and regional perspectives on graduate international collaborations. Washington, DC: Council of Graduate Schools. *Proceedings from the 2009 Strategic Global Summit on Graduate Education: Global Perspectives on Graduate International Collaborations.*

Western Michigan University. (2019). *Broncos Abroad: Cultural Connections Senegal Summer (Faculty Led).*

Kalamazoo, MI: Western Michigan University. Retrieved from https://broncosabroad.wmich .edu/index.cfm?FuseAction=Programs.View ProgramAngular&id=235

World Health Organization. (2001). *International classification of functioning, disability and health.* Geneva, Switzerland: Author. Retrieved from https://www.who.int/classifications/icf/en/

World Health Organization. (2011). *World report on disability.* Geneva, Switzerland: Author. Retrieved from http://www.who.int

Appendix 7–A

Proposed Competencies for Global Engagement

Competencies	Description
Dispositions	
Humility	Being humble enough to recognize values, beliefs, and world views different from one's own (Hyter, 2014; Ortega & Faller, 2011).
Self-reflectiveness	Having engaged in daily living experiences in cultures different than one's own (Longview Foundation, 2014).
Empathy	The ability to be aware and sensitive to others' needs, emotions, or perspectives (Jokinen, 2005).
Inquisitiveness	Curiosity; seeking information beyond what is required; being an active and engaged learner (Ebbeck, 2006; Gupta & Govindarajan, 2002; Jokinen, 2005).
Responsibility to promote equity and social justice	Taking the initiative to combat injustices and to improve the lives of others (AACU, 2015).
Knowledge	
Knowledge of one's own and others' culture and world view	The beliefs, values, and assumptions that determine daily practices (Ting-Toomey & Chung, 2011). Having knowledge of one's own culture and world view is an essential first step to moving along the continuum of global responsiveness (Green & Kreuter, 2004; Hyter, 2014; Lynch & Hanson, 2011; National Education Association [NEA], 2010).
Globalization's consequences around the world	The interconnectedness and interdependence among nation states, frequently resulting in uneven consequences (Green & Mertova, 2009; Hyter, 2014; Jogerst et al., 2015; Steger, 2013; Wilson et al., 2012).
Relations of power between different countries and different groups of people	The "ability to define goals and make decisions in the interests of one's own group" (Hyter, 2014, p. 114; Kahn & Agnew, 2015; San Jose State University, 2007).
Impact of privilege	Unmerited advantages (McIntosh, 2003).
Differences and similarities in economic, political, cultural, and ecological realities of high-, middle-, and low-resource countries	Economics (access to resources), politics (ability to exercise power), culture, and the ecology are social structures that impact daily life (Green & Whitsed, 2015; Hyter, 2014; Kahn & Agnew, 2015; Lustig & Koester, 2013). The term high, middle, and low-resource refers to the level of material resources available in a country (Murray, Wenger, Downes, & Terrazas, 2011).
Skills	
Self-awareness	The ability to know one's own beliefs, values, and assumptions (Hyter, 2014; Jokinen, 2005; Mansilla & Jackson, 2014; Pillay & Kathard, 2015).

Competencies	Description
Awareness of others	The ability to know the beliefs, values, and assumptions of others (Mansilla & Jackson, 2014; NEA, 2010).
Experiences with diverse cultures	Having engaged in daily living experiences in cultures different than one's own (Longview Foundation, 2014).
Ability to communicate in more than one language	Having the capacity to communicate (speak, read, write) in a language or other languages in addition to one's first language (Longview Foundation, 2014; NEA, 2010).
Ability to create an environment that is culturally and globally responsive	The ability to create an environment that demonstrates consideration of cultural and global diversity (Longview Foundation, 2014; Wickenden, 2013; Wylie, McAllister, Davidson, & Marshall, 2013).
Ability to engage in critical and dialectical thinking, and critical dialogue	Critical thinking is the precursor to dialectical thinking. Dialectical thinking and critical dialogue are important for being able to think of possibilities beyond what you believe is reality. In this way these are essential skills for becoming a more culturally and globally competent provider (Bean, 2011; Brookfield, 2012; Freire, 1990; Hyter, 2014; Marchel, 2007; Pillay & Kathard, 2015).
Ability to engage in international conversations	The ability to facilitate and participate in conversation across nations (Longview Foundation, 2014).
Ability to develop international partnerships (communities of practices) and sustainable practices	The ability to facilitate, develop, and maintain partnerships with colleagues around the world in ways that can be sustained by the local populations (Green & Kreuter, 2004; Green & Whitsed, 2015; Longview Foundation, 2014).
Attitudes	
Willingness to provide services and engage with others from a posture of reciprocity	Kalyanpur and Harry (2012) define reciprocity as a bidirectional exchange of knowledge, values, and perspectives (see also Hyter, 2014; Jogerst et al., 2015; Wilson et al., 2012).
Willingness to promote equity and social justice	The belief that communication is a human right and that all human beings have a right to be treated fairly and equally (Green & Whitsed, 2015; Jogerst et al., 2015).
Willingness to value ethical behavior	The practice of consistently adhering to moral and ethical principles (Green & Whitsed, 2015; Jogerst et al., 2015).

References Cited in this Appendix

Association of American Colleges and Universities. (2015). *Global learning VALUE rubric*. Washington, DC: Author.

Bean, J. C. (2011). *Engaging ideas: The professors guide to integrating writing, critical thinking, and active learning in the classroom* (2nd ed.). San Francisco, CA: John Wiley & Sons.

Ebbeck, M. (2006). The challenges of global citizenship: Some issues for policy and practice in early childhood. *Childhood Education, 82*(6), 353–357.

Freire, P. (1990). *Education for critical consciousness*. New York, NY: Continuum.

Green, L., & Kreuter, M. (2004). *Health program planning: An educational and ecological approach*. New York, NY: McGraw-Hill.

Green, W., & Mertova, P. (2009). Internationalization of teaching and learning at the University of Queensland: A report on current perceptions and practices. Retrieved September 15, 2016 from http://www.uq.edu.au/tedidev/docs/IoTL-at-UQ.pdf

Green, W., & Whitsed, C. (2015). Internationalising the curriculum in business: An overview. In W. Green & C. Whitsed (Eds.), *Critical perspectives on internationalising the curriculum in disciplines: Reflective narrative accounts from business, education and health* (pp. 3–24). Rotterdam, the Netherlands: Sense Publishers.

Gupta, A. K., & Govindarajan, V. (2002). Cultivating global mindset. *Academy of Management Executive, 16*(1), 116–126.

Hyter, Y. D. (2014). A conceptual framework for responsive global engagement in communication sciences and disorders. *Topics in Language Disorders, 34*, 103–120.

Jogerst, K., Callender, B., Adams, V., Evert, J., Fields, E., Hall, T., . . . Wilson, L. L. (2015). Identifying interprofessional global health competencies for 21st-century health professionals. *Annals of Global Health, 81*, 239–247.

Jokinen, T. (2005). Global leadership competencies: A review and discussion. *Journal of European Industrial Training, 29*, 199–216.

Kahn, H. E., & Agnew, M. (2015). Global learning through difference: Considerations for teaching, learning, and the internalization of higher education. *Journal of Studies in International Education*, 1–13.

Kalyanpur, M., & Harry, B. (2012). *Cultural reciprocity in special education: Building family professional relationships.* Baltimore, MD: Paul H. Brookes.

Longview Foundation. (2014). *The globally competent teaching continuum.* Retrieved from http://www.learnnc.org/lp/editions/global-continuum

Lustig, M. Q., & Koester, J. (2013). *Intercultural competence: Interpersonal communication across cultures* (7th ed.). Boston, MA: Pearson.

Lynch, E. W., & Hanson, M. J. (2011). *Developing cross-cultural competence: A guide for working with children and their families* (4th ed.). Baltimore, MD: Paul H. Brookes.

Mansilla, V. B., & Jackson, A. (2014). Educating for global competence: Learning redefined for an interconnected world. In H. Jacobs (Ed.), *Mastering global literacy: Contemporary perspectives* (pp. 5–29). Bloomington, IN: Solution Tree.

Marchel, C. (2007). Learning to talk/talking to learn: Teaching critical dialogue. *Teaching Educational Psychology, 2*(1), 1–15.

McIntosh, P. (2003). White privilege: Unpacking the invisible knapsack. In S. Plous (Ed.), *Understanding prejudice and discrimination* (pp. 191–196). New York, NY: McGraw-Hill.

Murray, J. P., Wenger, A. F. Z., Downes, E. A., & Terrazas, S. B. (2011). *Educating health professionals in low-resource countries: A global approach.* New York, NY: Springer.

National Education Association. (2010). *An NEA policy brief.* Retrieved from http://www.nea.org/assets/docs/HE/PB28A_Global_Competence11.pdf

Ortega, R., & Faller, K. (2011). Training child welfare workers from an intersectional cultural humility perspective: A paradigm shift. *Child Welfare, 90*(5), 27–49.

Pillay, M., & Kathard, H. (2015). Decolonizing health professionals' education: Audiology and speech therapy in South Africa. *African Journal of Rhetoric, 7*, 196–227.

San Jose State University. (2007). *School of Social Work transcultural perspective: A working definition.* Retrieved from http://www.sjsu.edu/socialwork/docs/Transcultural _Handout_xSJSU_SSWx.pdf

Steger, M. (2013). *Globalization: A very short introduction.* Oxford, UK: Oxford University Press.

Ting-Toomey, S., & Chung, L. C. (2011). *Understanding intercultural communication.* Oxford, UK: Oxford University Press.

Wickenden, M. (2013). Widening the SLP lens: How can we improve the well-being of people with communication disabilities globally? *International Journal of Speech-Language Pathology, 15*(1), 14–20.

Wilson, L., Harper, D. C., Tami-Maury, I., Zarate, R., Salas, S., Farley, J., . . . Ventura, C. (2012). Global health competencies for nurses in the Americas. *Journal of Professional Nursing, 28*, 213–222.

Wylie, K., McAllister, L., Davidson, B., & Marshall, J. (2013). Changing practice: Implications of the World Report on Disability for responding to communication disability in under-served populations. *International Journal of Speech-Language Pathology, 15*(1), 1–13.

SECTION II

Employment Issues

Appendix 7–B

◇◇◇

An MOU Checklist for International Collaborations

Memoranda of Understanding (MOUs) and Memoranda of Agreement (MOAs) for international collaborations vary considerably, depending on the scope and objectives of the partnership and the national and institutional contexts of the universities involved. The following checklist addresses general programmatic issues that should be considered when developing an MOU or MOA for a formal international partnership. The guidelines described in this checklist have been culled from sample memoranda and MOU checklists provided to the Council of Graduate Schools (CGS) by institutions that participated in the discussions and activities sponsored by the CGS Graduate International Collaborations Project. While this checklist is designed to cover a range of collaborations, components specific to international joint and dual degree programs are signaled with a "J/D" below. In addition to considering the guidelines below, institutions with experience overseeing collaborations recommend providing detailed information to faculty members about the process of submitting an MOU or other agreement for approval. Many institutions elect to include this information in online resources for faculty and/or with planning documents that must precede or accompany the MOU, such as an application to submit with a collaborative exchange proposal. It is recommended that these documents:

A. Define the types of possible agreements (MOU, Agreement of Friendship and Cooperation, etc.) and the purpose of each.

B. Describe the different types of documents that must be completed and approved. Explain the approvals process for different types of agreements, indicating routing and required signatures.

C. Provide an estimated timeline for approval once a proposed MOU and accompanying documentation have been submitted.

D. Provide names and contact information for senior administrators and staff members who can offer support and assistance for different types of questions.

VALUE

1. Establish the value of the collaboration to the university and to any other relevant groups of stakeholders. Refer to any documents that demonstrate the commitment of the institution and institutional leadership to internationalization and collaboration (for example, a vision statement or strategic plan).

2. Outline the rationale or objectives motivating the collaboration, outlining benefits to all groups of stakeholders.

3. Describe the potential for development of the collaboration across other departments, programs or schools.

4. Describe the potential of the proposed project to complement existing programs or to enhance areas of priority for the university.

PLANNING

5. Articulate concrete outcomes or actions that will result from the collaboration.

6. Summarize planning and communication activities that have already taken place between partners.

7. Define the program structure, including:

   a. The title of the program and the title of any degree(s) and certification(s) that will result (J/D)

   b. The duration of the program (with start date and end date, as applicable) and duration of the MOU, including provisions for early termination by mutual or single agreement (e.g., What happens to students who are already in progress at the time of termination?)

   c. The accreditation status of the partner institutions and programs, if appropriate (J/D)

   d. If applicable, the process of adding participating institutions

8. Define terms that may be interpreted differently between various academic contexts. ("academic year," "full-time enrollment," etc.) (J/D)

LEGAL ISSUES

9. Describe basic legal requirements for student mobility between the countries where partner institutions are located.

10. Define legal rights and liabilities of universities in relation to the program and its intellectual and material outcomes. (Issues to be considered would include, but would not be limited to, intellectual property, equal opportunity law, monetary exchanges or reimbursements between universities as the result of profits generated or expenses incurred.)

11. Establish which institutional rules and policies apply to students studying at the host institution, and terms of disciplinary action. (J/D)

ADMISSIONS (J/D)

12. Establish equivalencies for units of credit awarded by partner institutions.

13. Establish academic criteria for student participation in the program and mechanisms by which eligibility and admission to the program will be determined.

CURRICULUM (J/D)

14. Describe modes and mechanisms of delivering program content, including, as appropriate:

    a. The language(s) of instruction

    b. The curriculum, including courses and/ or instruction that will be provided by each institution

    c. Requirements for the thesis, dissertation, or capstone project, and mechanisms of supervision and defense of the project

15. Describe graduation requirements and mechanisms for awarding credit and certifying student work, i.e., transfer credit policy (including the number of credits, if any, that can be double counted at each institution), extenuating circumstances, and transcript release.

RESOURCES AND FINANCING

16. Outline the funding structure for the collaboration. Basic categories for funding sources may include: internal university budget; U.S. federal or state funding sources; private U.S. funders; and international sources (including the partner institution or self-supporting students). Basic categories of expenditures may include research expenses; facilities for faculty and administrative support staff; tuition/fees; housing; and travel.

17. Establish terms and resources for student advising and support, (i.e., visa support services, academic advising, terms of student access to academic, social, and health facilities). (J/D)

18. Establish student responsibilities and expenses, (i.e., registration, payment of tuition and living expenses, housing, immigration compliance, health insurance and medical expenses). (J/D)

ASSESSMENT AND REVIEW

19. Establish benchmarks for program success. (J/D)

20. Describe mechanisms and timeline for program evaluation and, if applicable, assessment of learning outcomes. (J/D)

21. Define period within which the MOU may be renewed or terminated with mutual consent of institutions. For agreements of indefinite length, describe university policy on inactive agreements.

Applying Evidence to Clinical Practice

Lizbeth H. Finestack, PhD and Stacy K. Betz, PhD

Introduction

This chapter focuses on the use of evidence in clinical practice. Although the American Speech-Language-Hearing Association (ASHA) emphasizes research methodology and evidence-based practice (EBP) across multiple accreditation standards for both speech-language pathology and audiology (Council on Academic Accreditation in Audiology and Speech-Language Pathology of the American Speech-Language-Hearing Association, 2019), you might still be wondering why this topic is included in a book about *professional* issues when the evidence for assessment and treatment methods is repeatedly emphasized in each disorder-focused course you have taken. The reason is simple. A client will come to you, the speech-language pathologist (SLP) or audiologist, because you are the *professional*. A client will seek out your services because you are the one who has the knowledge and expertise to provide effective services. In today's world anyone can search the internet for the signs and symptoms she is experiencing, make a self-diagnosis, and even determine what treatment she thinks she need. For example, a parent might decide her nonverbal 2-year-old doesn't need to see an SLP after reading a blog about another family whose child didn't start speaking until he was 3 years old and is now graduating valedictorian of his high school class. Someone else might decide the solution to her hearing difficulty is to purchase a hearing aid online without a professional evaluation or fitting. In each of these examples, neither individual is able to determine the quality of evidence she found online and whether that evidence validly applies to her communication needs.

As a professional you will be expected to use evidence as the foundation of your clinical decisions. In this chapter we frame the application of evidence to clinical practice around the three-pronged view of clinical evidence: external scientific evidence, clinical expertise, and client perspectives (Guyatt et al., 2000). After providing an overview of the evidence-based approach to clinical practice, the chapter primarily focuses on how you, as a professional, can incorporate research evidence into your practice. We first discuss how research informs clinical assessment, particularly the need for evaluation methods to be both reliable and valid. We then summarize types of treatment evidence, how the quality of treatment evidence should be evaluated, and how you can incorporate this evidence when planning treatment for a client. The ways in which research evidence interacts with clinician expertise and

client values will also be discussed. As you read through the chapter consider that your goal as a clinical professional is for the use of evidence to become second nature in all of your clinical decisions. Think not only about how you will apply evidence to making decisions for an individual client, but how you will become an evidence-based professional.

Evidence-Based Practice

Evidence-based medicine is traditionally defined as "the integration of best research evidence with clinical expertise and patient values" (Sackett et al., 2000, p. 1). With this in mind, ASHA further defines the goal of EBP as the integration of: "(a) clinical expertise/expert opinion, (b) external scientific evidence, and (c) client/patient/caregiver perspectives to provide high-quality services reflecting the interests, values, needs, and choices of the individuals we serve" (Robey et al., 2004, p. 1). Figure 8–1 displays the integration of these three key elements. EBP applies to clinical decisions regarding both the assessment and intervention of individuals with communication disorders. Below we define each of the three key components of EBP.

Clinical expertise refers to the clinician's experience and comfort level with a particular assessment or intervention. It includes the outcomes the clinician has previously experienced with the assessment or intervention. Clinical expertise allows the clinician to clearly understand the client's history and needs. Based on those identified needs of the client, clinicians can then use their clinical expertise to identify possible diagnos-

tic and intervention options and then seek out external scientific evidence for those clinical procedures. Clinical expertise also allows clinicians to judge the generalizability of external evidence to their particular client. It is important to note that along with clinical expertise and knowledge, for EBP to be successful, the clinician must display compassion, sensitive listening skills, and deep respect for their clients' culture and values (Guyatt et al., 2000).

Client perspectives comprise the experience, personalities, values, and culture of the client. The client perspective also includes the knowledge that the client brings to the treatment, their financial resources, and social supports. Often times, depending on cultural values, the client perspective also includes these features of the family who play key roles in the assessment and intervention of the client. When conducting evidence-based treatment, the clinician will have to educate the client and family on possible benefits, risks, and inconveniences associated with each treatment option. Ultimately, treatment decisions are made by the client and the client must decide if a particular assessment or intervention is a good fit; however, clinicians embracing EBP should gain a good understanding of their client's perspective so that they can effectively advocate for their client (Guyatt et al., 2000).

External scientific evidence refers to research that relates to the specific assessment or intervention method the clinician is considering using. Typically, this scientific evidence is patient centered and clinically oriented, as opposed to basic research. Clinicians must carefully evaluate the quality of external evidence to determine how much weight that evidence should have in their clinical decision making process. Locating and evaluating external scientific evidence is the main focus of the current chapter, although we will also discuss how the internal evidence (i.e., clinician expertise and client perspectives) should be integrated and used to conduct EBP. Table 8–1 presents one possible process for systematically engaging in EBP. These steps have been adapted from the strategies suggested by other researchers (e.g., Gillam & Gillam, 2006; Porzsolt et al., 2003).

Step 1 involves formulating a clinical question based on a specific clinical case. Traditionally this is in the form of a PICO question. A PICO question defines the clinical question which then helps focus the search for external scientific evidence. The acronym PICO stands for the following components: Patient (P), Intervention/Index Measure (I), Comparison (C), and Outcome (O). Example PICO questions include:

1. For a minimally verbal 5-year-old child with autism spectrum disorder (ASD), does a parent-implemented intervention or clinician-implemented intervention lead to greater requests

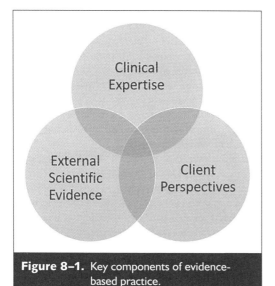

Figure 8–1. Key components of evidence-based practice.

Table 8–1. Process to Guide Evidence-Based Practice

1. Transform the clinical problem into a clinical question (PICO).
2. Evaluate the internal evidence based on clinical expertise.
3. Evaluate the internal evidence based on client and familial perspectives.
4. Find external evidence that addresses the question.
5. Evaluate the quality of the external evidence.
6. Evaluate the level of the external evidence.
7. Integrate the internal and external evidence to guide a decision.
8. Evaluate the outcomes of your decision.

and comments using augmentative and alternative communication (AAC)?

2. For a 75-year-old man with moderate bilateral hearing loss, does hearing aid use improve word recognition compared with no hearing aid use?

Patient refers to your client or the population to whom you will be delivering your services. In the above examples the patients are a 5-year-old child with ASD who is minimally verbal and a 75-year-old man with moderate bilateral hearing loss.

Intervention/index refers to the main intervention or assessment of interest. Often this is an alternative assessment or intervention approach that you are considering using. When developing a PICO question, it is necessary to identify a specific intervention or assessment method to investigate. Questions such as "What treatment should I use to improve the expressive language skills of a 5-year-old bilingual child with ASD?" and "How should I improve the auditory skills of a 75-year-old man with moderate hearing loss?" are too broad in scope. The interventions in the above examples are parent-implemented interventions and use of hearing aids.

Comparison refers to the treatment to which the main intervention is being compared or an alternative means for assessment. The comparison might be another specific approach, a traditional or "business as usual" approach, or even no treatment. In the first example, the comparison treatment is a traditional, clinician-implemented intervention; in the second example, the comparison treatment is no treatment.

Outcome is the primary behavior or measure of interest or the expected result. The outcome could be narrow such as performance on a specific probe or test or broad and more generalized such as overall improvement in quality of life. In the first example, the identified outcome is requesting and commenting using AAC; in the second example, the outcome is more broadly specified as improved word recognition abilities.

Steps 2 and 3 of the EBP process involve gathering internal evidence. This includes both the clinician and client perspectives described above. Considering the internal evidence prior to gathering external evidence can help guide the search to focus on viable and feasible approaches. Client perspectives should be gathered through conversations, interviews on history and background, and potentially surveys regarding the client's beliefs and treatment goals.

Step 4 involves gathering external evidence. Clinicians should use their PICO question to guide the search for external evidence. Broad-level searches can be completed using search databases such as ASHA Wire, Google Scholar, PsycInfo, and Ovid. Key words from the PICO question can be searched to identify primary research that addresses relevant topics. Such searches may prove to be onerous for full-time clinicians, however. Other databases exist that enable clinicians to more specifically search for research reviews that support EBP, such as ASHA's Evidence Maps (https://www.asha.org/Evidence-Maps/), which includes relevant research sorted by topic (e.g., dementia, speech sound disorders, tinnitus). Under each topic, clinicians can view the research by study type, including external scientific evidence, clinical expertise, and client perspectives. Other databases are available that contain systematic reviews, such as the Cochrane Library (https://www.cochranelibrary.com/cdsr/reviews). The Cochrane Library comprises more than 8,000 reviews that can be searched using keywords. The Institute of Education Science's What Works Clearinghouse (https://ies.ed.gov/ncee/wwc/FWW/Results?filters=,Children-Youth-with-Disabilities) also offers systematic reviews specifically focused on topics related to school-based clinical practice. Other collections are available from Campbell Collaboration (https://www.campbellcollaboration.org/library.html) and the Agency for Healthcare Research and Quality (https://www.ahrq.gov/research/findings/evidence-based-reports/search.html). If one or more

recent reviews exists that addresses the clinician's PICO question, this may be all of the external evidence needed. However, if a review does not exist or if the review is out of date, it may be necessary for the clinician to identify several relevant research studies to review and evaluate.

Steps 5 and 6 pertain to the evaluation of external evidence. To complete these steps, clinicians need to consider the level and quality of the evidence obtained in Step 4. In the following sections we provide more guidance on how external evidence should be evaluated for both assessment and intervention clinical questions.

Step 7 is the integration of the internal and external evidence to make a clinical decision. Not all evidence should be weighted equally. Each prong of EBP, including clinician expertise, client perspective, and external scientific evidence, must be carefully considered and integrated as a whole. For example, if the external evidence focused on parent-implemented AAC interventions did not suggest strong outcomes, but the family was incredibly motivated to play an active role in therapy and the clinician had limited availability for individual therapy, the integration of these pieces of evidence would warrant implementing a parent-implemented intervention. As another example, if a client is unwilling to wear a particular type of hearing aid because of feeling physically or socially uncomfortable despite strong external evidence and clinician expertise, the hearing aid intervention would not be an EBP approach.

Step 8, the final step of the evidence-based process, is evaluation of outcomes. Outcomes should be evaluated based on performance on the outcome measures defined in the PICO questions as well as the client's individual goals. Additionally when conducting treatment, the clinician's compliance implementing and the client's adherence to the intervention should be considered as well as their satisfaction with the approach.

EBP requires the clinician to carefully consider each of the three evidence components. In the following sections we describe all three aspects of evidence for both assessment and intervention clinical decisions; however, the greatest emphasis is on evaluating the scientific evidence (Steps 5 and 6). Each section includes descriptions of methods to evaluate external evidence as well as examples demonstrating how all three types of evidence can be integrated to conduct EBP for individuals with communication disorders.

Evaluating Assessment Evidence

Purposes of Assessment

Before evaluating the quality of assessment evidence or determining the intended outcome when develop-

ing a PICO question, you must identify your purpose for assessing a client. When we think of assessment the first thing that typically comes to mind is diagnosing a client. Making a diagnosis consists of two primary clinical decisions: first whether the client has a disorder and then if so, which disorder. Determining an initial diagnosis for a client is certainly one of the primary purposes of assessment, but not the only one. Another purpose is to conduct a formal re-evaluation for a client. This includes cases where a client has been receiving intervention services but also cases where a client was previously assessed and determined not to need services and now needs a re-evaluation because concerns about their communication have not resolved. Intertwined with the purpose of determining a diagnosis is the use of assessment information to determine eligibility for services or reimbursement. Screening is another purpose of assessment in which the aim is not to diagnose, but to evaluate whether the client should receive a more comprehensive evaluation to determine whether a disorder is present. Assessment can also have more qualitative purposes such as identifying the primary strengths and weaknesses of someone's communication abilities. Finally, assessment is used continually during the treatment process to document treatment progress.

These various purposes of assessment are not mutually exclusive. In many cases one assessment method might be used for multiple purposes. For example, an SLP might administer a formal aphasia test primarily to determine an individual's relative performance in each language domain and modality (i.e., identifying communication strengths and weaknesses) and subsequently use those results to determine the type of aphasia the client has (i.e., determining a diagnosis). Because the purposes of assessment are interrelated, using the same assessment method for multiple purposes is often beneficial; however, to evaluate the evidence for a particular assessment method you must know your purpose because one assessment method might be considered high quality for one purpose but not for another. For example, an SLP might use a portable audiometer in a non-soundproof room to assess hearing. This procedure might be an evidence-based way to *screen* hearing, but not to *diagnose* a hearing impairment.

External Evidence: Reliability

The external, scientific evidence for assessment methods typically addresses two essential factors: reliability and validity. In colloquial language, the terms reliability and validity are often used interchangeably with both intended to refer to the general quality of an assessment; however, within a professional context, these two terms should be used more precisely because the distinction

between the two helps to systematically evaluate the clinical evidence for a particular assessment method. Reliability reflects the consistency of results you obtain from an assessment, whereas validity reflects the accuracy with which an assessment measures what it claims to measure. An evidence-based assessment method will have both high reliability and validity for the purpose you are using it. From a clinical perspective, the evidence regarding an assessment method's validity is ultimately the most important to evaluate, however, because an assessment method cannot be valid if it is not reliable, external evidence for reliability is often evaluated first.

Multiple types of evidence can document an assessment method's reliability. One important clinical consideration is whether the method yields similar results regardless of when the assessment is administered or who administers the assessment. The consistency with which clinicians can administer the assessment is measured in two ways: intrajudge and interjudge reliability. *Intrajudge reliability* measures how consistent the same clinician is in using the assessment measure (i.e., in terms of both administering and scoring/interpreting the results). *Interjudge reliability* measures the extent to which different clinicians score an assessment measure in the same way. Low intrajudge and/or interjudge reliability can indicate that the procedures for administering and scoring the assessment are not clear enough to consistently obtain the same assessment result for a client. For example, a standardized assessment of child language might include questions that are rated on a 1 to 3 scale for accuracy without clear guidelines on what types of responses should receive each rating. This can lead to the same clinician scoring the child's response differently on different days (i.e., low intrajudge reliability). It can also lead to two clinicians scoring the same child's response differently (i.e., low interjudge reliability). The more an assessment involves subjective interpretation of client responses and the more complicated the administration procedures are, the more important it is for you to evaluate the intrajudge and interjudge reliability of the assessment. On the other hand, if an assessment method has extremely straightforward and objective scoring and administration procedures, it might not be essential for this information to be documented. For example, one common method for assessing receptive vocabulary is for the clinician to say a word, show the client a few pictures, one of which depicts the meaning of the word said, and then ask the client to select the picture that best matches the meaning of the word. In this case, the administration and scoring are straightforward with little chance that intrajudge and interjudge reliability would be low. Therefore, when evaluating the quality of reliability evidence, it is always important to ask how

likely it is for intrajudge and interjudge reliability to be low. If the potential is low, then the lack of documentation of this type of consistency should not be a primary concern, assuming other types of reliability document the consistency of the evaluation method.

Another type of reliability, *item reliability*, relates to the consistency of the items within the same assessment method. For example, a formal measure of receptive vocabulary typically includes numerous test items that are all intended to assess vocabulary. If those items do in fact all measure vocabulary, then there should be consistency in terms of how a client responds to each item. If there is not high consistency amongst items then the test might assess multiple and/or different skills rather than primarily vocabulary. Reliability of the test items can be documented through measures of internal consistency. Cronbach's alpha measures the consistency of all items in a test. *Split-half reliability* divides the test into two halves and then compares the scores of the two halves to determine their similarity. If the creator of the assessment measure has developed two different versions of the same test, then *alternate forms reliability* can be computed by administering both versions of the test to the same group of people and comparing performance on each version.

Another type of reliability that can be documented is *test-retest reliability*. When computing test-retest reliability, the examiner will administer the same test to a group of individuals on two different occasions within a time period when spontaneous change in performance would not be expected. The scores from each day of testing (i.e., the "test" and "retest") are compared to determine consistency. Test-retest reliability is usually interpreted as measuring how consistent the test is in assessing the client's performance. Assuming the underlying communication deficit is stable, you would expect a test to give the same results for the same client across multiple different test administrations. If it does not, then the results of the test might lead you to diagnose a disorder after one of the test administrations, but not the other!

Most measures of reliability are calculated as statistical correlations ranging from 0 to 1.0. A correlation of 1.0 indicates perfect consistency, whereas a value of 0 indicates a complete lack of consistency. Therefore, the closer the correlation is to 1.0, the more reliable the assessment method. A benchmark for acceptable levels of reliability that is used within the field of special education is requiring correlations higher than .90 if the assessment is to be used for a high-stakes decision, such as diagnosing a disorder. These values may be slightly lower with values down to .80 being acceptable for other types of evaluation such as screening (Salvia, Ysseldyke, & Witmer, 2013). Establishing the acceptable reliability of an evaluation method is essential because a measure must be reliable to be valid.

External Evidence: Validity

Once an assessment is determined to be reliable, its validity can be evaluated. Because validity refers to whether the assessment truly measures what it claims to measure, you cannot evaluate validity without first clearly identifying your purpose for using the assessment method. The most important aspects of validity are evaluated subjectively using your clinical expertise. After reviewing the procedures of the assessment, you should use your knowledge of typical communication and communication disorders to determine whether the procedures used are appropriate for the intended purpose. The review of the procedures should include analyzing each test item individually as well as how the entire set of test items function together. For example, if an assessment claims to assess receptive vocabulary, a valid measure would require the client's response to be nonverbal and include a wide range of test items representing different parts of speech, levels of concreteness, etc. This type of validity has traditionally been referred to as construct and content validity. If an assessment method includes the use of a procedure that is new to you, another source of external evidence is to search the literature for research studies documenting that the procedure is a valid measure for the disorder being evaluated.

Validity can also be evaluated statistically using criterion-related validity. For this type of reliability a second, "criterion," measure is selected. Both the criterion measure and the measure being evaluated are administered to a group of people. If a criterion whose purpose is similar to the assessment method being evaluated is used, then it is considered *convergent criterion-related validity* and you would expect people to perform similarly on both measures. For example, one could compare one standardized test of receptive language to another test of receptive language. If a criterion with a purpose that is different than that of the assessment method being evaluated is used, then the measure is *divergent criterion-related validity*. For example, comparing a measure of receptive vocabulary and a measure of expressive morphology would assess divergent criterion validity. In this case, the expectation is that the two assessments will not be highly related to each other.

Unlike the interpretation of reliability correlations, there is no specific benchmark for indicating high or low criterion-related validity. As with reliability correlations, values closer to 1.0 indicate a high similarity between the two measures. Thus, you would expect convergent validity measures to be closer to 1.0 than divergent measures. The exact interpretation will require clinical expertise on your part to determine how similar (or different) the intended purpose of the measures is to the criterion. For example, the authors of a single-word

receptive vocabulary measure might demonstrate convergent related validity by comparing their assessment to an existing standardized receptive language measure with the result being a correlation of .87. They might also demonstrate divergent criterion-related validity by comparing their assessment to a measure of expressive morphology and finding a correlation of only .51. Because criterion-related validity is assessed using a number, it can be easy to want to rely on this value as the main indicator of validity; however, criterion-related validity is not as important as construct and content validity. When evaluating evidence of validity, do not let statistical values be your guide; you must use clinical expertise to determine whether the assessment is an accurate method to meet your evaluation purpose.

The methods of measuring reliability and validity described above are based on the classical test theory approach. Item response theory is another method for designing and evaluating the quality of an assessment; however, it is beyond the scope of this chapter to describe the theoretical rationale for which approach is most appropriate for each assessment. The primary focus here is to stress that to adequately evaluate the quality of external evidence for an assessment measure, you must determine whether the assessment is reliable and valid.

External Evidence: Diagnostic Accuracy

If your assessment purpose is to determine the presence of a disorder then it will be essential to evaluate how accurate an assessment measure is in identifying that disorder. Evaluating this type of external evidence can be done statistically using a variety of mathematical measures of diagnostic accuracy. All of these statistics approach the concept of diagnostic accuracy from the perspective of the clinician's need to accurately diagnose both individuals without a disorder and individuals with a disorder. To understand how to evaluate diagnostic accuracy, imagine you are considering using a new assessment method which will be referred to as "New Assessment." Also assume that the currently available best method for diagnosing the disorder is "Best Method." The evaluation of diagnostic accuracy is considered part of the external scientific evidence component of the EBP model (see Figure 8–1); however, these calculations are not something you would determine as a clinician. They are a type of evidence that would be provided by the developer of the assessment or by other researchers conducting an independent analysis of the accuracy of the measure. To do this, the developers or the external researchers administer both the New Assessment and Best Method to a large group of people. This group of people will include people who have the

disorder that New Assessment is intended to diagnose as well as people who do not have the disorder. To compute measures of diagnostic accuracy a few quantitative values are needed: the number of people determined to have the disorder based on Best Method and of these, the number who have the disorder and the number who do not have the disorder based on New Assessment; the number of people determined not to have the disorder based on the Best Method and of these, the number who have the disorder and the number who do not have the disorder based on New Assessment.

In this example, pretend the developers of New Assessment included 1,000 people in their sample to determine the accuracy of New Assessment in diagnosing Disorder X. Each of the 1,000 people completed Best Method with the results showing that 155 have Disorder X and 845 people do not. All 1,000 people also completed New Assessment. According to New Assessment 150 people have Disorder X. Of those 150 people, 140 also were determined by Best Method to have Disorder X. Of the 850 people that New Assess-

ment found did not have a disorder, 835 of them also were determined by New Assessment to not have Disorder X. These numbers can then be organized in a table to easily compare each person's results on Best Method and New Assessment (Table 8–2).

Table 8–3 uses more technical terminology to present a general format for how to organize the information about diagnostic accuracy. The term "Index Measure" is used in the same way the term "Index" is used when developing a PICO question for diagnostic purposes: it is the measure you are considering using (i.e., New Assessment in Table 8–2). The term "Reference Measure" is used to refer to the existing way to diagnose the disorder (i.e., Best Method in Table 8–2). The terms positive and negative refer to an individual's assessment result. A positive result means the assessment method indicates the person is positive for the disorder (i.e., the person has the disorder according to that assessment). A negative result means the person is negative for the disorder (i.e., the person does not have the disorder). Because each person was administered both the index measure and

Table 8–2. Example of Diagnostic Accuracy

		Best Method		
		Based on the results from Best Method: Has disorder X	Based on the results from Best Method: Does not have disorder X	Total
New Assessment	Based on the results from New Assessment: Has disorder X	140	10	150
	Based on the results from New Assessment: Does not have disorder X	15	835	850
Total:		155	845	1000

Table 8–3. Terminology for Calculating Diagnostic Accuracy

		Reference Measure Result	
		+	–
Index Measure Result	+	True positives	False positives
	–	False negatives	True negatives

the reference measure they will have two results: whether they were positive or negative for the disorder based on the index measure and whether they were positive or negative for the disorder based on the reference measure. The terms true positive, true negative, false positive, and false negative refer to how an individual's result on the index measure compares to their result on the reference measure. A "true" result means those results are the same, which then implies that the result from the index test is accurate (i.e., "true"). A "false" result means the results of the index and reference measure are different. Because the reference measure is considered the best way to diagnose the disorder when the results of the index and reference measure differ, the reference measure is considered to be the accurate diagnosis.

Two measures of diagnostic accuracy that evaluate the overall quality of the assessment method are sensitivity and specificity. The formulas for each are given in Table 8–4.

Sensitivity can be interpreted as how accurate the index measure is in diagnosing a disorder. Mathematically it can be analyzed as either a proportion (i.e., a decimal value of 1.0 or below) or that proportion can be multiplied by 100 and evaluated as a percentage. In the example in Table 8–2, the sensitivity is .903 or 90.3% indicating that 90.3% of people with Disorder X (as determined by the reference measure) were correctly diagnosed by the index measure. Specificity is .988 or 98.8% indicating that 98.8% of people without Disorder X were correctly identified as not having a communication impairment based on the results of New Assessment. Clinical expertise is needed to determine how high sensitivity and specificity should be to consider an assessment accurate. One recommendation in the field is that values over .90 are preferred with values as low as .80 being acceptable (Plante & Vance, 1994).

Another set of measures to assess diagnostic accuracy are positive predictive power and negative predictive power. Table 8–5 includes the formulas for these measures.

Positive predictive power is interpreted as the percentage of people who are determined by the index measure to have a disorder who do have a disorder according to the reference measure. Vice versa, negative predictive

Table 8–4. Sensitivity and Specificity Formulas and Examples

	General Formula (from Table 8–3)	**Specific Example** (from Table 8–2)
Sensitivity	True Positives / (True Positives + False Negatives)	= 140 / 140 + 15 = 140 / 155 = .903 or 90.3%
Specificity	True Negatives / (False Positives + True Negatives)	= 835 / 10 + 835 = 835 / 845 = .988 or 98.8%

Table 8–5. Positive Predictive Power and Negative Predictive Power Formulas and Examples

	General Formula (from Table 8–3)	**Specific Example** (from Table 8–2)
Positive Predictive Power	True Positives / (True Positives + False Positives)	= 140 / 140 + 10 = 140 / 150 = .933 or 93.3%
Negative Predictive Power	True Negatives / (False Negatives + True Negatives)	= 835 / 15 + 835 = 835 / 850 = .982 or 98.2%

power identifies the percentage of people who the index measure identifies as not having a disorder who also do not have a disorder according to the reference measure.

Sensitivity, specificity, positive predictive power, and negative predictive power all quantify the diagnostic accuracy of the index measure, however none of these measures considers the accuracy in diagnosing all four cells in Table 8–3 simultaneously (i.e., true positives, true negatives, false positives, and false negatives). To do that, positive likelihood ratios and negative likelihood ratios are used. Table 8–6 includes the formulas for these measures.

A positive likelihood ratio can be broadly interpreted as indicating how much the likelihood a person has the disorder is increased if they get a positive result on the index measure whereas, a negative likelihood ratio indicates how likely a negative result on the index test is. When using likelihood ratios to evaluate the quality of an assessment, the higher the positive likelihood ratio the better, and the closer to 0 the negative likelihood ratio is the better. Current benchmarks to identify a high-quality test suggest that values near 1 are uninformative, positive likelihood ratios greater than 10 are informative, and negative likelihood ratios below .1 are informative (Guyatt, Rennie, Meade, & Cook, 2008; Haynes, Sackett, Guyatt, & Tugwell, 2006).

Using the example from Table 8–2, a positive result on New Assessment is 75.25% more likely to be the result of someone who has the disorder compared with someone who does not have the disorder. Similarly, a negative result on New Assessment is only .098% more likely to be from someone who has the disorder. Likelihood ratios have a statistical advantage because they combine sensitivity and specificity into a single measure.

When using any of these methods of diagnostic accuracy, it is important to keep two points in mind. First, the meaningfulness of any of these statistics is only as

useful as the quality of the reference measure. For all diagnostic accuracy measures, the index measure is compared with a reference measure. The intent is for the reference measure to reflect the best possible means to diagnose the disorder. However, if the reference measure that is selected has significant flaws, then any measure of diagnostic accuracy will not truly provide information about the accuracy of the index measure because the reference measure does not accurately diagnose people. You must use your clinical expertise to evaluate the quality of the reference measure. Also, it is important to remember that diagnostic accuracy provides information about the validity of an assessment in terms of its truthfulness in diagnosing a disorder. Therefore, if an assessment measure does not claim to diagnose a disorder and you do not intend to use the assessment for that purpose, then measures of diagnostic accuracy are not relevant. For example, if you collect a communication sample to document communication deficits in naturalistic situations but do not use your observations to diagnose a disorder, then there is no need to worry about the diagnostic accuracy of your observations because you are using the observations to characterize communication strengths and weaknesses, not diagnose a disorder. It is still important to document the validity of a communication sample for this purpose, but diagnostic accuracy measures are not needed.

Using Assessment Evidence

This section presents two hypothetical examples to demonstrate how to apply evidence to clinical practice when determining whether to use a specific assessment procedure. The combination of examples aims to highlight that, based on the situation, the scientific evidence, clinician expertise, and client perspectives, each can play a relatively different role in creating a PICO question and in the overall evaluation of the assessment.

Table 8–6. Likelihood Ratio Formulas and Examples

	General Formula (from Table 8–3)	**Specific Example** (from Table 8–2)
Positive Likelihood Ratio	Sensitivity / (1 – Specificity)	= .903 / (1 – .988) = .903 / .012 = 75.25
Negative Likelihood Ratio	(1 – Sensitivity) / Specificity	= (1 – .903) / .988 = .097 / .988 = .098

Assessment Example I: Evaluating a New Standardized Test

Imagine you are an SLP who needs to assess a child's single word expressive vocabulary. You know that a new standardized test is available which claims it can be used to assess expressive vocabulary. The test involves showing the child a picture and asking the child to either name the picture or describe what a person in the picture is doing. The first step in systematically evaluating assessment evidence is to create a PICO question that aligns with your clinical purpose. Imagine that you currently do not have a standardized expressive vocabulary test but you know that having such a test could improve your ability to diagnose language disorders in children. Based on the children on your caseload, the P in your PICO question could be phrased for a specific population such as children with a developmental language disorder. Because you are considering using the new standardized test it is the I. The C in the PICO question is a comparison evaluation that you believe is high quality. You can use your own clinical expertise to identify what an ideal comparison measure would be. For example, this might be an existing standardized expressive vocabulary test that you have experience with and know is valid. The O could also vary depending on your purpose which could be to identify word finding problems. Combined together, your question becomes: When evaluating children with a developmental language disorder (P), is the new standardized test (I) more accurate than the existing standardized test (C) in identifying word finding problems (O)?

Because this is a commercially available standardized test it is likely you will start your evaluation of the evidence by reading the test manual as a source of external evidence. When reading the manual you should evaluate both the reliability and validity information. In terms of reliability, you should investigate the reliability of raters. Because each test item requires the child to name a word, the test manual will likely include many of the most common responses that should be scored as correct as well as examples of incorrect responses; however, children will give other responses that are not listed. Therefore, it is important to know if there is consistency in how those other responses are scored in terms of both interjudge and intrajudge reliability. However, if the test directions state that only responses listed on the score form as possible correct answers should be awarded credit, even if the child's response indicates some knowledge of the word, then the scoring is very straightforward and interjudge and intrajudge reliability likely can be assumed to be high, even if the author of the test did not document this type of reliability. Test-retest reliability is important for you to evaluate because you need to ensure the child's abilities can be consistently measured using this new test.

After confirming that the test has adequate reliability, you can proceed to evaluating the validity of the test. The test manual will likely provide a qualitative description of why the authors of the test believe the individual items and the overall design of the test assess expressive vocabulary. This description is similar to an expert opinion level of evidence. You should also make your own determination of the validity of the test design based on your clinical experience. For example, as an expressive measure, ensure that the child is required to respond with a verbal response (e.g., not pointing or acting out the word). Because this test requires the child to name the picture associated with each test item, it does use a valid method for assessing expressive vocabulary. The test manual might also include information on why the authors believe the individual vocabulary items selected are valid to use for assessing vocabulary. Again, you should evaluate this type of validity using your own clinical experience and your specific needs for using this test. To start, review the test items that are used for each age. Based on your own clinical experience determine whether those test items are appropriate for your community. For example, if a test item for young children was the word "soda" but in your region the word "pop" was used and "pop" is not considered a correct answer, it might be invalid for that picture to be used to assess vocabulary in your community. Likewise if one of the pictures to name was a baler, children from urban areas might call it a "tractor" but children from farming communities might be more likely to name it more precisely. A standardized test that is created to be used (and purchased) by SLPs throughout the country has likely taken these regional vocabulary differences into account; however, you should not assume this. You need to use your clinical experience to verify this. If there are multiple test items that you think would bias the test for children in your community (including providing invalidly high or low scores), you should consider the test invalid for your needs. The PICO question for this scenario is to identify semantic weaknesses. In this case, your outcome is not to diagnose a disorder; therefore, diagnostic accuracy is not a relevant validity measure. However, you are interested in characterizing whether a child has semantic deficits. One source of evidence for this outcome can be criterion-related validity. Read the test manual to determine whether convergent criterion-related validity data is provided comparing this new standardized test to an existing expressive vocabulary measure. In addition, your subjective evaluation of the content and construct validity of the test will determine whether you believe the task provides useful information about children's word finding skills.

After evaluating the external evidence provided by the test manual, you should integrate this evidence with your clinical expertise and the perspectives of the children you typically assess. For example, if the test is so expensive that your budget does not allow you to purchase it, then it does not matter how reliable and valid the measure is; you will not be able to obtain it. You should also use your clinical experience to determine whether the children you assess are likely to engage in a task that requires them to look at books and name pictures.

Assessment Example 2: Evaluating New Technology to Supplement Existing Equipment

Imagine you are an audiologist who frequently assesses the hearing of children who will not wear headphones or enter a sound booth for hearing testing. You consider purchasing a new device that claims to assess hearing thresholds using procedures that only require insert earphones to be placed in a child's ear for two seconds and the testing can be conducted in any room. One PICO question you could ask is: For children who will not wear headphones or sit in a sound booth (P), can the new technology (I) compared with pure tone threshold testing in a sound booth (C) be used to accurately diagnose a hearing loss? The need for this PICO question largely centers on the need for accurate testing for a difficult to test population of children whose hearing cannot be assessed using traditional methods. Therefore, the client perspective component of EBP is extremely important. An accurate method to assess hearing exists, pure-tone audiometry; however, you cannot use it with this population. Therefore, regardless of the external evidence supporting the traditional method, it is not useful in this scenario. External evidence for the reliability and validity of this new technology can be obtained from the equipment manufacturer and possibly also from research studies that were conducted prior to this technology being commercially developed. Because your O in this question focuses on accuracy in diagnosing hearing loss, you should find and use diagnostic accuracy results to evaluate the quality of this new technology. Assume for this example that there is substantial high quality external evidence documenting the reliability and validity of this new technology including reliability correlations of higher than .90 and high diagnostic accuracy values such as sensitivity and specificity close to 1.0 using a reference measure you believe to be valid.

The next step is to evaluate the internal evidence related to your clinical experience. When considering using new technology for assessment, part of the clinical evidence will be your own expertise using the equipment. For example, imagine that your workplace purchases this new technology and the equipment manufacturer sends two audiologists to conduct an onsite training. Both of the training audiologists demonstrate how they can consistently and validly insert the needed test probe into a child's ear and complete the entire testing in under two seconds. They demonstrate this multiple times with the same child and obtain the same results (i.e., test-retest reliability). They also compare their results to each other's (i.e., interjudge reliability) and show they obtain consistent results.

When it comes time for you to try, it takes you more than a minute to get the accurate probe placement and even then you cannot get the correct probe insertion every time (i.e., low intrajudge reliability which will lead to poor validity). Even after practicing for three months, your timing does not get any faster than 50 seconds. Based on your clinical experience working with this difficult to test population, you know that 50 seconds is too long and the children who are the P in your PICO question will not allow having an insert earphone in for almost a minute. In this case, regardless of how validly someone else can use the equipment, it will not be a valid method for you to use with this specific population. You might find this technology useful for other populations, but not the one that was the focus of your PICO question.

The two examples above show how all three types of evidence (i.e., external, clinician, and client) are essential to consider when evaluating the quality of an assessment procedure. In addition, you cannot evaluate the quality of an assessment method without first identifying your purpose for using that assessment method. External research evidence will provide the data documenting whether a particular assessment method is reliable and valid when used according to the intended directions. You will also need to use your clinical expertise to determine whether you personally can reliably and validly administer that assessment. You must also consider whether your client is willing and able to participate in the assessment. If all three sources of evidence do not indicate an evaluation method will be reliable and valid, then you should start the process again by either continuing to investigate your PICO question or modifying your PICO question to identify the most effective assessment method available for your client.

Evaluating Intervention Evidence

External Evidence: Levels of Evidence

When evaluating external scientific evidence, it is important to consider that not all external evidence should be weighted equally. The study design differentially

weights the value of a study. Studies with more rigorous designs are weighted more heavily than those with less rigorous designs. Several hierarchies exist that provide weightings to study designs. For example, the Oxford Centre for Evidence-based Medicine (https://www.cebm .net/2009/06/oxford-centre-evidence-based-medicine-levels-evidence-march-2009/) offers evidence hierarchies focused on different clinical areas, including therapy, prognosis, diagnosis, differential diagnosis, and economic and decision analyses. Robey (2004) presents a hierarchy with five levels specifically tailored for research focused on communication disorders. Robey's levels are included in Table 8–7. In Robey's hierarchy, systematic reviews of randomized control trials are considered the highest level of evidence (1a). In general, a *systematic review* is a research study that integrates the findings of multiple peer-reviewed publications focused on a similar clinical question, which may take the form of a PICO question. Because they combine evidence from multiple sources, systematic reviews are considered a higher level of evidence than a single study. If the systematic review statistically analyzes the combined results of all those prior publications the review is considered a meta-analysis. Meta-analyses offer the advantage of being able to quantify outcomes across studies. The key component of a systematic review is the use of pre-specified, rigorous, and reproducible methodology that leads to comprehensive results (Bettany-Saltikov & Fernandes, 2010). Systematic reviews that only include randomized control trials (see below) are weighted more heavily than reviews that also include non-randomized trials, especially when there is homogeneity (i.e., consistency) across results across studies.

The next level of evidence (1b) comprises single *randomized controlled trials* (RCTs). The key feature of RCTs is that participants are randomized to a treatment group or a control group before the study begins. There may be more than one treatment group and the control group may receive no treatment, delayed treatment, or "business as usual," which is the intervention that would be delivered in the absence of the research study. Randomization adds rigor and integrity to the study design and helps to avoid effects due to biases. For example, if a researcher assigns participants to study groups in a non-randomized fashion, implicit biases may affect a participant's group assignment. Suppose that every other eligible participant is placed in the intervention group. Knowing that the next participant will be assigned to the intervention group, the researcher may schedule a potential participant who they think is likely to benefit from the study intervention prior to a potential participant with more severe impairments. Randomization also helps to ensure that the study groups are similarly heterogeneous.

Level 2 evidence includes well-designed, *non-randomized controlled trials*, which are also referred to as quasi-experiments. Studies are considered non-randomized if participants are not prospectively and randomly assigned to study groups. An example of a non-randomized study is one in which audiologists within a large health care network had the opportunity to participate in a study examining a new hearing aid. Half of the audiologists agreed to participate. All of the clients being served by these audiologists were eligible to participate in the study. These clients made up the treatment group and received the new hearing aid. Clients of the audiologists who did not want to be involved in the study were still eligible to participate in the study. However, these clients were all assigned to the control group and did not receive the new hearing aid. Instead, their progress was monitored without any additional intervention. A study of this nature is considered quasi-experimental because even though there is a control group, random assignment was not used. This example of non-randomization

Table 8–7. Robey (2004) Levels of Intervention Evidence

Level	Intervention Study Design
1a	Systematic review/meta-analysis of randomized controlled trials
1b	Individual randomized controlled trial
2	Well-designed non-randomized controlled trial (quasi-experiments)
3	Observational studies with controls (retrospective studies, case-control studies, cohort studies with controls)
4	Observational studies without controls (cohort studies without controls and case series)

can be a concern because there may be a factor associated with the audiologists who self-selected to be involved in the study and their clients that could impact the study outcomes, such as having smaller caseloads or practicing in areas in which clients are financially stable.

Level 3 evidence comprises *observational studies with controls*. Such studies include retrospective studies, case-control studies, and cohort studies with controls. Retrospective studies usually involve record reviews that document the outcomes of intervention approaches that were used with previous clients as well as the characteristics or those clients. Case-control studies are a specific type of retrospective study. To conduct a case control study, the researcher identifies a group of cases that demonstrates the outcome of interest and a group that does not demonstrate the desired outcome. The researcher then examines the case records to identify which cases received the target intervention and which did not. Cohort studies involve the observation of a large group, typically over a long period of time—for example, comparing the outcomes of a new reading program for struggling readers delivered to an entire school district for three years with the outcomes of another district that did not receive the reading program.

Level 4 evidence includes *observational studies without controls*. These may be case studies that include only individuals with desired outcomes or cohort studies that do not have a comparison group. Because they lack control groups and randomization, observational studies without controls are considered the lowest level of external evidence.

Another factor to consider when assessing the level of research for EBP is the state of conditions under which the study was conducted. Here, we make the distinction between *efficacy studies* and *effectiveness studies*. Efficacy studies evaluate treatment outcomes under highly controlled, ideal conditions. An example is a highly trained researcher providing language intervention to a child one-on-one in a laboratory setting. In contrast, effectiveness studies evaluate treatment outcomes under more typical everyday conditions. Consider, for example, training a paraprofessional to provide language interventions to small groups of children in the back corner of a classroom. Both types of studies serve important roles in the programmatic development and evaluation of interventions (Fey & Finestack, 2009). Efficacy studies generally precede effectiveness studies to establish a causal relationship between an intervention approach and the target outcome. Once this relationship has been established, the generalization of this effect to more typical conditions can be examined in effectiveness studies. Effectiveness studies can also be used to examine for whom the treatment is most beneficial and under what conditions. Thus, when characterizing the level of

evidence, it is also important to determine if the study examined efficacy or effectiveness. Effectiveness studies have greater external validity and should be weighted stronger than efficacy studies.

Beyond studies of efficacy and effectiveness are *implementation studies*. Implementation research is designed to identify and test possible barriers to the adoption and use of evidence-based approaches as standard care, with the ultimate goal to overcome barriers so that evidence-based approaches can be incorporated into community health policies and practices (Finestack & Fey, 2017). Implementation studies range in focus with the goal to change the practice of individual clinicians at one end and to change policies of national organizations at the other end. Once positive outcomes associated with effectiveness studies are established, clinicians, researchers, and policymakers need to work together to ensure adequate implementation of the approach.

External Evidence: Quality of Evidence

As is the case for levels of research, several systems exist for quantifying the rigor or quality of external scientific research. One such system is GRADE, which is an acronym for Grading of Recommendation, Assessment, Development, and Evaluation (Guyatt, Oxman, Vist, et al., 2008; Schünemann, Brożek, Guyatt, & Oxman, 2013). The GRADE approach considers the following study qualities: risk of bias (study limitations), inconsistency, indirectness, imprecision, and publication bias. Based on ratings related to these qualities, an overall score of high, moderate, low, or very low is assigned to the study. Next, we briefly define each of the GRADE study qualities to evaluate. It is not our assumption that, as professionals, you will need to systematically evaluate each of these qualities, but you should be aware of key qualities to help you generally evaluate external evidence and distinguish high quality studies from low quality studies.

Risk of bias evaluates how study limitations may bias estimates of treatment outcomes. The more study limitations, the greater the risk of bias, and the lower the quality of the study. Study limitations that are prone to exist in RCTs include:

■ Lack of Allocation Concealment—the person enrolling study participants knows the group assignment sequence. This bias is similar to the limitations mentioned above of using a non-randomized treatment study design, as the allocation concealment is a key component of randomization. If the person enrolling participants knows the randomization sequence, implicit biases may affect scheduling

or assessment. These biases may inadvertently influence study outcomes.

■ Lack of Blinding—clients, caregivers, assessors, or coders know to which study group they were enrolled. Blinding is necessary as much as possible to avoid placebo effects or expected results based on group assignment. Typically, in the fields of speech-language pathology and audiology, blinding of the client and clinician is difficult. The client will know that they are receiving treatment and the approaches used as will the clinician. For example, the client and their family would know if they are assigned to the treatment group that receives a parent-implemented AAC intervention or a clinician-implemented intervention. Likewise, the client will be aware if they are in a group receiving a new hearing aid, although it may be possible to disguise different hearing aid technologies to facilitate blinding. To mitigate biases due to lack of blinding, researchers may be vague regarding the primary study outcomes and include outcome measures on which they would not expect intervention-induced changes to function as a control measure. Although more expensive, researchers can hire assistants unaware of pre-intervention performance levels and group assignments to evaluate and/or code post-treatment performance.

■ Incomplete Accounting of Patients and Outcome Events—researchers not reporting the number of participants who did not complete the study and instead reporting outcomes only for those who completed the study. For various reasons, participants in a treatment study do not always complete the entire study. These reasons may not be tied directly to the study and therefore should not necessarily be interpreted as a reason for concern. For example, participants may relocate, their schedule may change, or they may no longer have necessary transportation to participate in the study. Other reasons for withdrawing from a study may be closely related to the study and can indicate weaknesses in the treatment. For example, participants may not like their group assignment, the intervention may be difficult or cause discomfort, they may no longer see benefit of the study, or they may meet their desired outcomes and no longer value their participation even though the study protocol requires additional sessions or follow-up. When evaluating outcomes, it is important to know how many participants in

each group did not complete the study and the reasons for withdrawal. If participants withdraw from a study, the researchers might statistically account for those withdraws when reporting their treatment outcomes (e.g., using "intention to treat" methods; see Hollis & Campbell, 1999).

■ Selective Outcome Reporting—researchers not reporting outcomes on all primary and secondary measures. Before conducting their study, researchers should identify the primary and secondary outcome measures they will use to evaluate the intervention. Ideally, they will also register their study protocol and plans for analyses prior to initiating data collection. This ensures that the outcomes published are not the result of "data mining," where the researchers examine multiple outcomes to find any significant results to report. Conducting multiple analyses increases the odds that analyses will reach a level considered to be of statistical significance and decreases the confidence consumers can have in the reported outcomes.

■ Other Limitations—including ending the trial early, using unvalidated outcome measures (e.g., patient-reported outcomes). One reason researchers may choose to end a trial prior to the time established in study protocol is due to loss of adequate study funding, which is likely out of the researchers' control. However, if researchers end a trial early because they believe they have enough data or have conducted unplanned analyses prior to the study's conclusion which indicate positive outcomes, this increases the risk of biases impacting outcomes. In this case, the ending of the trial may have been premature because analyses with additional participants or long-term measures may yield different outcomes. Thus, researchers should always follow their registered protocol to reduce biases. The use of unvalidated measures may also increase bias in study outcomes. Outcome measures based on self-report or family report are prone to be biased because the client and family are likely to be aware of group assignment. Those reporting on individuals who they know received the intervention may be more likely to rate themselves or the client higher than those reporting on individuals who they know did not receive the intervention. It is important for outcome measures, especially primary outcome measures, to be based on objective assessments as much as possible to mitigate such biases.

Inconsistency refers to inconsistency of the study's outcomes relative to outcomes of previous studies by the same or different researchers. When researchers cannot identify plausible reasons for inconsistent results, it suggests that the study's quality may have been compromised. One reason for outcome inconsistencies across studies may be differences in characteristics of study participants based on factors such as age, diagnosis, level of impairment, and socioeconomic status. Researchers can mitigate the impact of heterogeneous samples through statistical analyses that focus on outcomes relative to participant characteristics. If researchers cannot explain inconsistent outcomes based on differences in participant samples, intervention approaches, outcomes measures, or other study methods, the perceived quality of study should be reduced.

Indirectness occurs when features of the study under evaluation differ from the components defined in your PICO question. It likely will be difficult to find a systematic review, several studies, or even a single study that maps perfectly to your PICO question. For example, considering the example PICO questions presented at the beginning of the chapter, the study may include a slightly different population such as 5-year-olds with Down syndrome instead of 5-year-olds with ASD or men with moderate hearing loss above the age of 80 years instead of 75 years. The study may examine a teacher-implemented intervention instead of a parent intervention or use of a single hearing aid instead of bilateral hearing aids. The study may measure word combinations instead of comments and requests or conversational skills instead of word recognition skills. Some minor differences in study features may be acceptable, but significant differences limit the direct relevance of the study being evaluated. The weight of studies that do not offer direct application to your PICO question should be downgraded.

Imprecision reflects the degree of confidence surrounding a study's outcomes. Generally, studies that include few participants will have large confidence intervals associated with the treatment effect. Thus, small-scale studies with few participants generally have lower quality ratings because there is greater variability in treatment effects. Thus, studies with a large number of participants should be weighted more heavily than studies with a small number of participants.

Publication bias refers to the selective publication of studies. Not all studies are published. In some cases there may be fatal flaws in the research design or methodology that prohibit interpretation of study results. In other cases, the methodology may be sound, but the outcomes do not support a positive intervention effect (i.e., there is a "negative effect"). When studies with "negative effects" are not published, the remaining published outcomes may under or over estimate the potential benefits or harms of an intervention. Some reasons for the occurrence of publication bias in the publication process include: attempting to report small-scale studies with a "negative effect," authors uninterested or unmotivated to publish a study with a "negative effect," and authors choosing to submit manuscripts associated with a "negative effect" to non–peer reviewed journals. Thus, when evaluating systematic reviews, it is important to keep in mind that the studies included in the review likely do not reflect all research outcomes to date and their results should be interpreted with some caution.

If a study or review appears compromised based on any of the aforementioned factors, you should downgrade the weight of the study when evaluating the external evidence. It is important to note that there are also some study elements that may increase the weight of a particular study, such as when the study demonstrates a very large effect. For example, the quality of a nonrandomized trial should be upgraded if the treatment demonstrates very large effects.

External Evidence: Integrating Levels and Quality of Evidence

Levels of evidence and quality of evidence are both critical factors to consider when you are examining external evidence; however, it is necessary to consider these factors in tandem. Guyatt et al. (2011) suggest that evidence levels be used to establish an initial level of quality such that systematic reviews and RCTs are initially considered to provide high levels of evidence and observational studies are initially considered to provide low levels of evidence. Studies can be upgraded or downgraded based on previously defined features. Table 8–8 displays how level and quality of specific features can be integrated to establish a single quality descriptor.

Using Intervention Evidence: An Example

Imagine you are a school-based SLP working in a rural area. You are new to the area but worked for a large urban school district for five years. In your current position, you provide services for three elementary schools across two counties. One of your clients, Ronny, is a 5-year-old boy who was diagnosed with ASD at 4 years of age. Ronny's expressive vocabulary includes 10 words, most of which he uses to request food and drinks. Ronny's parents report that he becomes easily frustrated when his needs are not met and he does not engage in social interactions with them or his older brother. Ronny's mother

Table 8–8. Evaluating the Quality of Intervention Evidence

Level	Intervention Study Design	Quality of Evidence	Lower Quality	Raise Quality
1a	Systematic review/meta-analysis of randomized controlled trials	High	For presence of each of the following: ■ Risk of bias ■ Inconsistency ■ Indirectness ■ Imprecision ■ Publication bias lower quality –1 if serious; –2 if very serious	If large intervention effect, raise quality +1 for large effect; +2 for very large effect
1b	Individual randomized controlled trial			
2	Well-designed non-randomized controlled trial	Moderate		
3	Observational studies with controls			
4	Observational studies without controls	Low		

works part-time from home. She is highly motivated to support Ronny's communication skills.

After evaluating Ronny, you determine that his treatment goals should focus on increasing his requests and comments. Based on previous experience, you believe that Ronny would benefit from use of a picture-based AAC system that will allow him to make single-word requests and comments. Given the demands of your caseload and the high motivation level of Ronny's mother, you consider training Ronny's mother to implement the AAC-based intervention. However, you do not have much experience with parent-implemented interventions and the lead SLP wants you to justify the treatment approach. You decide to systematically evaluate the internal and external evidence using the principles of EBP. You begin by developing your PICO question. In this case, the PICO question is the same as the first example PICO question provided at the beginning of the chapter: For a minimally verbal 5-year-old child with ASD (P), does a parent-implemented intervention (I) or clinician-implemented intervention (C) lead to greater requests and comments using AAC (O)?

Next you consider the internal evidence: your clinical expertise and the client's perspectives. In this case, you do not have experience with parent-implemented approaches, but you are open to the approach and believe that it may be of greater benefit to Ronny than clinician-implemented intervention given that you will only be able to work with Ronny twice a week for 30 minutes each session. Additionally, you feel you have strong skills targeting communication using AAC that would help you in training Ronny's mother to develop the skills necessary to support her implementation of the

intervention. Through your conversations with Ronny's parents, you believe that Ronny's mother would be open to learning how to support his communication at home. Ronny's mother has offered to come to his school to attend sessions with Ronny to learn intervention strategies to use with Ronny at home.

Given that the internal evidence supports using a parent-implemented intervention approach with Ronny, you continue to pursue this approach by examining the external evidence. You begin by searching ASHA's Evidence Maps (American Speech-Language-Hearing Association, 2019). You search two maps: Spoken Language Disorders (94 articles) and Autism Spectrum Disorder (293 articles). On these maps you find several relevant systematic reviews, which were all published within the past three years. You identify two reviews on the Spoken Language Disorders map. The first is on parent-implemented interventions for children with developmental delays (Te Kaat-van den Os, Jongmans, Volman, & Lauteslager, 2017). The review includes 7 studies focused on children under 3 years of age and does not include children with ASD or use of AAC. The authors used standards put forth by the American Academy for Cerebral Palsy and Developmental Medicine to rank the levels and quality of the studies reviewed. All studies were ranked as small RCTs of moderate to high quality. The second review is focused on parent programs and includes 14 studies of children older than 2 years (Tosh, Arnott, & Scarinci, 2017). This study also excluded studies in which the child participants had ASD or focused on AAC. The authors of the review used the Crowe Critical Appraisal Tool (Crowe, Sheppard, & Campbell, 2011) to assess the quality of the evidence

All but one study was judged to be of low quality due to small sample sizes, lack of description of the intervention, and incomplete accounting of participants. Both of these reviews indicate that parent-implemented interventions are more beneficial than no intervention, although the quality of the studies were somewhat mixed. While both studies focus on parent-implemented intervention, neither includes participants who match the P in your PICO question or Ronny's specific profile. You decide to continue to search for more external evidence.

On the Autism Spectrum Disorder map, you find a review of RCTs focused on minimally verbal children with ASD (Brignell et al., 2018). This is a good match to Ronny's profile. Examination of the review indicates that it includes only two studies, both of which are RCTs. Both studies included children with ASD. One study (Siller, Hutman, & Sigman, 2013) included a verbally based intervention that trained parents to implement the intervention. This study included children under the age of 6 years. Results indicated no significant differences between the treatment group and control group, which received parent advocacy coaching, based on an assessment of verbal language. The other study (Howlin, Gordon, Pasco, Wade, & Charman, 2007) focused on improving communication using a low-technology AAC with children between the ages of 4 and 11 years. In this study, parents received 13 hours of training. Results indicated that children in the treatment group were 3.9 times more likely to use their low technology to communicate than children in the control group who did not receive treatment. Using GRADE, the authors of the systematic review judged both studies to be of low quality.

Although none of these reviews perfectly map onto your PICO question, you feel you have adequate external evidence to guide your clinical decision. There is fairly strong evidence supporting the general use of parent-implemented interventions; however, evidence for 5-year-olds who are minimally verbal is limited. One study that examined a low-technology AAC method with parent-implementation revealed positive treatment outcomes, although the study was judged to be of low quality. This evidence, combined with strong clinician and client internal evidence, supports the use of a parent-implemented treatment approach for Ronny.

For the past three months, you have been working with Ronny and his mother. For the first month, Ronny's mother attended every session you had with Ronny; for the past two months, Ronny's mother has been attending one session per week. During these sessions, you have Ronny's mother use basic strategies for encouraging Ronny to use AAC to request activities and to comment on things in his environment. You have been targeting similar goals in your individual sessions with Ronny with a focus on classroom activities and the

school environment. Using a clinician-designed probe administered in school, Ronny spontaneously used his AAC device to request 15 different activities and comment on 7 different events after 3 months of intervention. Ronny's mother reports that he currently uses his AAC device at home to request 7 different activities and comment on 8 different events. Ronny's mother reports that in the last month, Ronny has had fewer melt-downs and he appears to be less frustrated. You notice that Ronny enjoys having his mother attend sessions with him and that Ronny's mother appreciates learning strategies to use with him. Ronny's mother tells you that she wants to continue using the parent-implemented approach, but would like to focus on verbal requests and comments. Given all of this evidence, you decide to begin to integrate verbal communication into your goals and continue having Ronny's mother attend one of his intervention sessions each week. You will continue to monitor Ronny's treatment progress using your clinician-designed probes.

This example, admittedly, presented a clean illustration for using EBP to guide clinical decisions. In some cases, it won't be as easy as using the ASHA Evidence Maps as your only method for locating systematic reviews. There may not be a systematic review available on your topic requiring you to consult primary research; even then, there may not be evidence that is both high level and high quality available. Also, in this case the parent was enthused about being directly involved in the intervention and had flexibility in her schedule to attend sessions. This might not be the case for all families. Also, in the example, Ronny quickly made significant gains. Oftentimes, your client will not show significant improvement in a short amount of time. If treatment gains are not made, you will need to decide if you should modify the treatment and if so, how. This will likely require you to revisit the EBP steps outlined in Table 8–1.

Summary

The ASHA Code of Ethics states, "Individuals who hold the Certificate of Clinical Competence shall use independent and evidence-based judgment, keeping paramount the best interests of those being served" (ASHA, 2016). Therefore, it is essential for you, as a professional, to continually engage in identifying and evaluating the evidence for all of your clinical decisions. Using a focused approach to evaluate evidence will help ensure you meet this ethical obligation in an efficient manner. The EBP model can serve as a reminder that evidence can and should come from multiple sources: external, scientific evidence; your own clinical expertise; and the

client's perspective. Developing a PICO question and answering that question by systematically addressing all three components of the evidence-based approach to clinical decision making will focus your evaluation of the evidence in a way that will result in the best outcome for the client.

When evaluating clinical evidence for selecting specific assessment procedures, determining the reliability and validity of the assessment is the foundation for deciding whether to use that assessment. Validity can only be evaluated in terms of the purpose you have for choosing that assessment. If your purpose is to diagnose a disorder, then measures of diagnostic accuracy should be used to document validity.

In terms of treatment evidence, a PICO question can help identify the specific type of evidence needed to evaluate the impact an intervention might have. When evaluating the quality of research evidence it is important to determine what level of evidence a treatment study provides and the quality of the study methodology. Systematic reviews that include high-level, large-scale RCTs are considered the most useful evidence assuming the researchers used rigorous methodology.

Critical Thinking

1. Describe a time in your graduate program when the external evidence demonstrated high reliability and validity for an assessment method but your use of that assessment method in a clinical setting could not be validly used. What led to the disconnect between the external and internal evidence?

2. It can be expensive for test developers to document all the various types of reliability for a new measure. Which type/s of reliability do you believe would be most important and why?

3. Developing PICO questions and evaluating external and internal evidence can be time-consuming. Brainstorm ways you can integrate this evidence-based way of approaching clinical problems in a time efficient way. How do you think your use of evidence-based practice might change from now as a student, to the end of your first year of practice, and when you retire?

References

Alsayedhassan, B., Banda, D. R., & Griffin-Shirley, N. (2016). A review of picture exchange communication interventions implemented by parents and practitioners. *Child and Family Behavior Therapy*, *38*(3), 191–208.

American Speech-Language-Hearing Association. (2016). *Code of ethics* [Ethics]. Available from http://www.asha.org/policy/

American Speech-Language-Hearing Association. (2019, May 30). *Evidence Maps*. Retrieved from https://www.asha.org/Evidence-Maps/

Bettany-Saltikov, J. (2010). Learning how to undertake a systematic review: Part 2. *Nursing Standard*, *24*(51), 47.

Brignell, A., Chenausky, K. V., Song, H., Zhu, J., Suo, C., & Morgan, A. T. (2018). Communication interventions for autism spectrum disorder in minimally verbal children. *Cochrane Database of Systematic Reviews*, *2018*(11), CD012324.

Council on Academic Accreditation in Audiology and Speech-Language Pathology of the American Speech-Language-Hearing Association. (2019). *Standards for accreditation of graduate education programs in audiology and speech-language pathology*. Retrieved from https://caa.asha.org/wp-content/uploads/Accreditation-Standards-for-Graduate-Programs.pdf

Crowe, M., Sheppard, L., & Campbell, A. (2011). Comparison of the effects of using the Crowe Critical Appraisal Tool versus informal appraisal in assessing health research: a randomised trial. *International Journal of Evidence-Based Healthcare*, *9*(4), 444–449.

Fey, M. E., & Finestack, L. H. (2009). Research and development in children's language intervention: A 5-phase model. In R. G. Schwartz (Ed.), *Handbook of child language disorders*. New York, NY: Psychology Press.

Finestack, L. H., & Fey, M. E. (2017). Translation and implementation research in the development of evidence-based child language intervention. In R. G. Schwartz (Ed.), *Handbook of child language disorders* (2nd ed.). New York, NY: Psychology Press.

Gillam, S. L., & Gillam, R. B. (2006). Making evidence-based decisions about child language intervention in schools. *Language, Speech, and Hearing Services in Schools*, *37*(4), 304–315.

Guyatt, G. H., Haynes, R. B., Jaeschke, R. Z., Cook, D. J., Green, L., Naylor, C. D., . . . Evidence-Based Medicine Working Group. (2000). Users' guides to the medical literature: XXV. Evidence-based

medicine: principles for applying the users' guides to patient care. *JAMA, 284*(10), 1290–1296.

Guyatt, G., Oxman, A. D., Akl, E. A., Kunz, R., Vist, G., Brozek, J., . . . Jaeschke, R. (2011). GRADE guidelines: 1. Introduction—GRADE evidence profiles and summary of findings tables. *Journal of Clinical Epidemiology, 64*(4), 383–394.

Guyatt, G. H., Oxman, A. D., Vist, G. E., Kunz, R., Falck-Ytter, Y., Alonso-Coello, P., & Schünemann, H. J. (2008). GRADE: An emerging consensus on rating quality of evidence and strength of recommendations. *British Medical Journal, 336*(7650), 924–926.

Guyatt, G., Rennie, D., Meade, M. O., & Cook, D. J. (2008). *Users' guides to the medical literature: essentials of evidence-based clinical practice* (2nd ed.). New York, NY: McGraw-Hill.

Haynes, R. B., Sackett, D. L., Guyatt, G. H., & Tugwell, P. (2006). *Clinical epidemiology: how to do clinical practice research* (3rd ed.). Philadelphia, PA: Lippincott Williams & Wilkins.

Hollis, S., & Campbell, F. (1999). What is meant by intention to treat analysis? Survey of published randomised controlled trials. *British Medical Journal, 319*(7211), 670–674.

Howlin, P., Gordon, R. K., Pasco, G., Wade, A., & Charman, T. (2007). The effectiveness of Picture Exchange Communication System (PECS) training for teachers of children with autism: A pragmatic, group randomised controlled trial. *Journal of Child Psychology and Psychiatry, 48*(5), 473–481.

Plante, E., & Vance, R. (1994). Selection of preschool language tests: A data-based approach. *Language, Speech, and Hearing Services in Schools, 25*(1), 15–24.

Porzsolt, F., Ohletz, A., Thim, A., Gardner, D., Ruatti, H., Meier, H., . . . Schrott, L. (2003). Evidence-based decision making—the 6-step approach. *ACP Journal Club, 139*(3), A11–A12.

Robey, R. (2004, April 13). Levels of evidence. *The ASHA Leader*, p. 5.

Robey, R., Apel, K., Dollaghan, C., Ellmo, W., Hall, N., Helfer, T., . . . Lonsbury-Martin, B. (2004). *Report of the Joint Coordinating Committee on Evidence-Based Practice*. Retrieved from https://www.asha.org/uploadedFiles/members/ebp/JCCEBPReport04.pdf

Sackett, D. L., Straus, S. E., Richardson, W. S., Rosenberg, W., & Haynes, R. B. (2000). *Evidence-based medicine: How to practice and teach EBM* (2nd ed.). Edinburgh, Scotland: Churchill Livingstone.

Salvia, J., Ysseldyke, J. E., & Witmer, S. (2013). *Assessment in special and inclusive education* (13th ed.). Boston, MA: Cengage Learning.

Schünemann, H., Brożek, J., Guyatt, G., & Oxman, A. (Eds.). (2013). The GRADE Working Group. *GRADE handbook for grading quality of evidence and strength of recommendations*. Retrieved from https://gdt.gradepro.org/app/handbook/handbook.html

Siller, M., Hutman, T., & Sigman, M. (2013). A parent-mediated intervention to increase responsive parental behaviors and child communication in children with ASD: A randomized clinical trial. *Journal of Autism and Developmental Disorders, 43*(3), 540–555.

Te Kaat-van den Os, D. J., Jongmans, M. J., Volman, M. C. J., & Lauteslager, P. E. (2017). Parent-implemented language interventions for children with a developmental delay: A systematic review. *Journal of Policy and Practice in Intellectual Disabilities, 14*(2), 129–137.

Tosh, R., Arnott, W., & Scarinci, N. (2017). Parent-implemented home therapy programmes for speech and language: A systematic review. *International Journal of Language and Communication Disorders, 52*(3), 253–269.

9

The Future of Science

Raymond D. Kent, PhD

Introduction

Research is intrinsically futuristic, always directed to the next experiment, the next theoretical advance, the next challenge to the standard or popular view. Research is a frontier phenomenon, and its practitioners work on a horizon of possibilities. To dare any specific forecast into what research may bring is uncertain at best foolish or irrelevant at worst. Predictions about where science can take us are sometimes amusingly wrong, as described in *The Follies of Science* (Dregni & Dregni, 2006). Although it can be fun to look at predictions that went awry, science has spectacular accomplishments to its credit. In 1924, Bertrand Russell wrote, "The effect of the biological sciences, so far, has been very small." This may have been an accurate assessment a few decades ago. But what opinion would Russell have today about discoveries in genetics, biomolecular science, and nanomedicine? Thinking about the future of research (or any human enterprise) is more than an exercise in armchair speculation because designs for the future help to shape the research agenda of a discipline, project the needs for scientific expertise and research facilities, and develop strategies that have a high likelihood of success at a manageable cost. Because research is a human enterprise that rests on intellectual and economic resources, it is possible to make some general projections about the future of science, considering both the historic pattern and the present-day foundation for future development.

This chapter takes a general view of research with an emphasis on the discipline of communication sciences and disorders (CSD). The purpose is partly to predict some general directions of scientific effort in the field and to assay the socioeconomic trends and various factors that will govern funding for research and the parameters of its application. The expenditure for research on communication sciences and disorders is quite small compared with that for the major diseases such as cancer or heart disease, but all areas of research, whether large or small, are subject to the major forces of social policy. To put it in other words, "Science policy implements a social contract" (Pielke & Byerly, 1998, p. 42). For several decades, the social policy that undergirded research support was the Bush contract, named after Vannevar Bush, who in 1945 published a document of extraordinary influence. As noted by Pielke and Byerly (1998), the Bush contract is based on three fundamental assumptions: (1) It assumes that scientific advances are essential to meet national needs. Most citizens would agree with this contention, and the expectation that science will benefit society is critical to the public support of science. (2) The way in which science meets national needs can be described through a simple linear/

reservoir model. In this model, science creates a reservoir of knowledge that is tapped by society. (3) Science is practiced in relative autonomy, isolated from the direct influence of society. This isolation ensures a freedom and objectivity of scientific inquiry. In this model, society provides the resources for, but does not govern, the scientific enterprise. Ideally, science would grow continuously, and as it does, the reservoir of knowledge would expand, and society would benefit from this vast pool of information. But, as discussed later, all of these assumptions are being questioned by some segments of society. Whether or not the Bush contract survives in the future, it is certain that some kind of social contract is needed to ensure scientific progress.

The Committee on Science of the U.S. House of Representatives took a major step in defining the new federal science policy with its report "Unlocking Our Future: Toward a New National Science Policy" (U.S. House of Representatives Committee on Science, 1998; excerpts of the report appear in *Science Communication, 20,* 328–336). Some basic issues are summarized here. An important point is that the report affirms the importance of federal funding for fundamental scientific, or basic, research. It also endorses a program of research grants to individual investigators that offset indirect costs and are evaluated by a peer-reviewed selection process. The report recommends that funding be provided for creative, groundbreaking research that might be considered too risky in a conservative review process. Mention also is made of the Governmental Results and Performance Act, which mandates a review of outcomes of federally supported programs, including research. The report recommends that funding agencies evaluate outcomes by using a research portfolio rather than evaluating outcomes for individual research grants.

In meeting its obligations to society, science must accomplish a broad agenda of discovery and application. To accomplish this goal, science has a diversified nature, as described next.

The Research Landscape: Types of Research

Research is not a monolithic entity but rather a spectrum of investigative approaches that are complementary and potentially confirmatory. The following types are among the most widely recognized and are defined here in terms suitable for the CSD field. But it should be noted that these terms are defined in somewhat different ways by different authors and agencies and they may very well take different forms over time. Listed below are major types of research, which are not necessarily discrete and non-overlapping.

Basic Research

This type of research (also known as fundamental or preclinical research) is aimed at the study of mechanisms or processes that are universal in their application to scientific knowledge. Although basic research in CSD is often understood as research on normal processes of speech, language, hearing, and related functions, that is not necessarily the case because this kind of research can be conducted with a combination of typical and atypical behaviors and functions. Basic research is conducted to discover fundamental principles, often without an immediate clinical application. Basic research not only illuminates mechanisms and processes in communication but also establishes normative data that are critical to the assessment of communicative disorders (e.g., normative data on phonetic development, vocabulary size, syntactical structures). Basic biomedical research is a type of basic research directed to increase understanding of fundamental life processes, such as genetics, molecular biology, and functional patterns of neural activity. Much of this research focuses on normal or typical processes, such as the pattern of neural activation underlying processes of audition, language comprehension, or language expression. Proof-of-concept for the cochlear implant was accomplished in 1957 by scientist André Djourno and physician Charles Eyriès (Seitz, 2002). The use of transcranial magnetic stimulation in treating aphasia has its roots in the demonstration that this type of stimulation causes speech arrest (Pascual-Leone, Gates, & Dhuna, 1991).

But basic science includes a variety of research methods and objectives, some of which are closely linked to clinical issues. For example, research on epidemiology is critical in the understanding of the prevalence and incidence of disorders. These data are a gauge of the burden of disease or disorder, that is, the extent to which a particular condition endangers health and well-being. Among the most frequently occurring communication disorders are hearing loss (Stevens et al., 2013) and children's speech and language disorders (Rosenbaum & Simon, 2016). Knowing the impact of these disorders on human lives is key to securing financial support for research.

A demand for immediate applicability of all research could imperil the health of the research enterprise. Frequently, research on fundamental scientific problems yields enormous benefits, not all of which could be imagined at the time of the initial discovery. Funding agencies must take care that research into fundamental questions is not harmed by a drastic reallocation of funds to research that addresses applied problems of high priority. The value of a given research project cannot always be determined from a narrow set of immediate priorities.

Applied Research

Applied research seeks specific knowledge needed to improve the treatment of a disorder or to enhance function in some way. Frequently this research is couched in terms of a given disorder (e.g., hearing loss, stuttering, speech sound disorder, specific language impairment, voice disorder, dysphagia) or a communication difference such as dialect or second-language learning. Clinical research, considered later, is one branch of applied research.

Directed Research

This is research undertaken by an investigator in response to an outside request for study of a particular problem or question. This kind of research opportunity is often announced in a program announcement (PA) or a request for applications (RFA), which is one mechanism that the National Institutes of Health (NIH) uses to solicit applications for research on a given topic or problem. The NIH and several private organizations use this method to solicit research proposals that are congruent with the major aims of the funding agency.

Interdisciplinary Research and Team Science

These types are not defined consistently by those who use the term, but two common definitions are (1) the formation of research collaborations to focus on a common problem that is outside the boundaries of any one scientific discipline (e.g., the genetics of language impairment in children) and (2) the creation of hybrid disciplines such as biochemistry, psychoneuroimmunology, and neurolinguistics. Both the complexity of many research problems and the powerful benefits of hybrid expertise favor the continued development of inter-disciplinary research. Teams of investigators and technicians are often required in areas such as neuroimaging, prosthetics (mechanical and electrical), genetic studies, surgical monitoring, nanotechnology, tissue engineering, and many others. Collaborations and consortia will be the rule rather than the exception in certain kinds of research, and disciplinary specialists need to learn the skills of interdisciplinary and multidisciplinary communication and project management to be most effective.

It borders on the bromidic to say that the field of communication sciences and disorders draws from many different disciplines. But mere proclamation does not guarantee the desired result. The most sophisticated kind of interdisciplinary or multidisciplinary research requires an aggressive crossing of borders and

an enlightened understanding of what each discipline has to offer. The future of science will require scientific personnel to seek interdisciplinary and multidisciplinary projects. Multidisciplinary centers are being formed in several areas and are particularly suited to fields of study in which there are ample data but difficult problems. Ideally, the multidisciplinary center integrates scientists with different specialties to work on a complex problem.

One of the most important divides to be bridged in interdisciplinary or multidisciplinary initiatives is that between behavioral and natural sciences. Poor behavioral choices by individuals can induce, maintain, or exacerbate health problems. Just one behavioral issue—compliance with a clinical specialist's recommendations—is critical to the success of intervention. Behavioral and natural science can be mutually informative, but bringing them together in the desired symbiotic relationship is not as easy as one might hope. Glass and McAtee (2006) recommended three innovations to promote the integration of behavior and natural sciences. The first is an elaboration of the "stream of causation" metaphor along the two axes of time and levels of nested systems of social and biological organization. The second is an inquiry into the proposition that "upstream" features of social context (e.g., inequities in health care, poverty, and racism) are themselves causes of disease. It is well recognized by specialists in communication disorders that these features can contribute to disorders of speech, hearing, or language. The third is the concept of a risk regulator to advance the investigation of behavior and health in populations.

In their analysis of team science, Wuchty, Jones, and Uzzi (2007) reviewed 19.9 million research articles over five decades and examined 2.1 million patents. The data were grouped in three main areas: science and engineering (171 subfields), social sciences (54 subfields), and arts and humanities (27 subfields). The results indicated that teams increasingly dominate in knowledge production, and a strong shift toward collective research was evident in science and engineering, social sciences, and patents. A smaller shift was seen in the arts and humanities. In each area, work by teams dominated the top of the citation distribution. The National Research Council (2015) reported that over 90% of all publications in science and engineering are coauthored by teams of two or more. The report also noted that "team science can lead to results with greater scientific impact, innovation, productivity, and reach than single-investigator approaches" (p. 1 of report brief).

This transition to team science affects the way in which research is conceived and performed, while also redefining the roles of individual scientists, with implications for promotions and rewards in their own institutions. For example, it is becoming increasingly common

for coauthors of a published report to declare their individual roles in the design and conduct of the research. For further discussion of the far-reaching implications of team science, see the report of the National Research Council (2015).

Investigator-Initiated Research

This is a research project defined by the individual investigator or a team of investigators. Typically, this kind of research falls within broad parameters defined by the funding agency, but applicants have considerable latitude in selecting a particular topic of research. Both private and governmental agencies may support this type of research. Later in this section, attention is given to a major source of financial support, the NIH and the R01 funding mechanism.

Patient-Oriented Research

This broad category pertains to studies conducted with human subjects (or on material of human origin such as tissues, specimens, and behavioral phenomena) and addresses functional mechanisms in health and disease, developing and testing preventive and therapeutic principles or developing diagnostic tests.

Population Health Research

Work in this category focuses on the distribution and determinants of health status as influenced by social, economic, and physical environments; human biology; and health policy and services, with the general goal of prevention and health promotion at the population levels. A recent noteworthy example in CSD is an article by Raghavan et al. (2018) that discusses the concept of population health research as it pertains to pediatric speech and language disorders.

Clinical Research

This is a broad category of research that is conducted to learn about functions and disorders in human subjects, with the aim of informing the understanding, assessment, treatment, and prevention of disorders or risks to well-being. As the principles of evidence-based practice (EBP) sweep across professional specialties, levels of evidence have become the coin of the realm in guiding practice and justifying compensation. Figure 9–1 is a representation of the evidence pyramid, that is, a graphic view of the strength of evidence associated with various kinds of knowledge regarding clinical interventions. Strength of evidence increases with ascent through the levels of the pyramid. The pyramid is a transdisciplinary

standard, but disciplines are not necessarily homogeneous in their use of different research designs.

Outcome research is concerned with the end results of particular practices or interventions. This topic is too vast and complex to be discussed in detail here, but at least brief comments should be made on the subject of *clinical trials*. These trials include four phases of research. Phase 0 is a designation for exploratory research that is first used in humans. Phase I trials are the initial stage of testing in humans and are designed to assess safety, tolerability, and basic mechanisms of an intervention. Phase II trials are performed on larger groups of participants (usually in the range of 20 to 300) and are designed to assess how well the treatment works, as well as to continue Phase I safety assessments in a larger group of individuals. Phase III studies are randomized, controlled, multicenter trials on large groups of participants (in the range of 300 to 3,000 or more depending on the condition under study) and are aimed at offering a definitive assessment of how effective the intervention is compared with a current "gold standard" treatment. Phase III studies are expensive, with costs typically running into millions of dollars, and they are logistically demanding (requiring coordination across data collection sites). Phase III trials are considered to be the strongest evidence in support of a treatment.

Randomized controlled trial (RCT) designs are generally regarded as the top level of experimental research because they eliminate selection bias in assigning treatment and can potentially reveal causal relationships between interventions and consequent outcomes. However, RCT designs have characteristics that can limit their use in certain kinds of intervention research. For example, RCTs generally (1) take a considerable period of time from recruitment to dissemination, (2) can be costly to implement and may not be feasible in some circumstances, (3) have a rigid protocol that may confine generalizability of results to other settings, (4) tend to emphasize diagnosis-based treatments rather than individualized, patient-centric interventions, and (5) can raise ethical issues in the random assignment of participants when some individuals have a greater need for treatment.

Without question, RCTs are needed to substantiate treatment outcomes. However, several other designs can provide valuable data while offering advantages in implementation. In a field such as CSD, increasing attention is being given to designs such as case studies or individual subject designs (Byiers, Reichle, & Symons, 2012; Wilson, 2011), qualitative research designs (Tetnowski, 2015), mixed methods research (Glogowska, 2015), and others (Hahs-Vaughn & Nye, 2008). As these different types of research grow in number and sophistication, consideration will have to be given to their placement in the evidence pyramid.

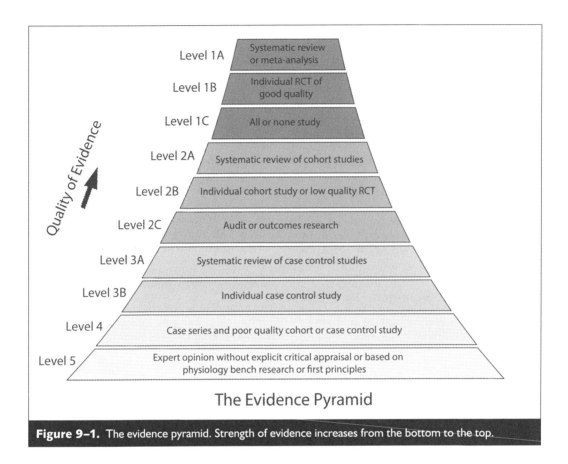

Figure 9–1. The evidence pyramid. Strength of evidence increases from the bottom to the top.

The top level of the evidence pyramid (see Figure 9–1) is occupied by *meta-analyses and systematic reviews*, which summarize and evaluate the evidence for a particular assessment, intervention, or prevention. Different studies on a given topic do not always lead to clear and convincing results. Sometimes different Phase III trials on the same treatment yield discrepant results, which can lead to frustration among the consumers of science, such as patients wanting a clear-cut remedy for their disorder or disease. When discrepant results are reported, a systematic review or meta-analysis can help to provide an overall assessment of the evidence. As defined by Haidich (2010), a systematic review "attempts to collate empirical evidence that fits prespecified eligibility criteria to answer a specific research question. The key characteristics of a systematic review are a clearly stated set of objectives with predefined eligibility criteria for studies; an explicit, reproducible methodology; a systematic search that attempts to identify all studies that meet the eligibility criteria; an assessment of the validity of the findings of the included studies (e.g., through the assessment of risk of bias); and a systematic presentation and synthesis of the attributes and findings from the stud-

ies used" (p. 30). Meta-analyses, a subset of systematic reviews, are quantitative, formal, epidemiological study designs that systematically assess the results of previous research to derive conclusions about that body of research. Robey and Dalebout (1998) provide a concise tutorial. Frequently, but not necessarily, a meta-analysis is based on randomized, controlled clinical trials.

Translational (or Translative) Research

These are efforts to take discoveries from basic science to applications in human health or well-being. In its very basic form, translational research consists of two components or stages. The first, T1, takes work from basic science to an application in a clinical problem (sometimes called "bench to bedside"). The second type, T2, takes a result from clinical research, such as a prevention or treatment strategy, and explores its use in population-based studies to define best practices in the community. The relationships can be summarized with the notation, Bench > Bedside > Population. Ideally, the flow would be bidirectional so that observations at bedside

(clinical application) can influence further work at the bench (basic research). A "translation gap" results from disproportionate efforts in basic research and clinical applications. Several factors contribute to this gap, including industry's preference for late-stage clinical trials, a static distribution of NIH support for basic and applied research, and the inclination of venture investors to seek companies that have products that are close to market (Moses et al., 2005).

As shown in Figure 9–2, translational research can be conceptualized in a more elaborated form, with five stages from T0 to T4. This elaborated view better captures the spectrum and continuity of research efforts needed to consolidate and transfer basic discoveries into personal and societal benefit. It also indicates the complexity of the overall effort, which involves several stages of planning, execution, and synthesis of data.

Implementation Research

This is the scientific study of methods to promote the integration of research results and evidence-based interventions into clinical practice and policy. Peters, Adam, Alonge, Agyepong, and Tran (2013) give an overview of the topic, and discussions relating to CSD are available in Douglas and Burshnic (2019) and Olswang and Prelock (2015). See also Chapter 8 in this volume.

Data Mining

Data mining is the analysis of large stores of data to discover patterns or trends. It exploits the data processing capabilities of computers to sort through large quantities of information to find relationships that are unlikely to be identified in simpler methods of analysis. Examples of the application of data mining to the field of CSD are the reports by Robles-Bykbaev, Quisi-Peralta, López-Nores, Gil-Solla, and García-Duque (2016) and Usip and Ekpenyong (2018) (the latter considers multilingual applications). A related concept is an ontology, which is defined as an explicit formal specification of the terms in a particular domain and the relations among them (Gruber 1993). An expert system uses the ontology to retrieve, analyze, and interpret data from the domain.

Balancing the Research Effort

The proportion of research activity in these categories can change over time. For example, an analysis of research grants on autism by Singh, Illes, Lazzeroni, and Hallmayer (2009) showed the following. First, the number of funded grants increased 15% per year from 1997 to 2006. Second, over the total period of the analysis, basic science accounted for 65% of the projects; clinical research, 15%; and translational research, 20%. Third,

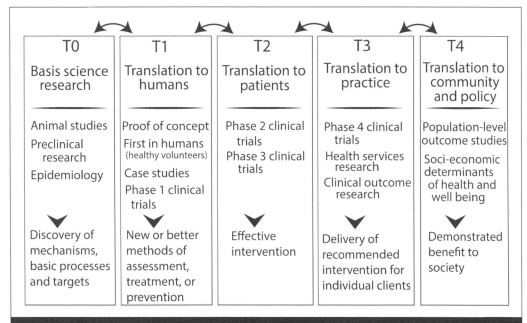

Figure 9–2. Types of translational research. This model shows several stages of research: basic science (T0), translation to humans (T1), translation to patients or clients (T2), translation to practice (T3), and translation to community and policy (T4).

the proportion of basic research grants decreased significantly per year while there was a significant increase in the proportion of translational grants per year. Such a pattern likely will be observed across other disorders. Frequently, basic research is needed to determine the parameters and variables needed for clinical investigations. For example, epidemiological studies provide data on incidence and prevalence, and basic research on mechanisms helps to identify the variables relevant to studies of clinical outcome.

Funding for Research

The future of research is inevitably tied to its funding. Financial support for science comes from primary two sources, private funds (from companies and foundations) or public funds (from a number of different government agencies but for CSD especially the NIH). The NIH is the world's leader in supporting health research. Its mission is "to seek fundamental knowledge about the nature and behavior of living systems and the application of that knowledge to enhance health, lengthen life, and reduce illness and disability." Several types of research support are available through the NIH. The main types are identified by an activity code, and the different types have an availability and purpose that vary somewhat among the various member institutes. The activity codes are found at https://grants.nih.gov/grants/funding/funding_program.htm. The R01 (Research Project Grant) is the original and historically oldest grant mechanism used by NIH. R01 projects can be investigator initiated or can be in response to a program announcement or request for application, as discussed earlier in this chapter.

Competition for federal funding of research is intense. The "payline" or "funding line" (the percentage of grants funded) recently has hovered around 10%, with variations across institutes within NIH, across areas of research, and depending on whether the grant was submitted by a new investigator, or as a first versus renewal application. The bottom line is that only about 1 in 10 proposals is funded in any given cycle of reviews, which are conducted three times annually. The risks are high, given that R01 proposals are the core of academic science and the keystone to individual research careers. But NIH, as important as it is, is not the only source of research funds. A helpful resource is maintained by ASHA: https://www.asha.org/research/grants-funding/Funding-for-Researchers/

Science is expensive. Research requires trained personnel, laboratory facilities, consumable supplies, participant reimbursement, and a variety of other items that come with a price. The actual cost of research includes both direct and indirect costs. Direct costs are those that can be identified specifically with a particular final cost objective, that is, an individual federal award, program, or project. Indirect costs are costs for a common or joint purpose within an organization and that benefit all programs or projects within that organization (e.g., costs related to administration, payroll processing and accounting, facilities maintenance, and utilities). Larger organizations typically negotiate an indirect cost rate, which is typically on the order of 50% to 75% of the direct costs. If a negotiated rate does not yet exist, then nonprofits can either request to negotiate a rate or elect the default rate of 10% of their modified total direct costs. The basic R01 research grant allows an applicant to request $250,000 annually without submitting an itemized budget. If the proposal requests support for five years (which is fairly typical), then the direct costs for the entire project period would come to $1,250,000. If the applicant's institution has negotiated an indirect cost rate of 50% (which is on the low side nationally), then the total costs of the five-year project would be $1,875,000.

Investigators are well advised to consider the mission and priorities of funding agencies in developing and submitting proposals. For example, the NIDCD strategic plan (National Institute on Deafness and Other Communication Disorders, 2017) is a helpful resource in understanding areas of research priority and opportunity. A given research proposal could conceivably receive funding from more than one agency (federal or private). For example, the NIH consists of a number of Institutes, Centers, and Offices (ICOs) that can be overlapping in some areas of research. The Voice, Speech, and Language Programs of NIDCD overlaps with mission areas of other NIH ICOs in the areas of language, literacy, and swallowing. Therefore, an investigator who seeks support for research in swallowing or swallowing disorders may be able to choose among ICOs, depending on the nature of the research and its relationship to the funding priorities of the individual ICOs.

Tensions, Pressures, and Opportunities

The Socio-Economics of Research

Like any human enterprise, science is subject to tensions, pressures, and opportunities, some of which come from outside forces, and some from within. Because the tensions and pressures can threaten the vitality and usefulness of science, it is important to be aware of them. Inevitably, science must compete for resources with other societal needs, such as national defense, health,

education, disasters, and a range of social services. Pew research (Funk, 2017; Kennedy, 2018) shows that approximately 80% of U.S. adults believe that government investments in research provide long-term benefits to society. However, the opinion on this issue differs markedly between Democrats and Republicans. About 90% of Democrats believe there is a long-term benefit, but only about 60% of Republicans feel that way. The political difference is even larger when it comes to the question of whether government support is essential for scientific progress. About 80% of liberal Democrats believe that government support is needed, compared with only 40% of conservative Republicans. The purpose of these comments is not to engage in partisan politics but rather to point out that public support of science cannot be simply assumed.

Even if there were general agreement that the reservoir of knowledge should be as large as possible, it may always be economically prohibitive to support vigorous programs of research in all specialties. Unharnessed growth of science is not sustainable. The conduct of science can also be affected by ethical issues, as in the case of reproduction science, the harvesting of fetal tissues for stem cell research, and genetic engineering. The social contract may change in favor of a model in which economic and moral priorities are established for the support of science. These priorities would determine the allocation of funds for various areas of research. Some sense of the difficulties involved can be gained from an examination of the factors that determine funding for research by the National Institutes of Health. It has been proposed that the funding for different areas and disorders can be gauged by the burden of disease (Gross, Anderson, & Rowe, 1999) or by the amount and effectiveness of lobbying (Gottlieb, 1999). See Curran, Effinger, Pantel, and Curran (1983) for further discussion of priorities and policy.

Public Awareness and Expectations of Science

Public opinion about the value of science can be affected by unfavorable news reports on issues such as scientific fraud, the crisis of replication, and discordant conclusions on matters such as climate change. It is incumbent on scientists to address these issues in an honest and serious manner. It is particularly important to educate the public on the self-policing and self-correcting nature of science. This is not to assert that science is perfect in its pursuit of knowledge but rather to say that scientists know that research is subject to errors, oversights, and even deceit. The so-called *crisis of replication* is a recent example. The headline in the *Washington Post* (August

27, 2018, column by Joel Achenbach) reads "Researchers replicate just 13 of 21 social science experiments published in top journals." Certainly, this statement is disconcerting, but it should be noted that this revelation comes from science itself, and not from outside agencies or schools of thought (Open Science Collaboration, 2015). Science is largely a self-perfecting and self-regulating human activity, one that always probes and analyzes the status quo. The word 'crisis' carries an alarmist tone and may erroneously suggest to those outside science that research is intrinsically untrustworthy. In fact, failure of replication is not new to science, and there has been a continuing struggle within science to ensure that replication (which is part of the essential nature of science) is pursued with vigor. After all, science is not a single piece of work but rather many pieces of work that are weaved together in an account that is mutually consistent and always open to further test. But the so-called crisis carries an important message: science must be diligent in pursuing replication. Certainly, efforts should be made to encourage replication—for example, by reducing publication bias against negative results or replication itself, and by refining statistical methods. Roettger (2019) offers several suggestions in this regard. He points out that one difficulty is that researchers have several "degrees of freedom" in designing and conducting a study; for example, decisions on what should be measured, which predictors and mediators should be specified, and which statistical models should be used. Any of these decisions can affect the outcome of a study and may result in a failure of replication. But some of the greatest obstacles to systematic replication studies are that they are not always rewarded in research careers (e.g., not an original line of research), may be difficult to publish, and may be given low priority by funding agencies (because they may not appear innovative).

Another obligation that falls to scientists is to inform the public and policymakers about what kinds of scientific advances are likely and at what cost. For example, Feigin (2005) considers how research may affect the prospects for child health. The NIH accomplishes a similar goal with the preparation of strategic research plans that typically summarize major research accomplishments and identify opportunities for new discoveries and their clinical application. The NIDCD Strategic Plan for 2017–2021 (National Institute on Deafness and Other Communication Disorders, 2017) discusses both research accomplishments and opportunities in CSD and related fields. Evidence-based practice places an urgency on research related to clinical assessment, treatment, and prevention. Clinical (and nonclinical) specialties have mounted efforts to increase the evidence base

of their practice. The term *evidence-based medicine* first appeared in Guyatt (1991). The growth of this concept has been nothing short of meteoric. For an informative oral history of EBP, see Smith (2014).

Science and Technology

Science and technology are almost inseparable insofar as scientific advances often come about by virtue of new or improved technologies, and the technologies themselves are frequently the products of leading-edge science. Trends in technology that are likely to influence research and practice in CSD over the near future include the following:

1. *Artificial intelligence* can provide expert opinions and guidance when a qualified professional is not available or when the question at hand demands processing of large and complex datasets. The ever-increasing sophistication and power of computational algorithms promises solutions to problems that could prove challenging to individual scientists or even teams of scientists.

2. *Augmented reality and virtual reality* offer both clinicians and their clients opportunities to visualize organs of the body, functions, behaviors, and relationships. These tools are likely to be increasingly used in educational and clinical programs.

3. *Telemedicine, telehealth, telepractice, telerehabilitation, e-rehabilitation, telemonitoring, mHealth* are the various terms attached to the practice of using electronic information and telecommunications technologies for a broad array of services and functions, including long-distance clinical health care, communication among specialists, patient and professional health-related education, and public health and health administration. These technologies are the means to a variety of clinical services including general approaches to telerehabilitation (Peretti, Amenta, Tayebati, Nittari, & Mahdi, 2017) and e-therapy and e-supervision in speech-language pathology (Houston, 2014). The purpose here is not to differentiate these terms but rather to emphasize their fundamental technological unity. The potential of these methods lies in large part in the ubiquity of the required digital technology. In 2013 the Pew Research Center reported that nearly half of all Americans have a tablet device, and 90% have a cell phone. The wide availability of these devices and the expanding range of their functions are a ready-made foundation for clinical and research applications reaching into multiple settings. The potential of mHealth is an ever-growing realm of mobile self-care in which consumer technologies like the smartphone and tablet apps can be used by clients and patients to collect their own health care data, without having a clinician to assist with procedures or interpret the results. Gaming techniques can be used in therapy to provide motivation, feedback, and structured progression through a treatment regimen. See Chapter 27 in this volume for further discussion of telepractice in CSD.

4. The *Internet of Things* (IoT) is a network of physical objects such as vehicles, machines, home appliances, and other devices that use sensors and application programming interfaces to connect and exchange data over the Internet. Given the proliferation of these objects, we are surrounded by interconnected devices that provide multiple opportunities to extend our human faculties (our senses, memory, and physical abilities). The widespread availability of these objects overcomes what has been a serious obstacle in harnessing technology for clinical services—the cost of dedicated technologies. The power of the IoT can support education, clinical services, and research in a variety of environments.

5. *Precision therapy* is identifying the intervention or interventions that will be most effective for individual clients or patients based on genetic, environmental, lifestyle, and motivational and temperament factors. Ultimately, the most effective treatment is one that accounts for individual differences. In medicine, precision therapy has been advocated especially in cancer treatment. Similar concepts are *personalized treatment* and *individualized treatment*. These are not technologies per se but they often rely on technologies as sources of information, such as the management and interpretation of data from different sources (e.g., genetics, psychological testing, speech-language assessments, audiologic tests). Precision therapy has been advocated for conditions such as Down syndrome, where there is substantial phenotypic variation within the genotype (McDaniel & Yoder 2016), but the concept has a general application in that treatment for individual clients and patients may be modified in factors such as dosage (frequency, amount, and duration), combination with other therapies, and definition of desired outcomes.

6. *Crowdsourcing* is the practice of obtaining services, ideas, opinions, or content by soliciting contributions from a large number of respondents, often by means of an online community, rather than from groups of employees, suppliers, or professional experts. It is a potential source of information on the effects of a variety of disorders (e.g., intelligibility, voice quality, naturalness of communication). Fernández, Harel, and McAllister (2018) discuss aspects of the statistical analysis for crowdsourced perceptual ratings of human speech.

7. *Three-dimensional printing* is a manufacturing technique that uses an additive process to build or form 3D objects in successive layers from a digital file derived from computer aided design (CAD) software. This technique can provide personalized implants and prosthetics that can be adapted as needed to physical growth or other changes in an individual patient. Particularly promising is the development of 3D printed biomaterials, already used successfully for printing tumor models, skeletal scaffolds, and human scale tissue products.

8. *Bioengineering* applies principles of engineering to the design and analysis of biological systems and biomedical technologies. The cochlear implant is a neural prosthesis that has had remarkable success in restoring auditory function in individuals who are deaf. Other opportunities include communication aids, tissue replacement or enhancement, and improved neural control.

Dissemination: The First Fruits of Research

The discovery of new information in any scientific domain is exciting and satisfying to the researchers involved, but unless the knowledge is disseminated, it may be of little or no real value to the general public, clinicians, or other researchers. Research is not only discovery but also the accurate and effective dissemination of the new knowledge. Dissemination of research information is changing quickly because of (1) new technologies such as the World Wide Web, (2) an increasingly active (but not always accurate) role of the media in presenting new results to the public, and (3) the urgent demands by third-party payers and others for certain kinds of data (e.g., data on the value of clinical interventions). Dissemination is not a simple pipeline between the scientific laboratory and the consumer of research. Rather, dissemination presents its own complex decisions about quality control, reliability, efficiency, and access. The ethical

burden on authors of scientific articles is considerable, as considered in the excellent papers by Benos and colleagues (2005) and Claxton (2005a, 2005b).

The main functions of a scholarly journal were identified in a seminal report by Ware and Mabe (2015).

1. *Registration:* journals are a vehicle for third-party establishment by date-stamping of the authorship's precedence and ownership of an idea or set of data. Credit for work done is important in establishing careers and obtaining funding for future research. As mentioned earlier, the increasing frequency of multi-authored research reports adds another level of registration, that is, the contributions made by individual authors.

2. *Dissemination:* a journal communicates research discoveries to their intended audiences through the journal's brand identity. The identity is based on several factors, including area of specialization, reputation, and readership.

3. *Credibility* (or certification): by virtue of its editorial processes and standards as typically accomplished through peer review, a journal ensures quality control and credibility. Peer review is not perfect but it is not likely to be overturned as the means to ensure credibility of scientific reports.

4. *Archival record:* in print or online formats, journals preserve a fixed version of a paper (called the article of record) that is maintained for future reference or citation. The archival record is available in digital form for most scholarly publications.

5. *Navigation:* especially through the technology of electronic publishing, journals provide filters and signposts to information in the ever-expanding universe of published material and related items such as datasets. The possibilities of navigation are enhanced by open access, which facilitates online access to scientific information by virtually any interested party.

A positive result of the new publishing technologies is that recently acquired knowledge can be accessed quickly by anyone with the technological resources. This includes the lay public. Clinical specialists frequently discover that patients and clients (or their caregivers) have searched the World Wide Web for information on diseases or disabilities. Consequently, consumers may be considerably better informed today than was the case even a decade or so ago. Another advantage of online publication is that it relaxes the problem of journal pages. For budgetary reasons, print-only journals typi-

cally fix limits on the number of pages in a given issue of the journal. But online publication readily accommodates lengthy articles that can include, either within the article itself or as supplementary information, such items as elaborate graphics, high-resolution images, large data sets, and audio or video recordings.

The media play an important role in announcing new scientific knowledge to the public. Many major discoveries attract the attention of the broadcast and print media almost as soon as they are released to the scientific community. Coverage by the media can be crucial to science because it demonstrates to the public the fast pace of discovery and the potential benefits to society. But at times, the advantages of such public dissemination are offset by inattention to limitations of the research or the need for corroboration of the findings. On occasion, clinical practitioners may feel caught between consumer demands for services (which may be fueled by powerful statements in the public media) and the need for scientific investigation into a type of intervention. The public may fail to understand that acceptance of a new intervention is not necessarily straightforward. Frequently, scientific studies may yield conflicting, or not entirely consistent, results. Some of the ways in which this problem is addressed are meta-analyses (mentioned earlier in this chapter) and consensus conferences, which convene a group of experts to consider the research on a particular topic (Ferguson, 1993).

Dissemination enables the vital step in the research-to-practice sequence, the application of evidence to clinical practice. The ultimate goal of clinical research is to improve clinical assessment and intervention. The vitality of research in a clinical discipline can be gauged by the responsiveness of clinical practice to new discoveries. Obviously, research by itself will not accomplish this goal. It is imperative that the results of research be disseminated to clinicians who have the discernment to use these results to modify clinical practice as indicated. This is not a simple process. It demands a breed of practitioner who is committed to a vigorous professional education that can be summarized as follows:

> Eventually, self-directed lifelong learning and the teaching of evidence-based medicine may take hold, so that practitioners learn during their training how to learn for the rest of their professional lives, becoming adept at keeping up with new evidence and applying it to the betterment of their patients' health. (Haynes, 1993, p. 220)

Dissemination of research should not only be in the technical language used by specialists but also in plain language that can be understood by nonscientists such as the general public, Congress, and members of the media.

President Barack Obama signed *The Plain Writing Act of 2010* on October 13, 2010, which requires federal agencies to write "clear Government communication that the public can understand and use." The President also emphasized the importance of establishing "a system of transparency, public participation, and collaboration" in his January 21, 2009 Memorandum on Transparency and Open Government. Some scholarly journals also have begun to include plain language abstracts in published articles to ensure a broad understanding of new discoveries.

Research on the Global Stage

Many scientific advances have a value that is not limited by cultural or national boundaries, so that a major scientific advance can have potential for worldwide benefit. Discovery of a new vaccine, a potent antibiotic, a new source of fuel, or an efficient means of waste management can affect people in every continent and every nation for generations to come. Research in communication sciences and disorders also can bring benefits to the international community, but these benefits are not always as straightforward as in other sciences. Particularly when a discovery is in some way specific to a given dialect or language, the application to other speech communities or languages cannot be immediately assumed. Nonetheless, it is clear from cross-language studies that important commonalities can exist and that language-related differences can illuminate important issues. Aside from the question of the immediate application of scientific discoveries, there is a fundamental issue concerning international cooperation. The issue is the education of scientists and the development of research facilities on the international stage. The United States is one of the world's leaders in research on communicative disorders, and it is not surprising that students from many other nations have come to the United States to study in the disciplines of speech-language pathology and audiology. Academic programs therefore have the potential for international influence. Thinking about communication and its disorders should become increasingly international in its character, even as the new communication technologies (e.g., machine translation) begin to erase linguistic barriers.

Educating the Next Generation of Scientists in CSD

Science is done by scientists, and the lifeblood of science in any discipline is the preparation and support of investigators. Unlike most academic specialties, CSD

has faced, and apparently continues to face, a shortage of trained research personnel. The shortage is measured not only against the potential benefits of research but also by the number of academic, research, and clinical positions that require a research degree—the PhD. This problem has been recognized for many years and has been addressed by initiatives within ASHA and the Council of Academic Programs in Communication Sciences and Disorders (CAPCSD). In 1997, ASHA and CAPCSD formed a joint committee, the Working Group on Recruitment, Retention, and Academic Preparation of Researchers and Teacher-Scholars. This working group made a number of recommendations, some of which were realized in the development of an ASHA-focused initiative in 2004 and 2005. A subsequent committee, jointly composed of representatives from ASHA and CAPCSD, prepared a report titled "Crisis in the Discipline: A Plan for Reshaping our Future" (Council of Academic Programs in Communication Sciences and Disorders, 2002).

The challenge of preparing future generations of researchers is formidable, but the attention given to this problem is the first step toward a solution. At least two points are clear: (1) newly graduated PhD students should find excellent professional opportunities in the field, and (2) educational programs must increase their generation of PhD students. With respect to the second point, the need is to recruit more PhD students into academic programs. The recruitment effort can be directed at two major groups of students: (a) those already enrolled in undergraduate, master's, or AuD programs (Myotte, Hutchins, Cannizzaro, & Belin, 2011; Osmelak, 2018) and (b) those with other kinds of academic backgrounds such as biology, computer science, linguistics, physics, and psychology. It is important also to attract and prepare PhD students who are capable of working in a research and scholarly environment that is increasingly multidisciplinary and international. Revamping graduate programs in the current economic climate is challenging, but realignment and pooling of resources may be one way of enhancing doctoral research education even though resources are basically static. An example of a new approach that specifically targets interdisciplinary collaboration was described by Humphrey, Cote, Walton, Meininger, and Laine (2005). The approach incorporates three major ways for students to learn about the value of interdisciplinary partnerships: (1) study of successful case studies of cooperation, (2) increased mutual interactions, and (3) experience in interdisciplinary approaches through team-based problem solving (collaborative problem-based learning). As applied to research education in CSD, these ideas would encourage interdisciplinary efforts with other academic units such as psychology, engineering, neuroscience, physics, and biology.

Financial support for research training is available from several sources, with two major sources being the NIH and the American Speech-Language-Hearing Foundation (ASHF), which offers a variety of educational and mentoring programs (see the ASHF website: http://www.ashfoundation.org/). A listing of various kinds of support is also available at http://www.scangrants.com, which is a public service listing of grants and other funding types to support health research, programs, and scholarship. General advice on research careers in CSD is available in Ludlow and Kent (2011).

Summary

The field of communication sciences and disorders is but one slice of a gigantic research enterprise. To some degree, the progress of research in any one discipline is affected by the overall vigor of science in its broadest scope. For example, the budgets for major federal funding agencies determine the number of research grants that will be funded in a given fiscal period. Directly or indirectly, budgets can also determine the amount and kind of preparation of new scientists. Different priorities for funding can enrich one area while impoverishing others. It is likely that there will be intense competition among scientific disciplines for financial support of research. Especially because there appears to be a major change in the social contract that underlies science policy, those who are concerned about the state of the science in the discipline should be prepared to take an active role in encouraging scientists and in providing the resources needed for a healthy research environment.

Critical Thinking

1. What is the Bush contract? Why is this contract important to understanding the public policy behind scientific research? What are the pressures that might cause a revision or rejection of this contract?

2. For what reasons might the proportion of grant funding for basic versus clinical or translational research on a given topic change over time?

3. Discuss the relationship between science and technology. How do they differ? How do they benefit one another? Think of some examples of the interaction between science and technology from communication sciences and disorders.

4. What experiences in your undergraduate or graduate education encouraged you to participate in research? Discouraged you? How and why should a practicing clinician participate in research?

5. What can graduate programs do to encourage students to participate in research opportunities during their graduate studies and prepare them for doing research once they become practicing professionals?

6. How do qualitative research, case studies, and individual research designs contribute to the need for evidence-based research? What types of research can practicing clinicians do in their everyday work?

References

Achenbach, J, (2018, August 27). Researchers replicate just 13 of 21 social science experiments published in top journals. *The Washington Post.*

Benos, D. J., Fabres, J., Farmer, J., Gutierrez, J. P., Hennessy, K., Kosek, D., . . . Wanget, K. (2005). Ethics and scientific publication. *Advances in Physiology Education, 29,* 59–74.

Bush, V. (1945; reprinted 1960). *Science: The endless frontier.* Report to the president on a program for postwar scientific research. Washington, DC: U.S. Government Printing Office.

Byiers, B. J., Reichle, J., & Symons, F. J. (2012). Single-subject experimental design for evidence-based practice. *American Journal of Speech-Language Pathology, 21,* 397–414.

Claxton, L. D. (2005a). Scientific authorship. Part 1. A window into scientific fraud? *Mutation Research, 589,* 17–30.

Claxton, L. D. (2005b). Scientific authorship. Part 2. History, recurring issues, practices, and guidelines. *Mutation Research, 589,* 31–45.

Council of Academic Programs in Communication Sciences and Disorders. (2002). *Crisis in the discipline: A plan for reshaping our future.* Joint Ad Hoc Committee on the Shortage of PhD Students and Faculty in Communication Sciences and Disorders. Retrieved from http://www.capcsd.org/reports/JointAdHocCmteFinalReport.pdf

Curran, A. S., Effinger, A. W., Pantel, E. S., & Curran, J. P. (1983). Public health: Priorities and policy setting in the real world. In F. S. Sterret (Ed.), Science and public policy III. *Annals of the New York Academy of Sciences* (Vol. 403). New York, NY: New York Academy of Sciences.

Douglas, N. F., & Burshnic, V. L. (2019). Implementation science: Tackling the research to practice gap in communication sciences and disorders. *Perspectives of the ASHA Special Interest Groups, 4,* 3–7.

Dregni, E., & Dregni, J. (2006). *Follies of science: 20th century visions of our fantastic future.* Denver, CO: Speck Press.

Feigin, R. A. (2005). Prospects for the future of child health through research. *Journal of the American Medical Association, 294,* 1373–1379.

Ferguson, J. H. (1993). NIH consensus conferences: Dissemination and impact. In K. S. Warren & F. Mosteller (Eds.), Doing more good than harm: The evaluation of health care interventions. *Annals of the New York Academy of Sciences* (Vol. 703, pp. 180–198). New York, NY: New York Academy of Sciences.

Fernández, D., Harel, D., & McAllister, T. (2018). Statistical considerations for crowdsourced perceptual ratings of human speech productions. *Journal of Applied Statistics,* 1–21. https://doi.org/10.1080/02664763.2018.1547692

Funk, C. (2017, May 1). Democrats far more supportive than Republicans of federal spending for scientific research. *Fact-Tank,* Pew Research Center (Washington DC). Retrieved from http://www.pewresearch.org/fact-tank/2018/07/03/americans-broadly-favor-government-funding-for-medical-and-science-research/

Glass, T. A., & McAtee, M. J. (2006). Behavioral science at the crossroads in public health: Extending horizons, envisioning the future. *Social Sciences and Medicine, 62,* 1650–1671.

Glogowska, M. (2015). Paradigms, pragmatism and possibilities: mixed-methods research in speech and language therapy. *International Journal of Language and Communication Disorders 46*(3), 1–10. https://doi.org/10.3109/13682822.2010.507614

Gottlieb, S. (1999). U.S. research funding depends on lobbying, not need. *British Medical Journal, 318,* 1715.

Gross, C. P., Anderson, G. F., & Rowe, N. R. (1999). The relation between funding by the National Institutes of Health and the burden of disease. *New England Journal of Medicine, 340,* 1881–1887.

Gruber, T. R. (1993). A translation approach to portable ontologies. *Knowledge Acquisition*, 5, 199–220. Retrieved from http://tomgruber.org/writing/ontolingua-kaj-1993.htm

Guyatt, G. H. (1991). Evidence-based medicine. *ACP Journal Club*, *114*, A16.

Hahs-Vaughn, D. L., & Chad Nye, C. (2008). Understanding high quality research designs for speech language pathology. *Evidence-Based Communication Assessment and Intervention*, *2*(4), 218–224.

Haidich, A. B. (2010). Meta-analysis in medical research. *Hippokratia*, *14*(Suppl. 1), 29–33.

Haynes, R. B. (1993). Some problems in applying evidence in clinical practice. In K. S. Warren & F. Mosteller (Eds.), Doing more good than harm: The evaluation of health care interventions. *Annals of the New York Academy of Sciences* (Vol. 703, pp. 210–225). New York, NY: New York Academy of Sciences.

Houston, K. T. (2014). *Telepractice in speech-language pathology*. San Diego, CA: Plural Publishing.

Humphrey, J. D., Cote, G. L., Walton, J. R., Meininger, G. A., & Laine, G. A. (2005). A new paradigm for graduate research and training in the biomedical sciences and engineering. *Advances in Physiological Education*, *29*, 98–102.

Kennedy, B. (2018, July). Americans broadly favor government funding for medical and science research. *Fact Tank*, July 14, 2005. Retrieved from https://www.pewresearch.org/fact-tank/2018/07/03/americans-broadly-favor-government-funding-for-medical-and-science-research/

Ludlow, C. L., & Kent, R. D. (2011). *Building a research career*. San Diego, CA: Plural Publishing.

McDaniel, J., & Yoder, P. J. (2016). Pursuing precision speech-language therapy services for children with Down syndrome. *Seminars in Speech and Language*, *37*(4), 239–251.

Moses, H., Dorsey, E. R., Matheson, D. H. M., & Their, S. O. (2005). Financial anatomy of biomedical research. *Journal of the American Medical Association*, *294*, 1333–1342.

Myotte, T., Hutchins, T. L., Cannizzaro, M. S., & Belin, G. (2011). Understanding why speech-language pathologists rarely pursue a PhD in communication sciences and disorders. *Communication Disorders Quarterly*, *33*, 42–54.

National Institute on Deafness and Other Communication Disorders. (2017). *Strategic Plan: FY 2017–2021*. Retrieved from https://www.nidcd.nih.gov/about/strategic-plan/2017-2021-nidcd-strategic-plan

National Research Council. (2015). *Enhancing the effectiveness of team science*. Washington, DC: The National Academies Press.

Olswang, L. B., & Prelock, P. A. (2015). Bridging the gap between research and practice: Implementation science. *Journal of Speech, Language, and Hearing Research*, *58*(6), S1818–S1826.

Open Science Collaboration. (2015). Estimating the reproducibility of psychological science. *Nature*, *349*, aac4716. https://doi.org/10.1126/science.aac4716

Osmelak, D. R. (2018). Undergraduate and graduate communication sciences and disorders students' views regarding the pursuit of a doctorate of philosophy degree. *Health Professions Education*. https://doi.org/10.1016/j.hpe.2018.10.001

Pascual-Leone, A., Gates, J. R., & Dhuna, A. (1991). Induction of speech arrest and counting errors with rapid-rate transcranial magnetic stimulation. *Neurology*, *41*, 697–702

Peretti, A., Amenta, F., Tayebati, S. K., Nittari, G., & Mahdi, S. S. (2017). Telerehabilitation: Review of the state-of-the-art and areas of application. *JMIR Rehabilitation and Assistive Technologies*, *4*(2), e7. https://doi.org/10.2196/rehab.7511

Peters, D. H., Adam, T., Alonge, O., Agyepong, I. A., & Tran, N. (2013). Implementation research: What it is and how to do it. *British Medical Journal*, *347*, f6753.

PEW Research Center (2013, June 6). Cell phone ownership hits 91% of adults. *Fact-Tank*. Retrieved from https://www.pewresearch.org/fact-tank/2013/06/06/cell-phone-ownership-hits-91-of-adults/

Pielke, R. A., Jr., & Byerly, R., Jr. (1998, February). Beyond basic and applied. *Physics Today*, 42–46.

Raghavan, R., Camarata, S., White, K., Barbaresi, W., Parish, S., & Krahn, G. (2018). Population health in pediatric speech and language disorders: Available data sources and a research agenda for the field. *Journal of Speech, Language, and Hearing Research*, *61*, 1279–1291.

Robey, R. R., & Dalebout, S. D. (1998). A tutorial on conducting meta-analyses of clinical outcomes research. *Journal of Speech, Language, and Hearing Research*, *40*, 1227–1241.

Robles-Bykbaev, V., Quisi-Peralta, D., López-Nores, M., Gil-Solla, A., & García-Duque, J. (2016, April). SPELTA-Miner: An expert system based on data mining and multilabel classification to design therapy plans for communication disorders. In *2016 International Conference on Control, Decision and Information Technologies (CoDIT)* (pp. 280–285). IEEE.

Roettger, T. B. (2019). Researcher degrees of freedom in phonetic research. *Laboratory Phonology, 10*(1), 1. https://doi.org/10.5334/labphon.147

Rosenbaum, S., & Simon, P. (Eds.) (2016). *Speech and language disorders in children: implications for the Social Security Administration's Supplemental Security Income Program.* Washington DC: National Academies Press. Childhood Speech and Language Disorders in the General U.S. Population. Retrieved from https://www.ncbi.nlm.nih.gov/books/NBK356270/

Russell, B. (1924). *Icarus: Or, the future of science.* Available from http://onlinebooks.library.upenn.edu/webbin/book/lookupid?key=olbp27562

Seitz, P. R. (2002). French origins of the cochlear implant. *Cochlear Implants International, 3,* 77–86.

Singh, J., Illes, J., Lazzeroni, L., & Hallmayer, J. (2009). Trends in U.S. autism research funding. *Journal of Autism and Developmental Disorders, 39,* 788–795.

Smith, R. (2014). Evidence based medicine—an oral history. *British Medical Journal, 348,* g371.

Stevens, G., Flaxman, S., Brunskill, E., Mascarenhas, M., Mathers, C. D., & Finucane, M. (on behalf of the Global Burden of Disease Hearing Loss Expert Group). (2013). Global and regional hearing impairment prevalence: An analysis of 42 studies in 29 countries, *European Journal of Public Health, 23,* 146–152.

Tetnowski, J. (2015). Qualitative case study research design. *Perspectives on Fluency and Fluency Disorders, 25,* 39–45.

U.S. House of Representatives Committee on Science. (1998). Unlocking our future: Toward a new national science policy (Document No. Y 4.SCI 2:105B, Item 1025-A-01). Retrieved from https://www.govinfo.gov/content/pkg/GPO-CPRT-105hprt105-b/pdf/GPO-CPRT-105hprt105-b.pdf

Usip, P. U., & Ekpenyong, M. E. (2018) Towards ontology-driven application for multilingual speech language therapy. In M. E. Ekpenyong (Ed.), *Human language technologies for under-resourced African languages: Design, challenges and prospects* (pp. 85–101). SpringerBriefs in Electrical and Computer Engineering. Heidelberg, Germany: Springer.

Ware, M., & Mabe, M. (2015). *The STM report: An overview of scientific and scholarly journal publishing.* The Hague, Netherlands: International Association of Scientific, Technical and Medical Publishers.

Wilson, K. P. (2011). Synthesis of single-case design research in communication sciences and disorders: Challenges, strategies, and future directions. *Evidence-Based Communication Assessment and Intervention, 5,* 1–12.

Wuchty, S., Jones, B. F., & Uzzi, B. (2007). The increasing dominance of teams in production of knowledge. *Science, 316,* 1036–1039.

10

Workforce Issues

◇◇

Cathy DeRuiter, MA

Introduction

The needs of a population as large and diverse as that of the United States should be reflected in its workforce. The occupations of audiologists (AuDs), speech-language pathologists (SLPs), and communication sciences and disorders (CSD) faculty-scholars and researchers contribute to the services and economy of our nation. This chapter addresses the current demographics and employment characteristics, including job and career satisfaction and salary information of those in our professions, with a focus on those who affiliate with the American Speech-Language-Hearing Association (ASHA).

The country is constantly evolving. Changes in the political climate, advances in medical and technological fields, and world events affect the global economy and can significantly impact the job market. Factors relating to future employment and the future of the professions such as personnel shortages and changes in population statistics that have informed our abilities to become more culturally aware in our practices will be addressed. This chapter is rich with data and many references are provided where readers can find continually updated resources of information.

The Current Workforce

ASHA is the professional, scientific, and credentialing association for more than 204,000 members and affiliates made up of audiologists, speech-language pathologists, speech, language, and hearing scientists, audiology and speech-language pathology support personnel, and students (ASHA, n.d.-a). ASHA's Certificate of Clinical Competence (CCC) is the internationally recognized voluntary professional credential for AuDs and SLPs. Students will likely have heard about this credential, and many may be striving for it. If you are a professional, it is likely that you work alongside many colleagues who hold the credential. One advantage to a national association for membership and certification is that there is a great deal of data available to you to learn about the demographics of your own discipline on the national level. The following sections on workforce issues are largely drawn from various ASHA reports. This chapter gives you the advantage of "one stop" for general information about your discipline. Note, however, things are subject to change, so it is important to monitor trends at the national, state and local levels.

ASHA Membership and Affiliation Data

At the end of 2018, ASHA represented 191,675 AuDs, SLPs, and speech, language, and hearing scientists (ASHA, 2019a). These numbers were through either memberships, certification, or both. When we consider this total, 172,805 are SLPs and 12,480 are AuDs (ASHA, 2019a). Figures 10–1 and 10–2 demonstrate the changes in certified AuDs and SLPs over the past 10 years, respectively. Overall, both AuDs and SLPs have continued to grow. However, the percentage of 10-year growth is greater for SLPs than AuDs.

Employment Characteristics

Where you work and how many hours you work per week are considerations for anyone in the profession. There are a wide range of environments and populations that are served by SLPs and AuDs. The data below are summarized from various reports on the national level. The following section summarizes data from ASHA regarding employment characteristics as reported by its membership/certificate holders and uses the association's terms and structure.

At the close of 2018, the majority of ASHA's membership and affiliation were employed full-time (71.7%), whereas 19.0% were employed on a part-time basis

(ASHA, 2019a). Less than 1% were unemployed and seeking employment. This number is below the December 2018 national unemployment rate of 3.9% reported by the U.S. Bureau of Labor Statistics (U.S. Department of Labor, Bureau of Labor Statistics [BLS], 2019a).

Where AuDs and SLPs work is another important variable that can be impacted by a variety of factors discussed in this book. In 2018, the majority of AuDs (73.6%) were employed in health care settings. These settings and the percentage of AuDs, respectively, included nonresidential health care facilities such as private physicians' or audiology offices (46.2%), hospitals (26.7%), and residential health care facilities such as skilled nursing facilities (0.8%; ASHA, 2019a). About 15.1% were employed in educational settings, including schools (8.1%) and higher education institutions (7.0%). Approximately one third (31.3%) were employed full or part time in private practice. This rate is somewhat higher than the rates of the past couple years.

As for speech-language pathologists, the percentages of those employed across the different settings varies from audiology. Roughly half of SLPs (54.2%) were employed in educational settings, including 51.4% in schools and 2.7% in higher education. Health care settings made up the employment site for 39.3% of SLPs, including 17.1% in nonresidential health care facilities, 12.5% in hospitals, and 9.7% in residential health care

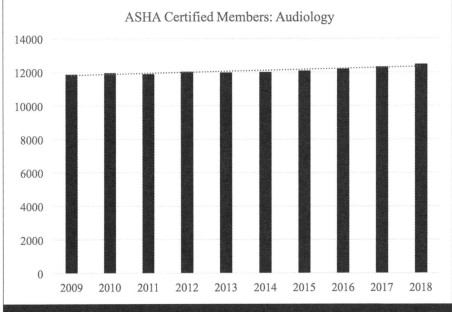

Figure 10–1. Number of ASHA certified audiologists over the past decade with associated trend line. Note: These data do not include dual certificate holders.

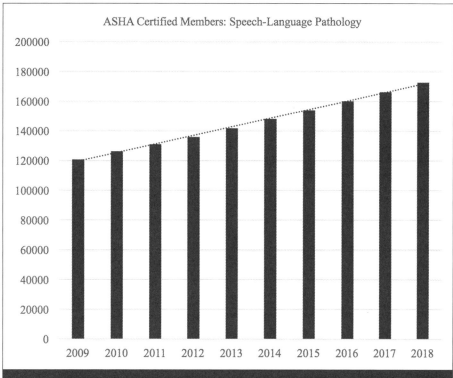

ASHA Certified Members: Speech-Language Pathology

Figure 10–2. Number of ASHA certified speech-language pathologists over the past decade with associated trend line. Note: These data do not include dual certificate holders.

facilities. The percentage of SLPs in private practice has remained stable over the past several years, at 21.1%.

In 2018, the majority of AuDs (77.7%) reported their primary work role as clinical service provider with 8% holding an administrative position (e.g., executive officer, department chair, or supervisor; ASHA, 2019a). A small percentage (5.5%) held a teaching position (0.6% held special education teacher roles and 4.9% were college or university professors), 2.1% were consultants, and 1.8% were researchers. Similar to AuDs, most SLPs (74.1%) reported their main work responsibility as a clinical service provider. In contrast to AuDs, more than one tenth (12.3%) held a teaching position (10.4% were special education teachers and 1.9% were college or university professors); and 6.8% held administrative positions. Only 1.5% were consultants and less than 0.2% were researchers. These percentages are consistent across the last several years.

Job and Career Satisfaction

Job satisfaction is an important consideration, especially as you are embarking on your new career path. In 2017,

ASHA conducted the CCCs, Jobs & Careers Mini-Survey gathering information about members' career and job satisfaction. The survey demonstrated that AuDs and SLPs have high levels of career and job satisfaction overall (ASHA, 2018a). The 2017 survey also asked participants how many years they had been in the professions. The mean across the professions combined was 18.4 years. The mean for AuDs was 21.1 years, 18.1 years for SLPs, and 31.7 years for those holding dual certification.

Note as you consider this career path, 92% of respondents reported that they were satisfied or very satisfied with their choice of career thus far. In addition, remember that there are a variety of reasons why you might be satisfied with your career. Respondents in the 2017 survey indicated that the most important factors for accepting or staying in a job were interesting/exciting/challenging work, good relationships with co-workers, and convenient work location.

Salary is an area where students have a great deal of interest. However, it is important to remember that salary is not the only factor in a satisfying career. Additionally, salary is a complex issue and depends upon many factors such as part- versus full-time employment, benefits eligibility, and region of the country and cost of living factors. The following section summarizes data from ASHA regarding salary as reported by its members and uses the association's terms and structure.

Salaries of Audiologists: 2018 Data. The majority of AuDs (72.0%) were paid an annual salary; 25% were paid on an hourly basis and 2% were paid via commission (ASHA, 2019b). Nearly all of the AuDs responding (95.0%) earned a salary over an 11- or 12-month calendar year. The remainder earned a salary for work that occurred over a 9- or 10-month period (i.e., an academic year). AuDs earned a median calendar year salary of $80,000 (this number excludes bonuses and commissions). They earned a median academic year salary of $83,843 (excluding bonuses and commissions). The median amount of a bonus was $2,000, for AuDs who earned a bonus. For those who received an *annual* commission, the median amount was $20,000 based on a median percentage of commission on product sales of 8%. The median commission was $12,270 for those receiving pay through an *hourly* wage. The salary was $82,872 for those who worked and received pay primarily by *commission* only based on a median percentage of commission on product sales of 27%. One quarter of AuDs (25.0%) worked for hourly pay. The median hourly wage was $40.00 (excluding bonuses and commissions). Those AuDs who worked for hourly pay who also had a bonus, received a median amount of $1,000. Of those hourly employees who received a commission, the median amount was $12,270. More than half (58.0%) of the AuDs who earned an hourly wage worked part time (ASHA, 2019c). Earnings can be affected by many different variables. These factors include: primary work setting and role, highest academic degree, years of experience in the profession, geographic region, and type of community (i.e., metropolitan/urban, suburban, or rural). Audiologists who worked greater than 26 hours/ week in the hospital setting earned $40.05/hour versus AuDs working greater than 26 hours/week from non-residential health care facilities who earned $37.00/hour (ASHA, 2019c).

Other factors that can impact earnings for AuDs included:

- AuDs who served as administrators earned a median calendar year salary of $104,293 compared with $79,095 for clinical service providers.

- The median calendar year salary of AuDs holding the PhD was $112,705, compared with $79,072 for those who hold the clinical doctorate (AuD) and $80,721 for those with a master's degree (ASHA, 2019b).

Salaries of Speech-Language Pathologists in Health Care Settings. Data from 2017 indicate that more than half (55.0%) of SLPs in health care settings were paid an hourly wage (ASHA, 2017a) versus approximately one third (34.0%) who were paid an annual salary (ASHA, 2017b). Over half (56.0%) worked full time (ASHA, 2017a). Around one-tenth (12.0%) were paid per home health visit (ASHA, 2017a). In 2017, the median hourly wage of SLPs who worked full time was $41.00 and those who worked part-time $48.00 in health care settings (ASHA, 2017a). The median annual salary for SLPs in health care was $78,000 (ASHA, 2017b). The median wage per home health visit was $65.00 (ASHA, 2017a).

Similar to audiology, numerous factors affected earnings for SLPs in health care.

- SLPs in home health settings reported a higher median hourly wage ($65.00) than those from other practice settings (ASHA, 2017a).

- Administrators, supervisors, and directors earned a median annual salary of $96,000, whereas clinical service providers earned $72,000.

- The median annual salary of SLPs was highest in the West region of the United States ($83,655) and lowest in the Midwest ($74,114) (ASHA, 2017b).

Salaries of Speech-Language Pathologists in School Settings. In 2018, most SLPs in school settings (87.0%) were paid an annual salary; the remaining 13% were paid an hourly wage (ASHA, 2018b). These data are in contrast to SLPs who work in health care, where the majority received an hourly wage. A large majority (90.0%) of school based SLPs worked 9 or 10 months per year with the remainder working 11 or 12 months annually. The median academic year salary of SLPs in school settings was $63,338 whereas the median calendar year salary was $72,000. A small percentage of SLPs

(13.0%) worked for an hourly wage. The median hourly wage was $51.00 (ASHA, 2018b).

Numerous factors can impact the salaries of SLPs in school settings.

- SLPs in secondary schools had a somewhat higher median academic year salary ($68,000) than those in other school settings (ASHA, 2018b).

- SLPs with 26–30 years of experience had a higher median academic year salary than those just starting out with 1–5 years of experience ($80,000 and approximately $52,000, respectively).

- SLPs in city/urban and suburban areas had a higher median academic year salary than those in rural communities ($67,087, $64,891, and $56,000, respectively) (ASHA, 2018b).

Salaries of Academic and Clinical Faculty in Colleges and Universities. The Council of Academic Programs in Communication Sciences and Disorders (CAPCSD) conducts a salary survey in higher education on a regular basis. Data are available on the CAPCSD website (http://www.capcsd.org) in a format enabling calculation and comparison of salaries by entering a year of interest (CAPCSD, 2018). The nine-month adjusted base mean salary for assistant professor *academic* faculty was $70,408 in 2018. Assistant professor *clinical* faculty earned a median salary of $58,756.

There are a variety of factors that influenced salaries in academia, regardless of professional area of focus. These included:

- highest academic or clinical degree earned,

- rank,

- tenure status,

- type of institution (i.e., public or private),

- Basic Carnegie classification of institution, and

- geographic region of institution (as defined by the Federal Reserve Classification).

Shortage of PhD Students and Faculty in CSD

Evidence-based practice is the foundation of clinical practice. A majority of the evidence base for our discipline has come from the research of faculty members appointed at universities throughout the country. Therefore, a sufficient pipeline of faculty and PhD students in CSD is critical.

Numerous reports over the past two decades have discussed the shortage of PhD students and faculty in CSD (CAPCSD, 2002; Eddins et al., 2016; Madison et al., 2004; McNeil et al., 2013; Oller, 2003). This situation is not new. In 1999, CAPCSD predicted that the number of doctoral graduates in audiology and speech-language pathology would not meet the needs for doctoral-level academic positions in the future.

There were numerous developments in response to CAPCSD's 1999 report, including:

- ASHA and CAPCSD established a Joint Ad Hoc Committee on the Shortage of PhD Students and Faculty in CSD in 2002. This group generated a report which developed an initial plan to address shortages in academia (2002–2007).

- A *Report of the 2008 Joint Ad Hoc Committee on PhD Shortages in Communication Sciences and Disorders* provided a strategic plan (2008–2011) addressing the shortage in academia (McCrea et al., 2008).

- In 2013, ASHA's Academic Affairs Board, in collaboration with CSD faculty, academic programs, and CAPCSD, developed a strategic plan for implementation between 2015 and 2018 to (1) address the PhD shortage and increase the quantity and quality of researchers and faculty-scholars and (2) facilitate an increase in the quantity and quality of the discipline's science base, especially with respect to research that advances clinical practice and improves patient/client outcomes (McNeil et al., 2013).

These efforts support a science base for the discipline and develop research scientists who will further support the foundation of scientific evidence in our field. This support is consistent with ASHA's Strategic Pathway to Excellence (ASHA, n.d.-b).

The Future: Factors Affecting Employment

Starting your new career is exciting and rewarding. It is important to consider what the future may hold as far as the ability to remain meaningfully and gainfully employed. The next section considers employment availability and what factors might impact your employment.

Bureau of Labor Statistics Projections

Total employment is expected to increase by 11.5 million jobs from 2016–2026 (U.S. Department of Labor, Bureau of Labor Statistics, 2017). About 23.6% of health care support occupations and 15.3% of health care practitioners and technical occupations, which includes public and private hospitals, residential health care facilities, and individual and family services, will contribute about one fifth of all new jobs by 2026.

Employment growth will be impacted by factors driving the demand for healthcare services such as:

- the aging baby-boom population,
- longer life expectancies,
- modern treatments and technologies,
- and growing rates of chronic conditions (U.S. Department of Labor, Bureau of Labor Statistics, 2017).

AuDs and SLPs are under the BLS category "health care." Employment of health care occupations is projected to grow 18% from 2016 to 2026, much faster than the average for all occupations, adding about 2.4 million new jobs. Health care occupations are projected to add more jobs than any of the other occupational groups. This projected growth is mainly due to an aging population, leading to greater demand for health care services. BLS projections indicate the employment of AuDs will grow much faster than the average for other occupations (21% from 2016 to 2026). As people age, hearing loss increases. Consequently, the aging population is therefore likely to increase demand for AuDs (U.S. Department of Labor, Bureau of Labor Statistics, 2019b). Additionally, the BLS projections indicate the employment of SLPs will also increase much faster than the average for all occupations (18% from 2016 to 2026). As the large baby-boom population grows older, there will likely be more instances of health conditions that can cause speech or language impairments, such as strokes and dementia (U.S. Department of Labor, Bureau of Labor Statistics (2019c).

An Aging Population

The U.S. Census Bureau is projecting that older adults (aged 65+) will outnumber children (under 18) by 2035 (U.S. Census Bureau, 2018a). In 2016, the U.S. population for older adults was estimated to be 49.2 million (15.2%), with projections to increase to 78 million by 2035, and 94.7 million by 2060 (23.5%). In comparison, the population of children in 2016 was estimated to be 73.6 million (22.8%), with projections to slightly increase to 76.4 million in 2035, and 79.8 million (19.8%) by 2060 (U.S. Census Bureau, 2018a). According to the U.S. Census Bureau's 2017 National Population Projections, by 2030, all baby boomers will be older than age 65. This will expand the size of the older population so that 1 in every 5 residents will be retirement age (U.S. Census Bureau, 2018a).

A Diverse Population

The majority of ASHA-certified AuDs, SLPs and those who are dually certified identify themselves as white (ASHA, 2019a). Therefore, the percentage of individuals in the professions from underrepresented ethnic and racial groups is far below that for the general population. According to the U.S. Census Bureau (2018b), the non-Hispanic white-alone population is projected to shrink over the coming decades, from 199 million in 2020 to 179 million in 2060—even as the U.S. population continues to grow. This decline is driven by falling birth rates and a rising number of deaths over time among non-Hispanic whites as that population ages. In comparison, the white-alone population, regardless of Hispanic origin, is projected to grow from about 253 million to 275 million over the same period.

For a 2017 survey, health care–based SLPs from a variety of facility types including general medical/VA/long term acute care hospitals, home health providers, outpatient clinics and offices, pediatric hospitals, rehabilitation hospitals, and skilled nursing facilities were asked to answer three closed-set questions related to cultural and linguistic diversity practices. The first question asked SLPs to identify which clinical approaches they had used to address cultural and linguistic influences on communication in the past 12 months (ASHA, 2017c). Nearly half (48.3%) used interpreters/cultural brokers; 34.5% modified assessment strategies or procedures; 27.5% acquired translated materials; 20.0% translated therapy tools; 19.1% translated written materials, including consumer information; 19.0% referred clients to bilingual service providers; and 28.3% had not used any of the above-mentioned approaches in the past 12 months. The second question asked SLPs if they had needed to request funding for interpreter or translator services in the past year. Participants stated "yes," they did have to request funds in 8.7% of responses. The third and final question then asked those who had responded "yes" to the previous question, if funding for interpreter or translator services had been reduced or denied based on the following listed reasons with calculated response percentages shown. Over one third (37.2%) indicated that family members provided interpreter or translator services; 21.6% made a referral to a bilingual service provider; 15.4% stated the budget was insufficient to cover interpreter or translator services; 14.8% indicated alternate service delivery models were required; 11.1% provided English-only services; 6.4% noted funding was denied for intervention; 3.1% indicated funding was denied for assessments; 1.8% stated funding was contraindicated by the patient's communication disorder; and 0.0% reported funding was contraindicated by patient's age. (Note, specific elements of bilingual service delivery will be discussed further in this chapter.)

⬦⬦⬦⬦⬦⬦⬦⬦⬦⬦⬦⬦⬦⬦⬦⬦⬦⬦⬦⬦⬦⬦⬦⬦⬦⬦

⬦⬦⬦⬦⬦⬦⬦⬦⬦⬦⬦⬦⬦⬦⬦⬦⬦⬦⬦⬦⬦⬦⬦⬦⬦⬦

In 2018, school-based SLPs were asked to use a 5-point scale (from *not at all important* to *very important*) to rate the importance of Language of Intervention for English Language Learners (ELLs) in relation to the Individuals with Disabilities Education Act (ASHA, 2018c). Overall, only 31.5% rated Language of Intervention for ELLs as *very important*. Less than one tenth (3.9%) rated this as *not at all important*.

⬦⬦⬦⬦⬦⬦⬦⬦⬦⬦⬦⬦⬦⬦⬦⬦⬦⬦⬦⬦⬦⬦⬦⬦⬦⬦

ASHA developed a web-based cultural competence assessment tool that provides the reader with a tutorial prior to taking a test that is scored. Results of the test are intended to assist in identifying areas where greater understanding is needed. Additionally, ASHA developed a series of self-assessment cultural competence checklists that can be used to enhance awareness of providing

services to culturally/linguistically diverse (CLD) populations including: personal reflection, policies and procedures, and service delivery checklists (ASHA, n.d.-c). See Chapter 25 for more discussion of cultural diversity.

Bilingual Service Delivery. Bilingual service delivery is a topic that warrants discussion. Based on earlier reported percentages of increasing numbers of minority populations in the U.S., particularly the Hispanic population, coupled with the information on cultural diversity, information on how the public will be served is needed. Those statistics already presented are meaningful to AuDs and SLPs. The numbers help to prepare recruitment initiatives and seek information related to grant funding for bilingual training programs so that there are culturally sensitive and culturally prepared providers to serve those in need.

Year-end 2018 (ASHA, 2019d) data indicated that there were 81 spoken languages other than English and of the 191,904 individuals represented by ASHA, 12,242 (6%) indicated they met the ASHA definition of bilingual service provider. The majority (64%) were Spanish-language service providers. There were 11,259 ASHA-certified SLPs (7,500 Spanish-language SLPs) and 738 were ASHA certified AuDs (283 Spanish-language AuDs). In addition, 702 individuals indicated that they were able to communicate using American Sign Language, 141 use Manually Coded English (including SE, SEE, Cued Speech, etc.), and 26 use "other sign languages." The majority (77%) of ASHA bilingual service providers worked full time; with 18% working part time. Nearly one half (49%) were employed in educational settings (44% in schools and 5% in colleges and universities), and 43% were employed in health care settings (23% in non-residential health care facilities, 13% in hospitals, and 7% in residential health care settings). Demographically, more than one third (42%) of ASHA bilingual service providers were of Hispanic or Latino descent, compared with 5% of ASHA's total membership and affiliation. The largest number of ASHA-certified SLPs and AuDs who lived in the United States and were bilingual service providers lived in Texas, New York, California, and Florida, which grossly coordinated with the U.S. Census Bureau's 2017 American Community Survey (ACS) data. The ACS data showed which states and percentage number within each state that individuals lived who spoke English less than very well, spoke a language other than English as their primary language at home, or spoke Spanish at home. In addition to the states listed above, New Mexico, New Jersey, New York, Nevada, Arizona, and Hawaii were also represented.

In response to issues related to cultural and linguistic diversity, some university programs have developed bilingual/multicultural tracks or certificate programs. These programs are often structured to increase the knowledge and skill of clinicians in training so that they can best meet the demands of a changing population.

Other Factors that May Impact the Future of the Professions

Other areas that will continue to shape the future covered in this text are changes in technology, federal policy, reimbursement, and interprofessional practice. These topics are all covered in this textbook with the reminder that our fields are anything but static. A professional in the discipline will continually monitor the landscape of the profession on the local, state, and national levels.

Summary

This chapter provided a description of the demographics and employment characteristics of individuals in the professions and discipline. It also presented salary and job and career satisfaction data. Steps taken to address the PhD shortage were also summarized. The chapter closed with employment projections and a discussion of factors that may affect future employment, including the changing demographics of the U.S. population related to the aging and cultural makeup of our nation. Data from ASHA and other organizations and agencies were used to evaluate the impact of these factors and our response as a discipline, to ensure the future supply of and demand for audiology and speech-language pathology professionals.

Critical Thinking

1. How has the number of ASHA-certified AuDs and SLPs, changed over the past decade? What are the advantages and disadvantages of having dual certification?

2. How does the ethnicity and race of ASHA certified AuDs and SLPs compare with that of the U.S. population as a whole? What strategies would you suggest to encourage more individuals from underrepresented ethnic and racial groups to enter the professions of audiology and speech-language pathology?

3. Suppose you are a human resources administrator in a health care or school setting. What would you do to recruit and retain qualified AuDs and SLPs in your setting?

4. What variables affect the earnings of AuDs, SLPs, and CSD faculty?

5. How might the forthcoming changes in the general workforce (using information from the BLS) affect the future number of AuDs and SLPs?

6. How might changes in the demographics of the U.S. population affect the supply of and demand for AuDs and SLPs in future years? How would you use demographic information to help you in deciding where you might like to work?

7. Why is the shortage of research-doctoral students in our professions so important? How does it affect our educational institutions? What could the schools of higher education do to make doctoral study more accessible and affordable for potential students?

References

American Speech-Language-Hearing Association. (n.d.-a). *Quick facts.* Retrieved from https://www.asha.org/About/news/Quick-Facts/

American Speech-Language-Hearing Association. (n.d.-b). *Strategic pathway to excellence: ASHA's strategic plan.* Available from http://www.asha.org/

American Speech-Language-Hearing Association. (n.d.-c). *Self assessment for cultural competence.* Retrieved from https://www.asha.org/practice/multicultural/self.htm

American Speech-Language-Hearing Association. (2017a). *ASHA 2017 SLP Health Care Survey: Hourly and per home-visit wage report.* Available from http://www.asha.org

American Speech-Language-Hearing Association. (2017b). *ASHA 2017 SLP Health Care Survey: Annual salary report.* Available from http://www.asha.org

American Speech-Language-Hearing Association. (2017c). *2017 SLP Health Care Survey summary report: Number and type of responses.* Available from http://www.asha.org

American Speech-Language-Hearing Association. (2018a). *2017 CCCs, Jobs, and Careers Mini-Survey. Summary report: Numbers and types of responses.* Available from http://www.asha.org

American Speech-Language-Hearing Association. (2018b). *2018 Schools Survey report: SLP annual salaries and hourly wages.* Retrieved from http://

www.asha.org/research/memberdata/schools survey/

American Speech-Language-Hearing Association. (2018c). *2018 Schools Survey. Survey summary report: Numbers and types of responses, SLPs.* Available from http://www.asha.org

American Speech-Language-Hearing Association. (2019a). *ASHA summary membership and affiliation counts, year-end 2018.* Available from http://www.asha.org

American Speech-Language-Hearing Association. (2019b). *2018 Audiology Survey report: Annual salaries.* Available from http://www.asha.org

American Speech-Language-Hearing Association. (2019c). *2018 Audiology Survey report: Hourly wages.* Available from http://www.asha.org

American Speech-Language-Hearing Association. (2019d). *Demographic profile of ASHA members providing bilingual services, year-end 2018.* Available from http://www.asha.org

Council of Academic Programs in Communication Sciences Disorders (CAPCSD). (2002). *Crisis in the discipline: A plan for reshaping our future.* Retrieved from http://www.capcsd.org/wp-content/uploads/2015/01/JointAdHocCmteFinalReport.pdf

Council of Academic Programs in Communication Sciences Disorders (CAPCSD). (2016). *2016 Salary Survey.* Retrieved from http://www.capcsd.org/salarysurvey.html

Eddins, A. C., & Rich Folsom, C. (2016). *PhD Programs in communication sciences disorders: Innovative models and practices.* Retrieved from https://www.asha.org/uploadedFiles/2016-PhD-Programs-in-CSD-Report.pdf

Madison, C. L., Guy, B., & Koch, M. (2004). Pursuit of the speech-language pathology doctorate: Who, why, why not. *Contemporary Issues in Communication Sciences and Disorders, 31,* 191–199.

McCrea, E., Creaghead, N., Goldstein, H., O'Rourke, C., Ryals, B., & Small, L. (2008). *Report of the 2008 Joint Ad Hoc Committee on PhD Shortages in Communication Sciences and Disorders.* Available from http://www.asha.org/

McNeil, M. R., Nunez, L., Armiento-DeMaria, M. T., Chapman, K. L., DiLollo, A., . . . Robertson, S. (2013). *Strategic plan to increase the student pipeline and workforce for PhD researchers and faculty researchers*; ASHA.

Oller, D. K. (2003). *The PhD Shortage in communication science disorders.* ASHA Special Interest Division 10, *Perspectives on Issues in Higher Education, 6*(1), 2–3.

U.S. Census Bureau. (2018a). *An aging nation: projected number of children and older adults.* Retrieved from https://www.census.gov/library/visualizations/2018/comm/historic-first.html

U.S. Census Bureau. (2018b). *Older people projected to outnumber children for first time in U.S. history.* Retrieved from https://www.census.gov/newsroom/press-releases/2018/cb18-41-population-projections.html

U.S. Department of Labor, Bureau of Labor Statistics. (2017). *Employment projections: 2016-26 summary.* Retrieved from https://www.bls.gov/news.release/ecopro.nr0.htm

U.S. Department of Labor, Bureau of Labor Statistics. (2019a). *Official unemployment rate was 3.9 percent in December 2018; U-6 was 7.6 percent.* Retrieved from https://www.bls.gov/opub/ted/2019/official-unemployment-rate-was-3-point-9-percent-in-december-2018-u-6-was-7-point-6-percent.htm?view_full

U.S. Department of Labor, Bureau of Labor Statistics. (2019b). *Occupational outlook handbook, Audiologists.* Retrieved from https://www.bls.gov/ooh/healthcare/audiologists.htm

U.S. Department of Labor, Bureau of Labor Statistics. (2019c). *Occupational outlook handbook, Speech-language pathologists.* Retrieved from https://www.bls.gov/ooh/healthcare/speech-language-pathologists.htm

Resources

Agency for Healthcare Research and Quality Patient-Centered Medical Home. Available from https://pcmh.ahrq.gov/

American Institute of Medical Sciences and Education (AIMS). (2018). *The impact of technology on healthcare.* Retrieved from https://www.aimseducation.edu/blog/the-impact-of-technology-on-

American Speech-Language-Hearing Association. (2011). *Explore the professions.* Available from http://www.asha.org/

American Speech-Language-Hearing Association. (2011). *Start a career: Job search tips.* Available from http://www.asha.org/

American Speech-Language-Hearing Association. (2012, May 15). ASHA members: 150,000 strong and growing. *The ASHA Leader.* Available from http://www.asha.org/

Centers for Medicare and Medicaid Services. (n.d.-a). *Quality Payment Program.* Retrieved from https://www.cms.gov/Medicare/Quality-Payment-Program/Quality-Payment-

Centers for Medicare and Medicaid Services. (n.d.-b). *Patient-driven payment models.* Retrieved from https://www.cms.gov/Medicare/Medicare-Fee-for-ServicePayment/SNFPPS/PDPM.html

Centers for Medicare and Medicaid Services. (n.d.-c). *Accountable Care Organizations.* Retrieved from https://innovation.cms.gov/initiatives/aco/

Council of Academic Programs in Communication Sciences and Disorders. Website: http://www.capcsd.org

U.S. Department of Health and Human Services. (n.d.-a). *Affordable Care Act overview.* Retrieved from https://www.hhs.gov/healthcare/index.html

U.S. Department of Health and Human Services. (n.d.-b). *Affordable Care Act essential health benefits.* Retrieved from https://www.hhs.gov/glossary/essential-health-

U.S. Department of Labor, Bureau of Labor Statistics. Website: http://www.bls.gov

11

Finding Employment

∞∞

Mark DeRuiter, PhD, MBA

Introduction

This chapter focuses on the process of and strategies for obtaining employment in speech-language pathology or audiology, with an emphasis on initial employment. It is followed by a chapter that discusses how to build your career in the professions once you have gained employment. This chapter begins with a discussion of the paths a career in speech-language pathology or audiology may take. Many aspects of finding employment have not changed greatly over time. For instance, a good cover letter and resumé are critical to the process. Therefore, many elements of this chapter remain true to its previous edition, written by Dr. Rosemary Lubinski. However, the job search and application processes continue to evolve as technology and other elements change. New to the chapter is information related to web-based applications, electronic interviews, using social media in employment searches, benefits, and specific interview tips. The chapter concludes with a discussion of how to accept a job.

Employment Settings

Speech-language pathologists and audiologists have a wide variety of options for employment. About 54% of ASHA-certified speech-language pathologists are employed in educational settings, including public and private schools, developmental learning centers, specialized schools such as schools for the deaf, language development programs, state schools for those with developmental disabilities, and colleges or universities (ASHA, 2018). This percentage has remained relatively stable over the past five years. About 39% of ASHA speech-language pathologists and about 74% of audiologists are employed in health care facilities, including hospitals, residential health care facilities, and nonresidential health care facilities (ASHA, 2018). Thirty-one percent of audiologists are employed in private practice settings, as are about 21% of speech-language pathologists (ASHA, 2018). Both of these percentages reveal a decrease since the previous edition of this book. (See Chapter 10 for more specific demographics of workforce characteristics of speech-language pathologists and audiologists.) The ASHA website has much more information regarding practice settings for audiologists and speech-language pathologists (https://asha.org).

Job Search

As you think about job settings, you will also need to consider the job search itself. Searching for a job will take time and energy. However, it is important because it is the first step in your career. In some instances, you may find employment through a current practicum or externship. However, in most cases, you will need to search for employment. On average, new graduates should plan on a minimum of a 90-day lead time when they seek employment, whereas audiology externs may need even more time.

The most frequently used source for finding jobs is the Internet. For example, you might use the American Speech-Language Hearing Association's Career Portal, the HearCareers site from the American Academy of Audiology, or a variety of job seeking sites such as Monster, ZipRecruiter, Indeed, and the like. Additionally, positions may be posted on the human resources pages of school districts, health centers, hospitals, and other agencies. You may also find positions through social media such as FaceBook and LinkedIn. What is most important to remember is that positions are fluid (particularly in health care) and you will need to continually check back for available positions. If you have the option to set alerts through a job search tool, you should do so.

One word of caution involves placing your resumé out on a website for many employers to see. Students often report that if they do this, they are inundated with erroneous calls for positions that do not fit their needs. Be advised to carefully consider where you post your resumé and what information you reveal about yourself through a posted resumé.

As you begin your search, think of some basic things:

- What environments and clinical populations interest you most?

- Do you need to work full-time? Or, are you seeking part-time employment?

- Is flexibility in scheduling critical to you?

Although only you can answer these questions, they get you thinking as you spend time looking at postings. Other sections of this chapter will provide you with information that might shape your answers to the questions above.

Consider What Information Is Available About You

Before you start officially applying for positions, you might want to consider your own electronic presence. Clabaugh (2018) reports that employers expect to find information about you online. However, you should closely monitor what information is available about you because it could bias an employer negatively. Begin by searching your name in various search engines. Also, check your social media sites and determine what is public versus private information. Are there objectionable pictures or posts? You will want to remove them. Have you blogged on controversial topics? You may want to take down these blogs. A proactive step can be to create some professional social media pages highlighting your skills as a clinician.

Resumé

The resumé or curriculum vitae (CV) is a critical tool for marketing yourself to an employer. Resumés can be constructed in a variety of styles such as: chronological, functional, targeted, or combination. Chronological resumés are most common. They display a reverse chronological order (most recent first) list of your education, employment/practicum experience, and other skills. A sample reverse chronological resumé is found in Appendix 11–A. Functional resumés separate your skills and accomplishments into categories that reflect your job objective. Often, functional resumés have education toward the end of the document because the assumption is that your educational credentials are the foundation of your skills. Functional resumés do not link skills to locations. Instead, all skills are defined in a broader skills section. However, you may list your practicum and employment sites later in the document. Targeted resumés emphasize your skills and achievements that meet the specific needs of the agency to which you are applying. Combination resumés combine chronological and functional styles.

A curriculum vitae is a "long form" of a resumé that is typically seen in academic environments. When you consider your resumé, think of displaying your competency and skills, primarily. When you consider a CV, think of displaying credentials, especially related to research and professional associations (Doyle, 2019). Most new graduates will use a one- to two-page resumé format.

Resumé Content Suggestions

The following suggestions will help you move forward with an initial draft of your resumé. Appendix 11–A will serve as a guide. However, note that the sample resumé is streamlined. Your final product may have more entries.

- **Identification section:** This section of your resumé provides your name, address, and contact information. Keep your email address professional and make certain that your outgoing voicemail message has a professional tone. If you are a student using a university email account, confirm with your university that you will have access to this email account after you graduate.

- **Job/career objective:** Advice varies on objective statements on resumés. An objective is an opportunity for you to state what you are seeking in employment. However, if the objective is obvious ("Obtain a Clinical Fellowship in a medical environment"), it may be best to leave it off.

- **Education:** List in chronological or reverse order your earned degrees, name of college or university where they were obtained, city and state, and dates. If you graduated with honors, you should state it. Audiology externs may be encouraged to include their GPA on the resumé. Other applicants may not need to include a GPA, as graduation from an accredited program is the most important element regarding education.

- **Certification and licensure:** State which certificates or licenses you hold. This will be a fast way for an employer to screen your application, should these credentials be required. You can state that you are "license eligible" if you believe you meet the requirements for a license in a given state. However, do not state that you hold

any credentials that you cannot immediately provide to an employer.

- **Clinical experience history:** This section lists your practicum experiences. You will want to state the name and location of where you were placed. Then, you will want to include relevant points about the experience so that the reader has a snapshot of what knowledge and skills you have gained at the rotation. Keep these entries fresh using action verbs wherever possible. A list of action verbs can be found in Table 11–1.

- **Publications:** Any published books, monographs, chapters, or articles should be included in American Psychological Association (APA) format. A dissertation or thesis can be included here as well.

- **Honors/Awards:** Include any honors and awards in this category. If you graduated summa cum laude (or other honors), you might want to include this near your degree designator versus in this category. Keep your honors category for other honors and awards (honors fraternities, scholarships, etc.).

- **Presentations:** Include any professional presentations using APA format. Remember to include all authors.

- **Professional affiliations:** This segment lists the name(s) of any professional local, state,

Table 11–1. Sample Action Verbs

administered	enhanced	programmed
aided	established	provided
analyzed	evaluated	recommended
appraised	examined	rehabilitated
assessed	facilitated	researched
assisted	formed	stimulated
communicated	generated	submitted
counseled	implemented	supervised
created	lectured	taught
demonstrated	managed	tested
designed	measured	trained
developed	monitored	undertook
directed	observed	utilized
documented	organized	
edited	performed	

national, or international associations to which the applicant belongs. If you held a specific role (e.g., Treasurer), make sure to state it here.

■ **Continuing education:** This section is reserved for professionals who have participated in postgraduate training or education. A new applicant may also use it if she has gone above and beyond typical graduate training.

■ **References:** Include references on a separate page. Make certain to include all information, including degree designator and title. There is no reason to state "References available upon request" on your resumé.

■ **Personal data:** Your professional resumé is not a place to include personal data regarding hobbies or interests.

Resumé Style Suggestions

There are multiple ways your resumé can look its best. Consider the following:

■ Do not use lines or pictures on your resumé

■ Use professional-looking fonts (avoid Comic Sans or scripted fonts) and keep the font size between 10 and 14

■ Make certain there is "white space" on the resumé so that it does not look busy or overwhelming

■ When printing your resumé, stick with standard white paper, 8.5 by 11 inches

Stahl (2016) provides some resumé style tips that may be useful to you. Her recommendations come to you from the business world. Therefore, always remember to have someone in your own discipline take another look at your resumé to make sure that it "fits" with the discipline of communication disorders.

Cover Letter

Your cover letter helps you "sell" yourself (Page, 2017). A simple internet search will provide you with many examples of effective cover letters. Overall, consider a cover letter like a brief introduction of yourself, your interests in the position, and how you might move forward to schedule an interview. These considerations will assist you in structuring the content of the letter.

The first paragraph should offer the reader information about you, how you found the position, and why you are interested in the opening. This paragraph can be relatively brief, containing about three or four sentences total. Make certain that this opening paragraph is tailored to the employer versus being generic in nature.

The second paragraph will provide you with the opportunity to discuss your fit for the position. What is important here is that you do not overwhelm the reader by recasting your entire resumé. Instead, look at the position posting and draw out the information that is most relevant to the position at hand. If you have special skills or certifications, you will want to highlight them in this section.

The third paragraph will be your closing. In this paragraph you reiterate your interest and indicate your desire to engage in an interview. Remember, you will want to learn things about the employer, just as the employer will want to learn about you. It is appropriate to state when you are typically available and that you will follow up within a given period of time. Monitor your tone in this paragraph to sound enthused yet professional.

You should use a block-style format for the cover letter and keep the tone of the letter appropriately assertive and positive. If possible, you might want to create a .jpeg file of your signature to give the letter a personal touch with an imported original signature.

Email Style Issues

Emailing cover letters and resumés is common. Make sure that you follow any directions you are given for emailing your resumé and cover letter. This includes any file naming conventions that may be required by an employer. Avoid using an ambiguous subject line and consider sending a resumé and cover letter with a read receipt where possible. Keep the text of the email formal and make sure that you address the recipient in a professional manner, using her name and title.

Often new job seekers will ask if they should copy the contents of their cover letter into the body of the email. Although this is not forbidden, it might be wise to send a briefer email that outlines your interest with the cover letter attached to the email as a formal application document. This way your documents can be forwarded without any concern about changes in format.

Web-Based Applications

Some employers will require you to fill out an application online. This can feel like a redundant task after you have worked diligently on your resumé. You might be tempted to fill in the fields with "See resumé" with the hopes that you will be able to attach a resumé at the end of the process. However, demonstrating that you can complete an entire application helps your future employer to see how you pay attention to detail and how you value their time in the review of your application materials. Complete these applications carefully!

Letters of Recommendation/ Verbal References

You will want to pull together a list of recommenders who can provide information about you in the search process. Usually three to five people are sufficient. Considering that most of the positions you will be applying for are clinical in nature, you should find people who can speak to your clinical skills. These can be preceptors, supervisors, and university faculty. You will want to avoid people who can only serve as a personal reference.

When asking for a reference, attempt to do it in a face-to-face meeting. You are asking for a serious commitment from someone and you should demonstrate that you respect their time and energies. Provide the recommender with a resumé, sample cover letter, list of classes taken, and any other information you feel would be helpful to them should they need to write a letter or speak with an employer on the phone. You should also provide a recommender with your targeted list of job locations and job descriptions, if you have them.

Your job search may be a fluid process. Do not forget to keep your recommenders up-to-date as to where you are applying.

Interviewing Success

You have searched for the perfect position and applied to postings that might launch your career. Now you have been invited to the interview. How do you prepare? This section provides you with tips for success. First, consider the following suggestions as you move forward with your job search.

Remain Flexible

Being asked to interview for a position is a privilege, not a right. You should remain as flexible as possible when scheduling an interview. This will be your future employer's first glimpse into your willingness to adapt and consider the needs of the others. While you should remain flexible in your timing, also be mindful of your needs. For instance, do not schedule an interview for a time when you know the timing will be tight for you to commute to the site or when you know you need to leave the interview at a very specific time.

Looking the Part

This will vary dependent upon the location and population you might potentially serve. Arriving underdressed conveys an image that you "don't care" and arriving very overdressed states that your expectations might be overwhelming.

Some general appearance guidelines include:

1. Think about the position. If it is in a school, consider what you might wear if you were already working in that environment and the Superintendent asked you to lunch. You would likely dress up for that occasion, right? You should treat the situation similarly for the interview. You can consider the same general rule in a medical setting; however, some medical settings may have a day-to-day dress code available to you with a basic internet search.

2. Women should consider skirts or dresses; men should wear long-sleeved collared shirts with a tie. All clothes should be clean and pressed, and clothes should fit appropriately. Often suits and jackets are best.

3. Hosiery for both men and women is a must, as well as closed-toed shoes.

4. Arrive clean and showered. Avoid excessive perfumes or colognes. If you are smoker, do not smoke after showering (and, consider quitting!). A patch or other smoking cessation technique will be very helpful to you on your interview day.

5. Avoid excessive jewelry, makeup, or nail colors that might be distracting to your interviewer.

6. An institution may have a policy about hair color, stating this needs to be a hair color typically found in nature. Your safest bet is to have a natural hair color.

7. Consider covering tattoos. Your interviewer may have an implicit bias against applicants with tattoos. Although this may not seem fair, it could stand between you and the position you desire.

8. Wear contact lenses or glasses if you need them. You may be looking at documents or websites with the employer or a human resources representative. You should be able to see them!

9. Look at yourself from all angles in a full-length mirror, or have a friend or family give one last look. Make certain all tags are removed from your clothing, no details have been missed (e.g., belt loops, collars are flat), and your clothing fits appropriately.

There are items to bring to your interview, and items to avoid. Many applicants will bring a small folio to the meeting. This simple system can contain a few extra print outs of your resumé, a pad of paper, and a working pen. When you consider the folio, a basic black or brown color is best. A simple pen with no logo is also recommended. This way you avoid any bias that an interviewer might have regarding affiliations you might display. Other items that might be useful in your folio include: lists of assessments you are familiar with, populations served, or hearing aid manufacturer programming software you are comfortable using. You should also have a written list of questions for your employer. You might also consider taking something to read to the interview. This can be useful should there be downtime and it may look more professional than engaging text messaging, email, or social media. You might want to print pages from the organization's human resource manual or other industry-related materials to look at while waiting. Finally, having the contact information for your references can be handy if you have not already submitted them to the employer.

If you bring your smartphone to the interview, it is best to have it turned completely off during the interview process. Phones that vibrate or light up are a distraction. If you forget and your phone makes a sound, do not look at the device. Looking at who is calling or texting you conveys one distinct message: there is someone else more important than your interviewer. Occasionally you may need to keep your phone and its notifications turned on (e.g., a sick child or elderly parent at home with a caregiver). Tell your interviewer that you may need to attend to a message at the beginning of the interview. If this is the case, silence all other notifications and only accept notifications from the one or two contacts who might reach out to you. If you make this type of request, you will have your first glimpse into how understanding a future employer might be in future situations.

Arriving at the Interview

Always arrive at least 10 to 15 minutes early to an in-person interview. If you are at risk of being late, make certain to call the employer and explain your situation and offer to reschedule the interview. If your reason for tardiness is a traffic incident, remember that these are easily verifiable online by the potential employer. Make certain that your reason is credible! When you arrive on site, be friendly and professional with any staff who might check you in for your appointment. Office staff are critical team members and may have more influence on the decision-making process than you know. A few kind words can go a long way. You may be offered water or coffee. Water is always a safe bet because it is not

likely to stain if you spill a bit and does not contribute to halitosis the way coffee might.

Things to Avoid

Avoid chewing gum or candy. If fresh breath is a concern, consider small mouthwash packets that can be used during a restroom break or dissolvable freshening strips. As mentioned previously, best practice will be to leave your cell phone at home or turned completely off in a bag or folio. You will also want to do your best to leave your problems at home. Occasionally we may have challenges with spouses, significant others, or our own health. The interview is a time to keep things in the positive and avoid conversations regarding your personal problems.

The Anatomy of an Interview

Interviews are relatively simply in their structure. Like most things, they involve a beginning, a middle, and an end. It is the beginning and ending that are often most challenging for those who are new to the interview process. Each of these sections will be discussed subsequently.

The Beginning of the Interview

The interview begins the moment you arrive. Remember to smile and greet your interviewer warmly. During this time, you will likely shake an interviewer's hand. Reach out with your right hand and grasp your interviewer's right hand firmly. Prepare to engage in three up-and-down "pumps" of your hand while you say "Hello" to the interviewer. Maintain eye contact during the handshake and do not waiver in your eye contact or glance away. This is an appropriate time to state your name (especially if you use a name that is different than what is on your resumé. For instance, an applicant whose full name is "Elizabeth" may state, "Please feel free to call me Liz"). During the handshake, you might also state that it is your pleasure to meet the interviewer and that you are doing well and are enthused to be invited for a formal meeting. Remember, your ability to engage in an appropriate greeting is part of what your employer is evaluating. How will you interact with clients and families? Are you confident? Your handshake will be the first impression.

One challenge point that occurs during the beginning for many new applicants is when you sit down with an interviewer. You may be asked, "Tell me a little bit about yourself." Although this may seem like an easy task, it might be one where you get lost without practice. Try and keep this response brief—to about 100 words with three to four talking points that you will easily remember. If you are beginning this statement with a phrase like, "I was born in . . . ," you are likely going to contain far too much information. Instead, consider what brought you to this profession and why you are excited about today's interview. Your "tell me a little bit" statement might vary slightly from interview to interview. This is acceptable as long as you are true to yourself.

After you engage in a few pleasantries and a description of yourself, you will quickly move to the "middle" of the interview.

The Middle of the Interview

The middle of the interview will typically be more technical and require answers to specific questions. Here your employer is looking for three "F's": fit, flexibility, and how you function.

When considering fit, the employer wants to understand how you meet the requirements of the position. Make certain that you have studied the job description and posting well. Have examples ready! If the posting reads, "Competence with a wide range of hearing aid software," be ready to state how you fit. Alternatively, if the posting is highly specific with a statement such as, "Experience with pediatric dysphagia a must," you should be ready to describe your experiences in detail.

Flexibility may be assessed by asking you general questions about what you enjoy about the environment where you are applying and what motivates you in your work. On a more specific level, an employer might look for confirmation regarding areas such as:

- What management style you prefer

- Confirmation of the working hours at the facility and what you might expect

- Commuting between facilities (as appropriate)

- How you might respond to interruptions during the day

- Your preferences for workspace and collaboration

- How you might respond to changes in your caseload (as appropriate)

- What you look for when working with a team

- Your aspirations for career advancement and leadership

It is important to be honest regarding your flexibility with your employer. For instance, if you are not able to be flexible with your working hours, you should not state that staying later on a given day and coming in later the next works for you. Instead, you should state what flexibility you do have, and where the challenges occur. For instance, regarding this flexibility example, you might state: "I can stay later on Tuesdays and Thursdays. However, the other days of the week are a challenge for me due to commitments after work." This lets your potential employer know what you *can* do, without interpreting your message as a complete "no."

Function is an area that is more critical to employers than most students or new graduates understand. You can be trained to perform assessments and use tools. However, how you function at work day-to-day may be less malleable. To get at function, employers will often ask questions using a "Behavioral Event Interview" strategy. Here the employer will ask questions and ask how you have responded in the past. There is a simple formula for answering these questions called "S.T.A.R."

- S: situation

- T: task

- A: action

- R: result

For instance, imagine the employer asks you, "Tell me about a time you worked with a team and you handled conflict." Your response can be framed using the STAR format.

S—"On one occasion at City Hospital, I was working with an interprofessional team. A situation evolved where we developed scheduling problems for the inpatients who needed our services. There were significant delays moving patients from room to room for the different treatments that they needed. It appeared that the staff responsible for patient transport was challenged in moving patients in a timely way."

T—"Our task was to meet as a team, both the providers and the transport staff, and have a productive conversation about the needs and limitations for the patients we served."

A—"My supervisor and I were called to action and scheduled a meeting with all of us at lunch. Of course, not everyone could make it, but over 90% of the team arrived because we all knew we were getting frustrated by the day-to-day problem. My supervisor and I led a guided conversation to determine where the bottlenecks and challenges fell in the process. It was important that everyone in the room used positive and non-blaming language. We made that one of our commitments to the conversation at the outset."

R—"The result was that we found three bottle-necks in patient transport as well as our inpatient rehab scheduling. We worked with the managers of our units to change scheduling and our process. It took about three working days, but soon we worked out the kinks and had a better experience for the patients."

Note how the example above uses the STAR format. Additionally, note how it avoids negative language or any strong focus on "negatives," and does not overstate the role that the student may have played in the situation.

When engaging in a STAR response, remember that you might want to avoid using the words "situation, task, action, result" over and over again. This will give your answers some variety!

Other STAR-based questions you might be asked include:

- Tell me about a time you handled conflict with your direct supervisor

- Tell me about a time you had many tasks to complete with similar deadlines

- Tell me about a time you disagreed with your direct supervisor

- Tell me about a time you addressed an unhappy patient/family

- Tell me about a time you failed to meet an obligation

- Tell me about a time you made a mistake in your work

- Tell me about a time you helped build a team

These statements may seem somewhat similar (e.g., conflict vs. disagreement). It is important to listen closely to the question at hand and answer as specifically as possible.

Again, it is critical to remember that there will be many areas of your position where you can be *trained* (e.g., administering a new assessment or operating new equipment). What is harder for your employer to change is your fit, flexibility, and function. What may seem like a dream job on paper may not be feasible for you because

of the three "F's." It is better to know this before accepting a position versus setting yourself up for failure on your very first job. Learning that a job is not a fit before you accept the position is actually a win for both you and the employer!

The End of the Interview

You will likely feel the interview will turn back to you at a certain point, signaling the final phase of the interview. Visual clues might be observing the interviewer looking at her watch or a clock on the wall. Verbal cues include the employer asking questions such as, "So, what questions do you have for me?" Or, "Is there anything you feel I should know about you and your application?" These types of questions signal that your interviewer is nearing the end and wants to be certain that no questions are left unanswered should they move to make you an offer.

Typical questions to ask toward the end of an interview include, but are not limited to, the following:

- What assistance will I have for completing licensure and certification requirements and applications?

- Who will mentor my first year of employment?

- Where will I work? (if more than one clinical site)

- What materials, tests, and equipment will be available to me?

- What opportunities are there for continuing education?

- What assistance is there for relocation?

Be sure to write down the answer to the questions and thank the interviewer for providing responses.

The end of your interview is a great time to go back to any list of questions that you have prepared as well. What is left unanswered? What would you need to make your decision, aside from salary information? You may have questions about benefits and many employers may direct you to a manual or website, rather than engage too deeply at this point in the conversation. This is normal.

As you close the interview, wrap up your final questions and make a positive statement about the interaction or organization. Even if the position is not the right fit for you, remember that the people at this organization

Questions you should *avoid* in the interview:

- When can I take my first vacation day?

- When am I eligible for sick time?

- Is it acceptable if I am late on Tuesdays?

- If I take this job, may I leave early on Fridays?

These types of questions signal to the employer that you are focused more on time away than time on the job. Of course, there may be times when this information is critical to you (e.g., you are responsible for picking a child up from childcare on Wednesdays and cannot be late). A question regarding this type of situation is best left to the final negotiation process.

are your professional colleagues. You will likely wrap up the final moments with a handshake. It is appropriate to thank the interviewer for her time and ask if she can tell you more about the decision timeline at this point. A simple question of, "Can you tell me more about your timeline for hiring?" is appropriate. You will want to avoid any statements that put pressure on the interviewer at this point, such as, "I've got several good offers, so, I really need to know soon." A statement about these needs is better left to a follow-up call or email.

Electronic Interview Formats

Many employers are screening candidates using web-based or teleconference communication technologies. Conducting interviews this way can be efficient for all parties involved. If you are asked to conduct a tele-interview, remember several things:

- For interviews that are conducted without visuals (audio teleconferencing):
  - ☐ Telephones can fail. At the outset of the call, determine who will return the call should there be a "drop" in the call.
  - ☐ Conduct a phone interview in a quiet space, free of distractions. Avoid making these calls in noisy, crowded spaces or while you are distracted. If your interviewer discovers you are multi-tasking it sends a message that this job is not important to you.
  - ☐ Speak clearly and ask for confirmation that everyone can hear you.

- ☐ Interviewers cannot see your facial expressions. You may need to tell your interviewer "That makes me smile" or "Your question is causing me to pause a bit and think of possibilities" so that you avoid any misunderstandings.

- ☐ Consider turn-taking during the call. Your interviewer won't have visual cues regarding when you are ready to move on from your answer. You can wrap up with summary statements such as, "Those are my thoughts on that question, what other questions do you have for me?"

- ☐ If you are being interviewed by a group, make certain to write down names and do your best to confirm who you are speaking to on the call. For instance, imagine an audiologist and a hiring manager are in the room. There could be instances where you change your language (either more or less technical) dependent upon the person who asks you a specific question.

- ☐ Maintain your sense of humor. If you make a mistake and call someone by the wrong name, apologize and move on. If the technology poses a challenge, acknowledge that the best-laid plans sometimes fail.

- For web-based video conferencing:
  - ☐ It is all about bandwidth. Make certain that you are in a space with a connection that can handle the demands of audio and video streaming. It is possible that a coffee shop or other area with public Wi-Fi cannot meet your demands.
  - ☐ Dress the same way that you would for a face-to-face interview. You might be tempted to wear formal clothes only on the top half of your body because "that's all they'll see." However, dressing the part completely will help you feel most confident!
  - ☐ Look into the camera. A common mistake can be to spend too much time looking at the screen. Although you want to monitor the expressions of your interviewer/s, you will also want to look directly into the camera to maintain eye contact with the interviewer/s.
  - ☐ Consider the position of your camera. Placing your camera where it is slightly higher than your forehead may provide a more flattering view of your face than a laptop placed on your desk or lap.

☐ Lighting is important. Play with lighting before the interview to make certain that there is adequate light on your face with few shadows. Your interviewer/s may need to use cues from your face just like our clients and patients do.

☐ What is happening in the room? Look carefully for what is in your background. Remove any pictures or items that may be busy or distracting. Also, keep pets out of the room. If there is the potential for extra noises to occur during the interview that you cannot control (e.g., a construction project that began minutes before your scheduled time), work to reduce the distraction and apologize to the person/people on the other end of the connection.

☐ Although you might be at home, do not allow yourself to become too relaxed. Maintain your posture during the interaction, just like you would in a face-to-face interaction.

☐ If you need to look down/look away, state why you are doing so. For instance, your interviewer asks which assessments you are comfortable using for a given population. It is appropriate to state, "That's a great question. I'm consulting a list that I have prepared in order to answer that question." This way your interviewer has an understanding as to why you are looking elsewhere.

☐ Practice! If the software platform is one you have available, practice with a friend. Make sure that your microphone and camera settings are working.

☐ Accept that it will likely take time to get connected. If your interview is at 9:00 AM, consider that, due to technology glitches, the actual interview might not start until 10 to 15 minutes later. This is a regular occurrence and should not reflect negatively on you. Instead, maintain a positive spirit and comply with any directions regarding settings on your computer. Also, avoid any negative statements regarding your personal technological prowess versus that of the interviewer. For instance, a statement such as, "I'm glad you *finally* figured out the technology problems on your end" could signal an unwanted attitude to your future employer. Instead, keep it positive with statements such as, "Sometimes technology takes a little extra time" or "What's most important is that we can see and hear each other. Thanks for your time and understanding to make that happen."

Meal Interviews

Interviews may include breakfast, lunch, or dinner with your primary interviewer and possibly a panel of other employees. Use your best etiquette at these meals and consider ordering foods that are easy to eat. If you need resources regarding etiquette, check with your university placement office; they may have workshops available to you. Another option is to search online resources and books. Be mindful of your food order so that you do not appear overly difficult to please with a long list of changes to menu items. Your interviewer will likely have many different questions during the meal, so, you can expect to spend a lot of time talking versus eating. Avoid criticizing the food or being rude if the service is inadequate. However, it is acceptable to be appropriately assertive should there be a problem with your meal. Follow the lead of your interviewer/other guests before ordering any alcohol. Most experts do not recommend ordering alcohol, even if your host elects to have a drink.

At the conclusion of the meal, make sure to thank the host. Also, determine if the restaurant environment was not conducive for you to talk with each member of the group (perhaps it was too noisy, or the table was too long). If this occurs, make certain to personally interact with each person immediately after the meal, thanking them for their time. This will provide your other tablemates with an opportunity to ask any last questions.

Second Interviews

Some employers might invite you to a second interview. Second interviews often signal that the employer is very interested in you and is seeking an opportunity for one last "look," or there is a short list of candidates and there is desire to make a ranked list of candidates who might receive an offer. You may not know exactly what your situation is; however, you might get hints by closely listening to the employer's invitation. Phrases such as, "We want you to have a chance to meet the team" or "We want to take a little more time to talk about the schedule and what the day-to-day might look like" are very positive signs. Phrases such as, "We've entered the second phase of the interviews and we'd like to spend more time with you" may signal that you are one of a few applicants invited to come back to the site.

The main issue about second interviews is this: *If you have no intention of accepting a position, do not engage in a second interview.* This wastes time and could be damaging to your professional relationships. Instead, state that you are very flattered, but you are pursuing other opportunities.

Prepare for the second interview just like you would the first. You will likely meet with different staff and be asked more detailed questions about yourself and your work style. Often second interviews focus on the "fit" portion of the three F's. They are often more relaxed than first interviews, but do not make any assumptions.

"Forbidden" Interview Questions

There are interview questions that are discriminatory and "off the table" during the interview process. These are questions related to age, race, color, gender, national origin, religion, and disabilities. There are several options you have if you are asked one of these questions.

1. Answer the question. This decision is entirely up to you. However, you may sense that the employer is not asking the question in a discriminatory manner. Instead, it is an error. An example might be that you discover your interviewer attended the same high school that you attended. If he/she asks, "What year did you graduate?" this could be taken as a method to determine your age. However, if you sense that it stems from a friendly and positive conversation, you could choose to answer it.

2. You can decline to answer the question and/or redirect the conversation. Perhaps your interviewer queries you about your plans to have a family. One option is to state, "I am not comfortable discussing my family planning in a job interview." Another that moves to redirection might be, "I'm reflecting on the posting for this job. The job posting deals with working as a pediatric audiologist. Let's talk about that." Making this form of statement tips your hand to the employer that you understand forbidden questions, but it keeps the conversation going and helps you redirect the discussion. (Note: You will have to determine whether or not you wish to engage with any offer from this employer.)

3. If you are deeply concerned or offended, you can close the interview with a polite but meaningful statement. "Thanks for taking the time to meet with me today. I'm uncomfortable discussing questions regarding my sexual orientation in this setting. I wish you the best in your search process."

This form of statement closes your time together in a polite way. You can then decide which, if any, further action you would like to pursue with the organization.

Post-Interview Follow-Up

You should plan to follow up with your interviewer within two days after the interview with a thank-you letter or email. Again, if you are sending a paper letter, appropriate business letter style should be used on 8.5 × 11 inch, good-quality bond paper. This letter gives you a chance to express your appreciation for the interview, renew interest in the position, briefly restate major qualifications, and explain any unresolved issues raised during the interview. Be sure to proof-read any follow-up correspondence before sending it. You could also send a handwritten thank-you card if you believe that a card fits the culture of the institution.

After you have sent your thank-you, you will spend some time waiting. Reflect back on what the employer told you about the timeline when you closed the interview. Give the employer an extra 24 hours after this timeline for follow-up. If you have not heard after waiting this period of time, it is appropriate to follow through with an email or phone call. Remember to keep your tone positive and upbeat during any follow-up interaction. Odds are your potential employer is very busy and there may be many demands on her time. Start any contact by briefly reminding the employer who you are, when you interviewed, and that you are following up to determine any next steps regarding the position. There are several outcomes of this phone call. One is that the potential employer will state that she needs more time to make the decision. You could then learn an approximate timeline for a decision. Another outcome could be that the potential employer has filled the position with another candidate. Although this may be disappointing to you, make sure to thank the potential employer for her time and energies. Also, it is reasonable to ask if she will keep you in mind for other opportunities. Another potential result of this call could be that you are offered a position. This will be covered later in the chapter.

Considering the Benefits That Might Be Available to You

You have done your homework and you are hoping for an offer! However, before moving to the specifics of receiving the offer, you should be considering what types of benefits may be provided to you. Some of this information might be available to you through an employee handbook or a website from the organization. Reviewing these benefits early, before receiving a final offer, can help you with the process when you receive an offer or multiple offers.

Salary and Benefits

Salary

Salary is often the focus for most people when they consider a job. Salary is important; however, you should consider salary in the context of many other factors. These include: cost of living, job satisfaction, work/life balance, and other benefits that an employer may be offering to you. The latter is very important. You might "trade away" a higher salary for a benefit that could be very important to you, simply because you are not examining all of the details carefully. Always look thoroughly at a benefits package and make comparisons where you can, if you have multiple job offers on the table.

Students are often primarily concerned about salary. Reliable information about salary exists at the Bureau of Labor Statistics. Other resources include salary surveys from the American Speech-Language-Hearing Association (ASHA) and the American Academy of Audiology (AAA). ASHA has sources that are specific to regions and practice locations that many students find helpful. It is important to remember, however, that most new graduates may not start at a "median" salary, simply due to a lack of years of experience.

Within salary, you need to consider the type of job for which you are applying. Some positions offer a higher salary with limited/no benefits. Other positions offer a full complement of benefits. What is important to you, and why? Always remember, forgoing benefits may sound like a good idea in the moment (for more pay). However, could there be instances where you need these benefits? Consider your future carefully.

Another important factor is to consider where you will be living. A given salary in the Midwest will require a significant adjustment if you are moving to a state like California or New York. There are several different salary tools available online to help you calculate differences across the country. Students are wise to check these, especially if you are conducting a national search for a position.

Another factor to consider is how your salary breaks down to an hourly rate. A common misconception is a clinician who works 9 to 10 months in the school but is paid over 12 months is "paid to work in the summer." This is not the case. Instead, this clinician is electing to be paid for work she has already performed during the summer months. This could mean that a clinician on a 9- or 10-month appointment may actually earn more per hour than her colleague who works in a setting where she is paid a similar salary for working all 12 months.

You will note that salary is considered in this chapter as something you will discuss *after* the first interview. However, you may find times that an employer will ask you about salary expectations in the first interview. You should study the aforementioned sites, confer with colleagues and university faculty, and use broad data from the Bureau of Labor Statistics in providing a salary range (www.bls.gov). Also, demonstrate your flexibility if you find an employer balks at your salary demand. A simple statement of, "I'm interested in this salary range; however, I am willing to negotiate for the right position" may keep you in the conversation longer than being very rigid.

Medical Insurance

For many new applicants, the health care market can be a challenging maze of information. Before you begin looking at health care options, consider your current health and any chronic conditions that you may have. Do you require frequent physician visits? Or, are you in good health? Do you have a spouse and children who may need health benefits? Or, are you planning to have a family in the near future? All of these decisions may impact your decisions around health care.

Small employers may have one option for health care. Larger employers may have several different plans to choose from, dependent upon your needs. In most instances (but certainly not all) employees subsidize some portion of the health insurance cost that is provided through the employer. This means that you are paying for part of the plan each month, and you may pay copays and other out-of-pocket costs as you use the health care system. Some broad examples of these plans include:

High-deductible plans. These plans may have lower costs to you on a monthly basis. However, should you need health care, you may pay a large portion of the cost up-front as you use care. In these plans, you might pay for entire visits and procedures until you reach a set limit (e.g., $10,000 annually). High deductible plans require an analysis on your part. How much care will you require? If you have a catastrophic need (e.g. accident or emergent health condition) can you afford to cover the deductible in a given calendar year?

Health Maintenance Organizations (HMOs): These plans typically require you to establish a primary physician who will manage your health care. This means that referrals to other providers come through your primary care physician, after you have seen this provider and been triaged for care. HMOs typically have a network of physicians and facilities that are your first point of referral. This means that you are restricted to these providers in order to receive the lowest cost of care out of pocket. Copays and deductibles may still be required; however, the deductibles are usually lower than a high deductible plan.

Preferred Provider Organizations (PPOs): These plans have published providers where you may not require a referral like an HMO. Often, as long as you use the providers in the network, you do not need to see a primary care physician for each referral to a specialist. Again, deductibles and copays may be required. Additionally, your portion of the subsidy for the cost of this type of plan is typically higher than the aforementioned plans.

Open access plans: These plans may be highly desirable, but costly. These plans give patients the widest range of options; however, copays and deductibles may still exist. Because these plans offer access to many providers, your portion of the cost of these plans may be very high.

WebMD offers resources that further describe health care plans. A link to this information can be found in the Resources section of this chapter. Remember, health care is fluid and subject to change in the United States. Also, some benefits may vary by the state or region of the country you are living in at the time. When in doubt, check with your employer and the associated health plan.

Retirement and Other Incentives

You should also consider retirement options with any employer.

401(K): These retirement plans involve you providing a portion of your salary (often pre-tax) and a complementary percentage paid by your employer as a match. For instance, your employer may match up to 5% of your net salary that you invest in a 401(K) plan. These plans are typically investment accounts where you make choices about the level of risk that you are willing to accept and the amount of return that you expect on the investment of your salary. It is important to understand that many of these plans are not guaranteed retirement plans. Instead, they depend upon how the accounts where they are invested perform in the financial markets. You could lose all or a portion of your money if the market is not doing well.

Defined Contribution Pension Plans: These plans are difficult to find, but they may exist in jobs that are funded as public service. For instance, some schools, universities, and other public positions may have this type of benefit. In these plans, you contribute to the retirement plan and work a given number of years until you are "vested." If you have worked the appropriate number of years and contributed appropriately, you will have a predictable income when you retire at the age stipulated by the plan. You will want to examine the terms of this type of plan carefully to make certain that you meet the requirements for the benefit.

Profit sharing or bonus plans: Some companies may have profit sharing plans that are available to you based on company performance. This type of plan may "pay out" annually, often at the close of a calendar year. As an employee and clinical service provider, you will want to confirm that a profit-sharing plan does not compromise your ability to make ethical decisions when treating patients or administrating in your role.

Paid Time Off (PTO)

Paid time off is something that many new employees are excited to learn about. This time is "vacation pay" or "sick pay" that the employee may earn where he/she is paid while not at work. You will want to look at an organization's PTO plan very carefully.

Look to answer questions about PTO such as:

- How much PTO do you earn? Is there a differential based on your years of service? Often, PTO is earned based on the number of hours you have worked in a given pay period. Some organizations may reward employees who have been working with them for multiple years with more PTO accrual than newer employees.

- When may you use your first days off? Some organizations will have a waiting period.

- What notice must you give for PTO? How is it reported? Is it approved first-come, first-served? Or is it based on seniority? This could impact your time away during peak vacation times, especially early in your career.

- Does your PTO "expire"? Alternatively, may any unused PTO be rolled into another year or period?

- May you donate PTO to another employee who is going through a hardship?

- Are personal days offered? These may be offered aside from "vacation" or "sick" time. The intention of these days is to give you time to conduct your personal matters.

Other Time Off

You will want to confirm with your employer what policies exist for other forms of time off as well. Different forms of PTO in this category might include:

- Bereavement time
- Any policies related to the birth of children or adoption (some organizations may be more liberal than any required federal policies)
- PTO for professional development, including time spent furthering your education, which may be necessary for licensure and any certificates you may hold
- Any other policies that an organization might have regarding time off, such as jury duty or other time away from work

Other Perquisites

Sometimes it may be easy to overlook other "perks" that an organization might have for you. However, these can add up. In some instances, a perk may be offered to you tax-free and so the advantage to you is that these benefits are not taxed as you earn them (of course, always check carefully).

Other perquisites to consider:

- *Parking:* Always verify parking costs and if they are subsidized in any way by the employer. Parking can be costly for those who commute to work on a daily basis.
- *Business partnerships:* Some organizations may have relationships that offer you discounts on gym memberships (these could be linked to the health plan that you choose), cell phone costs, tax preparation, and more. Check to see what benefits might exist by looking at the organization's benefits manual.
- *Professional fees/continuing education/ licensing:* Your new employer might be willing to cover some or all of the costs for professional credentialing and continuing education. You should examine these policies to determine how much funding is being offered, how it is requested, and how long you need to be with an organization to earn this type of benefit.

- *Employee assistance programs:* Some employers may have programs to assist you/ your family members with mental health, parenting skills, substance abuse, financial matters, or even adoption benefits. Although this type of benefit is not guaranteed, you should look at a benefits package carefully to determine whether these benefits exist and if they might be useful to you.
- *Educational assistance programs:* You might want to determine if an employer supports furthering your education. This might be in addition to something like funding your continuing education for licensing. In this case, perhaps an employer pays a portion of an additional degree, coursework, or certification that you might seek. This could have a great payoff for your future!

Receiving the Offer

You have engaged in the interview and reviewed potential benefits. Now your future employer contacts you to discuss the terms of an employment offer. This can be an exciting time. However, it can be stressful as well. Maintaining a clear mind during this process will be critical.

The First Contact

Many employers will contact you via telephone/teleconference to formally offer you a position. Make certain that you are in a place where you can take the call and focus on the conversation. Be ready to take notes and have any final questions answered. You should have these questions written down and readily available.

Remember, you are a professional interviewing and accepting a job in the real world. Although support from a parent or friend is comforting, asking for a third-party to be present during the offer reveals that you are not ready to handle the responsibilities of a clinician who needs to make independent decisions every day. Take this call independently knowing that you will gather all of the information without making a decision during the call. There will be many areas to consider, and these are covered in the section below:

- Remain enthused. Your future employer is moving forward with a big step for both of you. You may not be sure of the fit as you listen to the terms of the offer. Make sure to listen to the entire offer before being too negative or too positive. Avoid statements such as, "I can't believe this is happening!" or, "Is that all?" or, "Thank goodness, because I don't have any other offers." Statements such as these may limit your negotiating power with the future employer.

- Be mindful of your own research and how it fits the offer. It might be tempting to tell an employer about all the research you have done and how you believe the offer you are receiving can be better. Be mindful here, however. Your statements might be off-putting to the potential employer who may have this same information but have limitations. This is the time to determine what is most important to you versus passing along a vast amount of confusing information

- Receiving an offer is a confidence booster, be careful. You want to remain sensible during the call with an offer. Although receiving an offer is an affirmation for you, now is not the time to let your head get too big. You will want to be mindful and considerate as you negotiate with a future employer.

- Moving forward. Ask your future employer if you will receive the offer in writing, or, if the offer is a verbal offer. If the offer will be provided in writing, always ask for more time to review the written terms before saying, "Yes." If the offer is verbal, take detailed notes and ask your employer for the time you need to consider the offer. Written offers are always desirable over verbal offers. Note that employers may have a term during which the offer "expires." Some may give you a week, others may have a shorter term. If a future employer demands you make the decision on the spot, consider what working with this employer might be like in the future. Is this the type of pressure you prefer? Most employers will give you at least 24 hours if you confirm your interest and state clearly why you need a little time to consider the situation. If you have a spouse or significant other, stating that you would like to confirm the offer with your family is a reasonable first step.

Negotiating

On some occasions, you will look at the offer and possibly wish for something better. Consider the following tips:

- If you have another offer that appears "better" to you, consider talking about how the other

meets your needs without conveying an attitude that "educates" your future employer about the competitive market. Instead, state why the other offer you have may be a good fit for you and determine how the employer can meet your needs.

- If you have solid data (i.e. Bureau of Labor Statistics, cost of living calculators), and wish to further negotiate salary, let your future employer know where you are drawing your information from during the conversation.

- Sometimes there is no negotiation. It is possible that some positions will have little room for negotiation. An example might be positions where there are published salary schedules/negotiated contracts such as public schools. In these instances, attempting to make large demands regarding salary negotiation will reveal your naiveté more than anything else.

- Be clear about your requirements for the position. Many applicants are advised to aim slightly higher than what they require in order to land somewhere in the middle. Often employers will negotiate for "one round." This means that you need to treat your negotiations all in one event, in contrast to something iterative that moves the process across days and days. So, if you are seeking to negotiate around salary and funding for continuing education, you need to do so all in the same negotiation discussion.

- Remember that some elements of a position may be established around policy. For instance, if a large employer has a policy in place regarding vacation, it might not be malleable due to parity with other employees in the organization. You will want to consider the size of your employer here, as well. Sometimes a small business may have more flexibility than a larger corporation or agency.

- Think back to your conversations with your potential employer. Did she provide you with any clues? For instance, hearing something like, "We've been waiting to fill this position for quite awhile now" may reveal that you have additional bargaining power. In contrast, if you know that you are one of many applicants, your ability to negotiate may be reduced.

- Finally, think about your special knowledge and skills. Do you bring something to the table that others do not? Highlighting this during the interview and negotiating process is important!

Making the Decision

As you prepare to accept a position, confirm with your employer what the final terms of the employment will look like. Will you be signing a contract? Or, will you be giving your word? If there is a contract to sign, always read it carefully. There may be hidden elements in a contract that require further legal review before you sign them. This is particularly true of non-compete clauses that might exist in any contract. Non-compete clauses may state that you will either not take patients with you should you accept a different position, or, that you will not accept a position within a given radius of your current employer. You should look closely at non-compete clauses to avoid legal headaches down the line. It is best to have non-compete clauses reviewed by a lawyer.

Is This Where I Want to Work?

Although it may seem that an interview is one-sided and the interviewee is the only person being judged, an interview ought to allow an applicant to judge the qualities of the organization that will influence his or her determination of *is this where I want to work?* (Golper & Brown, 2004).

When determining where you want to work, consider factors such as the following:

- What is the reputation of this program? Will I be proud to say I work here?

- What is the financial stability of the program?

- What are the program's vision, mission, and values?

- Is the facility clean and well maintained?

- Are there sufficient supplies and materials?

- Will I have my own computer?

- Will I have sufficient privacy to do my desk work?

- Do people seem happy?

- What is the staff turnover?

- Are the support and clinical staff friendly, respectful, and welcoming?

- Do people appear to behave and dress in a professional manner?

- Are there others in the program who are a part of my ethnic or cultural group?

- Does the staff work as a team or independently?

- Can I see myself making friends here?

- Is there someone who could be a good mentor for me?

- Is the supervisor someone I can trust? Does he or she demonstrate good leadership?

Red Flags

While you are interviewing or considering the offer, you may get a "feeling" that this job has problems. Common red flags may include issues such as the following:

- The interviewer is rude, abrupt, or ignores staff as you visit the agency.

- The interviewer challenges you rather than inviting your responses.

- The interviewer takes numerous calls or accesses media during your interview without apologizing.

- You need to find your own clinical fellow (CF) or fourth-year experience mentor.

- The salary is comparatively higher than you would expect for your experience and the position.

- The person who previously worked in the position left after a very short time.

- You are not invited to speak with current employees or given other access to them.

- You are asked to take a personality assessment before you are allowed to interview for the position.

You should weigh all red flags carefully and determine whether the position is the right fit for you. Occasionally, positions that may appear the most prestigious or offer the highest salary may not be the best fit for you.

Getting Started

Once you have made your decision and signed any necessary contracts, it is time to make sure that you are fully credentialed and ready to begin your new job. This will involve providing all elements necessary to start work such as: copies of transcripts/diplomas, licensure, payer credentials, background clearances, fingerprint studies, and any other required documentation. Remember, your employer is monitoring you and your enthusiasm for the job, even before you start your clinical work. Make sure to comply with credentialing and paperwork requirements diligently!

Summary

The focus of this chapter has been on how to secure employment. Key concepts can be summarized in single words: research, networking, preparation, practice, style, and follow-up. Finding employment can feel stressful. However, the rewards are great with thoughtful and detailed preparation. Remember that your role as an employee starts upon submitting your accurate credentials upon application to the job. Chapter 12 continues with how to build your career once you have secured employment.

Critical Thinking

1. What makes for a "good" resumé or cover letter? Why?

2. What skills and experiences do you have that will be attractive to an employer?

3. Consider what questions might be asked of you based on a review of your resumé and cover letter. What stands out as most notable where a reader would seek more information?

4. What is the STAR method of responding to behavior event interview questions? Why are these questions important?

5. What are the differences in the job search process for someone seeking first employment versus an experienced professional?

6. What could the ramifications be of exaggerating an element of your resumé?

7. What would you do if an interviewer asked you a question and you did not have an answer?

8. What types of benefits are valuable to you at this stage of your life? What benefits might you want or need in 10 years?

9. After an interview, you felt that you really "blew it." How would you know this? What would you do now?

10. Prepare a hard copy of your resumé and have a peer and a professional colleague critique it. What needed improvement?

References

American Speech-Language-Hearing Association. (2018). *ASHA membership and affiliation counts, year-end 2018.* Retrieved from https://www.asha .org/research/memberdata/

Clabaugh, J. (2018). *Clean up your 'digital dirt': bosses check your social media profile.* Retrieved from https://wtop.com/business-finance/2018/08/ checking-you-out-online-is-now-sop-for-the-boss- so-clean-up-your-digital-dirt/

Doyle, A. (2019). *The difference between a resume and a curriculum vitae.* Retrieved from https://www .thebalancecareers.com/cv-vs-resume-2058495

Golper, L., & Brown, J. (Eds.). (2004). *Business matters: A guide to business practices for speech- language pathologists.* Rockville, MD: ASHA Publications.

Page, M. (2017). *Why cover letters are important.* Retrieved from https://www.michaelpage.com/ advice/career-advice/cover-letter-and-resume- advice/why-cover-letters-are-important

Stahl, A. (2016). *8 resume style mistakes you're probably making.* Retrieved from https://www.forbes.com/ sites/ashleystahl/2016/02/08/8-resume-style- mistakes-youre-probably-making/#a0875485 62da

Resources

Securing Employment

- **American Academy of Audiology.** In addition to job listings and opportunities for interviews at the annual convention, check for current job listings at http://www.audiology.org

- **ASHA Publications and Website.** The monthly publication *The ASHA Leader* has a section on employment opportunities. The ASHA Career Portal (https://www.asha.org/ careers/ has numerous resources for job tips, finding jobs, resumé writing, interviewing, and salary negotiations. You may also post a job resume and search available jobs online.

- **College Department Listings.** Most college or university departments receive notices of job vacancies. These may be posted or available in a department administrator's office or in student areas. Check your local communication disorders department for such information.

- **Local Library and Bookstores.** Check your local library or online bookstore for the section on employment or business. There are dozens of texts on topics such as interviewing, resumé preparation, and follow-up methods.

- **Professional Conventions.** Check state and national conventions for any placement and networking opportunities that may exist.

- **United States Department of Defense.** See the contact information at: https://www.usa.gov/federal-agencies/u-s-department-of-defense for positions and requirements related to the Department of Defense.

Benefits

- WebMD provides information regarding health plans. See: https://www.webmd.com/health-insurance/types-of-health-insurance-plans#1

- Money Magazine provides general information about retirement accounts at: https://money.usnews.com/money/retirement/articles/retirement-accounts-you-should-consider

- Vacation Counts offers considerations for Paid Time Off at: https://www.vacationcounts.com/vacation-days-paid-time-off-work-policies-top-10-questions-ask-hr/

Internet Sources

Allied Healthcare Professionals
- http://www.AlliedVIP.com

American Hearing Aid Associates
- http://www.ahaanet.com/

America's Health Care Source
- http://www.healthcaresource.com

America's Job Bank
- http://www.jobsearch.org

ASHA
- http://www.asha.org/careers/

Audiologyonline.com
- http://www.audiologyonline.com

CareerBuilder.com
- http://www.careerbuilder.com

iHireTherapy.com
- http://www.ihiretherapy.com

MedHunters
- http://www.medhunters.com

MedSearch
- http://www.medsearchcorp.com

MiracleWorkers
- http://www.miracleworkers.com

Monster.com
- http://www.monster.com

Rehab.Career.com
- http://www.rehabcareer.com

Rehabworld.com
- http://rehabworld.com

SLPJOB.com
- http://www.slpjob.com

SpeechPathology.com
- http://www.speechpathology.com

Therapy Jobs
- http://www.therapyjobs.com

Sample Interview Questions

http://www.best-interview-strategies.com/questions.html

https://www.indeed.com/career-advice/interviewing/how-to-prepare-for-a-behavioral-interview

Internet Resumé Preparation Sources Examples

CollegeGrad.com
- http://www.collegegrad.com/jobsearch/Best-College-Resumes

The Damn Good Resume
- http://www.damngood.com

My Perfect Resume
- https://www.myperfectresume.com/lp/mprrwzlp06.aspx

Susan Ireland's Resume Site
- http://susanireland.com/resume

State and Local Association Resources

Contact your state or local professional association to determine if it has a job listing or matching service. For state association contact information, visit ASHA's website, https://www.asha.org

Appendix 11–A

◇◇

Sample Resumé

Samuel Smith
123 Harbor Lane
Lakeville, KY 23414
samuel@university.edu
(555) 555-5555

EDUCATION

University of the Lakes, Lakeville, KY
Master of Arts in Speech-Language Pathology,   May 2020
Speech-Language Pathology Outstanding Student Scholarship 2019

Hope College, Holland, MI
Bachelor of Arts in Communications,   May 2018
Summa Cum Laude, Phi Beta Kappa

PRACTICUM EXPERIENCES

Graduate Student Clinician

Lakeville Elementary School, Lakeville, KY   January–May 2020

- Provided assessment and treatment services to children with speech, language, fluency, voice, and literacy disorders
- Led social thinking group for children with autism in 4th and 5th grades
- Conducted hearing screenings for K–5th grades, directed parent volunteers
- Documented services, wrote Individualized Education Plans (IEP), attended IEP meetings

Mooresville Hospital, Mooresville, KY   August–December 2019

- Assessed and treated a variety of patients with speech, language, and swallowing disorders secondary to stroke, neurodegenerative conditions, and traumatic brain injury
- Conducted supervised bedside and videofluoroscopic swallow evaluations and provided appropriate recommendations
- Engaged in group treatment with patients with a variety of types of aphasia as well as cognitive communication disorders
- Documented all services using electronic medical records system

University of the Lakes Speech & Hearing Clinic, Lakeville, KY   September 2017–August 2018

- Provided comprehensive diagnostic and treatment services for patients with fluency, voice, motor speech, and phonological disorders
- Conducted hearing screenings for all pediatric patients upon intake to the clinic
- Participated in 4-week augmentative and alternative communication (AAC) camp for children using a variety of high-tech devices

continues

Appendix 11–A. *continued*

VOLUNTEER

Washington Elementary School, Ames, IA   June–August 2015
  • Literacy Buddy for 8–9-year-old children in a 9-week intensive program

PRESENTATION

Smith, S. (2018). *Providing Literacy Enhancement in the Group Setting.* Paper presented at the annual convention of the Kentucky Speech, Language, and Hearing Association, Lexington, KY

SPECIAL ABILITIES/CERTIFICATIONS

  • Conversational fluency in Spanish and American Sign Language
  • CPR and Healthcare BLS Certified

12

Building Your Career

◇◇

Marva Mount, MA and Melanie W. Hudson, MA

Introduction

This chapter has been written by two professionals who have more than 60 years of combined professional experience in a variety of settings in addition to volunteer service to professional associations. Professional experience reveals particular issues that are as important to building your career as your clinical expertise and knowledge. We begin with your first year of professional practice and the issues you will face. We then move to what it is like to be a mentor/preceptor, ethical practice, organization, time management and work–life balance, productivity, teamwork, politics in the workplace, networking, performance evaluations, advancement, continuing education and specialization, and factors to consider when changing employment. We examine how each of these issues plays a distinct part in professional growth and success.

Your First Year of Clinical Practice

You should be very pleased that you have obtained employment in your first professional position as a speech-language pathologist or audiologist. It is now your responsibility to know the laws in your state regarding licensure, educator's certificate, or other professional credential(s) you should have specific to your work setting. Keep in mind that no matter what setting you have selected to begin your career, you may not stay in the same position or work setting for your entire career, and thus, it is best to consider all your current options regarding licensure and certification. See Chapter 3, "Establishing Competencies in Professional Education, Certification, and Licensure," for more information.

If you are a candidate for certification from the American Speech-Language-Hearing Association (ASHA), this is also the time to sit down with your mentor or preceptor and discuss the plan to meet those requirements, including documentation of on-site visits and timely completion of required forms. Further discussion on the topic of working with a mentor/preceptor is provided later in this chapter. You may also see Chapter 26, "Supervision and Mentoring," for more information.

You should also review your schedule, specific responsibilities, materials, equipment, computing and communication systems, and anything else that will help you get started. Review your employer's policies and procedures manual and take a look at sample diagnostic protocols and reports; observe others working; and get a real feel for what the job entails. Meet the other professionals with whom you will be working and administrative/support staff so that you know who can help you when you have questions. You are no longer a student, and you will be expected to be "ready to go" with less direct supervision.

Mentoring

Mentoring works best when it focuses on the entire person versus focusing on skill development alone.

—Harvard Business Review

As you begin your career in the field of speech-language pathology or audiology, you will require the support and guidance of a mentor or preceptor as you work toward establishing yourself as an accomplished professional. Your mentor or preceptor serves as a coach or guide, employing less of a "hands-on" but more of an indirect style of supervision than you experienced as a student clinician.

Effective mentors/preceptors provide a support system during critical stages of career development. They are good listeners, knowledgeable, nonjudgmental, candid, and honest. They provide constructive feedback and networks to find and provide resources to assist you with gaining personal success. Finally, a mentor is one who is willing and able to devote the time required to develop skills in others while being eager to learn themselves.

A mentor may be assigned to you within your work setting, or you may be required to identify one. The ASHA website has information on how to find a mentor, if necessary. You will find that the ASHA website will be more specific to mentorship in a general sense, since preceptorship in audiology will be negotiated by the university program. A mentor or preceptor is typically a more senior, respected professional in your field who will take a personal interest in your career development. It is important that you establish a good working relationship with your mentor or preceptor to gain the maximum benefit from this worthwhile relationship, which is collaborative in nature (ASHA, 2008a).

You and your mentor/preceptor should discuss how often you will be communicating and what modes of communication work best for each of you. Frequent contact, at least initially, is important to build trust and establish a mutual respect. This contact will gradually allow for each person to respect the experiences and views of the other, even when not in agreement. It will also serve to establish the relationship as a two-way street to promote flexibility and enjoyment.

At the first meeting, you and your mentor/preceptor will work together to establish goals that offer you a challenge as you grow professionally. As you tackle these goals together, ASHA (2008b) recommends that you describe and measure your own progress and achievement to promote independence and confidence in your work. You may need to develop a tool for self-assessment to serve this purpose, or there may be a ready-made tool available from your employer or professional organization. See Chapter 26 for more information about setting goals and assessment.

The focus of the relationship with your mentor/preceptor will be on sharing information that requires critical thinking while maintaining an open line of communication. You may be discussing how you can take better data, what strategies you could utilize to improve client outcomes, or how you and your mentor/ preceptor can improve your communication with one another. Both you and your mentor/preceptor must possess good interpersonal communication skills and be able to openly share ideas, suggestions, and concerns as part of this process.

Effective communication is a critical component of any supervisory relationship, and it is important to remember the role that both verbal and nonverbal communication plays in all of our relationships. Because much of our communication with another person is through tone of voice, appearance, and interpersonal and/or written interactions, we must be ever mindful of the message we send to others. Open communication will assist with navigating through problem areas when they arise and in the negotiation of resolutions to potential areas of conflict.

At times, you and your mentor/preceptor may be required to have a *difficult conversation*. For instance, you may need to tell your preceptor that you think he is interfering during your diagnostic sessions, causing you to feel inadequate in front of your patients. Or your mentor may be of the opinion that an aspect of your clinical treatment is inadequate. These types of situations require a dialogue that is based upon a predetermined plan. Maintaining open lines of communication is supported by deciding ahead of time in what manner this type of conversation will take place.

During these conversations, each party must invite joint problem solving and be willing to consider and understand both points of view. Good communication skills require the separation of the problem from the person. Effective communicators will listen first and talk second, to assist with establishing facts necessary to explore all options in a nonjudgmental way. The goal in this collaborative relationship is to work together to find solutions to all situations that arise and to utilize conflict as an additional way to promote both personal and professional growth.

Both you and your mentor/preceptor must recognize that the relationship will evolve over time as you become more proficient and move from a novice to a proficient speech-language pathologist or audiologist. This relationship is an excellent opportunity for you to examine your response to constructive feedback and for you to learn how to not only listen to and accept guidance but to offer your suggestions to others in a positive way. Your relationship with your mentor/preceptor sets the stage for your professional growth as a clinician and as a leader in your chosen profession.

Work Ethic and Professional Code of Ethics

In the professions of speech-language pathology and audiology, the landscape is ever changing, and the most competitive jobs can be difficult to find and to keep. To remain competitive in this type of work environment, you must instill in yourself a good work ethic where you are committed to holding yourself to the highest standards within the profession. Terms that are often synonymous with work ethic include diligence, dedication, enthusiasm, energy, focus, initiative, reliability, honesty, and steadfastness, to name a few. You want to become "indispensable." So how does one begin to develop these characteristics within the work setting?

Work Ethic

Instilling a good work ethic is a process that develops during your growth as a professional. Learning about employer expectations is the first step in this process. Within your work setting, you will have an employee policies and procedures manual, which contains information regarding a variety of topics specific to your facility. Work topics that may be covered in a facility policies and procedures manual include attendance and punctuality, discrimination, sexual harassment, confidentiality, disability accommodations, conflict of interest, substance abuse, misconduct regarding technology (including the use of email and social media), and federal and state laws and regulations such as FERPA, IDEA, HIPAA, and Medicaid, to name a few. In addition, you will need to familiarize yourself with all state licensure and/or certification rules and requirements regarding scope of practice, delegation of work, and ethical conduct. You should learn about these policies and procedures early on in order to be educated and fully informed and to prevent problems that could arise from your lack of knowledge and experience.

The Council of Academic Programs in Communication Sciences and Disorders (CAPCSD) (Schwartz, Horner, Jackson, Johnstone, & Mulligan, 2007) document *Eligibility Requirements and Essential Functions*

describes a set of knowledge and skills requisite to the practice of speech-language pathology to function in a broad variety of clinical situations. Although written for students in graduate programs, it established guidelines that may be applied to working professionals, including both speech-language pathologists and audiologists. The document identified five areas of focus necessary to be effective as a professional: communication, motor, intellectual-cognitive, sensory observational, and behavioral/social.

The behavioral/social area plays an important role in any discussion of work ethic, as it addresses the display of mature professional relationships. The requirements and essential functions included in this section of the CAPCSD document are displaying respect for others; conducting oneself in an ethical and legal manner, to include upholding the ASHA Code of Ethics as well as all federal privacy policies; maintaining general good physical and mental health and self-care; the ability to adapt to changing and demanding environments; managing time effectively; the acceptance of suggestions and constructive criticism; and appropriate professional dress. Each of the areas described and discussed within this document is an essential ingredient in the development of a good work ethic.

Code of Ethics

In addition to developing a solid work ethic, you should be cognizant of the code of ethics of your professions and maintain ethical standards for yourself in every aspect of your job. ASHA (2016) explains that a code of ethics is the fundamental principles and rules considered essential for the preservation of the highest standards. Therefore, it is imperative that you are familiar with the ethical standards that govern your practice, including the ASHA Code of Ethics, the AAA Code of Ethics, the ethical code and rules established for the state in which you work, and the ethical code of conduct required for your place of employment and any other professional association that you are affiliated with.

If you are faced with an ethical dilemma, what should you do? For instance, your employer has asked you to submit a billing statement to an insurance provider for client hours for which you have no documentation. You should begin by informing your employer that you do not have the necessary documentation for submission. In situations such as these, always be sure to explore what the possible courses of action are and what the outcomes could be for each of those actions. In your place of employment, it is a good idea to be familiar with what is permissible (can be done or not done), impermissible (must never be done under any circumstance), obligatory (cannot change and must always be done, regardless of circumstance or personal feeling), or necessary. Having this foundation will assist you in your decision-making process and prevent you from making decisions that are contrary to ethical standards within the workplace.

Let us explore what the potential benefits and burdens are for each action that you investigate. Sue Hale (2006) describes an ethical decision-making process that is as powerful as it is simplistic. She suggests that you follow a four-step decision-making process that requires that you (1) recognize that you may have an ethical issue, (2) gather information on the issue, (3) evaluate the situation, and (4) make a decision and test it using your definition of ethics and your knowledge of ethical practices. You should also familiarize yourself with what the outcomes could possibly be for ethical misconduct, should it occur. Violations such as falsification of documents and/or records or violation of laws associated with professional regulations, or felony or misdemeanor convictions for matters involving moral turpitude, for example, may result in sanction or revocation of your credentials.

Developing and maintaining a solid work ethic and adhering to principles of professional ethical conduct are as important to your success as knowledge of clinical skills. The choices we make in our personal lives can affect our professional lives in ways that we may not have even considered until it is too late to repair the damage. Employee personnel policies and procedures and your professional code of ethics are important tools. They are there to serve as your road map and compass as you navigate your career. See Chapter 5 for more information on professional ethics and Chapter 6 for discussion of professional accountability.

Being Organized

Did you know the average human being in our society loses an hour per day due to disorganization and poor time management? That is more than 14 individual 24-hour days per year. As you develop your career path, you will need to learn how to work efficiently in order to best serve the needs of your clients and to maintain a healthy work–life balance. Employing strategies of organization and time management will also help in the prevention of job burnout.

Many believe being organized is the foundation of success. Being organized typically means keeping things in predictable places or arranging things in an orderly or structured manner. An organized workspace is one in which materials can easily be located and where distractions are minimal. It is not as easy as being neat, which may simply mean maintaining cleanliness in a state of disorganization. Knowing where all items are on a consistent basis helps to maintain the flow of your workday and eliminates the need to waste time searching for what you need. We will examine several strategies for organization.

Start by scheduling a specified amount of time for organizing your space and begin by organizing your desk. Look through everything initially and make decisions about what to discard and what to keep. For those items you choose to keep, make a clearly labeled file immediately for those items. As you locate tasks that are in process, make a to-do file to place those items in so you can find them readily and complete them on time. Do not be afraid to throw things away. Find a box to place items in that require shredding and place those items there for shredding at a later time. Do the same with file cabinets, desk drawers, bookshelves, and any other area where disorder abounds.

You also need to organize the information you are required to obtain and maintain in your work environment. By organizing your information, you will ensure that time lines are kept and compliance is maintained. Organizing your information properly will also help you remember critical information. Information can be organized by utilizing filing systems (paper or digital) that make sense to you personally, where you can physically manipulate your information when necessary. In the age of technology, many choose to organize their information on the computer for easy access so they do not have to find a location to store and file information within their limited office space. Organize your computer files for your information there as well so you do not have to spend valuable time searching for information due to disorganization of your computer filing system.

There are two sobering statistics from time management experts Dodd and Sundheim (2005), authors of *The 25 Best Time Management Tools and Techniques*:

1. We use only 20% of the papers we file.

2. We spend at least 75 hours per year looking for lost papers, which averages out to about 13 minutes per day.

They suggest three types of files to organize the "paper" in your life. This system may also be applied to your computer filing system. One file should be an Action file. This file is for projects you are currently working on. The Reference file is the second type of file, and this file should include those things you need to keep for future reference. The third and final file type is the Reading file. These files are filled with those things you wish to read. Every paper you choose to keep should fit into one of these file types. If it does not, you should consider discarding it.

According to Silber (2004), author of *Organizing from the Right Side of the Brain*, we all have different styles that guide how we organize ourselves. Understanding your individual style can assist you as you employ strategies for organization. The manner in which you organize your information will be dependent on many factors, including if you are a "right brainer" or a "left brainer."

"Right brainers" are creative and visually oriented, with a need to see things in order to make sense of them. They usually get totally caught up in the moment and completely lose track of time. Filing papers and clearing desk space can make them feel as if they are being suffocated and as if their creativity is stifled. For "right brainers," many organizational strategies typically suggested will not be effective tools for them. They will need to try a wide variety of strategies to see what is most effective.

"Left brainers," on the other hand, like to feel in control of everything, particularly the environment around them. They are linear and structured and must compartmentalize to feel organized. They must finish things at regular intervals and put things away in order to feel that sense of accomplishment. Work environments tend to try to force individuals into a "left brain" way of doing business because, in the work environment, neatness and punctuality are highly valued. For "left brainers," many organizational strategies typically suggested will be effective tools for them.

Having an organized workspace with easy access to information and materials will save you time, energy, and frustration. It is a good idea to have specific places where items are always kept, and therefore easily accessible to you. Once you have initiated an organizational system that meets your needs and works for you, make an effort to maintain that system, even if it requires a few extra minutes of your day. You will reap the benefits of working smarter, not harder.

Time Management and Work–Life Balance

Many events in our day rob us of our time. Most often, our time is lost due to the three major factors of *disorganization*, *procrastination*, or *interruptions*. As we have already discussed, disorganized work spaces and disorganized information systems rob of us valuable time. Follow the guidelines for organization explored earlier in this chapter to avoid having disorganization rob you of your valuable time.

We can add *procrastination* to the list of time robbers. Why do we procrastinate? If we can answer that question, we can avoid the pitfalls procrastination will cause. Usually, we procrastinate because we are overwhelmed, because we do not estimate correctly the amount of time

a project will take us, because we would much prefer to be doing something else, because we fear failure or the inability to complete a task, or because we strive for perfection that is not required or necessary. If you find that you are procrastinating, examine the possible reasons. Once you find out why you are procrastinating at a particular time and on a particular project, you can follow some simple rules to move forward.

First, have a realistic sense of time, and work within the time frame that you have available. Work from a to-do list and tackle challenging projects first. Set small deadlines for yourself along the way and share those deadlines with colleagues in order for them to encourage and support your progress. Find what motivates you (reward, sense of accomplishment) and expect problems along the way so you are not disappointed or frustrated when they occur. Have reasonable expectations for yourself and for others. Expect the unexpected, and plan accordingly.

Dodd and Sundheim (2005) explain that we live in a world of *urgent*. They say if something demands our attention, it usually gets it, no matter what we are doing. They go on to explain that occasional urgency is not a problem. However, a steady diet of it can become a huge drain on your time and other resources. They suggest making lists of some type, such as a weekly to-do list, a daily to-do list, a master list that has everything you need to do, or some type of checklist for frequently occurring activities. When making lists, they suggest you think strategically, cut out the excess, and focus on main priorities.

They also suggest utilizing the "ABC System" as a way to prioritize. Using this system, you rank each item on your list as *A = high priority, B = medium priority, C = low priority*. This system is designed in order for you to complete all of your "A" activities each day, and fill in with "B" and "C" activities as time permits. This system is designed to assist you with crossing things off your list that really matter in the overall scheme of your day.

The final area for us to explore in terms of good time management is the issue of *interruption*. Most interruptions occur when the priorities of someone else are in conflict with what you have planned. You can minimize interruptions in order to improve time management by having a schedule planned for your daily activities and by sticking to it. Within that schedule, look at all the activities you are required to complete as a part of your current position as a speech-language pathologist or audiologist in your current work setting.

Scheduling suggestions include flex scheduling, where you change your schedule as new duties and responsibilities find their way to you. Incorporate the use of calendars, day planners, online calendar systems, wall calendars, desk calendars, and to-do lists to adequately schedule, maintain, and plan for all aspects of your day.

Because time with your clients/students/patients is typically the most important part of your day, you should plan your schedule for that first. In addition, schedule time for the planning of your sessions, for consultation and collaboration with family members and with colleagues, for the completion of diagnostics, for completion of paperwork and compliance issues, and for time to review and answer email and voice mail.

When reviewing your emails, decide if the email is something you can delete, if it is something you need to act on, or if you need to file it. If you do not need to delete it or act on it, then you should file it. When setting up electronic files, remember it is better to have fewer large files than it is to have many small ones. Finally, make an appointment with yourself to clean out your email, text messages, and voice mail on a regular basis.

Plan for designated "office hours" and make conscious decisions regarding when you will be available to colleagues. Even if you are in a shared work space, try not to encourage interruptions by always making yourself available to others. Develop a system whereby your colleagues know that you are unavailable, such as wearing headphones, a sign on your desk, and so forth. Understand that lack of planning on the part of someone else should not constitute an emergency for you. Suggest to colleagues that you schedule a designated time with them rather than have a conversation with them when you are unable to provide them with your undivided attention. By doing this, you enable your coworkers to work independently as well.

As a last resort, remove yourself from areas or activities where the interruptions seem to occur most often. Expect that interruptions will occur throughout the workday, and plan accordingly. Above all, do not use interruptions as a way to avoid your work. Sometimes, this will be tempting, particularly if you have an unpleasant or challenging task to complete. You may be tempted to allow interruptions to delay beginning those projects. And try to take advantage of those unexpected bits of time that become available to you to tackle unfinished and/or ongoing tasks.

To be effective time managers, we must also learn to set boundaries. Setting boundaries assures that we are not only achieving excellence in our professional lives, but that we are also achieving a level of excellence in our personal lives. Make a conscious effort to establish boundaries so your quality time can truly be quality time. People who are constantly reactive feel less in control of their lives, and are more prone to stress (Brooks, 2004).

The bottom line is to start small and build those boundaries little by little. It is understandable, particularly when you are new to something, to give it your all

and then some. We want to be noticed by our employers. We want to give the impression that we are willing to do anything to succeed and to excel to the top of our craft.

To achieve a solid work–life balance, identify what is most important to you, right now, in your life. Establishing priorities may require you to take an inventory of your daily work activities, to identify what tends to waste your time during the day as well. Is it constantly checking your email? Answering your phone every time it rings? Or is it dealing with those less constructive individuals that seem to devour your time before you know it? Allow what you identify as important to truly reflect your present set of priorities. By mapping out your priorities, it will be much easier for you to see how your present schedule will need to be modified in order to accommodate those identified priorities. Keep in mind this may change frequently over time, and may require that you revisit your priorities often.

By taking an inventory of your time, you will be able to determine what you waste time on, so you can eliminate those things. This will allow you to focus on the people and/or activities that add the most value to your day, and that make you the most productive. By focusing on the daily items that bring the most value to your professional life, you will be continuing to establish those boundaries that will assist you with a better work–life balance.

Keep in mind that employers place the highest value on individuals who are not simply workaholics, but those who are intelligent and bright, and who show up to work ready to give the absolute best they have to give every day. Of course, there will be times in our professional lives when we must dig deep and give more time and attention to our job than is usually expected. For example, when we are new to a job, the learning curve is typically steep for a time. Or, when we have been given a project with a deadline that does not allow us the luxury of extended time, we may be expected to spend more time at work until the project is complete.

However, for the majority of our work lives, the fact that we spend far too much time at work may simply be the result of self-imposed expectations. It is a habit we may easily fall into, and one that can be quite detrimental to both our mental and physical health, as well as our professional and personal relationships. We cannot give excellence to our clients if we do not first give excellence to ourselves in terms of work–life balance. When beginning your career, begin with and maintain healthy habits. Give yourself permission. Be kind to your mind and body.

Ultimately, effective time management that allows you to establish and maintain a healthy work–life balance is all about your plan. A plan gives you an overall view of what must be accomplished, and it saves you valuable time in the long run. Making a plan and sticking to it will ensure that your work life has balance and that you are productive in your job.

Productivity

Now that we have explored the importance of organization and time management, we will discuss productivity in the workplace. Productivity is important for both personal and professional growth. When you are productive in your work, you obtain more enjoyment from your job and are less likely to be complacent or unhappy with where you work. Your confidence in your performance typically results in positive work behaviors, positive work relationships, superior work performance, better performance evaluations, and higher compensation. When you are more productive, you are more efficient and more creative and have more energy.

It is important to implement your treatment effectively and efficiently to achieve the highest levels of success with those you serve in the least amount of time possible. In some work settings, specified *productivity standards* are in place that you must meet in order to maintain employment. In those settings, productivity is usually described in percentage amounts, such as 80%. That figure translates into the amount of time during your total working hours in which you are expected to be providing direct services or accruing "billable" hours. You need to know what those standards are in your work setting and comply accordingly.

To begin your road to productivity, you may want to look at a few things to focus your attention as you begin your new job. First, you will want to set target goals for each day, with some "mini" goals built in so that you can identify, more efficiently, time requirements for the tasks that you have to complete. Break those larger tasks into smaller tasks, and then stick with the task until it is completed. You will find that by doing so, you can also group like tasks together in order to complete them in less time.

In addition, it is necessary for you to be able to problem solve and make decisions efficiently in order to remain productive. Time wasted in the decision-making process can erode your productivity. Have a set amount of time for the decision-making process, a plan for how you will make decisions, and then stick with that plan. Force yourself to make important decisions within the time frame that you set. Recognize that your problem is your responsibility until it is solved, and "own" the problem until you resolve it. You may have to solicit the

assistance of others to help you solve the problem; however, you are ultimately responsible for the resolution.

At the end of each workday, identify the task that you will begin the next day, and prepare for that task in advance by readying the materials you will need to complete the task (Pavlina, 2007). The next day, you will be able to begin working on that task immediately. If you are interrupted at the beginning of the day with unplanned events, you will be less likely to get "off track" if you have planned ahead and have a clear vision for the new day.

You are paid to do a specific job based on your specific skill set, within a specified time frame. In your job as a speech-language pathologist or audiologist, multitasking is necessary on a daily basis. Steve Pavlina (2007) has a blog with many helpful suggestions regarding productivity. He states that in order to multitask and maintain productivity, we must handle our jobs with flexibility and decreased distraction. Setting deadlines is crucial in order to prioritize tasks and remain highly productive for long periods of time.

Being productive in the workplace improves your performance as you become more self-sufficient in organizing your daily tasks. Productivity goes along with developing a good work ethic, and it goes hand in hand with time management and organization. By organizing your daily tasks, prioritizing your tasks, and keeping track of your progress, you can maintain a very productive schedule and meet employer productivity expectations, if required. Just as with organization and time management, we must utilize such strategies to assist us with being and remaining productive.

Heathfield (2011), a management and organization development consultant, suggests that you maintain a portfolio that demonstrates your productivity. The portfolio may document assignments, projects, and personal achievements. She also recommends that you keep copies of appraisals and/or evaluations, samples of your work, and written feedback from employers and colleagues, organized in chronological order. This effective strategy will demonstrate your productivity as you take on and complete new tasks and assignments. You should ask team members for letters of recommendation and add those to your growing portfolio for future career conversations.

The satisfaction derived from a "job well done" fuels us on to do more, be more, accomplish more. When you are productive, you gain more mastery of yourself and your work environment and are more likely to achieve both your professional and personal goals. By achieving these goals, you are more aligned with the goals of your coworkers and employer and therefore better able to obtain success personally and make a significant contribution to the workplace.

Teamwork

Teamwork is paramount in the professions of speech-language pathology and audiology. In a team environment, you find shared values, shared vision, inspiration, and energy. Team members must be able to empower, coach, and reward themselves as well as their colleagues. In successful work settings, you find shared credit for accomplishments, ideas, and contributions. In environments where individuals embrace the team concept, you find those capable of rewarding themselves rather than those who have the expectation that others will reward them. True team environments help all parties find their own personal rewards on the way to "greatness."

As you begin your career, you will be assigned a number of tasks commensurate with your job description. Some of those assigned tasks may not be ones you will find appealing. However, it is important to understand that most assignments serve as potential growth opportunities and will require that you engage in them willingly. Be the employee that asks for new assignments that will challenge you, both personally and professionally, and allow others to see the extent of your diversity as a team member.

When taking on a new assignment, particularly one that is more challenging, try to create a vision of how you will accomplish it, and share that vision with your fellow team members. Through this vision, and a sense of shared values, you and your team members can establish goals that will benefit all parties while you energize and inspire one another. In this kind of collegial environment, you assist each other with achieving those goals as you coach and reward one another.

As your confidence and skills continue to grow, request more challenging work, ask for assignments that require increased responsibility, and exhibit over time that you deserve them. Contribute to the workplace by offering your unique qualifications in order to enhance the work setting and contribute to the effectiveness of the team as a whole. To perform well, be certain you understand the project you are undertaking, as well as all deadlines associated with it. Meet deadlines without fail, and ask for assistance if you require it. It is imperative that you check and recheck your work before providing it to your supervisor, mentor, or fellow team member. Ask for constructive feedback from colleagues as you complete tasks together, and keep a positive attitude when that feedback is provided.

Heathfield (2011) discusses building relationships with your coworkers. Being friendly and supportive of coworkers contributes to your success and visibility. Show your creative talents, mediate conflicts, demonstrate your willingness to experiment, and take advantage of opportunities to participate in seminars, training events, and classes. As you learn new things, *share* them. Forget the "them versus me" attitude. Your ability to work well with other team members is the key to your success. The goals of your workplace become your goals, and you need to fully understand how your work complements the work of others, and vice versa.

In today's workplace, jobs are demanding, and much is required of you as a professional. Remember that success is attributable to a pattern of mutually beneficial interpersonal relationships, and this includes being part of a team. Being part of a true team environment allows you to celebrate shared victories while examining defeats in an environment rich with trust and respect for one another.

Politics in the Workplace

Before you step inside the building where you will begin your new job, you need to do some homework. Do some research and find out everything you can about your new employer, including the employer's philosophy or mission statement, goals and strategic plans, and corporate structure or staff roster. Make an attempt to meet someone who works there before you start, as it is nice to see a familiar, friendly face on your first day. Learning as much as possible before that first day will keep you from feeling overwhelmed and possibly unwelcome.

During the first few weeks, do your best to make a positive, lasting impression. When it comes to interacting with your coworkers, spend more time observing rather than offering opinions, and planning rather than acting. There will be plenty of opportunities for you to demonstrate your talents, skills, and personality attributes. Show how eager you are to learn and not how eager you are to instruct.

Keep in mind that you are the "new kid in town" and that relationships among your new coworkers were formed before your arrival. It will not go unrecognized that you have the power to destabilize some of those relationships before you have even found out where the restrooms are located. So tread carefully as you begin to form working and, certainly, personal relationships with your coworkers.

Rosenberg McKay (2010) shares four rules that will help you grasp the importance of understanding the politics within your new setting. First, she stresses the importance of listening and observing before suggesting any changes. You may have some great ideas and see a better way to do things, but until you are able to appreciate the dynamics of your surroundings, your suggestions may be met with negative reactions. Suppose a clinical fellow (CF) working in an elementary school observes what appears to be unused office space in a much more desirable location than the room to which she has been assigned. She approaches the principal in the hallway as he is speaking with a parent and mentions the "unused, wasted office space" that would be better utilized if she were permitted to relocate. As it turns out, the parent to whom the principal is speaking is the PTA president and the "unused, wasted office" is the PTA office. The CF has not only offended the PTA president but has made a negative impression on the principal.

Second, she suggests that you be aware of the "office troublemaker," adding that every office has one. This is the individual who will try to warn you about other employees and stirs up trouble only to later pretend to have nothing to do with it. Listen to what this person tells you but refrain from making a comment. For example, the AuD extern has just met a coworker who proceeds to warn him about the mean-spirited clinic director. He tells him that the clinic director, among other negative things, always assigns the most difficult patients to the newest person hired. Mr. Talkative adds that this is how the director is able to make an early determination as to the competence of any new employee. The extern now faces with dread the first patient encounter, assuming that it will be a very difficult case and that the director is prepared to give him a poor evaluation. Be aware that even though there may be some truth in what he says, it may be greatly exaggerated, or based upon only his personal experiences. In time, you will be able to form your own opinions based upon your own experiences, and you will not need Mr. Talkative to help you in this process.

The third rule is to mind your manners, as people may not remember your politeness but they are sure to remember rude behavior. The CF who heard a funny but off-color story on the radio while driving to work cannot resist the temptation to share it with his coworkers during the lunch break at the skilled nursing facility. What made it even funnier to the CF was that it had to do with an elderly individual, with striking similarity to one of the patients in the facility. When he told the joke, no one laughed and one individual even left the room to finish her lunch elsewhere. Such stories have no place in the workplace, especially if you are the new employee and do not know how your coworkers would react.

The last rule is to keep your ear to the grapevine but do not contribute to it. Although you can gain valuable insight into office dynamics by paying attention to what is being said, you may also damage your reputation by making statements that have no substance. Suppose a new employee heard the news that a coworker was leaving. This news came soon after she overheard a patient complaining loudly about the poor manner in which the coworker had fitted a hearing aid. The new employee concluded that this was the reason for the coworker's

departure and added to the story by saying that the coworker was probably fired. The coworker was in fact not fired but was moving to another city to take care of an ailing family member. Furthermore, the angry patient was known to be unreasonably difficult and had always expressed his displeasure with any audiologist who fitted his hearing aids. Contributing to the grapevine is never good practice, particularly when you are new.

Every work setting has its own culture, its own set of unwritten rules, and its own climate for developing professional and personal relationships. It is important to take time to understand and appreciate how these factors may influence and contribute to your own professional growth and development. Remember that it is a small world and your reputation can follow you for years. Your willingness to listen, observe, discourage unproductive interactions, avoid gossip, and show consideration for others will go far in helping you achieve success in the workplace.

Networking

The true measure of a man is how he treats someone who can do him absolutely no good.

—Samuel Johnson

You have probably heard people say, "It's not what you know, it's who you know." That may be especially true in today's culture of being connected to one another in so many ways. Your friends, acquaintances, and professional colleagues are a vast resource for you as you navigate the professional world. Having the knowledge and skills to perform your job well is your primary focus, but having the ability to demonstrate your knowledge and skills to your professional colleagues is also a very important part of building your career.

There are many benefits that come with professional networking, including sharing knowledge, finding new approaches to the way you do your job, and creating new opportunities that contribute to your professional growth and development. Networking allows you to meet with other speech-language pathologists and audiologists who might have had similar challenges in the past that you are facing today. By sharing knowledge, they are able to help you demonstrate possible solutions to these challenges while also learning to appreciate your individual talents and skills.

Many audiologists and speech-language pathologists have used networking to supplement their ability to do things well and to expand their careers in directions that go beyond the clinical setting. They have, in essence, developed networking into an art form and would offer the following tips:

1. When starting a new job, try to get to know as many people as possible, particularly the "key players." Do not isolate yourself and be sure to take advantage of non-work-related activities to be with your colleagues, such as lunch, after-hours activities, and so on.

2. Join your professional associations and become active by signing up for a committee, helping out at a conference or meeting, editing a publication, and so on.

3. Make yourself noticeable by volunteering for responsibilities at your worksite and in your professional organizations, particularly the ones that may be the most unpopular, and follow through with them.

4. Approach someone who appears to be "well connected" and ask how you can help them with their projects, and so forth, thereby having them serve as an informal mentor.

5. Establish specific networking goals, such as making important contacts, establishing and advancing professional relationships, and widening your professional contact base.

6. Do not exhibit blatant self-promotion by trying to be the star of the show. Make a genuine effort to include others in your activities, be a true team player by learning how to share responsibility and adopt a "share the wealth" philosophy. (These are also key elements in developing leadership skills.)

7. Show a genuine and sincere interest in those individuals within your network by focusing on building a relationship with them that relates to goals you share in common.

Your place of employment and your professional associations offer the best opportunities for you to develop your professional networking skills. Attending staff meetings and informal get-togethers, eating lunch in the employees' break room, and volunteering at professional conferences are just a few of the ways your knowledge, interests, skills, and talents will be recognized by your colleagues. There are also opportunities for networking within your university alumnae associations, religious groups, civic associations, political organizations, and special interest/hobby clubs, to name a few. These can serve as excellent opportunities for you to meet and establish relationships with individuals with whom you share common interests that extend beyond the worksite, while enabling you to practice your networking skills.

Social networking sites on the Internet such as Facebook, Instagram, and LinkedIn provide additional ways to network with fellow professionals. These sites are an effective way to stay in touch with people you already know and want to get to know better. ASHA and several other professional organizations have a strong presence on these networking sites, so take advantage of following them and interacting, as appropriate. Keep in mind that when you take advantage of these sites for the purpose of networking, your communication exchanges should only reveal information about you that is appropriate for all readers. Therefore, you must pay careful attention to confidentiality, your choice of topics, language style, and photos in order to project a professional image.

ASHA members may join one or more of the Special Interest Groups for specialized networking opportunities, also allowing access to educational programs, research, publications, and dialogue with members with similar interests. There are 18 Special Interest Groups that address the diverse areas of language learning, neurogenic disorders, voice disorders, fluency disorders, orofacial disorders, hearing research and diagnostics, aural rehabilitation, hearing conservation, hearing disorders in childhood, issues in higher education, administration and supervision, augmentative and alternative communication, swallowing and swallowing disorders, communication issues in culturally and linguistically diverse populations, gerontology, school-based issues, global issues, telepractice, and speech science (ASHA, 2019).

Networking plays a significant role in the growth and development of the new professional. Opportunities for establishing networking relationships exist both in and out of the workplace. Successful networking results in the establishment and maintenance of long-term relationships that are mutually beneficial. These relationships are built on confidence and trust, and require planning, time, effort, nurturing, diplomacy, integrity, and good judgment. Professional networking becomes an integral component of building a career that is both productive and meaningful over the course of time.

Performance Evaluations

Evaluations of employee performance are a component of any job. The purposes of performance evaluations are typically to provide a system of accountability, promote quality assurance, support professional growth and development, and promote performance improvement. They should also provide an opportunity for feedback and serve to rejuvenate and renew the employees' approach to their work. Most employers have an evaluation system in place for employees at all levels.

Some frequently used types of performance evaluations include top-down, peer-to-peer, performance development plans, and self-assessment performance reviews.

The top-down evaluation involves the assessment of the employee by the direct supervisor. The supervisor is typically someone who works closely enough with the employee to be familiar with the employee's specific strengths and weaknesses. This form of assessment often includes a rating scale or a narrative, or a combination of both. Most graduate student clinicians would have experienced being evaluated with an assessment tool of this type. An offshoot of this type of performance evaluation is referred to as a "matrix" evaluation. This is used when an employee works for multiple supervisors or managers, perhaps in several facilities, and is thereby evaluated by several of these individuals.

The peer-to-peer evaluation requires employees at the same level to review each other. The rationale for this type of evaluation is that no one is in a better position to observe performance than a coworker. There are some obvious problems with this type of evaluation, including level of experience and qualifications for assessing performance, personality issues, and the possibility of negative reviews getting back to fellow workers. This can be an effective format in certain situations—for example, a team of clinicians co-treating a patient where specific content knowledge is required.

The U.S. Office of Personnel Management (2017) describes a performance development plan using an eight-step process. It is designed to develop elements and standards that measure employee and work unit accomplishments rather than to develop other measures that are often used in appraising performance, such as measuring behaviors or competencies. The first five steps of this process focus on how supervisors and employees measure results to develop a performance development plan. The final three steps focus on developing standards, monitoring performance, and checking the performance plan in keeping with developed standards of performance.

Self-assessment performance reviews are effective when combined with other types of performance assessments, including the previous three presented. With this type of assessment, employees are asked to rate their performance, often using the same form that a supervisor uses to review them. Having employees complete the assessment performance prior to the supervisor's review can set a positive tone for the evaluation session. An example of this type of performance review is used for ASHA certification for speech-language pathologists during their clinical fellowship experience, as described in the following section. Because the mentoring relationship is a collaborative one, the CF and the CF mentor complete this rating scale together, and they discuss further action for improvement as part of the process.

Your employer will most likely have an established performance appraisal process in place upon your arrival. As part of your orientation to the job, it is important that you become acquainted with the manner in which your performance will be evaluated. The types of performance appraisals are varied and your employer may use one or any combination of appraisals, depending on your setting, responsibilities, pay grade or level, or even the culture of your individual working environment. Your participation in the performance appraisal process provides you with an opportunity to help you improve your skills and promote your own professional growth and development.

Continuing Education and Advanced Education

Once employed, you will be expected to keep abreast of advances and changes within your profession. Your employer will want you to have the latest assessment and intervention skills and use evidence-based practice. Maintenance of certification and licensure will also require documentation of continuing education (CE). Be sure to know these requirements for the credentials you hold. You do not want to jeopardize your credentials because you did not fulfill continuing education mandates or to feel pressured to find an appropriate program to meet your goals. Your employer may offer on-site educational opportunities or you may participate in local, state, or national conferences that provide live, on-site continuing education sessions. There are also a number of online CE programs available, many with minimal cost. It is important to keep a log of your completed continuing education activities and proof of completion and attendance. Your employer may contribute to the cost of required continuing education, and in all cases, you should keep receipts for reimbursement or tax purposes.

In addition to the continuing education requirements for maintenance of licensure and certification, you may want to consider developing your expertise in a specific area and seek formal recognition of your advanced skill and knowledge. The American Academy of Audiology (AAA), ASHA, and other professional organizations have created specific credentials that recognize specialized areas of practice. Such a credential is a demonstration of your advanced expertise and will likely set you apart from your colleagues in the eyes of both employers and consumers. See Chapter 3 for more information on certification related to specialty recognition.

If you are considering advancing your education by obtaining a PhD, there are a number of considerations to take into account. The structure of a PhD degree program focuses on preparation for careers in research, teaching, and other scholarly activities. Therefore, the majority of people in communication sciences and disorders (CSD) who have a PhD pursue a career within a college or university. If you expect to continue your career exclusively in clinical practice, pursuing a PhD may not be the best decision for you given the cost and the time commitment of typically five years.

CSD programs are currently experiencing a shortage of people with PhDs to assume faculty positions, so there are many employment opportunities should you decide to earn your PhD. In addition to opportunities within a college or university, individuals with PhDs may be employed as clinical researchers in hospitals and clinics. PhD audiologists may be employed in industry—for example, by hearing aid companies, for product research and development (ASHA, 2019). There is more information about obtaining the PhD on the ASHA website.

Promotion and Advancement

Once employed, you may find that opportunities are possible for advancement within the current program, within the larger organization, or even within other settings. Individuals become aware of available positions through professional publications, networking, or direct solicitation to apply for a position. Advancement can take the form of moving upward to positions of more direct program responsibility such as supervisory roles, or it can take place laterally with the individual remaining in a similar position but assuming new responsibilities or a new type of caseload. For example, in some programs, individuals may become team leaders or have special duties such as coordinator of quality improvement or continuing education. Increasingly, programs have "career ladders" intended to promote staff development and leadership and provide opportunities for new challenges, without employees having to be "promoted" to a supervisory position. Advancement both vertically and laterally can be challenging and contribute to a more fulfilling career.

Before advancement, some basic questions arise. What duties does the new position entail? What are prerequisite technical and personal skills and credentials for fulfilling the position? Will the new responsibilities be challenging or constitute a professional or personal burden? Will the prestige or financial reward be adequate to compensate for new responsibilities? For example, if promotion entails increased travel, is this possible within

your current lifestyle? What personal accommodations, such as the need for child care, would be required? A major difference in seeking an advanced position within a present organization is that the interview will be with familiar individuals. Careful preparation is no less important for a longtime employee. In some cases, a current employee may be competing with individuals from both within and outside the organization whose credentials and experiences are equal or superior to your own.

If you decide to apply for advancement within your present organization, you need to be prepared psychologically for a rejection. Some individuals may perceive this as an overwhelming personal rebuff by colleagues, and it may affect their ability to work productively in that setting. This is an important concept to consider as you apply for promotions within your setting. Having a positive support network is vital to helping you cope if such a rejection occurs. While rejection does not usually mean that your current position is in jeopardy, this may be a good time to reevaluate your goals and have a frank discussion with trusted colleagues about your options at this time. See Chapter 11 for further discussion on this topic.

Changing Employment

An employee may change employment settings for any number of reasons. These reasons include job loss, relocation, unreasonable demands in the current position, lack of opportunities for professional growth, infrequent raises, boredom or burnout, lack of employer appreciation, or readiness to assume new or increased responsibilities associated with a different position. Regulatory policies pertaining to reimbursement for long-term care and outpatient rehabilitation services have significantly affected employment in medical settings. Thus, some professionals may make a job change by choice, whereas others will find this an unwelcome event in their lives.

The new job search may begin while you are currently employed, or the process may begin after resignation or termination from a position. Securing a new position while currently employed presents some challenges. If you are currently employed, you may not want your employer to know that you have begun a job search. If the job search becomes public, how will this knowledge affect your current position? How available can you be for interviews? If you feel that you do not want your current employer to know about a potential move, you will need to change options for references. You also must be prepared to take time off from work to attend interviews, either on the phone or in person.

In the case of relocation or a mutually agreeable job change, your current employer will be the best possible reference in securing new employment. In the situation in which a position has ended before beginning a job search, you again have to evaluate the helpfulness of a former employer. Targeted employers will want to know the circumstances of why you left the last position and generally will want some reference from that employer. It is important to consider that a current employer is the most important reference for the future; therefore, conditions under which the applicant leaves should be positive—"a graceful exit" (Kroner, 1989). When an employee leaves, employers are sometimes asked to indicate on the termination documentation if they "would" or "would not" rehire this individual. That is a question often asked by future employers when calling for references on a terminated employee. An ungraceful exit, such as leaving without reasonable notice for your employer to find a replacement, or leaving without completing required paperwork, is not likely to get a "would rehire" response.

Before you resign from a current position, be sure to have the new offer in writing. Check your current employer's policies and procedures manual for contractual information on what time period constitutes sufficient notice of termination. Your present employer must then receive notification of your intended departure. Include in this letter your exit date, the title of your new position and employer, and the last date of work. It is also dignified to inform your boss before telling coworkers and meet with this person in a formal exit interview. Exit interviews should be positively focused on making an orderly and courteous transition between you and your replacement (Kennedy, 1998). Before leaving a current position, all work should be summarized for a successor, and all required paperwork must be updated, completed, and filed. Some employers will require you to help train a replacement, so an overlap time may be necessary. How a departure is handled can positively or negatively affect the tone of future references from the employer.

Many speech-language pathologists and audiologists have felt the impact of changes in Medicare and other insurance reimbursement in medical settings. Some have lost their jobs while others have had positions changed or hours reduced. Although this is likely to be a time of anger, despair, and frustration, it is also an important time to know what your options are financially and vocationally. Be sure to consider psychological support during this time of unwelcome transition. Some human resources departments will have such support available to assist you.

Financial Considerations

If you are faced with an impending loss of a job, as a result of changing employment or otherwise, it is critical to plan for the time when you may be without a regular income. To be prepared:

1. know your financial assets and monthly expenses and make a realistic financial plan,

2. reduce all unnecessary expenses,

3. build a three- to six-month cash reserve,

4. reduce debt,

5. know the rules regarding any 401(k) or retirement plans to which you have contributed,

6. discuss mortgage and insurance coverage with qualified professionals,

7. investigate your agency's severance package options and negotiate the best one,

8. plan for health insurance while unemployed (e.g., COBRA option), and

9. claim your unemployment benefits.

The Interval Between Jobs

It may take you more time than you had anticipated finding new employment. This is an important time to review your skills and update them as this demonstrates a commitment to learning and self-improvement. For applicants who have been unemployed for an extended time, the prospective employer will want to know if and how you have kept your clinical skills up to date. Applicants need to provide clear, concise, and honest answers to these questions. All attempts should be made to redirect the interviewer to the applicant's interest in and qualifications for the present position. It is prudent to maintain your professional certification, licensure, and continuing education requirements during any extended periods from active work. You should also use this opportunity to maintain contact with other professionals. This is an excellent example of the value of professional networking that you have hopefully established prior to this time.

Changing jobs is never an easy prospect, whether or not by choice. Careful planning must be a part of any job change. The conscientious professional will ensure a smooth transition for the successor, leaving the former job site in "turnkey" condition. Financial considerations are also part of this planning and should always play an important role in your career choices. Particularly if the job change is related to stress or burnout, you may want to consider psychological support and/or career counseling during this time of transition. Networking relationships should continue to be developed and maintained both during the transition period and upon entering the new employment setting. Finally, once you have entered the new setting, treat it as you would any new job, remembering that first impressions do count and that your reputation, although it may precede you and will certainly follow you, is always a work in progress. See Chapter 11 for further discussion of this topic.

Summary

Your decision to enter the profession of audiology or speech-language pathology requires more than the acquisition of clinical knowledge and skills. Many important issues affect your ability to build your career in a positive direction, leading to job fulfillment and professional success. You must understand the nature of the collaborative relationship you have with your mentor/preceptor and develop effective communication skills as part of that and all relationships in your work setting. In addition to having a solid appreciation for a good work ethic, you will need to adhere to a professional code of ethical conduct established by your professional association. Effective time management and good organizational skills will help you prioritize and keep you motivated as you perform your day-to-day tasks while increasing productivity. Being an effective member of a team, understanding the political culture of your workplace, and maintaining a supportive professional network will also help you as your career develops. Performance evaluations are a required component of any job, and you should play an active role in the assessment process as you make advances in your career path. The Clinical Fellowship and the audiology externship serve as launch pads for the beginning professional, and it is important to be familiar with the requirements leading to certification. Finally, when changing employment, either by choice or not, you need to consider many factors as you continue to build your career with confidence, competence, and success.

Critical Thinking

1. What are some of the dynamic differences you should anticipate as you move from working with a clinical supervisor in a university setting to a mentor in your professional workplace? What role do interpersonal communication skills play in this relationship?

2. Your preceptor has made a comment in front of your patient that you perceived as calling into question your competence. You are embarrassed and would like to have a difficult conversation with your preceptor to address the situation. What is the predetermined plan that you and your preceptor have decided upon for such a dialogue? What factors should you keep in mind during the conversation to make it a productive one for both of you?

3. You are preparing to discharge a client from services at a private clinic where you work. The clinic director has asked you to keep the client on your caseload in order to ensure revenue for the practice. What steps should you take to address the situation? Why is ethical behavior important as you build your career?

4. You have been too busy to keep up with the amount of paperwork that seems to be piling up on your desk. How can you tackle this problem immediately, and what strategies can you employ to avoid this situation in the future?

5. Your colleague has told you that he stays in his office during lunch and avoids non-mandatory staff functions because he has "too much work to do." His clinical knowledge and organizational skills appear to be excellent, so he is frustrated that many of his coworkers do not include him when discussing caseload management issues. He is also disappointed that his director recently overlooked him for a promotion for which he thought he was well suited. He has asked you for advice, so what would you tell him?

6. Your employer has informed you that due to budget cuts, your position has been eliminated and you will need to find employment elsewhere. Develop a "game plan" that will ensure some financial stability while you seek new employment. What role will your professional networking play during this time period? What factors should you consider during your search for a new position?

7. What is meant by having a "work ethic"? Why is it important to develop a realistic work ethic as you begin your first professional position? How is work ethic related to time management?

8. You need to take a leave from your job for family reasons. How would you go about this? What should you do to prepare your replacement until you return to your position?

9. As a professional, you will be evaluated each year by a supervisor. What performance criteria will go

into this evaluation? Should performance criteria for a first-year professional be the same as those for a seasoned professional? Suppose you do not agree with the evaluation your supervisor has given you. What would you do?

10. You are the director of a large clinical program that has few opportunities for your staff to get promoted. What could you do to encourage and reinforce innovation, dedication, and service among your staff without promoting them?

References

American Board of Audiology. (2011). *Board certification in audiology.* Retrieved from http://www.boardofaudiology.org/board-certified-in-audiology/

American Speech-Language-Hearing Association. (2018). *ASHA membership and certification handbook.* Rockville, MD: Author.

American Speech-Language-Hearing Association. (2008a). *Clinical supervision in speech-language pathology* [Technical report]. Available from http://www.asha.org/policy

American Speech-Language-Hearing Association. (2008b). *Knowledge and skills needed by speech-language pathologists providing clinical supervision.* Available from http://www.asha.org/policy

American Speech-Language-Hearing Association. (2010). *Code of ethics.* Available from http://www.asha.org/policy

American Speech-Language-Hearing Association. (2019). *Special interest groups.* Rockville, MD: Author. Retrieved from https://www.asha.org/SIG/About-Special-Interest-Groups/

Brooks, D. (2004). *Stressed for success.* Retrieved from https://www.nytimes.com/2004/03/30/opinion/stressed-for-success.html

Dodd, P., & Sundheim, D. (2005). *The 25 best time management tools and techniques: How to get more done without driving yourself crazy.* Orlando, FL: Peak Performance Press.

Hale, S. (2006). *Ethics: It's more than common sense.* Retrieved from http://www.asha.org/uploadedfiles/practice/ethics/NSSLHAEthicspresentation.pdf

Heathfield, S. (2011). *Human resources and career planning.* Retrieved from http://humanresources.about.com/cs/perfmeasurement/a/pdp.htm

Kennedy, J. L. (1998, September 12). When it's time to resign, do it with savvy. *Buffalo News,* A14.

Kroner, K. (1989). Take the gamble out of changing jobs. *Nursing, 20,* 111–118.

Pavlina, S. (2007). *Personal development for smart people.* Retrieved from http://www.stevepavlina.com/

Raudsepp, E. (1990). Knowing when to look for a new job. *Nursing, 20,* 136–140.

Rosenberg McKay, D. (2010). *Your first job. Making a good impression.* Retrieved from http://careerplanning.about.com/cs/firstjob/a/first_job.htm

Schwartz, I., Horner, J., Jackson, R., Johnstone, P., & Mulligan, M. (2007). *Eligibility requirements and essential functions.* Minneapolis, MN: Council of Academic Programs in Communication Sciences and Disorders.

Silber, L. (2004). *Organizing from the right side of the brain: A creative approach to getting organized.* New York, NY: St. Martin's Press.

U.S. Office of Personnel Management. (2017). *A handbook for measuring employee performance.* Retrieved from https://www.opm.gov/policy-data-oversight/performance-management/measuring/employee_performance_handbook.pdf

Resources

American Speech-Language-Hearing Association. (2019). *Building your professional brand.* Retrieved from https://careers.asha.org/on-the-job/

American Speech-Language-Hearing Association. (2019). *Frequently asked questions about pursuing a PhD.* Retrieved from https://www.asha.org/Students/faq-pursuing-phd/

Covey, S. (1989). *The 7 habits of highly effective people.* New York, NY: Simon & Schuster.

Covey, S. (1995). *The 7 habits of highly successful people* [DVD series]. Retrieved from http://www.enterprisemedia.com/product/00038/habits_highly_successful_people.html

Hudson, M. W. (2010). Supervision to mentoring: Practical considerations. *Perspectives on Administration and Supervision, 20,* 71–75.

Silber, L. (1998). *Time management for the creative person.* New York, NY: Three Rivers Press.

Internet Sources

Note: The following sources are fluid and should be checked periodically for their availability and current internet addresses.

American Speech-Language-Hearing Association. Building Your Professional Brand https://careers.asha.org/on-the-job/

Personal Development for Smart People (Steve Pavlina) http://www.stevepavlina.com/

Thedigeratilife.com http://www.thedigeratilife.com/blog/ index .php/2008/12/05/got-laid-off-lose-your-job/

whatithinkabout.com http://www.whatithinkabout.com/8-starting-a-new-job-tips/

Wikihow.com http://www.wikihow.com/Network

13

Support Personnel in Audiology and Speech-Language Pathology

Diane Paul, PhD, Tricia Ashby, AuD,
Lemmietta G. McNeilly, PhD, and Steven D. Ritch, CRMT

Introduction

Many individuals help to support the work of audiologists and speech-language pathologists (SLPs) including families, administrators, teachers and instructional aides, psychologists, social, workers, other professional staff, interns, and volunteers. This chapter focuses specifically on those individuals who are hired in a professional capacity and have some degree of training and supervision to extend audiology and speech-language pathology services. They perform services that are prescribed, directed, and supervised by licensed and/or certified audiologists or SLPs. The chapter also will include information about credentialing of audiology and speech-language pathology assistants (SLPAs) at the national level.

Support personnel in audiology and speech-language pathology have been employed in a variety of work settings since the 1960s. They are support staff that are used to extend and expand clinical services and do not substitute or replace qualified audiologists or SLPs. Several terms are used to designate individuals who provide support services in audiology and speech-language pathology (e.g., *aides, assistants, extenders, paraprofessionals, technicians*). The American Speech-Language-Hearing Association (ASHA) uses the term "assistant" (ASHA, 2016b). The employment of support personnel has been a topic of debate, particularly in the field of speech-language pathology, with passionate views on both sides. Those favoring the use of support personnel, or more specifically audiology assistants and SLPAs, believe that access to care is improved, frequency and efficiency of service are increased, and the skills of clinicians are better used. From this perspective, the judicious use of assistants facilitates practice at the top of the license for clinicians. Those opposing the use of assistants in clinical practice argue that the quality of care may be compromised, and the services of professionals devalued. Proponents say use of assistants is in the best interest of consumers; opponents say consumers may be misled (Breakey, 1993; Werven, 1993). Consumers may mistakenly think that assistants have the education and training to provide all services. Or they may not realize they are working with an assistant who has a more limited scope of practice.

The dynamics of the service delivery system, in tandem with cost controls and personnel needs, have led to the development of new and changing state and national policies related to the training, supervision, credentialing, and responsibilities of assistants in the professions of audiology and speech-language pathology (American Academy of Audiology [AAA], 2010a; n.d.; ASHA, 1992, 1998, 2004g, 2013, n.d.-a, b, e).

In many health care and education settings across the country, audiologists and SLPs are experiencing escalating caseloads and increasing paperwork in conjunction with shrinking budgets and personnel shortages (particularly for school-based SLPs) (ASHA, 2018c). In response, some facilities and institutions have chosen to employ assistants to support their clinical staff.

The purpose of this chapter is to provide information about the training, responsibilities, supervision, and effectiveness of support personnel in audiology and speech-language pathology. Specifically, the chapter includes information on the rationale, challenges, professional policies, state regulations, current use, training recommendations, national credentialing, supervision requirements, job responsibilities, reimbursement, research, and future directions related to support personnel in audiology and speech-language pathology. A glossary of key terms used in this chapter is provided in Appendix 13–A.

Rationale for Use of Support Personnel

Service delivery for individuals with communication disorders continues to evolve. When audiologists and SLPs practice at the "top of the license," an essential option includes using extenders to participate in the service delivery process. Assistants who are educated to participate in the service delivery process are supervised by audiologists and SLPs who are competent to design intervention plans that include extension of their services with the engagement of assistants. The audiologists and SLPs are qualified and competent to assess the communication functioning of individuals; they also design intervention plans, monitor the individual's progress, and make decisions regarding entry and exit from treatment. Assistants can provide guided practice of targeted behaviors, document progress of functional goals, and select therapeutic resources. The intervention plan for a patient/student/client is the responsibility of the audiologist or SLP. Practicing at the top of the license means that the audiologist and the SLP are engaging in those activities that require their level of expertise and skills. Appropriately delegating activities to assistants, monitoring the progress on functional goals, and intervening

periodically are options for practicing at the top of the license (McNeilly, 2018).

The growing and diverse needs of individuals with communication and related disorders are increasing the demand for audiology and speech-language pathology services (Bureau of Labor Statistics, 2018a, b). This increasing demand for these services is one of the converging factors leading to the use of assistants by audiologists and SLPs. Other influences include federal legislation sustaining the education rights of students with disabilities, the Individuals with Disabilities Education Improvement Act of 2004 (IDEA, 2004), including the right of students to be assessed in their native language, and increasing caseloads due to (1) recognition of the value and need for early intervention services (ASHA, n.d.-b.; Guralnick, 2011, 2019; Joint Committee on Infant Hearing, 2007); (2) aging of the population with concomitant health needs (Administration on Aging, 2017; National Academies of Sciences, Engineering, and Medicine, 2016); (3) need to care for individuals with hearing loss resulting from occupational noise (AAA, 2003; ASHA, 2004a); and (4) expanding scopes of practice in audiology and speech-language pathology (AAA, 1997, 2004; ASHA, 2001, 2004d, 2004e, 2016b, 2018d). Thus, because of the growing need for services, combined with the rising health care and education costs and personnel shortages, some audiologists and SLPs have identified roles for assistants in the delivery of service for children and adults with communication disorders. First, we will consider the rationale for three of the roles, participating in telepractice (ASHA. n.d.-i, j), serving as interpreters/translators in bilingual/bicultural environments, and working on collaborative teams in classrooms. Following the discussion of these roles, we will address policy, practice, training, and research issues related to the use of support personnel in audiology and speech-language pathology.

Role of Telepractice

Telepractice is an appropriate model of service delivery for both audiologists and SLPs (ASHA, n.d.-b, e, i, j). In audiology, tele-audiology clinical technicians (TCTs) are appropriately trained and competent to provide support for patients and equipment while being supervised by ASHA-certified audiologists (ASHA, n.d.-f, g). Currently, TCTs are only used in the Veterans Administration health care system. SLPs engaging in telepractice can train and use support personnel appropriately to deliver services. Assistants can work with clients/patients/students in their homes, classrooms, or other settings while the SLP supervises either synchronously or asynchronously. State licensure laws must be adhered to for practice within states or across state lines (ASHA, n.d.-g, i, j).

Roles of Assistants: Interpreters/Translators

The need to use bilingual/bicultural assistants in audiology and speech-language pathology has increased as the United States population continues to diversify with respect to language and culture (U.S. Bureau of the Census, 2010). Because only 7.0% of ASHA members, certificate holders, international affiliates, and associates are non-white, 4.6% are Hispanics or Latino (ASHA, 2017a), and less than 6% are bilingual (ASHA, 2018b), it often is not possible to match a clinician to a client's cultural and linguistic background (ASHA, 2004c). Consequently, the assistance of professional interpreters and cultural brokers is often necessary to provide culturally and linguistically appropriate services (ASHA, 2004e, 2016b; Lynch & Hanson, 2004). ASHA has a profile of individuals who have self-identified that they are bilingual service providers (ASHA, 2018b).

Executive Order 13166 that reinforces Title VI of the Civil Rights Act (U.S. Department of Justice, 2000) reminds facilities that receive any type of federal funds, including Medicaid/Medicare, that they must develop a plan to provide equal access to services for people with limited English proficiency. IDEA 2004 also requires that assessment be conducted in a child's native language. Assistants who share the same language and/or culture with a client may be asked to fill these roles to help meet the needs of a multilingual population (ASHA, 1985a; Langdon & Cheng, 2002; ASHA, n.d.-a, e, f). However, the role of an interpreter and assistant is decidedly different. Therefore, ongoing training, planning, and communication are needed. As discussed in the section on "Challenges Using Support Personnel," adequate training for each role is critical when one person plays multiple roles. In the 2012 ASHA Schools survey SLPs were asked how they provided services to English language learners—2.0% of respondents indicated they use bilingual SLPAs (ASHA, 2012). In the 2009 ASHA Membership survey, 12% of respondents indicated that they employ support personnel to provide services to users of other languages (ASHA, 2009a, b, 2010). In the ASHA 2015 Work Life Survey, 13.2% of SLPs across all settings reported support personnel acting as interpreters (ASHA, 2016d).

Roles of Assistants: Classroom Teams

IDEA 2004 recognizes the use of paraprofessionals and assistants as adjuncts to the team of service providers in the schools. In accordance with state law, paraprofessionals and assistants who are appropriately trained and supervised may be used to assist in the provision of special education and related services for children with dis-

abilities. In addition, the state must adopt a policy that requires local educational agencies to take measures to recruit, hire, train, and retain highly qualified personnel, including paraprofessionals, to provide special education and related services to children with disabilities. Special education paraprofessionals who provide instructional support in Title I programs (Improving the Academic Achievement of the Disadvantaged) also must meet the requirements of the Elementary and Secondary Education Act.

The use of alternative service delivery models for SLPs in the schools also has prompted the use of SLPAs. Although the prevailing speech language pathology service delivery model in the schools has been and continues to be a "pull-out" model (ASHA, 1995a, 2010), it may not be the most ideal model for fostering natural, contextually-based communication interactions. In recent years, the recognition of the need for more functional outcomes has led to an extension of service into the classroom (Cirrin et al., 2010; Paul-Brown & Caperton, 2001). The use of SLPAs who work directly in the classroom has been a means to integrate speech and language goals into the curriculum, generalize learned concepts, enhance carryover of functional skills, and reinforce SLP goals in the student's natural setting (Gerlach, 2000; Goldberg & Paul-Brown, 1999; Pickett, 1999; Pickett & Gerlach, 1997).

The appropriate use of trained, supervised, and less costly assistants may be one way to meet the growing service needs of persons with communication disorders and still maintain the role of the fully qualified audiologist and SLP (Paul-Brown & Goldberg, 2001). The use of assistants in various roles (e.g., interpreters/translators, classroom collaborators) may provide a means to supplement services for a diverse population, extend services in natural settings, free clinicians to dedicate more time to those individuals with more complex conditions, and fulfill increasing managerial responsibilities (ASHA, n.d.-a, b, f).

Challenges Using Support Personnel

Some audiologists and SLPs have expressed concerns about the impact of using assistants on service delivery. Some believe that assistants (1) may be hired in lieu of qualified providers, (2) may be used to increase caseload size, (3) may be asked to provide services for which they are not trained, or (4) may receive inadequate supervision. Audiologists are concerned about otolaryngologists hiring support personnel, specifically otologic technicians (OTO techs), instead of hiring or referring to audiologists.

In many school settings, demand for educational audiologists and SLPs outweighs supply. Indeed, 25% of audiologists and 54.3% of SLPs responding to ASHA's 2018 Schools survey (ASHA, 2018c) indicated that job openings were more numerous than job seekers in their facility. According to the ASHA Schools survey (ASHA 2018c), 16.2% of audiology respondents and 23.1% of SLP respondents reported that personnel shortages were among the greatest challenges of a school-based clinician. Employers may be tempted to hire assistants to fill a persistent vacancy. There is a concern about quality of services when the motivation for using support personnel is to respond to a personnel shortage rather than to extend and enhance service (Paul-Brown & Goldberg, 2001). As ASHA recognized more than 30 years ago, "limited professional resources do not constitute a justification for applying lower standards in either the employment or utilization of supportive personnel" (ASHA, 1988, p. 56).

Another area of concern is when a bilingual assistant is asked to work with clients without adequate supervision or support. Although using a bilingual assistant may be beneficial, there is the potential for misuse or overuse if the assistant has not been trained appropriately or is asked to go beyond an assistant's job responsibilities (e.g., inappropriately expected to conduct evaluations and create treatment plans for bilingual clients). Furthermore, the ability to speak a second language does not automatically qualify someone to be a translator or interpreter, nor does it mean that the individual has the skills necessary to serve as an audiology assistant or SLPA (ASHA, 1985a, 2004c, 2013, n.d.-b, e, f; Langdon & Cheng, 2002).

Clearly, inappropriate use of assistants could have far-reaching and negative effects on the professions (ASHA, n.d.-a, e, f). One way to ensure that the quality of care is not compromised is for audiologists and SLPs to adhere to state and national laws and follow professional ethics statements and guidelines, so that assistants receive appropriate training and supervision and only provide services within a limited scope of practice. Even in the absence of mandatory state requirements, audiologists and SLPs are responsible for adhering to professional guidelines that delineate appropriate use and supervision of assistants.

Another way to promote the appropriate use of assistants is through education and awareness initiatives, such as providing information to administrators, principals, school boards, hospital boards, otolaryngologists, and others responsible for personnel or hiring decisions about the role of supervised assistants and their job responsibilities in comparison to the scope of practice of the supervising audiologists and SLPs.

In 2009, ASHA established an affiliation category for support personnel in audiology and speech-language pathology to give ASHA and its members a stronger, more credible voice in explaining the proper use of assistants with defined boundaries for how they are used. ASHA supports the use of assistants to ensure both the accessibility and the highest quality of care while addressing productivity and cost-benefit concerns. The professional continuum concept, affirmed by ASHA's Board of Directors (BOD), includes SLPAs and master's level SLPs within the service delivery process. SLPAs can play a critical role in the service delivery process (McNeilly, 2009). Starting in 2011, ASHA began to offer associate status to assistants who work under the supervision of an ASHA-certified audiologist or SLP. Applicants are required to adhere to ASHA's guidance for audiology assistants or SLPAs, perform only tasks that are appropriate for assistants, adhere to state laws and state licensure requirements for assistants, and pay the requisite annual fees (McNeilly, 2010).

Benefits for associate status for assistants through ASHA are networking opportunities (e.g., joining special interest groups), continuing education programs, ASHA online and print resources, and participation on ad hoc committees. They are not able to vote or hold elected office within ASHA.

Recently, ASHA has taken another step toward setting a national standard for the use of assistants in audiology and speech-language pathology, a credentialing program for assistants. In November 2017, ASHA's Board of Directors approved funding and implementation of an Assistants Certification program for audiology assistants and SLPAs. Currently, ASHA is developing and validating standards and a national examination. ASHA anticipates starting the credentialing program and examination by the end of 2020.

Evolving Professional Policies and Practices

State licensure boards and professional organizations have responded to the concerns about misuse of support personnel by providing regulations, policies, and reports with specific guidance. ASHA (1998, 2004b, 2013, 2016b, 2018d, n.d.-a, b, e), AAA (1997, 2006, 2010a), the Council for Exceptional Children (Consortium of Organizations on the Preparation and Use of Speech-Language Paraprofessionals in Early Intervention and Education Settings, 1997), and the National Joint Committee on Learning Disabilities (1998) are among the professional organizations representing audiologists and/or SLPs that have developed documents to provide guidance for the appropriate use and supervision of support personnel in those education and health care settings in which they are employed. All of the professional policies rely on the clinical judgment and ethics of qualified professionals. This includes decisions regard-ing the delegation of tasks and the amount and type of supervision to provide. Table 13–1 presents a chronology of the policies that professional organizations have developed over the last 50 years to guide the practice and performance of support personnel in audiology and speech-language pathology.

Table 13–1. Policy Timeline for Support Personnel in Audiology and Speech-Language Pathology

Time Frame	Policies by Professional Organizations
1960s	**1967**—ASHA's Executive Board established the Committee on Supportive Personnel. **1969**—ASHA developed the document *Guidelines on the Role, Training, and Supervision of the Communicative Aide.*
1970s	**1973**—Council for Accreditation in Occupational Hearing Conservation started training and certifying hearing conservationists. **1979**—ASHA referenced *supportive personnel* in the Code of Ethics and issued an Issues in Ethics statement highlighting the professional and ethical responsibilities of the supervising professionals and emphasizing the dependent role of the *communication aide.*
1980s	**1981**—ASHA revised its guidelines for supportive personnel. **1988**—ASHA developed a technical report about the use of support personnel in speech-language pathology with underserved populations.
1990s	**1990**—ASHA revised the Code of Ethics and included a proscription about service delegation. **1992**—ASHA developed a technical report on issues and the impact of support personnel in audiology and speech-language pathology and the **1992** and **1994** revised Code of Ethics dealt with the delegation of support services. **1994**—ASHA approved a position statement supporting the establishment and credentialing of categories of support personnel in speech-language pathology. **1995**—ASHA approved guidelines for the training, credentialing, use, and supervision of SLPAs. **1996**—ASHA convened a consensus panel to develop a strategic plan for approving speech-language pathology assistant programs and credentialing SLPAs. The plan was used as a framework to develop a training approval process and credentialing process for SLPAs. **1997**—Consortium of Organizations on the Preparation and Use of Speech-Language Paraprofessionals in Early Intervention and Education Settings developed guidelines for three levels of paraprofessionals in education settings: aides, assistants, and associates. The assistant category paralleled the ASHA SLPA guidelines. Consortium organizations included ASHA; Council for Exceptional Children/Division for Children's Communication Development and Division for Early Childhood; Council of Administrators of Special Education; and Council of Language, Speech, and Hearing Consultants in State Education Agencies. **1997/1998**—AAA and ASHA published separate position statements and guidelines for support personnel in audiology. **1998**—National Joint Committee on Learning Disabilities developed a report on the use of paraprofessionals with students with learning disabilities.

continues

Time Frame	Policies by Professional Organizations
	Table 13–1. *continued*
2000 to 2009	**2000**—Council on Academic Accreditation in Audiology and Speech-Language Pathology (CAA) developed criteria and procedures for approving technical training programs for SLPAs, the Council on Professional Standards in Speech-Language Pathology and Audiology developed criteria for registering SLPAs, and the Council for Clinical Certification in Audiology and Speech-Language Pathology (CFCC) developed the implementation program.
	2001—ASHA revised its Code of Ethics, added terms (e.g., assistants, technicians) to the term support personnel, and mandated informing persons served about the credentials of providers.
	2002—ASHA developed knowledge and skills statements for supervisors of SLPAs.
	2002—ASHA developed an approval process for SLPA training programs.
	2003—ASHA established a registration process for SLPAs.
	2003—ASHA voted to discontinue the approval process for SLPA training programs and the registration program for SLPAs as of December 31, 2003, due primarily to financial concerns.
	2003—ASHA revised its Code of Ethics and elaborated on delegation and supervision of support personnel.
	2004—ASHA issued a new Issues in Ethics Statement on support personnel.
	2004—ASHA revised its position statement for support personnel in speech-language pathology and its guidelines for SLPAs to remove references to SLPA credentialing.
	2006—AAA published a new position statement to define the function of the audiologist's assistant.
2010 to 2019	**2010**—ASHA revised its Code of Ethics and continued to set forth rules concerning accurate representation of credentials, delegation of tasks, and supervision for assistants, technicians, and support personnel.
	2010—AAA updated its position statement about the use of an audiology assistant. The rationale was provided in a 2010 task force report.
	2011—ASHA revised its guidelines for support personnel in audiology and speech-language pathology.
	2011—ASHA established an Associates Program for audiology assistants and SLPAs. The Associates Program provides an affiliation category entitling approved applicants' access to ASHA benefits and discounts (such as professional liability insurance) without full ASHA membership (Associates may not vote or hold office but may be appointed to committees). The program is open to individuals who: <ul><li>are currently employed in support positions providing audiology or speech-language pathology assistant services, and</li><li>work under the supervision of an ASHA-certified audiologist (CCC-A) or speech language pathologist (CCC-SLP).</li></ul>
	2012—ASHA added provisions related to audiology assistants and SLPAs to its model bill for the state licensure of audiologists and SLPs. The model bill, updated in 2014, provides a prototype for state regulation of audiologists, SLPs, and audiology assistants and SLPAs. It is designed as an example to be modified to reflect individual state's needs.
	2013—ASHA developed the *Speech-Language Pathology Assistant Scope of Practice* to address the way SLPAs should be used and the specific responsibilities that fall within and outside their clinical practice roles.
	2013—ASHA Practice Portal pages include "audiology assistants" and "speech-language pathology assistants."

Time Frame	Policies by Professional Organizations
2010 to 2019 *continued*	**2014**—ASHA issued an Issues in Ethics statement on Audiology Assistants. **2014**—ASHA updated its *Model Bill for State Licensure of Audiologists, Speech-Language Pathologists, and Audiology and Speech-Language Pathology Assistants.* **2015**—ASHA Board of Directors (BOD) voted to make the Associates Program an ongoing program of ASHA. Also, the BOD thought that there should be some standardization of requirements for audiology assistants and SLPAs and thus it approved a feasibility study regarding the potential of credentialing assistants. **2017**—The Board of Ethics revised the Issues in Ethics: Audiology Assistants and Issues in Ethics: Speech-Language Pathology Assistants to be consistent with the 2016 ASHA Code of Ethics. **2017**—The ASHA BOD voted 14–0 in favor of approving funding and implementation of an Assistants Certification Program. **2018**—ASHA published the Audiology Assistant Exam Blueprints and the Speech-Language Pathology Exam Blueprints to help identify core competencies for assistants. **2019**—The CFCC determined eligibility pathways for assistants in audiology and speech-language pathology.

Table 13–1. *continued*

Chronology of Ethical and Professional Practice Policies Related to the Use of Support Personnel by Audiologists and Speech-Language Pathologists

Ethical Responsibilities

ASHA's Code of Ethics and Issues in Ethics statements have provided a general framework for the supervision of support personnel in the professions of audiology and speech-language pathology. The first reference in the ASHA Code of Ethics was in the 1979 Code, specifically, Principle of Ethics II, Ethical Proscription 4, which stated: "Individuals must not offer clinical services by supportive personnel for whom they do not provide appropriate supervision and assume full responsibility." The first ASHA Issues in Ethics statements to address support personnel highlighted the professional and ethical responsibilities of the supervising clinicians and emphasized the dependent role of the "communication aide" (ASHA, 1979). The 1990 ASHA Code used the same language and had the first reference to "delegation" with its proscription not to delegate "any service." The 1992 ASHA Code and its revision in 1994 both dealt with the delegation of "support services." The 2001 ASHA Code added terms (e.g., *assistants, technicians*) to

the term *support personnel* and mandated that members had an affirmative requirement to "not misrepresent the credentials of assistants, technicians, or support personnel and shall inform those they serve professionally of the name and professional credentials of persons providing services."

The 2003 revision of the ASHA Code maintained this requirement pertaining to representation of credentials and added requirements pertaining to delegation of tasks and supervision. The 2010 revision of the ASHA Code continued to set forth rules concerning accurate representation of credentials, delegation of tasks, and supervision. The 2016 revision of the ASHA Code continues to address representation of credentials, delegation of tasks, and supervision of assistants (ASHA, 2016a). ASHA Issues in Ethics statements discuss a variety of training options and tasks and indicate that support personnel should be supervised by ASHA-certified audiologists and/or SLPs (ASHA, 2017b, 2017c). The statements identify principles and rules in the Code that are applicable to supervision in clinical practice and use of assistants.

Consistent with its prior Code of Ethics (AAA, 2009), AAA's Code (AAA, 2018) puts forth a rule pertaining to delegation and supervision of support personnel by its audiology members. Specifically, Rule 2d states: "Individuals shall provide appropriate supervision and assume full responsibility for services delegated to supportive personnel. Individuals shall not delegate any service requiring professional competence to unqualified persons" (AAA, 2018).

Chronology of Professional Practice Policies

In addition to the policies related to ethical use of support personnel, professional organizations developed documents to guide professional practice. In 1970, ASHA published its first professional practice guidelines on the use of support personnel in audiology and speech-language pathology. These guidelines, revised in 1981, delineated training needs, scope of responsibilities, and amount of supervision for support personnel in audiology and speech-language pathology (ASHA, 1970, 1981). The following two sections address professional practice policies specific to either audiology or speech-language pathology support personnel.

Support Personnel in Audiology. Multiple professional organizations are involved in the use of audiology support personnel. In 1997, a Consensus Panel on Support Personnel in Audiology was convened with members of the Academy of Dispensing Audiologists, AAA, Educational Audiology Association, Military Audiology Association, and National Hearing Conservation Association and developed a position statement and guidelines (AAA, 1997). ASHA developed its own audiology support personnel position statement and guidelines (ASHA, 1998) that differed only in its requirement for supervisors to hold the ASHA Certificate of Clinical Competence in Audiology.

Currently, ASHA outlines specific guidelines for the use of support personnel assisting audiologist as follows (ASHA, n.d.-b):

- The roles and tasks of audiology assistants are assigned *only* by supervising audiologists.

- Supervising audiologists provide appropriate training that is competency based and specific to job performance.

- Supervision is comprehensive, periodic, and documented.

- The supervising audiologist maintains the legal and ethical responsibilities for all assigned audiology activities provided by support personnel.

- Services delegated to the assistant are those that are permitted by state law, and the assistant is appropriately registered/licensed if the state so requires.

- The needs of the consumer of audiology services and protection of that consumer are always

paramount (AAA, 2010a, 2010b; ASHA, 2010; National Hearing Conservation Association, 2018).

The AAA also developed a position statement to guide audiologists on the education and job responsibilities of "audiologist's assistants" in 2006 and updated it in 2010 (AAA, 2006, 2010a). The updated position statement was based on the rationale articulated in an Audiology Assistant Task Force Report (AAA, 2010b). The AAA statement indicates that audiology assistants may be assigned duties at the discretion of an audiologist, provided that the assistant has a minimum of a high school diploma and competency-based training (AAA, 2010a). AAA also addresses use of support personnel for newborn hearing screening (AAA, n.d.).

Support personnel in audiology are trained and used in a variety of employment settings, such as industry, schools, private clinics, and Veterans Administration hospitals and other military hospitals and medical centers. In industrial and military settings, assistants may help with the prevention of hearing loss resulting from noise. Occupational hearing conservationists have been trained and certified by the Council for Accreditation in Occupational Hearing Conservation (CAOHC) since 1973. They may be audiometric technicians, occupational health nurses, engineers, and others who do audiometric testing and help to fit hearing protection devices for employees (Suter, 2002). The CAOHC is an interdisciplinary group that currently includes representatives from nine organizations. Its mission is to provide education about noise in the workplace and to prevent noise-induced hearing loss in industry. A certificate program for otolaryngology personnel (CPOP) has been promoted by the American Academy of Otolaryngology-Head and Neck Surgery (AAO-HNS) and the American Neurotology Society to train otolaryngology office personnel to become OTO techs and conduct hearing testing. The program includes a self-study reading component, a 2½-day workshop, and six months of supervision by an otolaryngologist. The list of tasks these groups delegate to an OTO tech closely matches the scope of practice of audiologists. Such overlap of responsibilities is a concern to professional audiology organizations such as AAA and ASHA about the blurring of professional and technical level boundaries, particularly when otolaryngologists hire OTO techs rather than audiologists and bill for the services. Those endorsing the use of OTO techs suggest that their use can free up time for audiologists to perform more complex hearing and balance services.

Some audiologists have argued that the move to the doctoral level for the profession of audiology may lead to increased use of audiology support personnel to have a less costly option for the more technical aspects of the profession (Thornton, 1993). One of the reasons that audiologists decided not to require a higher education degree or credential for support personnel is to have the educational level and scope of responsibilities as distinct as possible between technical-level and professional-level personnel. Rather than have prescriptive policies related to education and tasks, audiologists prefer to determine independently what support personnel should do and how they should be trained.

Support Personnel in Speech-Language Pathology.
In a 1995 position statement, ASHA endorsed the use of support personnel in speech-language pathology for the first time, rather than only providing guidance for their use (ASHA, 1995b). In 1996, the earlier ASHA guidelines from 1981 were revised to address one category of support personnel, *speech-language pathology assistants,* defined as "support personnel who perform tasks as prescribed, directed, and supervised by certified SLPs, after a program of academic and/or on-the-job training" (ASHA, 1996, p. 22). SLP assistants were differentiated from SLP aides, who usually have a narrower training base and more limited responsibilities relative to the duties of assistants. Like the first two ASHA guideline documents, the 1996 guidelines specified a scope of responsibilities and outlined the type and amount of supervision required. Some of these decisions were influenced, in part, by the less restrictive policies developed by other professions with a longer history using support personnel, such as occupational therapy and physical therapy (ASHA, 1992). The ASHA guidelines were more prescriptive than those of the other professions to avoid the risk of assistants working outside of their limited scope of responsibilities or being hired in the place of SLPs (ASHA, 1996).

The ASHA guidelines also called for training at the associate degree level rather than just on-the-job training and recommended a credentialing program for assistants and for assistant-level training programs. ASHA's plan to credential SLPAs and approve training programs started with the 1995 position statement supporting the establishment and credentialing of categories of SLP support personnel (ASHA, 1995b). In 2000, criteria for approving technical training programs and for registering SLPAs were developed by the Council on Academic Accreditation in Audiology and Speech-Language Pathology (CAA) (ASHA, 2000a) and the Council on Professional Standards in Speech-Language Pathology, respectively (ASHA, 2000b). Recommendations for assistant-level tasks, knowledge required, and where this knowledge could and should be obtained were based in part on a job analysis of SLPAs conducted by the Educational Testing Service (Rosenfeld & Leung, 1999). ASHA established implementation dates of January 2002 for the approval process for training programs and January 2003 for the SLP assistant registry process. The CAA was responsible for implementation of the technical training approval

process and the Council for Clinical Certification in Audiology and Speech-Language Pathology (CFCC) was responsible for implementation of the assistant registration program. ASHA's commitment to these programs was linked to the receipt of sufficient fees to cover administrative costs paid by training programs and individuals seeking registration. When those revenues fell well short of what was required, the decision was made to discontinue the approval process for SLPA training programs and the registration program for SLPAs as of December 31, 2003. In 2004, the ASHA position statement for SLP support personnel and guidelines for SLPAs were revised to remove references to SLP assistant credentialing. Relevant portions of the criteria for SLPA technical training programs and assistant registration that related to training, use, and supervision were folded into the 2004 SLPA guidelines (ASHA, 2004b, 2004g).

The guidelines documents were superseded in 2013 by the ASHA *Speech-Language Pathology Assistant Scope of Practice* and provide guidance for SLPAs and their supervisors (ASHA, 2013). Recognizing that standards, licensure, and practice issues vary from state to state, the document delineates specific responsibilities that ASHA considers to be within and outside an SLPA scope of clinical practice.

With respect to the training of SLPAs, several academic training programs for support personnel have evolved (and continue to develop) over the years. ASHA has a self-reported list of Technical Training Programs for Speech-Language Pathology Assistants (ASHA, n.d.-e). Additionally, the opportunities for training and life-long learning for SLPAs do not end with the various degree programs available. Indeed, there are several learning opportunities, such as in-service seminars, that are presented in the various work settings. Similarly, as supervisors learn new techniques and practices in the profession evolve, they can convey ideas and information on how their assistants can best work with them to ensure the highest quality outcomes for their clients/patients/students.

ASHA has developed other documents and products over the years to assist professionals who choose to employ support personnel in various settings. These include a report on using support personnel with underserved populations (ASHA, 1988), knowledge and skills for supervising SLPAs (ASHA, 2002a), and practical tools and forms for supervising SLPAs (ASHA, 2009c) and for using and supervising SLPAs working in school settings (ASHA, 2000c).

State Regulations

Support personnel in audiology and speech-language pathology may or may not be regulated by state laws and regulations (ASHA, n.d.-a, e). Supervising audiologists and SLPs are responsible for determining the applicable requirements in their state and work setting. Laws and regulations for support personnel in audiology and speech-language pathology in educational and other practice settings vary from state to state. Differences may be reflected in a number of requirements, including the following: education, supervision, continuing education, titles used for support personnel, and regulation or laws or lack thereof. State licensure boards and/or departments of education provide the most current information about the requirements for specific practice settings.

As of September 2019, 31 states regulate (license, register, or certify) audiology and speech-language pathology support personnel in school settings and 41 states regulate (license, register, or certify) support personnel outside of school settings. Of the states that regulate the use of support personnel, a wide range of educational requirements is found. A few states have different requirements for different levels of support personnel, ranging from a high school diploma or equivalent to a bachelor's degree in communication sciences and disorders (CSD) with enrollment in a master's degree program. Continuing education for support personnel is required in 20 states for those in school settings and in 26 states for those regulating outside of school settings. A variety of titles is used to designate support personnel in the professions, with *assistant and aide* being the most common. State agencies (licensure boards) currently regulating support personnel also have a variety of differing supervision requirements (see ASHA's website for state specific information).

Supervisory Requirements

To ensure that support personnel do not exceed the boundaries of their education and experience, most of the states that regulate support personnel have imposed one or more supervision requirements. Some states limit the number of support personnel that one licensed SLP or audiologist may supervise. Some states specifically prescribe the amount of direct and indirect supervision that a supervisor must provide to the support personnel. Some states specifically define what activities may or may not be performed by support personnel, and others simply provide a general statement that support personnel are the responsibility of the licensed audiologist or SLP and should be appropriately supervised given their individual education and experience.

In addition to state regulatory agencies, state education agencies may credential support personnel to work solely in schools to support service delivery provided by qualified professionals. Some school districts hire assistants under the classification of teacher assistants. If a state regulates support personnel (i.e., under the term of *assistant, aide, paraprofessional,* or *apprentice*), then individuals

who wish to become employed in that state must meet the state requirements for practice under a licensed professional. ASHA also requires that audiologists and SLPs hold the Certificate of Clinical Competence to supervise support personnel (ASHA, n.d.-a, d). Information about the regulation of support personnel in schools in all states and contacts for state licensure boards or departments of education is available at the ASHA website.

State regulations may differ from ASHA's standards and policies (e.g., in terms of number of hours of direct supervision required per week). In those states where there is a conflict, members and certificate holders must abide by state requirements including applicable laws, regulations, and policies (ASHA, n.d.-e). As a general rule, it is best to adhere to the strictest requirements to be in compliance with the Code of Ethics, national certification standards, and state licensure.

Employment Trends of Support Personnel

Survey data were reviewed to determine the use of audiology support personnel in audiology and speech-language pathology in educational and health care settings. Having more time to work with clients/patients/students with more complex needs (71% of audiologists and 36% of SLPs) and having fewer clerical duties (64% of audiologists and 33% of SLPs) were two of the primary effects reported from the use of support personnel (ASHA, 2009b). Other effects reported for using support personnel were to increase frequency or intensity of service and respond to personnel shortages. The main reasons reported for not using support personnel were that they were not budgeted or not needed. Also, approximately one-quarter of audiologists and SLPs indicated that larger caseloads or workloads were an effect of using support personnel. Changes in the employment rates of support personnel over time were explored for each profession and are discussed below.

Employment of Support Personnel in Audiology

Survey data have been collected to determine the average number of support personnel that audiologists supervise, the tasks that they perform, and the percentage of audiologists who use support personnel. ASHA survey data from 2009, 2016, and 20018 show that audiologists who use assistants or aides supervise an average of one or two (ASHA, 2009b; 2016c; 2018c), with the use highest in hospital settings (mean of 2.3).

The activities in which audiology assistants are most commonly used are in performing administrative tasks, followed by information sharing with patients, families, and/or staff. Other activities include preparing for an audiology session/appointment; hearing prevention activities; therapy services; and serving as an interpreter (ASHA, 2018c). Karzon, Hunter, and Steuerwald (2018) analyzed data from questionnaires to audiologists who employ assistants. Their data suggested the use of assistants to assist with conditioned play audiometry, visual reinforcement audiometry, infection control, mail management, disposing of protected health information, ordering supplies, calling families, fielding family phone calls, stocking supplies, troubleshooting equipment, and doing auditory brainstem response (ABR) screening.

In terms of the numbers of audiologists who employ support personnel, a 2001 survey of audiologists showed that 45% hired assistants or previously hired assistants in their practices (Hamill & Freeman, 2001). A 2004 survey of AAA members showed that approximately 28.4% of audiologists employed assistants (AAA, 2006). A 2005 report from the United States Department of Veterans Affairs by Robert Dunlop revealed a 619% increase in the number of audiology support personnel in Veterans Administration hospitals from 1996 to 2004 with a decrease in the ratio of audiologists to support personnel from 24:1 in 1996 to 5.26:1 in 2004 (as cited in AAA, 2006). ASHA's 2009 Membership survey showed that 43% of audiologists reported that one or more support personnel were employed at their facility (ASHA, 2009b).

Employment of Support Personnel in Speech-Language Pathology

Forty-one percent of school-based SLPs and 32% of health care–based SLPs reported that there was one or more SLP support personnel employed at their facility (ASHA, 2009b). In the 2015 Work Life Survey, of those using one or more support personnel, the median number reported was 1.2 for school-based SLPs and 1.1 for SLPs based in health care settings (ASHA, 2016d). Consistent data were found in 2016 and 2018 for SLPs in schools: Of the SLPs who supervised assistants or aides, the median number that they supervised was 1 (ASHA, 2016c; 2018c). The average number of SLPAs in the schools and health care settings appears to have remained stable over time.

SLPs indicated that support personnel assist primarily in the following five ways: (1) providing therapy services (77%); (2) making preparations for a session (61%); (3) sharing information with patients, their families, or staff (40%); (4) performing administrative tasks (38%); (5) engaging in prevention activities (23%); and (6) acting as interpreter (13.2%) (ASHA, 2016d).

Consistent with 2016 Schools Survey data, most of the SLPs who supervised assistants or aides and who responded to the 2018 ASHA Schools Survey reported an impact on their workload or caseload: 46% said that they increased workload and 27% said that they increased caseload; 30% said that they decreased workload and 36% reported that they decreased caseload (ASHA, 2016c, 2018c).

Training for Support Personnel

Support personnel should not be permitted to work with individuals unless the supervising audiologists or SLP is confident that the support person has obtained a reasonable amount of training and possesses appropriate skills (ASHA, n.d.-a, e).

Training Support Personnel in Audiology

Support personnel in audiology are expected to have at least a high school diploma or equivalent and competency-based skills needed to perform assigned tasks (AAA, 2010a; ASHA, n.d.-b, c). The CFCC will launch a new credential for Audiology Assistants in 2020. Candidates that are eligible to take the audiology assistants exam must complete one of three pathway options that best fit their education and experiences. The need for three pathway options stems from the high variability in training for audiology support personnel. ASHA will require all applicants to complete the following (ASHA, n.d.-b):

- 1-hour of ethics course
- 1-hour course in universal safety precautions
- 2-hour patient confidentiality training course (HIPPA, FERPA, etc.)

One example of a training program for audiology support personnel is the program of study for audiologist's assistants at Nova Southeastern University. This distance learning program offers self-paced training modules in the areas of diagnostic testing and amplification. Students go to a website for course materials, tests, and tutorials.

There is a training program offered by CAOHC for occupational hearing conservationists that involves successful completion of a practical and written exam after a 20-hour course on a variety of topics such as social and legal ramifications of noise on people and pure-tone audiometric procedures. CAOHC also offers an 8-hour recertification course; recertification is required every five years. CAOHC also certifies course directors, the majority of whom are audiologists (ASHA, 2004a).

Training Support Personnel in Speech-Language Pathology

Training requirements for support personnel in speech-language pathology vary across the country. ASHA's 2004 guidelines were developed to promote greater uniformity in training requirements across the country (ASHA, 2004b). The 2004 ASHA guidelines recommended completion of an associate degree from a technical training program with a program of study specifically designed to prepare the student to be an SLPA. The guidelines suggested that SLPAs complete course work, field work, and on-the-job training.

The ASHA Speech-Language Pathology Assistant Scope of Practice (ASHA, 2013) extended the training paths to include an associate degree in an SLPA program or a bachelor's degree in a speech-language pathology or CSD program.

The CFCC developed three eligibility pathways for SLPAs. Applicants must complete the following mandatory requirements as well as one of three education options to be eligible to take the SLPA certification exam.

- A 1-hour course in ethics
- A 1-hour course in universal safety precautions
- A 2-hour patient confidentiality training course (HIPAA, FERPA, etc.)
- Clinical field work: A minimum of 100 hours, to include
  - □ 80 hours of direct patient/client/student services under the supervision of an ASHA-certified SLP)
  - □ 20 hours of indirect patient/client/student services under the supervision of an ASHA-certified SLP

Education Option 1

Completion of a minimum 2-year SLPA program degree from an accredited institution (e.g., associate degree from a community college, technical training program, certificate program, or bachelor's degree).

Education Option 2

- Bachelor's degree in CSD from an accredited institution
- Complete ASHA's Online SLPA Training Modules or equivalent

Education Option 3

- College degree (associate or bachelor's) from an accredited institution

- Pass coursework from an accredited college institution in the areas below:
  - □ Introductory or overview course in communication disorders
  - □ Phonetics
  - □ Speech sound disorders
  - □ Language development
  - □ Language disorders
  - □ Anatomy and physiology of speech and hearing mechanisms

- Complete ASHA's Online SLPA Training Modules or equivalent

As of September 2019, ASHA is aware of 28 operational associate degree programs for SLPAs in 16 states (ASHA, n.d.-e). Some of these programs have training opportunities through distance learning and collaborations between community colleges and universities. The course work and field work experiences required in the SLPA training programs typically differ from those at the bachelor's, preprofessional, or master's professional levels. It is a challenge for SLPA training programs in community colleges to locate textbooks that are written specifically for SLPAs. Often the programs must use more advanced textbooks that are written for SLP students and omit the sections that do not apply, such as those related to assessment and diagnosis and detailed theoretical discussions.

Assistant-level training programs are not specifically intended to be the start of a career ladder to professional level positions; however, some programs lend themselves to such opportunities. Assistant training programs also may be another avenue for students, including bilingual and bicultural students, to seek their bachelor's and master's degrees in CSD. Universities do not always accept course work from the SLPA training program to transfer to the bachelor's degree programs. Knowledge and skills needed to be an SLPA are distinctly different from those needed to be an ASHA-certified SLP. Academic programs/institutions have the discretion to determine which academic course work completed in technical training programs will be accepted for transfer to a bachelor's degree program. Students interested in pursuing a career as an SLP are encouraged to verify the transferability of credits between assistant training programs and bachelor's programs. Students also are encouraged to investigate the requirements of graduate educational programs to ensure that basic science courses taken at the undergraduate level will be acceptable to the graduate program (ASHA, n.d.-e, f).

Credentialing Assistants

ASHA's proposed national credentialing programs recognize that there are a variety of ways of transmitting knowledge and acquiring the knowledge, skills, and abilities for assistants. The credentials will recognize multiple training paths to becoming an audiology assistant or an SLPA. Rather than expecting all assistants to have the same training or degree, the credentialing process instead will expect applicants to pass a national exam to assess the acquisition of competencies related to practice as an assistant in audiology or speech-language pathology.

In November 2018, the CFCC approved exam blueprints for audiology assistants and SLPAs (ASHA, 2018a, f). The blueprints outline the duties and tasks and assigns weighted percentages for the content. The certification exam for audiology assistants will test an applicant's knowledge, skills, and abilities on tasks related to providing patient care, performing hearing device maintenance, and maintaining the audiology clinic. Tasks for SLPAs pertain to providing services, providing administrative support, and participating in prevention and advocacy activities.

ASHA describes a variety of benefits for certifying assistants: aid assistants in maintaining current knowledge; enhance confidence that they have met nationally recognized standards; demonstrate professional commitment; and help potential employers, clients, and other professionals. Additionally, it is expected that credentialing will improve access to care by creating an opportunity for a cost-effective and reliable means of identifying qualified professionals who can provide the skills expected of a trained assistant (ASHA, n.d.-a). National credentialing standards also may help states determine licensure standards without the costly burden of each state conducting independent job analyses and exams.

Supervision of Support Personnel

Audiologists and SLPs may delegate services to support personnel only with appropriate supervision (ASHA, 2016b, 2018d). It is essential that the supervising professional has the knowledge and skills needed to provide such supervision (ASHA, n.d.-a, b, d). Supervisors who do not speak the same language as the assistant are still responsible for his or her supervision. Ideally an interpreter would be provided.

Management and supervision skills are not synonymous with the skills needed to be a highly qualified audiologist or SLP. Many professionals have not received specific supervisory training during their preservice education programs. To become a competent supervisor and manager, professionals may consider taking continuing education courses that target these areas. The amount and type of supervision provided should be based on the skills and experience of the support person, the needs of clients/patients/students served, the service delivery setting, the tasks assigned, and other factors such as initiation of a new program, orientation of new staff, and change in client/patient/student status (ASHA, n.d.-a, d, e). The goal for the supervising professional is to ensure that support personnel restrict their clinical activities to prescribed tasks in contrast with the goal of independent clinical practice for supervision of students and clinical fellows (ASHA, 1985b; Paul-Brown & Goldberg, 2001).

The supervising audiologist or SLP is responsible for the actions of support personnel. Specifically, the supervisor would be held responsible and could be subject to sanctions if an assistant performed activities beyond the scope of his or her job responsibilities. Thus, any alleged violation of the Code(s) of Ethics governing the supervising professionals should be reported to the AAA Ethical Practices Board or the ASHA Board of Ethics for adjudication. ASHA members and certificate holders have a responsibility to ensure that support personnel under their supervision behave in an ethical manner (ASHA, 2017b, c). Thus, although ASHA currently does not have jurisdiction over support personnel, ASHA members and certificate holders are vicariously liable for the unethical conduct of support personnel they supervise and can sanction them if they are found in violation.

State laws pertaining to supervision vary and may differ from professional policies. This means that audiologists and SLPs need to check specific state regulations to determine minimum amounts of supervision required and qualifications for supervisors of assistants in a particular state. Audiologists, SLPs, and support personnel are legally bound to follow licensure laws and rules that regulate them and their practice in the state in which they work. Use of support personnel is not permitted in every state.

Concerns are ever present about the potential for inappropriate actions by support personnel and the lack of consequences when there are no state regulations to govern the use of support personnel in audiology or speech-language pathology. Currently, no professional organization has direct oversight of the actions of support personnel in audiology or speech-language pathology. This is of particular concern when an audiology assistant or SLPA is working under the supervision of a professional who is not required to be ASHA-certified and/or is employed in a state where there is no law that addresses the use of support personnel in audiology or speech-language pathology.

Supervision of Support Personnel in Audiology

Neither ASHA nor AAA has prescribed supervisory requirements for training support personnel in audiology; nor are there professional policies that set a specific amount of supervision after training or that specify a maximum number of support personnel to be employed. The supervising audiologist has the sole responsibility for these decisions (AAA, 2010a; ASHA, n.d.-b).

Regarding supervision of occupational hearing conservation personnel, the Hearing Conservation Amendment (HCA), administered by the United States Department of Labor's Occupational Safety and Health Administration (OSHA), specifies who may perform certain audiological procedures and indicates where the responsibility resides (U.S. Department of Labor, n.d.).

With regard to supervision of OTO techs, an otolaryngologist is responsible for providing supervision during the 6-month portion of the training period. Thereafter, the OTO tech works loosely under the supervision of the physician. However, this is like a physician providing supervision to anyone in the physician's office who provides patient care as governed by the state's medical practices act. Presumably, a credentialed audiologist also may supervise the OTO tech consistent with the Code(s) of Ethics governing the audiologist and provided the physician accepts this role for the audiologist (AAO-HNS, 2006).

Supervision of Support Personnel in Speech-Language Pathology

ASHA provides specific guidance related to the amount and type of supervision for support personnel in speech-language pathology. For an SLPA in training, ASHA recommends no less than 50% direct supervision (ASHA, 2013). The minimum amount of supervision suggested for a trained assistant is 30% weekly (at least 20% direct) for the first 90 workdays and 20% (at least 10% direct) after the initial work period. Direct supervision means "onsite, in-view observation and guidance by the SLP when a clinical activity is performed by the assistant" and includes supervision via telecommunication technology because the SLP can provide ongoing immediate feedback. Indirect supervision "may include demonstration tapes, record review, review and evaluation of audio- or videotaped sessions, and/or supervisory conferences that may be conducted by telephone and/or live, secure webcam" (ASHA, 2013, n.d.-e, f). The ASHA SLPA

scope of practice recommends that an SLP supervise no more than two SLPAs at the same time (ASHA, 2013).

The supervising SLP has responsibility for establishing a means of documenting the supervision of the SLPA. Even when faced with time and workload pressures, the SLP is expected to adhere to these supervision guidelines. Although state and national guidelines are available to guide decisions about the amount of direct and indirect supervision, it remains the supervising SLP's responsibility to determine the type and exact amount (beyond the minimum) of supervision that each SLPA requires. For example, some SLPAs may require more guidance and oversight to complete the required documentation. Another SLPA may need mentoring to ensure adherence to the rules and regulations of the facility. The SLP makes these decisions based on the SLPA's individual strengths and technical proficiency.

Job Responsibilities of Support Personnel in Audiology

The supervising audiologist is responsible for planning and delegating tasks that a support person may perform (ASHA, n.d.-b). Examples of tasks that have been delegated over the past 20 years to support personnel by supervising audiologists include daily visual and listening checks on hearing aids and auditory trainers for children in public schools (Johnson, 1999); assisting with hearing screenings, hearing aid monitoring, and use of assistive listening devices in rehabilitation hospitals (Johnson, Clark-Lewis, & Griffin, 1998); learning ways to optimize communication during interactions with persons with hearing loss (Johnson et al., 1998); and assisting with hearing conservation programs at work sites (ASHA, 2004a; Suter, 2002).

Currently, the ASHA Practice Portal on Audiology Assistants delineates services an audiology assistant may perform—if permitted by state law and after the assistant has demonstrated competence (ASHA, n.d.-b). ASHA also provides ethical guidance for those performing tasks as an audiology assistant and for those supervising the assistants (ASHA, 2017b).

The audiologist has exclusive responsibility for a variety of clinical activities. Audiology support personnel may not interpret data; determine case selection; transmit clinical information, either verbally or in writing, to anyone without the approval of the supervising audiologist; compose clinical reports; make referrals; sign any formal documents (e.g., treatment plans, reimbursement forms, reports); discharge a patient/client from services; or communicate with the patient/client, family, or others regarding any aspect of the patient/client status or service without the specific consent of the supervising audiologist (ASHA, n.d.-b).

Job Responsibilities of Support Personnel in Speech-Language Pathology

Because the assistant must be supervised by a licensed and certified SLP, it seems reasonable that the SLP should make decisions about the specific tasks and activities assigned to the SLPA (ASHA, 2013). The SLP should advise the administrator of a facility or school principal that it is the supervising SLP's responsibility to select the clients/patients/students, assign responsibilities, and determine the amount and type of supervision needed. Viewed collectively across states, support personnel have a broad scope of responsibilities ranging from clerical duties to clinical activities. ASHA has delineated a restricted set of tasks in the areas of service delivery, administrative support, and prevention and advocacy, which an SLP may delegate to an SLPA, and those responsibilities that only an SLP can provide (ASHA, 2013).

It is the responsibility of the supervising SLP to make certain that SLPAs engage only in those activities that are within their scope of practice. The SLP assigns clients/patients/students to an SLPA based on the student's needs and the SLPA's level of experience. The SLPA may be assigned to work with clients/patients/students on previously learned, less clinically challenging, or more rote or repetitive skills. For example, the SLP may assign an SLPA to work on increasing generalization after the SLP has worked with a student to establish a specific sound. Support personnel also may work as members of a team in health care and education settings (Longhurst, 1997). In schools, IDEA has institutionalized the practice of using teams to determine the most appropriate course of action for each student and to collaborate and develop the Individualized Family Service Plan (IFSP) or the Individualized Education Program (IEP).

Reimbursement of Services Provided by Support Personnel

Medicare policy currently does not recognize support personnel in audiology or speech-language pathology regardless of the level of supervision. An otolaryngologist, however, can bill for work performed by OTO techs.

Private insurers may cover licensed or registered SLPAs. One must query each payer to verify coverage.

Private insurers may or may not provide a different rate of reimbursement for services provided by an audiologist or SLP compared with an audiology assistant or SLPA. Most private insurers do not cover services that do not require the skills (directly or indirectly) of an audiologist or SLP.

Each state has considerable latitude in administering its Medicaid program. The federal regulation indicates that services may be rendered "by or under the direction of" a qualified SLP, but a state may still prescribe the qualifications of the subordinate practitioners. A state would be more likely to assign a Medicaid provider number to SLPAs if they were registered or licensed in the state.

The federal regulations for Medicaid specifically recognize services provided by audiology support personnel if such services are provided under the direction of a qualified audiologist. According to regulations, the supervising audiologist must have face-to-face contact with the client in the beginning and periodically throughout the treatment. An audiologist must provide adequate supervision of support staff as well as keep documentation of the supervision and ongoing involvement in the case. If an audiologist is employed by a Medicaid agency, clinic, or school, the federal regulations require that the audiologist's employment terms allow for adequate supervision of support personnel. Although specific supervision ratios are not stated, regulations do require that these ratios be "reasonable and ethical and in keeping with professional practice acts" (Preamble to Federal Regulations).

The key point with respect to reimbursement of support personnel in audiology or speech-language pathology is that for Medicaid and private insurers, each payer makes its own decisions about what is covered and who is the qualified provider. For Medicaid, this will vary by state, and with the infusion of Medicaid Managed Care Plans, may even vary within a state, defined by the specific plan.

Research Related to Support Personnel

To determine the effectiveness of using support personnel to extend the clinical work of audiologists and SLPs, a systematic literature search of published English language studies was conducted searching electronic databases (the search methodology is available upon request of the first author). The studies, which spanned several decades, needed to be relevant to two clinical questions and contain original data or purport to be systematic reviews of the literature. A summary of the studies is provided below.

Have Any Studies Compared Support Personnel in Audiology or Speech-Language Pathology with Professionals?

No studies were identified that compared support personnel in audiology with clinical service provision. Some studies compared treatment outcomes by support personnel and SLPs, primarily with elementary schoolchildren with articulation disorders and adults with aphasia.

Studies with Children. A large scale, blinded, randomized controlled trial was designed to compare language outcomes following direct versus indirect and individual versus group treatment for 161 children (6–11 years) with primary language impairment (Boyle, McCartney, Forbes, & O'Hare, 2007; McCartney, O'Hare, & Forbes, 2009). The study also had a control group of children that received "usual levels of community-based speech and language therapy." The authors provided an intervention manual with suggested procedures and activities, which focused primarily on comprehension monitoring, vocabulary, grammar, and narratives (McCartney et al., 2004). Speech-language therapists conducted the direct interventions and speech-language therapy assistants conducted the indirect interventions with individuals or small groups of children attending inclusive schools in Scotland, UK. The study found no significant differences in language outcomes between direct and indirect treatment or between individual and group treatment based on post-intervention testing. All groups showed short-term improvements in expressive language outcomes. Receptive language skills proved to be more intractable and did not show improvements regardless of the intervention group (Boyle, McCartney, O'Hare, & Law, 2010). The authors suggested that the assistants acted effectively with these children because of the lack of differences in language outcomes across groups. Language outcomes did not improve for a cohort intervention group when "school staff" rather than SLPs or speech and language assistants conducted indirect, consultative language treatment (McCartney, Boyle, Ellis, Bannatyne, & Turnbull, 2011). A cost analysis of the different modes of treatment revealed that indirect assistant-led group therapy was the least costly option and therapist-led individual therapy was the costliest (Dickson et al., 2009).

Additional studies involving children, most conducted in the mid-1970s, found no significant differences in the articulation outcomes of children with mild-to-moderate speech disorders when comparing treatment by *trained paraprofessionals* (also called *supportive personnel* or *speech therapy aides*) and professional clinicians; children in both groups showed improvements in articulation (Alvord, 1977; Costello & Schoen, 1978; Gray & Barker, 1977). Sounds that were not targeted for treatment showed no change for children in either the aide or clinician group (Gray & Barker, 1977).

One study reported no significant differences between groups of children with learning disabilities with "perceptual deficits" treated by trained "perceptual-aides" and "therapists" (including occupational, physical, recreational, and language); improvements were noted in motor skills, visual, and somatosensory perception, language, and educations skills in children from both treatment groups (Gersten et al., 1975). One study reported that four out of five young children made more progress on computer-based language tasks when a parent volunteer provided the training compared with an SLP (Schery & O'Connor, 1997). Small sample size and lack of statistical comparison make these results difficult to interpret.

A mother–child home program administered by paraprofessionals was compared with interventions by professionals that were tailored to the cognitive and language needs of 2-year-old children. Children in both groups showed similar improvements; however, the children were still delayed in cognitive and language functioning at age 4 in both groups (Scarr, McCartney, Miller, Hauenstein, & Ricciuti, 1996).

Studies with Adults. Studies comparing volunteers and professionals providing clinical services for adults focused primarily on volunteers working with individuals with aphasia. Patients showed improvement in communication, and no differences were found in the amount of progress made for adults who received services from professionals compared with those receiving services from untrained volunteers (David, Enderby, & Bainton, 1982; Meikle et al., 1979). In a study with trained volunteers, men with aphasia showed improvement in their communication during treatment but not when treatment was discontinued. These results were similar to patients with aphasia who received treatment from SLPs (Marshall et al., 1989). In a study that compared three different treatment approaches and a no-treatment condition, two of the treatments for patients with aphasia were administered by professionals, and one was administered by "trained nonprofessionals" (Shewan & Kertesz, 1984). The two approaches administered by professionals showed significant differences compared with the nontreatment condition; the treatment method used by nonprofessionals approached significance. It is not possible to determine whether the difference in significance level was due to the treatment approaches themselves or to differences between nonprofessionals and professionals. In another study with patients with aphasia, comparisons were made among clinic treatment by an SLP, home treatment by a trained volunteer, and deferred treatment. No significant differences were found among the three groups after the deferred-treatment group received treatment by a professional (Wertz et al., 1986).

Studies Comparing Service by Professionals and Support Personnel.
Ideally, supervising professionals should only assign tasks to support personnel that can be performed with the same level of quality as professionals. The studies available reveal no differences in treatment outcomes for children or adults when the services provided by support personnel in speech-language pathology are compared with those provided by professionals. The consistency between outcomes for professionals and support personnel is encouraging for those who employ or wish to employ assistants. Clearly, more research, with a large enough sample for adequate statistical power and sound methodology, is needed (see summary by Greener, Enderby, & Whurr, 2000).

Do Any Studies Show the Effectiveness of Support Personnel in Audiology or Speech-Language Pathology?

The studies described for the first clinical question (i.e., comparing clinical service by support personnel with professionals) also address the second question of the effectiveness of support personnel in speech-language pathology. All previously cited studies showed that children and adults made improvements when support personnel in speech-language pathology were used. Other studies have been conducted that show the effectiveness of support personnel in audiology or speech-language pathology but did not have a comparison group.

Effectiveness of Support Personnel in Audiology.
A study was identified that addressed the use of support personnel for individuals with hearing loss. A Canadian consumer organization trained seniors with hearing loss to serve as peer models and provide support for other seniors with hearing loss in long-term health care facilities or in the community (Dahl, 1997). The volunteers were trained to assist with hearing aid care, use of assistive listening devices, and strategies for coping with hearing loss. Within a five-month period, the volunteers totaled 288 weekly half-day visits. The seniors receiving support found the visitor program to be helpful. An informal follow-up evaluation one year after the project showed continued visits by some of the volunteers and the addition of new trained volunteers.

A report by the National Academies of Sciences, Engineering, and Medicine (2016) suggested that community health workers (CHWs) could be used to address issues surrounding access to hearing care. Audiologist-trained CHWs were used in two pilot programs focused on addressing the public health issue of hearing loss by providing access to services in underserved communities. A study by Mamo, Frank, and Korczak (2019) was completed to identify whether CHWs might be accepted as extenders of audiology services and in what ways. Their study was not focused specifically on the effectiveness of a CHW but it identified audiologists' involvement was necessary to recognize patient needs and to provide focused training for the CHWs. Additionally, use of CHWs allowed for improved efficiency for the audiologist and better access to services for those in communities lacking access to hearing care.

Four studies were identified that addressed whether audiometric technicians could determine which patients could be fitted with a hearing aid without the need for a medical referral. One study was conducted to determine if "physiological measurement technicians" could safely prescribe hearing aids without medical supervision. The technicians reportedly failed to mention the presence of active inflammatory ear disease in the referral letter for three of eight cases where middle ear disease was present. The authors concluded that review by ear, nose, and throat (ENT) medical staff was needed before prescription of a hearing aid (Bellini, Beesley, Perrett, & Pickles, 1989). In the other studies, the authors concluded that the audiology technicians made accurate assessments of patients to determine if they required a hearing aid referral to an ENT (Koay & Sutton, 1996; Swan & Browning, 1994; Zeitoun, Lesshafft, Begg, & East, 1995). For example, a "senior audiology technician or higher grade" working in a general practitioner's office determined that 23% of the 135 patients required medical referral before being fitted for a hearing aid. The ENT review of the same patients showed 100% agreement with the audiology technicians (Koay & Sutton, 1996).

Additional data are available from De Wet Swanepoel, an audiologist using support personnel globally to aid in hearing care service delivery in underserved areas of South Africa. Swanepoel (2010) documented that the use of community-trained hearing support personnel within a telehealth service delivery model has yielded "clinically equivalent results for remote, telehealth-enabled tests compared to conventional face-to-face versions" (p. 187).

Effectiveness of Support Personnel in Speech-Language Pathology.
The few studies conducted on the effectiveness of support personnel in speech-language pathology focus primarily on their use with children with articulation and expressive language disorders and adults with aphasia or dementia.

Studies with Children. Support personnel in speech-language pathology have been used to conduct speech and language screening programs for children. In a pilot program, existing school personnel serving as "aides" were trained to screen the speech and language skills of elementary-age children. The aides were reported to administer the screening tests accurately to make appropriate referrals for those children with a high probability of having speech and language problems (Pickering & Dopheide, 1976). In another pilot screening program, "paraprofessionals" screened young children between 19 and 21 months during home visits for language delay. Screening data from the administration of a standardized screening test were found to be reliable, valid, and sensitive in identifying children for further assessment (Pickstone, 2003).

Children with speech sound disorders showed improvement when they received speech services from SLP support personnel. A study of articulation treatment for elementary-age children by trained paraprofessionals reported that 83.5% of the treated sounds were used correctly in a conversational sample (Galloway & Blue, 1975). Improvements in speech production were reported for children treated by students (Hall & Knutson, 1978), "communication aides" (Van Hattum et al., 1974), and paid aides and volunteers (Scalero & Eskenazi, 1976).

Studies focused on improving language skills in children also demonstrated improvements when services were provided by support personnel in speech-language pathology. A single-participant study reported increases in communication (e.g., percentage of correct information and words per minute) when a "nonprofessional" provided a structured maintenance program for an individual with epilepsy and language and cognitive impairments (Wright, Shisler, & Rau, 2003). Teachers in another study reported that 41% of their 22 kindergarten students showed improvement after receiving computer-aided language enrichment by volunteers, although the outcomes were not quantified (Schetz, 1989). "Nonprofessional tutors" were used to help first-grade children develop phonological and early reading skills (Vadasy, Jenkins, & Pool, 2000). Tutors provided one-to-one instruction for 30 minutes, four days a week, for one school year in phonological skills, letter–sound correspondence, decoding, rhyming, writing, spelling, and reading. Tutored children received significantly better reading, spelling, and decoding scores than students who did not receive tutoring. The tutored children continued to do better than non-tutored children in decoding and spelling after second grade. An exploratory study used "specialist teaching assistants" to conduct speech and/or language intervention for 35 children (4–6 years) for four one-hour sessions over 10 weeks. The children, from an inclusive school in the UK, showed improve-

ment in targeted language outcomes and on a standardized language test. Differences also were noted on a questionnaire comparing speech and language performance at school and at home before and after intervention (Mecrow, Beckwith, & Klee, 2010).

Positive outcomes in speech and language also were shown when children with severe disabilities received services from support personnel in speech-language pathology. In one study, two psychiatric aides who served as "paraprofessional teachers" were trained to use a structured language training program with children with severe disabilities. In this study, matched pairs of children were randomly assigned to an experimental or control condition. Results showed that the children in the experimental group who received language training by the aides for two months showed improvement in language (e.g., identifying and labeling objects) and social skills (Phillips, Liebert, & Poulos, 1973). Another study trained undergraduate students to use behavioral principles to develop the verbal behavior of young children with severe disabilities with limited verbal repertoires (Guralnick, 1972). Five of the eight children showed progress in their development of communication skills (e.g., imitating sounds, sustaining eye contact, using gestures). Another article reported on the use of blind and partially sighted high school students who were trained and paid to serve as "speech assistants" in a residential school to provide extra class practice for younger children with visual impairments who had speech problems (Briggs, 1974). Although data were not collected on the speech outcomes of the students receiving services, the author reported that most appeared to benefit from the additional practice provided by the assistants.

A systematic review of different service delivery models demonstrated that trained SLPAs could provide effective services for children with language disorders (Cirrin et al., 2010).

Assistants also have been used with positive outcomes in countries and communities where speech-language pathology services are scarce. For example, "speech assistants" were found to be an efficient way to extend speech correction services for children with a cleft lip and palate in Thailand and other developing countries (Hanchanlert, Pramakhatay, Pradubwong, & Prathanee, 2015; Makarabhirom, Prathanee, Suphawatjariyakul, & Yoodee, 2015; Pradubwong, Prathanee, & Patjanasoontorn, 2016). Supervised student speech-language pathology students worked in rural communities in Australia with school-age children who demonstrated improved communication skills (Kirby, Lyle, Brunero, Purcell, & Dettwiller, 2018).

Studies with Adults. Adults with aphasia showed communication improvements when treatment was provided by support personnel, including relatives (Lesser, Bryan, Anderson, & Hilton, 1986), untrained volunteers (Eaton Griffith, 1975; Griffith & Miller, 1980; Lesser & Watt, 1978), and "community volunteers" (Lyon et al., 1997). Similarly, adults with "communication handicaps" showed increased responsiveness, verbalizations, and social interactions when trained volunteers were used as an adjunct to professional treatment (Mueller, 1990). Trained volunteers were judged to be better conversational partners for adults with aphasia than were untrained volunteers (Kagan, Black, Duchan, Simmons-Mackie, & Square, 2001). The individuals with aphasia showed significant improvements in social skills and message exchange skills when interacting with volunteers who received supported conversation training. These changes were not seen in the adults with aphasia who interacted with the untrained volunteers.

Support personnel also have been used successfully with adults with dementia. One article described a "partnered volunteering" language and memory stimulation program for adults with Alzheimer's disease. The study reported positive changes in language and memory on pre- and posttests after two semesters of service by student volunteers from speech-language pathology or psychology (Arkin, 1996). Another study used nursing assistants to enhance discourse skills of nursing home residents with dementia. In this study, one group of nursing assistants was trained and supervised using communication techniques and memory books with the residents. A control group paired nursing assistants with residents with dementia but did not use specific communication or memory tools. The conversational skills of residents in the treatment group were more coherent and had fewer vague "empty phrases" compared with the no-treatment control group. The nursing assistants in the treatment group also used more "facilitative discourse strategies" (e.g., encouragement, cuing) than assistants in the control group (Dijkstra, Bourgeois, Burgio, & Allen, 2002).

Effectiveness of Support Personnel in Audiology and Speech-Language Pathology. The effectiveness of support personnel in audiology and speech-language pathology remains an open question. Only a few studies are available, and most studies were conducted in the 1970s and 1980s. The methodological quality of many of the studies was poor (e.g., no control group, few participants, no randomized groups, few statistical comparisons) or not accessible, with the exception of a more recent 2007 study (Boyle et al., 2007). Audiometric technicians appear capable of determining which patients need a medical referral before being fitted for a hearing aid. The available studies using support personnel in speech-language pathology appeared to show that they could be effective in improving speech production

for children with articulation disorders or conversational skills for adults with aphasia or dementia. Support personnel also appear to have positive benefits in extending services in countries and rural communities where audiologists and SLPs are not widely available.

Future Research Issues

In 1977, Gray and Barker wrote that "there is little substantive information about whether or not [aides] can reliably and effectively provide services" (p. 534). More than 40 years later, this same statement can still be made. There is a paucity of high-quality efficacy research on the use of support personnel in audiology or speech-language pathology. Among the few studies conducted, there is some evidence of comparable outcomes between supervised SLPAs and SLPs, particularly when services are limited to more repetitive treatment activities. Although some studies demonstrate that support personnel in audiology and speech-language pathology can carry out assigned tasks, most are descriptive rather than empirical. Except for a controlled trial in the UK (Boyle et al., 2007), few research designs go beyond a low level of evidence using case studies with no randomization or control group. Research also is needed pertaining to the optimal amount and type of supervision necessary for assistants with various amounts of experience and to determine the effectiveness of different types of training programs for support personnel. The use of appropriately trained, supervised, and credentialed support personnel may be a viable option in some settings to enhance the frequency and intensity of service delivery in the professions of audiology and speech-language pathology. However, more evidence, and better-quality evidence, is needed before the value of support personnel in audiology and speech-language pathology can be ascertained. Future research questions could address the value of using credentialed assistants, comparisons in efficacy in different work settings, and the benefits of using support personnel in maintenance programs and highly scripted programs.

Summary

The intended use of support personnel is to supplement and extend the work of audiologists and SLPs. The audiology assistant and SLPA may be hired to increase the frequency, intensity, efficiency, and availability of services by following a specific set of job responsibilities. However, the licensed and certified professional ultimately remains responsible for the training, selection, management, and supervision of the assistant. It is also the clinician's obligation to inform the consumer of the level of training and expertise of the assistant, so that at no time is the assistant represented as an audiologist or SLP. The clinician retains the legal and ethical responsibility for all services provided or omitted. The clinician and the assistant need to work as a team to support the communication needs of the individuals they serve. ASHA is starting a national credentialing program for assistants and several states regulate their use. In these states, the use of assistants can be monitored, ensuring that the assistants are used in a legal manner in terms of education and supervision. Adherence to professional guidelines also serves as a means of monitoring ethical clinical practice. The limited research available suggests that services provided by assistants are effective, although much more quality research is needed to determine the degree of effectiveness and optimal amount of supervision and to make comparisons with services by audiologists and SLPs. Additionally, studies are needed that involve audiologists and SLPs who are systematically educated to use support personnel appropriately as an extension of their services.

Critical Thinking

1. What are some of the factors that have led to the use of audiology assistants and SLPAs?

2. What specific job responsibilities are appropriate for audiology assistants and SLPAs? What are some activities/tasks that are not appropriate for assistants?

3. What are some of the possible advantages and risks to using assistants? How might the possible negative effects be alleviated?

4. How have our state laws and national associations addressed the issue of assistants? Consider issues such as training, regulating, certifying, supervising, and ensuring that standards and ethics are not being compromised.

5. How might the inclusion of audiology assistants and SLPAs help to address the needs of our linguistically diverse community? When using assistants as interpreters or translators, how should training and supervision issues be addressed?

6. According to the available research, does the use of assistants diminish or enhance the effectiveness of treatment? What additional information do we need to make a more objective analysis of the effectiveness of assistants and ensure comparability with service by audiologists and SLPs?

7. As the supervisor of an assistant, list and describe your responsibilities and necessary knowledge and skills.

8. Consider the following: As an SLP, who is a monolingual English speaker, you work in a school district with many students whose primary language is Spanish. Your administrator hires and assigns an assistant to you. The assistant has a bachelor's degree in CSD and is fluent in Spanish. The administrator states that the assistant will be doing all of the Spanish language testing as well as writing and managing the IEPs and working with the families of all students on your caseload whose primary language is Spanish. What are the ethical and legal implications? How might you address them in this scenario?

Acknowledgments

The authors gratefully acknowledge the expertise, attention to detail, and care of the following ASHA National Office staff in the preparation of this chapter: Eileen Crowe, Janet Deppe, Laurie Alban Havens, Brooke Hatfield, Andrea Moxley, Sarah Slater, and Sarah Warren. The authors also extend their appreciation to Beverly Wang and Tracy Schooling for their assistance with the literature review.

Dedication

In loving memory of our dear friend, Steve Ritch (1964–2019), whose light, love, and joy touched everyone who knew him and whose dedication and commitment advanced the development of the ASHA Audiology Assistants and Speech-Language Pathology Assistants program.

References

Administration on Aging. (2017). *2017 Profile of older Americans. Future growth.* Retrieved from https:// acl.gov/sites/default/files/Aging%20and%20 Disability%20in%20America/2017OlderAmericans Profile.pdf

Alvord, D. J. (1977). Innovation in speech therapy: A cost-effective program. *Exceptional Children*, *43*, 520–525.

American Academy of Audiology. (1997, May/June). Position statement and guidelines of the consensus panel on support personnel in audiology. *Audiology Today*, *9*(3), 27–28.

American Academy of Audiology. (2003, October). *Preventing noise-induced occupational hearing loss.* Retrieved from http://www.audiology.org/

American Academy of Audiology. (2004, January). *Audiology: Scope of practice.* Retrieved from http://www.audiology.org/

American Academy of Audiology. (2006). Position statement on audiologist's assistants. *Audiology Today, 18*(2), 27–28. Retrieved from http://www.audiology.org/publications-resources/document-library/audiologists-assistant/

American Academy of Audiology. (2009). *Code of ethics.* Retrieved from http://www.audiology.org/

American Academy of Audiology. (2010a). *Audiology assistants.* Retrieved from https://audiology-web.s3.amazonaws.com/migrated/2010_Audiology Assistant_Pos_Stat.pdf_539978b1321499 .80405268.pdf

American Academy of Audiology. (2010b). Audiology assistant task force report. *Audiology Today, 22*(3), 68–73.

American Academy of Audiology. (2018). *Code of ethics.* Available from www.audiology.org/

American Academy of Audiology. (n.d.). *Considerations for the use of support personnel for newborn hearing screening.* Retrieved from www.audiology.org/publications-resources/document-library/considerations-use-support-personnel-newborn-hearing/

American Academy of Otolaryngology–Head and Neck Surgery. (2006). *Certificate program for otolaryngology personnel launched.* Retrieved from http://www.entnet.org/education/CPOP.cfm/

American Speech-Language-Hearing Association, Committee on Supportive Personnel. (1970). Guidelines on the role, training, and supervision of the communication aide. *Asha, 12*, 78–80.

American Speech-Language-Hearing Association. (1979). *ASHA policy regarding support personnel.* Rockville, MD: Author.

American Speech-Language-Hearing Association. (1981, March). Guidelines for the employment and utilization of support personnel. *Asha, 23*, 165–169.

American Speech-Language-Hearing Association. (1985a, June). Clinical management of communicatively handicapped minority language populations. *Asha, 27*(6), 3–7.

American Speech-Language-Hearing Association. (1985b, June). Clinical supervision in speech-language pathology and audiology. *Asha, 27*(6), 57–60.

American Speech-Language-Hearing Association. (1988, November). Utilization and employment of speech-language pathology supportive personnel with underserved populations. *Asha, 30*, 55–56.

American Speech-Language-Hearing Association. (1992). *Technical report: Support personnel: Issues and impact on the professions of speech-language pathology and audiology.* Rockville, MD: Author.

American Speech-Language-Hearing Association. (1995a). *ASHA Omnibus survey.* Rockville, MD: Author.

American Speech-Language-Hearing Association. (1995b, March). Position statement for the training, credentialing, use, and supervision of support personnel in speech-language pathology. *Asha, 37*(Suppl. 14), 21.

American Speech-Language-Hearing Association. (1996, Spring). Guidelines for the training, credentialing, use, and supervision of speech-language pathology assistants. *Asha, 38*(Suppl. 16), 21–34.

American Speech-Language-Hearing Association. (1998). Position statement and guidelines on support personnel in audiology. *Asha, 40*(Suppl. 18), 19–21.

American Speech-Language-Hearing Association. (2000a). *Council on Academic Accreditation in Audiology and Speech-Language Pathology: Criteria for approval of associate degree technical training programs for speech-language pathology assistants.* Rockville, MD: Author.

American Speech-Language-Hearing Association. (2000b). *Council on Professional Standards in Speech-Language Pathology and Audiology: Background information and criteria for registration of speech-language pathology assistants.* Rockville, MD: Author.

American Speech-Language-Hearing Association. (2000c). *Working with speech-language pathology assistants in school settings.* Rockville, MD: Author.

American Speech-Language-Hearing Association. (2001). *Scope of practice in speech-language pathology.* Rockville, MD: Author.

American Speech-Language-Hearing Association. (2002a). *Knowledge and skills for supervisors of speech-language pathology assistants.* Retrieved from http://www.asha.org/policy/

American Speech-Language-Hearing Association. (2002b). *Speech-language pathology health care survey.* Retrieved from http://www.asha.org/

American Speech-Language-Hearing Association. (2002c). *A workload analysis approach for establishing speech-language pathology caseload standards in the schools.* Retrieved from http://www.asha.org/policy/

American Speech-Language-Hearing Association. (2003a). *ASHA Omnibus survey.* Retrieved from http://www.asha.org/

American Speech-Language-Hearing Association. (2004a). *The audiologist's role in occupational hearing conservation and hearing loss prevention programs: Technical report.* Retrieved from http://www.asha.org/policy/

American Speech-Language-Hearing Association. (2004b). *Guidelines for the training, use, and supervision of speech-language pathology assistants.* Retrieved from http://www.asha.org/policy/

American Speech-Language-Hearing Association. (2004c). *Knowledge and skills needed by speech-language pathologists and audiologists to provide culturally and linguistically appropriate services.* Rockville, MD: Author.

American Speech-Language-Hearing Association. (2004d). *Preferred practice patterns for the profession of speech-language pathology.* Retrieved from http://www.asha.org/policy/

American Speech-Language-Hearing Association. (2004e). *Scope of practice in audiology.* Rockville, MD: Author.

American Speech-Language-Hearing Association. (2004f). *Support personnel.* Rockville, MD: Author.

American Speech-Language-Hearing Association. (2004g). *Training, use, and supervision of support personnel in speech-language pathology.* Rockville, MD: Author.

American Speech-Language-Hearing Association. (2006). *Preferred practice patterns for the profession of audiology.* Retrieved from http://www.asha.org/policy/

American Speech-Language-Hearing Association. (2009a). *Demographic profile of ASHA members providing bilingual and Spanish-language services.* Retrieved from http://www.asha.org/uploadedFiles/Demographic-Profile-Bilingual-Spanish-Service-Members.pdf

American Speech-Language-Hearing Association. (2009b). *2009 Membership survey summary report: Number and type of responses.* Retrieved from http://www.asha.org/uploadedFiles/2009MembershipSurveySummary.pdf

American Speech-Language-Hearing Association. (2009c). *Practical tools and forms for supervising speech-language pathology assistants.* Rockville, MD: Author.

American Speech-Language-Hearing Association. (2010). *2010 Schools survey summary report: Number and type of responses, SLPs.* Retrieved from http://www.asha.org/uploadedFiles/Schools10Frequencies.pdf

American Speech-Language-Hearing Association. (2012). *2012 Schools survey. Survey summary report: Number and type of responses, SLPs.* Retrieved from http://www.asha.org/

American Speech-Language-Hearing Association. (2013). *Speech-language pathology assistant scope of practice* [Scope of practice]. Retrieved from http://www.asha.org/policy/

American Speech-Language-Hearing Association. (2014). *Model bill for state licensure of audiologists, speech-language pathologists, and audiology and speech-language pathology assistants.* Retrieved from http://www.asha.org/uploadedFiles/State-Licensure-Model-Bill.pdf

American Speech-Language-Hearing-Association. (2016a). *Code of ethics* [Ethics]. Retrieved from http://www.asha.org/code-of-ethics/

American Speech-Language-Hearing Association. (2016b). *Scope of practice in speech-language pathology* [Scope of practice]. Retrieved from http://www.asha.org/policy/

American Speech-Language-Hearing Association. (2016c). *2016 Schools Survey report: SLP workforce/work conditions.* Retrieved from http://www.asha.org/research/memberdata/schoolssurvey/

American Speech-Language-Hearing Association. (2016d). *2015 Work life survey. CCC-SLP survey summary report: Number and type of responses.* Retrieved from http://www.asha.org/

American Speech-Language-Hearing Association. (2017a). *Highlights and trends: Member and affiliate counts, year end 2017.* Retrieved from http://www.asha.org/uploadedFiles/2017-Member-Counts.pdf

American Speech-Language-Hearing Association. (2017b). *Issues in ethics: Audiology assistants.* Retrieved from http://www.asha.org/policy/

American Speech-Language-Hearing Association. (2017c). *Issues in ethics: Speech-language pathology assistants.* Retrieved from http://www.asha.org/policy/

American Speech-Language-Hearing Association. (2018a). *Audiology assistant exam blueprint*

speech-language pathology assistants. Rockville, MD: Author.

11-1-2018. Retrieved from http://www.asha
.org/uploadedFiles/ASHA/associates/Audiology-
Assistant-Exam-Blueprint.pdf

American Speech-Language-Hearing Association.
(2018b). *Demographic profile of ASHA members
providing bilingual and Spanish-language services.*
Retrieved from http://www.asha.org/uploadedFiles/
Demographic-Profile-Bilingual-Spanish-Service-
Members.pdf

American Speech-Language-Hearing Association.
(2018c). *2018 Schools survey summary report:
Number and type of responses, SLPs.* Retrieved from
http://www.asha.org/uploadedFiles/Schools10Fre-
quencies.pdf

American Speech-Language-Hearing Association.
(2018d). *Scope of practice in audiology* [Scope of
practice]. Retrieved from http://www.asha.org/
Practice-Portal/Professional-Issues/Audiology-
Assistants/

American Speech-Language-Hearing Association.
(2018e). *SLPA exam blueprint 11-1-2018.* Retrieved
from http://www.asha.org/uploadedFiles/ASHA/
associates/SLPA-Exam-Blueprint.pdf

American Speech-Language-Hearing Association.
(n.d.-a). *ASHA assistants.* Retrieved from http://
www.ashaassistants.org/

American Speech-Language-Hearing Association.
(n.d.-b). *Audiology assistants* [Practice portal].
Retrieved from http://www.asha.org/Practice-
Portal/Professional-Issues/Audiology-Assistants/

American Speech-Language-Hearing Association.
(n.d.-c). *Audiology assistants certification: Eligibility
pathways.* Retrieved from https://www.ashaassis
tants.org/pathways-audiology-assistant/

American Speech-Language-Hearing Association.
(n.d.-d). *Early intervention* [Practice portal].
Retrieved from http://www.asha.org/Practice-
Portal/Professional-Issues/Early-Intervention/

American Speech-Language-Hearing Association.
(n.d.-e). *Frequently asked questions: Speech-language
pathology assistants (SLPAs).* Retrieved from http://
www.asha.org/associates/SLPA-FAQs/

American Speech-Language-Hearing Association.
(n.d.-f). *Speech-language pathology assistants*
[Practice portal]. Retrieved from www.asha
.org/Practice-Portal/Professional-Issues/Speech-
Language-Pathology-Assistants/

American Speech-Language-Hearing Association.
(n.d.-g). *Speech-language pathology assistants*

certification: Eligibility pathways. Retrieved from
https://www.ashaassistants.org/pathways-speech-
language-pathology-assistant/

American Speech-Language-Hearing Association.
(n.d.-h). Technical training programs for *speech-
language pathology assistants.* Retrieved from http://
www.asha.org/associates/SLPA-Technical-Training-
Programs/

American Speech-Language-Hearing Association.
(n.d.-i). *Teleaudiology clinical technicians.*
Retrieved from http://www.asha.org/practice-
portal/professional-issues/audiology-assistants/
teleaudiology-clinical-assistants/

American Speech-Language-Hearing Association
(n.d.-j). *Telepractice* [Practice portal]. Retrieved
from http://www.asha.org/Practice-Portal/
Professional-Issues/Telepractice/

Arkin, S. (1996). Volunteers in partnership: An
Alzheimer's rehabilitation program delivered by
students. *American Journal of Alzheimer's Disease
and Other Dementias, 11*(1), 12–22.

Bellini, M. J., Beesley, P., Perrett, C., & Pickles, J. M.
(1989). Hearing-aids: Can they be safely prescribed
without medical supervision? An analysis of patients
referred for hearing-aids. *Clinical Otolaryngology
and Allied Sciences, 14,* 415–418.

Boyle, J. M., McCartney, E., O'Hare, A., & Forbes, J.
(2009). Direct versus indirect and individual versus
group modes of language therapy for children with
primary language impairment: Principal outcomes
from a randomized controlled trail and economic
evaluation. *International Journal of Language and
Communication Disorders, 44*(6), 826–846.

Boyle, J., McCartney, E., O'Hare, A., & Law, J.
(2010). Intervention for mixed receptive-expressive
language impairment: A review. *Developmental
Medicine and Child Neurology, 52*(11), 994–999.

Boyle, J., McCartney, E., Forbes, J., & O'Hare, A.
(2007). A randomized controlled trial and economic
evaluation of direct versus indirect and individual
versus group modes of speech and language therapy
for children with primary language impairment.
Health Technology Assessment, 11(25), iii–iv, xi–xii,
1–158.

Breakey, L. K. (1993, May). Support personnel: Times
change. *American Journal of Speech-Language
Pathology, 2*(2), 13–16.

Briggs, B. M. (1974). High school speech assistants in
a residential school for the blind. *Education of the
Visually Handicapped, 6*(4), 119 124.

Bureau of Labor Statistics, U.S. Department of Labor. (2018a). *Occupational outlook handbook, Audiologists.* Retrieved from http://www.bls.gov/ooh/healthcare/audiologists.htm#tab-6/

Bureau of Labor Statistics, U.S. Department of Labor. (2018b). *Occupational outlook handbook, Speech-language pathologists.* Retrieved from http://www.bls.gov/ooh/healthcare/speech-language-pathologists.htm#tab-6/

Cirrin, F. M., Schooling, T. L., Nelson, N. W., Diehl, S. F., Flynn, P. F., Staskowski, M., . . . Adamczyk, D. F. (2010). Evidence-based systematic review: Effects of different service delivery models on communication outcomes for elementary school-age children. *Language, Speech, and Hearing Services in Schools, 41*(3), 233–264.

Code of Federal Regulations, Title 42, Section 440.110(c)

Consortium of Organizations on the Preparation and Use of Speech-Language Paraprofessionals in Early Intervention and Education Settings. (1997, January). *Report of the consortium of organizations on the preparation and use of speech-language paraprofessionals in early intervention and education settings.* Reston, VA: Author.

Costello, J., & Schoen, J. (1978). The effectiveness of paraprofessionals and a speech clinician as agents of articulation intervention using programmed instruction. *Language, Speech, and Hearing Services in Schools, 9,* 118–128.

Dahl, M. O. (1997). To hear again: A volunteer program in hearing health care for hard-of-hearing seniors. *Journal of Speech-Language Pathology and Audiology, 21,* 153–159.

David, R., Enderby, P., & Bainton, D. (1982). Treatment of acquired aphasia: Speech therapists and volunteers compared. *Journal of Neurology, Neurosurgery, and Psychiatry, 45,* 957–961.

Dickson, K., Marshall, M., Boyle, J, McCartney, E., O'Hare, A., & Forbes, J. (2009). Cost analysis of direct versus indirect and individual versus group modes of manual-based speech-and-language therapy for primary school-age children with primary language impairment. *International Journal of Language and Communication Disorders, 44*(3), 369–381.

Dijkstra, K., Bourgeois, M., Burgio, L., & Allen, R. (2002). Effects of a communication intervention on the discourse of nursing home residents with dementia and their nursing assistants. *Journal of Medical Speech-Language Pathology, 10*(2), 143–157.

Eaton Griffith, V. (1975). Volunteer scheme for dysphasic and allied problems in stroke patients. *British Medical Journal, iii,* 633–635.

Galloway, H. F., & Blue, C. M. (1975). Paraprofessional personnel in articulation therapy. *Language, Speech, and Hearing Services in Schools, 6,* 125–130.

Gerlach, K. (2000). *The paraeducator and teacher team: Strategies for success.* Seattle, WA: Pacific Training Associates.

Gersten, J. W., Foppe, K. B., Gersten, R., Maxwell, S., Mirrett, P., Gipson, M....Grueter, B. (1975). Effectiveness of aides in a perceptual motor training program for children with learning disabilities. *Archives of Physical Medicine & Rehabilitation, 56*(3), 104–110.

Goldberg, L., & Paul-Brown, D. (1999). *Strategies for the effective use of speech-language pathology assistants in the classroom.* Proceedings of the Seventh Annual Comprehensive System of Personnel Development Conference, National Association of State Directors of Special Education, Alexandria, VA.

Gray, B. B., & Barker, K. (1977). Use of aides in an articulation therapy program. *Exceptional Children, 43,* 534–536.

Greener, J., Enderby, P., & Whurr, R. (2000). Speech and language therapy for aphasia following stroke *Cochrane Database of Systematic Reviews, 2000*(2). http://doi.org/10.1002/14651858.CD000425

Griffith, V. E., & Miller, C. L. (1980). Volunteer stroke scheme for dysphasic patients with stroke. *British Medical Journal, 281,* 1605–1607.

Guralnick, M. J. (1972). A language development program for severely handicapped children. *Exceptional Children, 39,* 45–49.

Guralnick, M. J. (2011). Why early intervention works: A systems perspective. *Infants and Young Children, 24*(1), 6–28.

Guralnick, M. J. (2019). *Effective early intervention: The developmental systems approach.* Baltimore, MD: Brookes.

Hall, P. K., & Knutson, C. L. (1978). The use of preprofessional students as communication aides in the schools. *Language, Speech, and Hearing Services in Schools, 9,* 162–168.

Hamill, T., & Freeman, B. (2001). Scope of practice for audiologists' assistants: Survey results. *Audiology Today, 13*(6), 34–35.

Hanchanlert, Y., Pramakhatay, W., Pradubwong, S., & Prathanee, B. (2015). Speech correction for children with cleft lip and palate by networking of community-based care. *Journal of the Medical Association of Thailand, 98*(Suppl. 7), S132–S139.

Individuals with Disabilities Education Improvement Act of 2004, Pub. L. No. 108-446, 20 U.S.C. § 1400 *et seq.*

Johnson, C. E. (1999). Dimensions of multiskilling: Considerations for educational audiology. *Language, Speech, and Hearing Services in Schools, 30*, 4–10.

Johnson, C. E., Clark-Lewis, S., & Griffin, D. (1998). Experience, attitudes, and competencies of audiologic support personnel in a rehabilitation hospital. *American Journal of Audiology, 7*, 1–6.

Joint Committee on Infant Hearing. (2007). *Year 2007 position statement: Principles and guidelines for early hearing detection and intervention.* Retrieved from http://www.asha.org/policy/

Kagan, A., Black, S. E, Duchan, J. F., Simmons-Mackie, N., & Square, P. (2001). Training volunteers as conversation partners using "supported conversation for adults with aphasia" (SCA): A controlled trial. *Journal of Speech, Language, and Hearing Research, 44*, 624–638.

Karzon, R, Hunter, L, & Steuerwald, W. (2018). Audiology assistants: Results of a multicenter survey. *Journal of the American Academy of Audiology, 29*(5), 405–416.

Kirby, S., Lyle, D., Jones, D., Brunero, C., Purcell, A., & Dettwiller, P. (2018). Design and delivery of an innovative speech pathology service-learning program for primary school children in Far West NSW, Australia. *Public Health Research & Practice, 28*(3), e28231806.

Koay, C. B., & Sutton, G. J. (1996). Direct hearing aid referrals: A prospective study. *Clinical Otolaryngology and Allied Science, 21*, 142–146.

Langdon, H. W., & Cheng, L. L. (2002). *Collaborating with interpreters and translators.* Eau Claire, WI: Thinking Publications.

Lesser, R., Bryan, K., Anderson, J., & Hilton, R. (1986). Involving relatives in aphasia therapy: An application of language enrichment therapy. *International Journal of Rehabilitation Research, 9*, 259–267.

Lesser, R., & Watt, M. (1978). Untrained community help in the rehabilitation of stroke sufferers with language disorder. *British Medical Journal, ii,* 1045–1048.

Longhurst, T. (1997). Team roles in therapy services. In A. L. Pickett & K. Gerlach (Eds.), *Supervising paraeducators in school settings: A team approach* (pp. 55–89). Austin, TX: Pro-Ed.

Lynch, E. W., & Hanson, M. J. (Eds.). (2004). *Developing cross-cultural competence: A guide for working with children and their families* (3rd ed.). Baltimore, MD: Brookes.

Lyon, J. G., Cariski, D., Keisler, L., Rosenbek, J., Levine, R., Kumpula, J., . . . Blanc, M. (1997). Communication partners: Enhancing participation in life and communication for adults with aphasia in natural settings. *Aphasiology, 11*, 693–708.

Makarabhirom, K., Prathanee, B., Suphawatjariyakul, R., & Yoodee, P. (2015). Speech therapy for children with cleft lip and palate using a community-based speech therapy model with speech assistants. *Journal of the Medical Association of Thailand, 98*(Suppl. 7), S140–S150.

Mamo, S. K., Frank, M. R, & Korczak, P. (2019). Exploring community health worker (CHW) models for delivering audiology services. *Hearing Review, 26*(1), 12–17.

Marshall, R. C., Wertz, R. T., Weiss, D. G., Aten, J. L., Brookshire, R. H., Garcia-Bunuel, L., . . . Goodman, R. (1989). Home treatment for aphasic patients by trained nonprofessionals. *Journal of Speech and Hearing Disorders, 54*(3), 462–470.

McCartney, E., Boyle, J., Bannatyne, S., Jessiman, E., Campbell, C., Kelsey, C., . . . O'Hare, A. (2004). Becoming a manual occupation? The construction of a therapy manual for use with language impaired children in mainstream primary schools. *International Journal of Language and Communication Disorders, 39*(1), 135–148.

McCartney, E., Boyle, J., Ellis, S., Bannatyne, S., & Turnbull, M. (2011). Indirect language therapy for children with persistent language impairment in mainstream primary schools: Outcomes from a cohort intervention. *International Journal of Language and Communication Disorders, 46*(1), 74–82.

McNeilly, L. (2009). Speech-language pathology assistants Current state of affairs. *Perspectives on School-Based Issues 10*(1), 12–18.

McNeilly, L. (2010, November 23). ASHA will roll out Associates program in 2011. *The ASHA Leader.*

McNeilly, L. (2018). Using the International Classification of Functioning, Disability and Health Framework to achieve interprofessional functional outcomes for young children: A speech-language pathology perspective. Pediatric speech and language: Perspectives on interprofessional practice. *Pediatric Clinics of North America, 65*(1), 125–134.

Mecrow, C., Beckwith, J., & Klee, T. (2010). An exploratory trial of the effectiveness of an enhanced consultative approach to delivering speech and language intervention in schools. *International Journal of Language and Communication Disorders, 45*(3), 354–367.

Meikle, M., Wechsler, E., Tupper, A., Benenson, M., Butler, J., Mulhall, D., & Stern, G. (1979). Comparative trial of volunteer and professional treatments of dysphasia after stroke. *British Medical Journal, 2,* 87–89.

Mueller, P. B. (1990). A volunteer speech-language facilitation program for communicatively handicapped elders in long-term care facilities. *Adult Residential Care Journal, 4,* 217–225.

National Academies of Sciences, Engineering, and Medicine. (2016). *Hearing health care for adults: Priorities for improving access and affordability.* Washington, DC: The National Academies Press. Retrieved from http://nationalacademies.org/hmd/reports/2016/Hearing-Health-Care-for-Adults.aspx

National Hearing Conservation Association. (2018). *Working together to prevent noise induced hearing loss (NIHL).* Retrieved from http://www.hearingconservation.org/

National Joint Committee on Learning Disabilities. (1998). Learning disabilities: Use of paraprofessionals. In *Collective perspectives on issues affecting learning disabilities* (2nd ed., pp. 79–98). Austin, TX: Pro-Ed.

Paul-Brown, D., & Caperton, C. J. (2001). Inclusive practices for preschool children with specific language impairment. In M. J. Guralnick (Ed.), *Early childhood inclusion: Focus on change* (pp. 433–463). Baltimore, MD: Brookes.

Paul-Brown, D., & Goldberg, L. R. (2001). Current policies and new directions for speech-language pathology assistants. *Language, Speech, and Hearing Services in Schools, 32,* 4–17.

Phillips, S., Liebert, R. M., & Poulos, R. W. (1973). Employing paraprofessional teachers in a group language training program for severely and profoundly retarded children. *Perceptual and Motor Skills, 36,* 607–616.

Pickering, M., & Dopheide, W. R. (1976). Training aides to screen children for speech and language problems. *Language, Speech, and Hearing Services in Schools, 7,* 236–241.

Pickett, A. L. (1999). *Strengthening and supporting teacher/provider–paraeducator teams: Guidelines for paraeducator roles, supervision, and preparation.* New York, NY: City University of New York Graduate Center.

Pickett, A. L., & Gerlach, K. (Eds.). (1997). *Supervising paraeducators in school settings: A team approach.* Austin, TX: Pro-Ed.

Pickstone, C. (2003). A pilot study of paraprofessional screening of child language in community settings. *Child Language Teaching & Therapy, 19,* 49–65.

Pradubwong, S., Prathanee, B., & Patjanasoontorn, N. (2016). Effectiveness of networking of Khon Kaen University community-based speech model: Quality of life. *Journal of the Medical Association of Thailand, 99*(Suppl. 5), S36–S42.

Preamble to Federal Regulations. (2004, February 28). *Federal Register,* p. 30585.

Rosenfeld, M., & Leung, S. (1999, July). *A job analysis of speech-language pathology assistants: A study to aid in defining the job of speech-language pathology assistants. A job analysis study conducted on behalf of the American Speech-Language-Hearing Association.* Princeton, NJ: Educational Testing Service, Education Policy Research Division.

Scalero, A. M., & Eskenazi, C. (1976). The use of supportive personnel in a public school speech and language program. *Language, Speech, and Hearing Services in Schools, 7,* 150–158.

Scarr, S., McCartney, K., Miller, S., Hauenstein, E., & Ricciuti, A. (1996). Evaluation of an islandwide screening, assessment and treatment program. *Early Development & Parenting, 3,* 199–210.

Schery, T., & O'Connor, L. (1997). Language intervention: Computer training for young children with special needs. *British Journal of Educational Technology*, *28*, 271–279.

Schetz, K. F. (1989). Computer-aided language/ concept enrichment in kindergarten: Consultation program model. *Language, Speech, and Hearing Services in Schools*, *20*, 2–10.

Shewan, C. M., & Kertesz, A. (1984). Effects of speech and language treatment on recovery from aphasia. *Brain and Language*, *23*, 272–299.

Suter, A. H. (2002). *Hearing conservation manual* (4th ed.). Milwaukee, WI: Council for Accreditation in Occupational Hearing Conservation.

Swan, I. R., & Browning, G. G. (1994). A prospective evaluation of direct referral to audiology departments for hearing aids. *Journal of Laryngology and Otololgy*, *108*, 120–124.

Swanepoel, D. W., & Hall, J. W. (2010). A systematic review of telehealth applications in audiology. *Telemedicine and E-Health*,*16*(2), 181–200.

Thornton, A. (1993). The Cheshire profession. *American Journal of Audiology*, *2*, 5.

U.S. Bureau of the Census. (2010). *Census 2010 data*. Retrieved from http://2010.census.gov/2010census/ estimates/nation/intfile3-1.txt

U.S. Department of Justice. Civil Rights Division. (2000, August 11). *Executive Order 13166, Title VI of the Civil Rights Act of 1964 (Title VI): Improving access to services for persons with limited English proficiency*. Retrieved from http://www.justice.gov/ crt/about/cor/13166.php

U.S. Department of Labor. Occupational Safety and Health Administration. (n.d.). *Occupational noise exposure*. Retrieved from www.osha.gov/laws-regs/ regulations/standardnumber/1910/1910.95/

Vadasy, P. F., Jenkins, J. R., & Pool, K. (2000). Effects of tutoring in phonological and early reading skills on students at risk for reading disabilities. *Journal of Learning Disabilities*, *33*, 579–590.

Van Hattum, R. J., Page, J. M., Baskervill, R. D., Duguay, M. J., Conway, L. S., & Davis, T. R. (1974). The Speech Improvement System (SIS) taped program for remediation of articulation problems in the schools. *Language, Speech, and Hearing Services in Schools*, *5*, 91–97.

Wertz, R. T., Weiss, D. G., Aten, J. L., Brookshire, R. H., Garcia-Buñuel, L., Holland, A. L., . . . Goodman, R. (1986). Comparison of clinic, home, and deferred language treatment for aphasia. A Veterans Administration cooperative study. *Archives of Neurology*, *43*, 653–658.

Werven, G. (1993). Support personnel: An issue for our times. *American Journal of Speech-Language Pathology*, *2*(2), 9–12.

Wright, H. H., Shisler, R. J., & Rau, B. (2003). Maintenance of communication abilities in epilepsy: A clinical report. *Journal of Medical Speech-Language Pathology*, *11*, 157–167.

Zeitoun, H., Lesshafft, C., Begg, P. A., & East, D. M. (1995). Assessment of a direct referral hearing aid clinic. *British Journal of Audiology*, *29*, 13–21.

Appendix 13–A

◇◇◇

Support Personnel in Audiology and Speech-Language Pathology: Key Word Definitions

Aides: Support personnel who have a narrower training base and more limited responsibilities relative to the duties of assistants.

Assistants: Support personnel who perform tasks as prescribed, directed, and supervised by certified and licensed (where applicable) professionals after a program of academic and/or on-the-job training.

Cultural broker: A person who is knowledgeable about the client's/patient's culture and/or speech community and who provides this information to the clinician for optimizing services. Also referred to as cultural guides, cultural informants, or cultural-linguistic mediators.

Direct supervision: On-site, in-view observation and guidance by the clinician while an assigned activity is performed by support personnel.

Indirect supervision: Activities performed by the clinician that may include demonstrations, record review, review and evaluation of audio- or videotaped sessions, and/or interactive television.

Interpreter: Individual who conveys information from one language to another for oral messages.

Support personnel: Provide activities adjunct to the clinical efforts of certified and licensed (where applicable) professionals with appropriate training and supervision.

Telepractice Types

    Asynchronous services (store-and-forward): Images or data captured and transmitted for viewing or interpretation by a professional.

    Synchronous services (client interactive): Services are conducted with interactive audio and video connection in real time to create an in-person experience similar to that achieved in a traditional encounter.

Translator: Individual who conveys information from one language to another for written messages.

SECTION III

Setting-Specific Issues

14

Health Care Legislation, Regulation, and Financing

Jeffrey P. Regan, MA

Introduction

As the end of the second decade of the twenty-first century draws to a close, the political environment of the United States has become complex. Several contributing factors are behind this complexity, such as enduring partisan gridlock, sharpening ideological division, and never-ending election and campaign fundraising cycles. Within this environment the foundational institutions of governing and policymaking are being challenged in new ways. Consequently, legislative and regulatory processes—both in Washington and in state capitals nationwide—have acquired a degree of uncertainty.

Despite the current political environment, recent health care legislation and regulation have had a profound impact on the professions of audiology and speech-language pathology. This impact has been chiefly caused by the paradigmatic shift under way in health care reimbursement policy.[1] Over the past decade the nation has moved away from provider-centered payment models that are based on service volumes and fragmented care toward patient-centered payment models that incentivize health outcomes and high-quality coordinated care. This emerging policy landscape offers both challenges and opportunities for audiologists and speech-language pathologists in the years ahead.

This chapter begins by providing an overview of Medicare, Medicaid, and private health insurance—the three major drivers behind health care reimbursement policy for audiologists and speech-language pathologists. Next, the chapter provides an overview of coding systems, which collectively form the bedrock for reimbursement policy. Finally, the chapter discusses recent health care legislative and regulatory issues of particular importance to audiology and speech-language pathology. Questions that facilitate further thinking and discussion are provided at the end.

Medicare

Established in 1965 as Title XVIII of the Social Security Act, Medicare is federal health insurance principally for individuals 65 years or older, and is managed by the Centers for Medicare and Medicaid Services (CMS). Medicare currently has four parts that provide specified benefits.

---

[1]The sections on Medicare, Medicaid, private health insurance, and coding systems complement resources developed and routinely updated by the American-Speech-Language-Hearing Association for members. https://www.asha.org/practice/reimbursement/

Medicare Part A provides hospital and medical benefits. Certain audiology and speech-language pathology services provided in inpatient hospital, skilled nursing facility (SNF), home health, and hospice settings are covered by Part A, and included in the facility payment.

Medicare Part B provides supplemental medical insurance. Part B is optional and includes a monthly premium. Certain audiology and speech-language pathology services provided in outpatient hospital and non-institutional settings, including private practice settings, are covered by Part B. Part B also covers services provided in inpatient hospital and SNF settings when a Medicare beneficiary is determined ineligible for Part A or has exhausted Part A benefits.

Audiologists who bill under Medicare Part B currently require a physician referral prior to diagnostic testing. Speech-language pathologists who bill under Medicare Part B must have a physician approve a plan of care within 30 days of the beneficiary's first visit. Audiology and speech-language pathology services covered by Part B (excluding audiology services provided in hospital outpatient settings) have reimbursement rates set annually by the Medicare Physician Fee Schedule. Audiology services provided in hospital outpatient settings have reimbursement rates set annually by the Outpatient Prospective Payment System.

Medicare Part C, or Medicare Advantage, provides supplemental medical insurance through private managed care organizations. Managed care organizations, or MCOs, must offer benefits and coverage at least on par with Medicare Part B. Audiologists and speech-language pathologists may contract directly with MCOs. Medicare Part C currently covers over 20 million Medicare beneficiaries.

Medicare Part D provides a prescription drug benefit. Offered under both traditional Medicare and Medicare Advantage, Part D plans vary significantly in coverage and cost.

Medicare is locally administered by Medicare Administrative Contractors, or MACs. There are currently 15 MACs nationwide. MACs are private entities responsible for processing claims and issuing payments under Parts A and B. Each MAC develops and disseminates Local Coverage Determinations, or LCDs, for selected services. LCDs are based on national coverage policies issued by CMS. They are designed to give greater clarity about coverage and coding procedures to providers, including audiologists and speech-language pathologists. In addition to MACs, Recovery Audit Contractors review claims for inappropriate payments or fraud.

Medicare currently covers only diagnostic testing provided by an audiologist when a physician (or non-physician practitioner in certain states) orders the testing for the purpose of informing the physician's diagnostic medical evaluation, or determining appropriate medical or surgical treatment. Treatment services, rehabilitation services, hearing aids, and other neurologic assessments are not currently covered by Medicare when performed independently by an audiologist.

Audiology services that are recognized in the Medicare Benefit Policy Manual at Chapter 15, Section 80.3, include evaluation of the cause of disorders of hearing, tinnitus, or balance; evaluation of suspected change in hearing, tinnitus, or balance; determination of the effect of medication, surgery, or other treatment; reevaluation to follow up regarding changes in hearing, tinnitus, or balance that may be caused by established diagnoses that place the patient at probable risk for a change in status, including but not limited to otosclerosis, atelectatic tympanic membrane, tympanosclerosis, cholesteatoma, resolving middle ear infection, Meniére's disease, sudden idiopathic sensorineural hearing loss, autoimmune inner ear disease, acoustic neuroma, demyelinating diseases, ototoxicity secondary to medications, or genetic vascular and viral conditions; failure of a screening test (note that the screening test itself is not covered); diagnostic analysis of cochlear or brainstem implant and programming, and audiologic diagnostic tests before and periodically after implantation of auditory prosthetic devices.[2]

Medicare currently covers medically necessary assessment and treatment services provided by a speech-language pathologist when a physician (or non-physician practitioner in certain states) approves a plan of care within 30 days of a beneficiary's first visit. Speech-language pathology services provided under Part B are subject to special requirements designed to ensure medical necessity. When the cost of speech-language pathology and physical therapy services combined reaches $2,040, a special modifier must be used to justify the medical need for continued services. When the cost of speech-language pathology and physical therapy services combined reaches $3,000, a targeted medical review by CMS may occur. Services may continue beyond the $3,000 threshold provided there is documented justification for why such services are medically necessary.

Medicaid

Established in 1965 as Title XIX of the Social Security Act, Medicaid is an initiative funded in partnership between the federal government and states to provide medical care to individuals who meet defined low-

---

[2]Centers for Medicare and Medicaid Services, *Medicare Benefit Policy Manual.* (Rev. 256, 02-01-19). https://www.cms.gov/Regulations-and-Guidance/Guidance/Manuals/Downloads/bp102c15.pdf

income or disability thresholds. The federal government establishes broad guidelines for the program while the states have significant latitude to establish eligibility requirements, service coverage, and reimbursement rates. Each state is required to submit a State Medicaid Plan which must be approved by CMS.

Federal guidelines do not require that audiology and speech-language pathology services be covered by Medicaid for individuals 21 years of age or older; however, most states provide some coverage of services. For individuals under the age of 21, federal guidelines mandate comprehensive audiology and speech-language pathology services through the Early and Periodic Screening, Diagnostic, and Treatment (EPSDT) Program. EPSDT services include: identification of children with speech or language impairments, diagnosis and appraisal of specific speech or language impairments, referral for rehabilitation of speech or language impairment, provision of speech and language services, and hearing aids and augmentative and alternative communication devices when deemed to be medically necessary.

Federal guidelines require that audiologists and speech-language pathologists meet certain qualifications in order to receive payments under Medicaid.

Under the Code of Federal Regulations, Title 42, Section 440.110, a "qualified audiologist" means an individual with a master's or doctoral degree in audiology that maintains documentation to demonstrate that he or she meets or exceeds state licensure requirements, and that the individual is licensed by the state as an audiologist to furnish audiology services. In states that do not license audiologists, or if an individual is exempted from state licensure based on practice in a specific institution or setting, the individual must meet one of the following conditions: maintains Certificate of Clinical Competence (CCC) in Audiology granted by the American Speech-Language-Hearing Association (ASHA); successfully completes a minimum of 350 clock-hours of supervised clinical practicum; performs at least nine months of full-time audiology services under the supervision of a qualified master or doctoral-level audiologist after obtaining a master's or doctoral degree in audiology, or a related field; or successfully completes a government-approved national examination in audiology.

Federal guidelines define a "speech-language pathologist" as an individual who must meet one of the following conditions: maintains a CCC from ASHA, successfully completes the equivalent educational requirements and work experience necessary for the certificate, or successfully completes the academic program and is acquiring supervised work experience to qualify for the certificate.

Federal guidelines grant significant latitude to states in determining payment rates and payment methodologies. Payment rates and methodologies vary widely.

Rates must be adequate to support enough participating providers so that Medicaid beneficiaries have appropriate access to Medicaid services. What constitutes "appropriate access" is not defined explicitly in federal law or regulation. Both payment rates and payment methodologies must be included in each state's Medicaid plan.

Private Health Insurance

Private health insurance plans offer coverage of audiology and speech-language pathology services, but coverage varies significantly. Inpatient services are often included in basic hospital coverage. Outpatient services are often covered with utilization restrictions. Coverage varies for early intervention, prevention, wellness, and hearing aid services.

Payment rates and methodologies for audiology and speech-language pathology services vary widely between private health plans. Private insurers generally set rates using a market-driven approach, a relative value approach, or a combination of market-value and relative value approaches. Market-driven approaches tie payments to service delivery or utilization trends in local areas or regions. Relative value approaches tie payments to the provider's competence, time, and risk for each procedure. Payment methodologies may include fee-for-service, discounted fee-for-service for patients enrolled in a health plan, or capitation, in which fixed payments are made in advance on a "per patient per unit of time" basis.

Coding Systems

Appropriate coding forms the bedrock of health care reimbursement policy. Audiologists and speech-language pathologists utilize coding systems when submitting claims to Medicare, Medicaid, or private health plans. Codes specifically identify what diagnoses are made, what procedures are performed, and what devices are supplied by a provider. Appropriate coding ensures that audiologists and speech language-pathologists are accurately paid for time given and services rendered.

There are currently two coding systems commonly used by audiologists and speech-language pathologists: Healthcare Common Procedures Coding System (HCPCS) and the International Classification of Diseases, 10th Revision, Clinical Modification (ICD-10).

The HCPCS was first established in 1978 as a means by which to standardize the delivery of health care procedures and devices. Managed by CMS, HCPCS currently consists of two distinct levels of codes.

Level I of HCPCS comprises the Current Procedural Terminology (CPT) codes maintained by the American

Medical Association (AMA). The CPT codes capture a wide array of health care procedures and services across six separate categories. The CPT Editorial Panel is responsible for making sure that the codes and accompanying information are updated annually to comport with current practice standards and evidence-based care. The CPT Editorial Panel comprises 15 physicians and two non-physician providers. Each year, the CPT Editorial Panel convenes three meetings during which health care providers, device manufacturers, and other stakeholders provide comments on new codes or changes to existing codes. The CPT Editorial Panel is supported by the CPT Advisory Committee, which also comprises physicians and non-physician providers. The process of approving new codes or changing existing codes is highly structured. Medical societies and non-physician provider associations, such as ASHA, play critically important roles in the CPT process. These roles include proposing new codes or making changes to existing codes, and preparing audiologists and speech-language pathologists to serve as designated CPT advisors.

Once the CPT Editorial Panel makes decisions on new or existing CPT codes, AMA's Specialty Society Relative Value Scale Update Committee (RUC), meets and recommends CPT code valuations to CMS, which are set using Relative Value Units, or RVUs. The RUC comprises 31 members, the majority of whom are physicians. The RUC is supported by a larger RUC Advisory Committee, which is composed of physicians and non-physician providers. A core component of the RUC's work is collecting survey data on the CPT codes under review for valuation. These data are used to develop recommendations to the RUC. The RUC's recommendations, in turn, are forwarded to CMS's Medical Officers and Contractor Medical Directors for final review. Ultimately, CMS's reviews of the RUC recommendations are contained in the annual Medicare Physician Fee Schedule, which is published in July and finalized after stakeholder input in November. The Medicare Fee Schedule finalizes RVUs for each CPT code. As with the CPT process, medical societies and non-physician provider associations, such as ASHA, play critically important roles in the RUC process. These include conducting code surveys, compiling survey data, making valuation recommendations to the RUC based on the survey data, and preparing audiologists and speech-language pathologists to serve as designated RUC advisors.

Level II of HCPCS comprises codes that capture devices, supplies, and other equipment which are provided to patients. There are also a small number of health care procedures captured under Level II. These code sets are updated annually and administered by CMS in cooperation with private insurers, medical soci-

eties, and non-physician provider associations. HCPCS Level II includes codes for speech generating devices, augmentative and alternative communication devices, voice amplifiers, voice prosthetics, and hearing services (excluding services related to hearing aids).

The ICD-10 is the current revision of the International Classification of Diseases coding system used by the United States. ICD is managed globally by the World Health Organization; the Centers for Disease Control and Prevention and the National Center for Health Statistics have joint responsibility for maintaining ICD in the United States. ICD codes principally capture diagnoses, disorders, conditions, symptoms, and morbidities. Audiologists and speech-language pathologists are required to use ICD-10 codes when billing Medicare, Medicaid, or private health plans for payment. Revisions to the ICD codes happen relatively infrequently; however, when new revisions take place, they are often significant in scope and require a lengthy period of transition for providers, manufacturers, and payers alike.

Key Health Care Legislative and Regulatory Issues

Health care coverage and payment policy remains of utmost importance to the professions of audiology and speech-language pathology. This policy has undergone a paradigmatic shift over the past decade, the significance of which cannot be overstated. The nation's health care system has largely moved away from provider-centered payment models that are based on service volumes and fragmented care, towards patient-centered payment models that incentivize health outcomes and high quality coordinated care. This shift has significant impacts on audiology, speech-language pathology, and the 40 million Americans who have communication disorders.

There are three legislative and regulatory issues of current and principal importance to the professions of audiology and speech-language pathology: the Affordable Care Act, the Medicare Access and Children's Health Insurance Program (CHIP) Reauthorization Act, and—more recently—the Patient Driven Payment Model.

Affordable Care Act

The Patient Protection and Affordable Care Act (P.L. 111-148), or ACA, is fundamentally designed to reduce the number of uninsured Americans and curtail the rising cost of health care. Enacted into law in 2010, the ACA accomplishes its objectives in four principal ways. First, it mandates that Americans obtain health insurance at the risk of a tax penalty, and facilitates the sale of private health plans on regulated state-based exchanges. Second, it mandates that private health plans cover pre-existing conditions. Third, it mandates that private health plans cover ten so-called Essential Health Benefits (those specifically pertaining to speech-language pathology and audiology services are further explained below) without any annual or lifetime caps on coverage. Finally, it requires states with limited federal assistance to expand state Medicaid programs by raising income-based eligibility thresholds.

The ACA has been politically controversial since its enactment. During the administration of President Barack Obama, Republicans in Congress made numerous and unsuccessful attempts to repeal the ACA or replace it with weaker coverage mandates. In 2012, the Supreme Court upheld most of the law in the landmark decision in *National Federation of Independent Business v. Sebelius* (567 U.S. 519). The Court found that the individual mandate to purchase health insurance was an appropriate exercise of Congress' taxing power; however, the requirement to expand Medicaid was an inappropriate exercise of Congress' spending power. During the administration of President Donald Trump, Republicans in Congress—even while enjoying a majority in both the Senate and House of Representatives—failed to secure sufficient support to repeal or replace parts of the ACA. However, in late 2017, Republicans were successful in repealing the individual mandate and its associated tax penalty.

Of particular relevance to audiologists and speech-language pathologists are the ACA's Essential Health Benefits. Habilitative and rehabilitative services and devices must be covered by health plans sold on state-based exchanges. The terms "habilitation" and "rehabilitation" have been defined in federal regulation since 2016 using language initially recommended by the National Association of Insurance Commissioners.

Habilitation is defined as "health care services that help a person keep, learn or improve skills and functioning for daily living. Examples include therapy for a child who isn't walking or talking at the expected age. These services may include physical and occupational therapy, speech-language pathology and other services for people with disabilities in a variety of inpatient and/or outpatient settings."

Rehabilitation is defined as "health care services that help a person keep, get back or improve skills and functioning for daily living that have been lost or impaired because a person was sick, hurt or disabled. These services may include physical and occupational therapy, speech-language pathology and psychiatric rehabilitation services in a variety of inpatient and/or outpatient settings."

Habilitative services establish skills that have not yet been acquired at an age-appropriate level. Rehabilitative services and devices help individuals reestablish skills that were acquired at the appropriate age but have been lost or impaired. For example, speech-language treatment for a child with autism spectrum disorder is habilitative; speech-language treatment for an adult with aphasia following a stroke is rehabilitative. A child born with severe to profound hearing loss who is fit with hearing aids receives audiologic habilitation to develop speech and language skills. An adult with hearing loss and tinnitus who is fit with hearings aids equipped with sound generators receives audiologic rehabilitation to improve listening skills and to cope with tinnitus.[3]

Identifying habilitative and rehabilitative services and devices as Essential Health Benefits under the ACA has clearly improved patient access to services provided by audiologists and speech-language pathologists. However, two recent regulatory developments have threatened to undermine the progress gained by the ACA.

The first development concerns state flexibility in defining Essential Health Benefits. Beginning in 2020, states have the authority to change or modify the list of services and devices covered under each Essential Health Benefit category. States also have the authority to substitute benefits both within and between Essential Health Benefit categories provided such substitutions cause no change in value to the overall benchmark plan (i.e., the model benefit that serves as a standard for health plans sold on a state's ACA exchange). This development essentially puts each Essential Health Benefit category in competition with each other, and may lead to a weakening of covered habilitation and rehabilitation services in the coming years, especially if states grapple with budgetary shortfalls or other fiscal challenges.

The second development concerns so-called Short-Term Limited Duration (STLD) plans. STLD plans are primarily designed to provide basic levels of coverage to individuals transitioning between health plans. As such, they provide far less robust coverage and are exempt from coverage mandates promulgated by the ACA, such as covering pre-existing conditions and Essential Health Benefits.

In the wake of the congressional repeal of the ACA's individual mandate in 2017, President Trump issued an Executive Order that directed the Department of Health and Human Services to expand the availability of STLD

---

[3]See American Speech-Language-Hearing Association, *Speech, Language, and Hearing Services: Essential Coverage of Habilitation and Rehabilitation*, (2019). https://www.asha.org/uploadedFiles/ASHA/Practice/Health-Care-Reform/Habilitation-Talking-Points-and-Fact-Sheet.pdf

plans. This action clearly indicated a desire of the President to encourage more Americans to purchase STLD coverage instead of insurance coverage under the ACA-regulated state exchanges. In 2018 the Department of Health and Human Services issued a final rule that expanded STLD coverage to a maximum of 12 months, with an option to renew for an additional 36 months.

The recent development around STLD plans may lead to a weakening of covered habilitation and rehabilitation services in the coming years, as STLD plans are exempt from ACA coverage mandates, and as current federal policy encourages more Americans to purchase STLD coverage at the expense of ACA-compliant health plans.

Medicare Access and CHIP Reauthorization Act

The Medicare Access and CHIP Reauthorization Act (P.L. 114-10), or MACRA, makes sweeping changes to health care reimbursement policy. Enacted into law in 2015, MACRA serves as a principal driving force behind the paradigmatic shift from provider-centered payment models that are based on service volumes and fragmented care toward patient-centered payment models that incentivize health outcomes and high-quality coordinated care.

MACRA established a new policy framework called the Quality Payment Program that sets Medicare payments under Part B to physicians and specified non-physician providers in outpatient and non-facility settings based on high quality and coordinated care. There are two components to the Quality Payment Program: the Merit-based Incentive Payment System (MIPS) and Advanced Alternative Payment Models (AAPMs).

MIPS is Medicare's provider reporting system on high quality and coordinated care. It consolidates three previous reporting systems: the Physician Quality Reporting System (reports quality of care), the Value-based Payment Modifier (reports cost of care), and Meaningful Use (reports utilization of electronic health records). It also adds a new reporting activity on practice improvement. All physicians and specified non-physician providers, including audiologists and speech-language pathologists, are required to report into MIPS if they meet certain patient volume thresholds (see below).

Providers may report into MIPS as individuals or as part of a group in a variety of ways, including claims, a qualified clinical data registry, and electronic health records. Each year, reports generate a score for the quality, cost of care, interoperability, and practice improvement categories. These scores are subsequently combined and weighted to create a final score that is measured against a performance threshold. This deter-

mines a positive or negative payment adjustment. The maximum positive and negative payment adjustments are 9% beginning in 2021. Payment adjustments are distributed on a sliding scale and must remain budget neutral. The adjustments are applied two years after the performance score. In other words, scores achieved by providers in 2019 determine payment adjustments made in 2021.

Reporting into MIPS may be involuntary or voluntary. As of 2019, involuntary or required reporting applies to physicians and non-physician providers, including audiologists and speech-language pathologists, who bill $90,000 or more to Medicare annually, treat 200 or more distinct Medicare beneficiaries annually, and provide 200 or more distinct procedures annually. This current threshold excludes nearly all audiologists and speech-language pathologists from involuntary reporting; however, it is quite possible that this threshold will be progressively lowered in the coming years. Audiologists and speech-language pathologists who meet one or two of the threshold criteria may voluntarily report into MIPS and compete for payment adjustments. Others who meet none of the criteria may voluntarily report into MIPS, but are ineligible for any payment adjustment. As of 2019 audiologists and speech-language pathologists only report into the quality and practice improvement categories.

AAPMs comprise the second component of MACRA's Quality Payment Program. AAPMs are Alternative Payment Models (APMs) endorsed by Medicare that seek to enhance quality and value of services. AAPMs may include a number of existing and emerging APMs, such as Accountable Care Organizations (ACOs), Patient-Centered Medical Homes (PCMHs), and episode-based bundled payments. In order to qualify as an AAPM under Medicare, an APM must demonstrate utilization of quality measures comparable to measures under MIPS, utilization of certified electronic health record technology, and assumed financial risk. Audiologists and speech-language pathologists are eligible to participate in AAPMs as qualifying or partially qualifying participants.

As of 2019, physicians and non-physician providers must receive at least 50% of payments under Medicare Part B through the AAPM or see at least 35% of Medicare beneficiaries through the AAPM in order to be designated as a qualifying participant. Eligible providers may be considered partial qualifying participants if they receive at least 40% of payments under Medicare Part B through the AAPM or see at least 25% of Medicare beneficiaries through the AAPM. Qualifying participants are exempt from MIPS reporting requirements. Partial qualifying participants may voluntary report into MIPS and compete for payment adjustments.

Qualifying participants of a successful AAPM receive an annual 5% lump sum bonus until 2024. Partial qualifying participants will receive a 0.75% positive payment adjustment beginning in 2026.

Patient Driven Payment Model

APMs are not just limited to Medicare Part B. Efforts to identify innovative ways by which to improve the quality of care and reduce costs are taking place across the public and private reimbursement landscape. Notably, the ACA supports the development of APMs, such as ACOs and PCMHs. Audiologists and speech-language pathologists have the ability to participate in ACO entities and PCMH practices as ancillary providers. To date, the overall effectiveness of APMs in achieving quality and cost targets have been mixed. Some APMs have successfully improved health outcomes while lowering overall costs relative to fee-for-service payment models. Other APMs have been less successful. As of 2019, ongoing efforts are underway to identify what APMs are most suitable for audiologist and speech-language pathologist participation.

Beginning in 2019, an APM with significant impact to speech-language pathology services is the Patient Driven Payment Model (PDPM). Developed by CMS, the PDPM radically changes how speech-language pathology services are paid for in SNFs.[4]

Prior to October 2019, speech-language pathology services, along with occupational and physical therapy services, were paid under the Resource Utilization Group, Version IV (RUG-IV). RUG-IV was a prospective payment system that based payments on a case-mix model that favored volume and quantity of services over the value and quality of services. CMS determined that RUG-IV was providing inappropriate financial incentives to SNF providers by not taking into consideration a patient's unique clinical characteristics, needs, or goals. The PDPM was consequently developed as a way to remove this incentive and improve the overall value and quality of care.

As an APM, the PDPM bases payments on a patient's unique clinical characteristics. Payments for patients who demonstrate a need for speech-language pathology services are based on the presence of five case-mix factors: the patient's primary diagnosis, the presence of at least 1 of 10 identified comorbidities, a mechanically alternated diet, a swallowing disorder, and a cognitive impairment. These case-mix factors are used in part to score the patient. A patient who meets the criteria for all five factors receives a higher score than a patient who meets the criteria for three factors and so forth. The higher score translates into higher payments for speech-language pathology services.

The PDPM model also addresses the provision of concurrent (treatment of two patients at the same time) and group therapy (treatment of at least four residents at the same time) in SNFs. Under the RUG-IV model, the amount of group therapy provided to a patient was capped at 25% per discipline while there was no cap on the provision of concurrent therapy. The PDPM model retains the 25% cap of group therapy, and also applies a 25% cap on concurrent therapy. This cap is designed to ensure that individualized therapy is appropriately provided to patients when deemed clinically appropriate.

The PDPM promises to improve the overall quality and value of services provided to a SNF patient. It is too early to ascertain whether the model is successful at the time of this publication. Nevertheless, it is critically important that speech-language pathologists remain employed by SNFs to provide the services that fall within the profession's scope. It is equally important that the PDPM ensures the provision of speech-language pathology services that are both clinically necessary and appropriate to the patient.

Summary

As the end of the second decade of the twenty-first century draws to a close, the political environment of the United States has become complex and uncertain. Despite the current political environment, recent health care legislation and regulation, particularly around reimbursement policy, have had a profound impact on the professions of audiology and speech-language pathology. This impact has been chiefly caused by the paradigmatic shift under way from provider-centered payment models that are based on service volumes and fragmented care towards patient-centered payment models that incentivize health outcomes and high-quality coordinated care. This shift is most apparent in Medicare, Medicaid, and private insurance. The Affordable Care Act, the Medicare CHIP Reauthorization Act, and the Patient Driven Payment Model are three principal legislative and regulatory issues of particular importance to audiologists and speech-language pathologists, and how the professions provide and bill for health care services. Ongoing work is needed to ensure that audiology and speech-language pathology services are appropriately delivered and properly valued in these emerging health care delivery and payment services.

---

[4]See American-Speech-Language Hearing Association, *The Medicare Patient-Driven Payment Model (PDPM) Toolkit*. (2019). https://www.asha.org/Practice/reimbursement/medicare/Medicare-Patient-Driven-Payment-Model

Critical Thinking

1. How has health care legislation and regulation principally impacted the professions of audiology and speech-language pathology over the past decade?

2. What are the four parts of Medicare? What parts of Medicare do audiologists and speech-language pathologists principally participate in?

3. What audiology services does Medicare cover? What audiology services are not covered?

4. What qualifications are required of audiologists and speech-language pathologists to participate in Medicaid?

5. What approaches do private insurers generally use to set payment rates?

6. Why are coding systems important to the professions of audiology and speech-language pathology?

7. What are the principal objectives of the Affordable Care Act? What part of the Affordable Care Act bears particular relevance to the habilitation and rehabilitation services?

8. What was the main objective of the Medicare and CHIP Reauthorization Act? What are the two principal components of the MACRA's Quality Payment Program, and why are they each important?

9. What are the changes being implemented to payments for speech-language pathology services in skilled nursing facilities?

10. What professional opportunities do you see in the current health care policy landscape? What challenges do you see?

References

Agency for Healthcare Research and Quality—Patient-Centered Medical Home. Retrieved from https://pcmh.ahrq.gov/

American Medical Association—Current Procedural Terminology (CPT). Retrieved from https://www.ama-assn.org/amaone/cpt-current-procedural-terminology

American Medical Association. Retrieved from https://www.ama-assn.org/

American Medical Association—RVS Update Committee (RUC). Retrieved from https://www.ama-assn.org/about/rvs-update-committee-ruc

American Speech-Language-Hearing Association. Billing and Reimbursement Resources. Retrieved from https://www.asha.org/practice/reimbursement/

America's Health Insurance Plans. Retrieved from https://www.ahip.org/

Center for Consumer Information and Insurance Oversight—Affordable Care Act Essential Health Benefits. Retrieved from https://www.cms.gov/cciio/resources/data-resources/ehb.html

Centers for Disease Control and Prevention—ICD-10. Retrieved from https://www.cdc.gov/nchs/icd/icd10cm.htm

Centers for Medicare and Medicaid Services—Accountable Care Organizations. Retrieved from https://innovation.cms.gov/initiatives/aco/

Centers for Medicare and Medicaid Services—EPSDT. Retrieved from https://www.medicaid.gov/medicaid/benefits/epsdt/index.html

Centers for Medicare and Medicaid Services—Healthcare Common Procedure Coding System. Retrieved from https://www.cms.gov/medicare/coding/medhcpcsgeninfo/index.html

Centers for Medicare and Medicaid Services—ICD-10 (specific to Medicare and Medicaid). Retrieved from https://www.cms.gov/medicare/coding/icd10/

Centers for Medicare and Medicaid Services—Local Coverage Determinations. Retrieved from https://www.cms.gov/Medicare/Coverage/DeterminationProcess/LCDs.html

Centers for Medicare and Medicaid Services—Medicaid. Retrieved from https://www.medicaid.gov/

Centers for Medicare and Medicaid Services—Medicare. Retrieved from https://www.medicare.gov/

Centers for Medicare and Medicaid Services—Medicare Administrative Contractors. Retrieved from https://www.cms.gov/Medicare/Medicare-Contracting/Medicare-Administrative-Contractors/What-is-a-MAC.html

Centers for Medicare and Medicaid Services—Medicare Benefit Policy Manual. Retrieved from https://www.cms.gov/Regulations-and-Guidance/Guidance/Manuals/Internet-Only-Manuals-Ioms-Items/Cms012673.html

Centers for Medicare and Medicaid Services—Medicare Physician Fee Schedule. Retrieved from https://www.cms.gov/medicare/medicare-fee-for-service-payment/physicianfeesched/

Centers for Medicare and Medicaid Services—Patient-Driven Payment Models. Retrieved from https://www.cms.gov/Medicare/Medicare-Fee-for-Service-Payment/SNFPPS/PDPM.html

Centers for Medicare and Medicaid Services—Quality Payment Program. Retrieved from https://www.cms.gov/Medicare/Quality-Payment-Program/Quality-Payment-Program.html

Centers for Medicare and Medicaid Services—Recovery Audit Contractors. Retrieved from https://www.cms.gov/Research-statistics-data-and-systems/monitoring-programs/medicare-FFS-compliance-programs/recovery-audit-program/index.html

Families USA. Retrieved from https://familiesusa.org/

Henry J. Kaiser Family Foundation. Retrieved from https://www.kff.org/

Medical Billing and Coding Certification. Retrieved from https://www.medicalbillingandcoding.org/

U.S. Department of Health and Human Services—Affordable Care Act Essential Health Benefits. Retrieved from https://www.healthcare.gov/glossary/essential-health-benefits/

U.S. Department of Health and Human Services—Affordable Care Act Overview. Retrieved from https://www.hhs.gov/healthcare/index.html

15

Service Delivery in Health Care Settings

◇◇◇

Alex Johnson, PhD and Jeffrey Johnson, PhD

Scope of Chapter

This chapter addresses key professional issues that impact speech-language pathologists (SLPs) and audiologists in health care settings. Professionals from these disciplines serve patients with a variety of health conditions, lead and teach other practitioners and learners, promote best and evidence-based practice, advocate for patients and their discipline, and deal with a variety of unique ethical and regulatory issues. At the center of the various activities associated with service delivery in health care settings is the primary responsibility of the clinician to provide excellent, safe, affordable care for those being served. Beyond the core commitment to the patient are collaboration with the health care team and service to the profession.

The first section of this chapter summarizes the various locations and settings in which health care is delivered: acute care, rehabilitation, specialty focused hospitals, extended settings, and outpatient settings. Because the nature of the work and its primary focus and goals change by setting, it is important for current and future practitioners to understand these differences. Much of the information provided applies to both SLPs and audiologists.

The second part of the chapter summarizes several complex and dynamic foci of modern health care. Interprofessionalism is an emerging topic of discussion that affects preparation of professionals and behavioral aspects of service delivery by members of various disciplines (including our own), and it competes with traditional (and more simplistic) concepts of autonomy with a collective focus on best practice and patient care. Health care disparities represent yet another special concern that is well documented in the literature. Issues of patient safety, health literacy, and documentation are discussed in this chapter as well.

The concept of evidence-based practice (EBP) is central to almost every discussion of clinical service delivery in audiology and speech-language pathology. Reviewed thoroughly in Chapter 8 of this text, the principles of EBP (using relevant scientific data, focusing on the wishes and needs of the patient, and aligning the data and patient wishes with the expertise and experience of the clinician) underlie the discussion that follows. In every clinical situation across the health care continuum, the principles and strategies of EBP are relevant and should be applied. Using the highest level of evidence available goes far to protect patients, clinicians, and institutions from faddish or unproven approaches, while ensuring quality, patient-centric care.

Finally, this chapter examines trends that will affect and/or drive the future of service delivery in these settings. Preparation of competent and qualified clinicians, degree status and certification programs, and the status of research are some of the topics briefly discussed with the emerging professional in mind.

Health Care Settings and Key Responsibilities

Settings

Speech-language pathologists and audiologists work across a continuum of health care settings. For the individual unfamiliar with some of the specific characteristics of each of these settings, this brief introductory description is provided and summarized in Table 15–1.

The key point for consideration here is appreciation of the unique purpose of each setting within the overall health care enterprise. A secondary point is consideration of the skill and/or knowledge set that may be most useful in that particular type of setting. It is important to note that experience in one setting may not serve as adequate preparation for service in another setting. Clinicians who move across the continuum need significant flexibility, extensive and appropriate background preparation, and essential orientation and competency in program development to be effective and successful. The American Speech-Language-Hearing Association (ASHA, 2019) reported that 39.3% of members were employed in health settings. An additional 19% were employed in private practice and it can be assumed that a significant portion of these individuals provide in-patient services on a contractual basis to patients in health care facilities or to outpatients with rehabilitative needs.

The ASHA membership survey (ASHA, 2019) also provides data regarding audiology members of ASHA: 73.6% of audiologists work in health care, and of this group 26.7% work in hospital settings, 17.1% in nonresidential health care facilities, and 9.7% in skilled nursing settings in other residential facilities.

Acute care hospitals can be differentiated across a number of criteria, which are important for prospective clinicians to understand. In general, *acute care hospitals* are those hospitals in which patients are admitted for care (typically short term) for an acute illness or for management of problems of such complexity that they cannot be diagnosed or treated in outpatient or other settings. Within the broad category of acute care, several

additional descriptors can be helpful in appreciating various roles and differences. Some acute care hospitals provide the most advanced levels of life support, advanced procedures, and surgeries and are able to handle patients with the most complex diseases. These *tertiary care hospitals* are usually located in large metropolitan areas, may be university affiliated (i.e., academic medical centers), have a significant physician education component, and are staffed and technologically designed to handle the most complex medical cases. These hospitals are typically large, to accommodate a large specialty staff of physicians. Typically, these hospitals have a staff of SLPs who are employed to handle the volume of inpatients and outpatients. When otolaryngology, neurology, or neurosurgery are key specialty components, audiologists may also be employed to provide inpatient and outpatient hearing assessment, vestibular testing, and/or intraoperative monitoring, as well as habilitation/rehabilitation of hearing.

A second type of acute care hospital is the *more general community* or *rural hospital*. General hospitals vary in size depending on the geographic area and population served. They may emphasize some aspects of specialty care, are more likely to be staffed by primary care physicians and general surgeons, and have a number of specialists on call. The emergency departments of these hospitals are designed to manage common illnesses and traumas and are typically not organized to receive the most complex cases. A common staffing pattern for speech-language pathology in this setting would be one or two staff SLPs (more in larger institutions). Audiologists may also be on staff to provide assessment and rehabilitation services, often on an outpatient basis.

Another example of an acute care hospital is the *long-term acute care hospital (LTACH)*. These hospitals are designed to provide specialty care to patients with acute illnesses who require a longer stay (more than 25 days) than the average of 4 to 5 days that is typical of many tertiary care hospitals. Many of these specialty hospitals focus specifically on two populations of great interest for SLPs: ventilator-dependent individuals and those who have sustained traumatic brain injury. When these are predominant patient populations, skilled SLPs are required to assist in dysphagia and communication management and rehabilitation.

Two more types of acute specialty hospitals should be mentioned: *pediatric specialty hospitals* and *designated cancer hospitals*. Most pediatric specialty hospitals in the United States operate in a manner similar to the tertiary care hospitals described previously, serving acute patients with complex diseases and staffed by a variety of specialists. Pediatric hospitals also have the specific mission of being child-centric and family-centric. They are particularly attuned to the illnesses of childhood and

Table 15–1. Unique Characteristics of SLP Practice by Health Setting

Setting	Brief Description	SLP Caseload Medical Diagnosis	Most Common SLP Diagnoses	Essential Clinical Skills
Acute care	▪ Hospitalization for management of complex medical problems ▪ Requires specialized medical, nursing, surgical, and extensive availability of other services	▪ Respiratory Diseases (24%) ▪ Cerebrovascular Diseases (20%) ▪ Head Injury (5%) (*Source:* "National Outcomes Measurement System. Adults in Healthcare–Acute Hospital National Data Report 2017," 2017)	▪ Dysphagia (83%) ▪ Cognitive-Comm Disorder (22%) ▪ Aphasia (11.2%) ▪ Dysarthria (7.6%) (*Source:* "National Outcomes Measurement System. Adults in Healthcare–Acute Hospital National Data Report 2017," 2017)	▪ Differential diagnosis ▪ Interpretation of medical information on communication disorders ▪ Advanced interprofessional skills ▪ Consultative communication skills ▪ Competency in MBS, FEES, trach/vent management skills, bedside language, speech, voice assessment
Inpatient rehabilitation	▪ Hospitalization for immediate post-hospital rehabilitation needs ▪ At least 3 hours per day of rehabilitation treatment	▪ Respiratory Diseases (29%) ▪ Cerebrovascular Diseases (21%) ▪ Head Injury (5%) (*Source:* "National Outcomes Measurement System: Adults in Healthcare–Inpatient Rehab National Data Report 2017," 2017)	▪ Dysphagia (63%) ▪ Cognitive-Comm Disorder (43.4%) ▪ Aphasia (11%) (*Source:* "National Outcomes Measurement System: Adults in Healthcare–Inpatient Rehab National Data Report 2017," 2017)	▪ Comprehensive assessment and treatment skills ▪ Skills in outcomes and change measurement ▪ Management of complex language, cognitive, and dysphagia disorders ▪ Family and team communication skills ▪ Advanced collaboration and interprofessional skills ▪ Post-discharge planning and management skills

continues

Table 15–1. *continued*

Setting	Brief Description	SLP Caseload Medical Diagnosis	Most Common SLP Diagnoses	Essential Clinical Skills
Outpatient	■ Variety of settings including hospitals, clinics, medical offices, and independent private SLP practice	■ Cerebrovascular Disease (32.6%) ■ CNS Diseases (11.7%) ■ Head Injury (11.3%) ■ Respiratory Diseases (8.9%) (*Source:* "National Outcomes Measurement System. Adults in Healthcare-Outpatient National Data Report 2017," 2017)	■ Cognitive-Comm Disorder (40%) ■ Aphasia (25%) ■ Voice (21.8%) ■ Dysphagia (21.5%) ■ Dysarthria (18%) (*Source:* "National Outcomes Measurement System. Adults in Healthcare-Outpatient National Data Report 2017," 2017)	■ Long-term patient management skills ■ Additional skills in both group and individual therapy ■ Skill in educating, counseling, and assuring follow-up with families ■ Outcomes measurement ■ Efficiency in management of therapy termination ■ Business-related skills, especially in private practice
Skilled nursing	■ Offers subacute rehabilitation services for patients with complex medical conditions, unable to tolerate more intensive rehabilitation ■ At least 1–2 hours of daily rehabilitation treatment	■ Mental Disorders (12.5%) ■ Cerebrovascular Disease (10.5%) ■ Respiratory Diseases (8.7%) ■ CNS Diseases (8.6 %)	■ Dysphagia (61.9%) ■ Cognitive-Comm Disorder (49%) ■ Aphasia (5.9%)	■ See inpatient rehabilitation skills (above) ■ Communication and advocacy skills focused on elderly persons ■ Competence in independent clinical decision making ■ Ability to deal with larger corporate structures
Hospice/palliative	■ Addresses either end of life or quality of life issues in persons with severe or terminal illnesses	■ Any severe or chronic condition that affects communication of basic needs or swallowing, particularly after medical treatments have been decreased	■ Dysphagia ■ Neurogenic Language or Speech Disorders ■ Cognitive Disorders	■ Application of ethical and clinical reasoning ■ Ability to adapt tools and resources to achieve maximum functionality with least patient/family effort ■ Use of communication technologies ■ Adaptive feeding/swallowing skills

the stressors that are common when a child is ill, and usually have programs and staff customized to address this very important group of patients and their families. Because of the common intersection of communicative/swallowing disorders with childhood illness and disease, it is common for SLPs and audiologists to be employed as part of a large outpatient or inpatient service in this setting. A second setting, designated *cancer hospitals*, provides care to patients with focus on treatment, management, and end-of-life issues associated with cancer. The federal government has designated a number of cancer centers throughout the country, and it is common for these to be associated with other large medical institutions. SLPs in these settings are typically employed in order to serve patients with head and neck cancer, brain tumors, or other cancers that affect communication or swallowing in children and adults.

Several *post-acute settings* may also employ SLPs and audiologists. These include *rehabilitation hospitals*, where patients typically have a short post-acute period of rehabilitation, as well as *skilled nursing facilities* where patients may receive rehabilitation, but with less intensity than in the acute rehabilitation setting. In each of these settings, SLPs and audiologists may be involved in assessment and treatment, although audiologists are less likely to be included while SLPs are almost always utilized in an attempt to help patients restore function. These settings can be described along continua of acuity, complexity of cases, and prognosis. For example, patients admitted from the acute care setting to the rehabilitation hospital will have significant remaining complications, may have multiple problems needing skilled rehabilitative *and* medical/nursing care, and will have a prognosis that is more positive, even when it is not for full recovery. When patients cannot tolerate the required three hours per day of rehabilitation, or if they have factors that negatively contribute to their prognosis but could still benefit from rehabilitation, they are typically admitted to a skilled nursing setting that has a rehabilitation component, including speech-language pathology services. It is rare for audiologists to have a full-time appointment in this setting, although contractual arrangements may be in place for individual patient consultation. Patients in skilled nursing settings are seen for post-acute convalescent recovery, with a plan for discharge to home or for transfer to a long-term care environment. In these settings, rehabilitation activities may be slower paced than in the rehabilitation hospital, but this is not necessarily the case and the goals of treatment, as always, are based on the patient's personal goals and capacity. A larger number of patients in these settings are likely to have dementia, and many will have dysphagia and its associated complications with nutrition and feeding.

Another location of post-acute care that is quickly growing is *home care*. Now, more than at any time in the past, clinicians can serve patients in the home who are more ill or have complex illnesses. Through the use of new protocols and with advanced technology, patients are being discharged from the hospital earlier than ever. Many SLPs now work primarily in the home setting. Home care organizations may be aligned with specific hospitals or may be independent and accept referrals from many acute or rehabilitation settings. Speech-language pathologists are frequently employed by these agencies as either independent contractors or employees who provide skilled rehabilitation in the home. It is not uncommon for SLPs in this environment to also be required by the employing home health agency to provide some routine health services (e.g., blood pressure monitoring, suctioning).

A final post-acute setting is that of *hospice care*. Hospice is provided for patients for whom the goals have changed to comfort rather than cure or prolongation of life. Most hospice care is provided in the patient's home, but approximately 20% is provided in inpatient settings (National Hospice and Palliative Care Organization, 2009). The role of speech-language pathologists or audiologists in hospice is limited, given that rehabilitation is not a goal. However, given that comfort and quality of life are particular foci in hospice, the SLP or audiologist has a role in ensuring that communication is maintained with family and staff via external supports and technology, that caregivers understand helpful ways to communicate with the patient, and that the eating process is comfortable and safe. Family and staff may also need education about communication and/or swallowing. Pollens (2004) provides guidance for the SLP interested in working in palliative hospice care.

The third general category of care is the *outpatient setting*. Patients may be seen as outpatients after a hospitalization if further inpatient care is no longer indicated. Commonly, the SLP or the audiologist may see patients with clinical conditions that do not require hospitalization for evaluation and treatment. Examples include patients with a variety of conditions (e.g., dementia, head injury, voice disorders, neurodegenerative diseases). Some outpatient settings are multidisciplinary, rehabilitation-focused programs, while others have services limited to SLP or audiology. In these outpatient settings, it is possible for services to be delivered via a hospital or agency where the clinician is an employee or by a private practitioner who is self-employed.

A final point about the setting in which services are provided should be acknowledged. Regardless of the physical setting where the patient is seen, it is likely that *every* SLP or audiologist will see patients with communication disorders that are health related. Frequently, an assumption is made that school-age children have communication disorders that are educationally relevant and that health concerns are handled by the medical SLP. In recent years, however, school-based speech-language pathologists have seen increased school participation by children with serious health-related conditions (Ballard & Dymond, 2018; Lefton-Greif & Arvedson, 2008). Thus, all speech-language pathologists need to develop expertise in serving individuals with health-related communication disabilities, regardless of the setting of their employment. This role is not new for school-based clinicians, however the increased frequency and complexity of children with health concerns places considerable demands on the work of already busy SLPs in school settings. It is incumbent on clinicians from medical settings to assure that school based SLPs have access to necessary information and resources to support the children they serve.

Routine Considerations for Speech-Language Pathologists and Audiologists in Health Care

As noted, individuals with health-related conditions that affect communication and swallowing may be seen in any of the settings in which clinicians practice. There are a specific set of considerations that impact the way SLPs and audiologists can and should practice. This section focuses on these concerns and their effect on the nature of service delivery in the health care setting.

Health Status of the Patient

For every patient seen in a given health setting, the primary concern is the health status of the patient. When a patient comes for diagnostic services, accurate and timely diagnosis is a critical factor in managing the patient's condition. When a patient comes for audiology, speech, language, or swallowing treatment, the clinician should ensure that the patient is safe, make note of any significant changes in behavior that could have medical significance, and be cognizant of the overarching medical diagnosis and understand its implications for rehabilitation. The general medical diagnosis and prognosis are key factors in determining the purpose of the evaluation or treatment referral and contribute to decision making about the nature of any approach to intervention that will ensue. For example, the young patient with a traumatic brain injury or post-stroke aphasia may be an excellent candidate for rigorous rehabilitation provided by the speech-language pathologist. An approach that is quite different may be appropriate for the individual

with progressive deterioration in neurological function, for whom a more palliative approach to assistance may be in order. Thus, the speech-language pathologist is obligated to understand the implications of the patient's health status on communication and swallowing, and understand the impact of that condition on the communication/swallowing prognosis and potential benefit for rehabilitation.

Safety

A second issue of great concern in all health settings today is patient safety (Institute for Health Care Improvement, 2011). The implications of disorders of speech-language or hearing on patient safety are not well documented. The effects of language impairment and cognitive, perceptual, or sensory difficulties on compliance with medical or nursing instructions remain undocumented with specific regard to patient safety issues. A growing literature summarizes the effect of low health literacy on patient compliance with such tasks as following medication instructions or other directions from care providers (Davis, Jacklin, Sevdalis, & Vincent, 2007). A logical extension of this literacy concern suggests that the SLP or audiologist should ensure that patients understand and can participate in decision making about their own care. This is especially important in inpatient settings where the pace can be fast, and a patient's misunderstanding or lack of hearing can be misinterpreted as cognitive impairment. In these situations, SLPs and audiologists should be conscious of the need for advocacy, provide assistive devices to augment communication or hearing, and advocate for these needs for patients under their care. When patients are knowledgeable about their condition and can obtain the information needed for informed decision making, they are safer. Woods (2006) cites six factors that make communication challenging for patients: gender, cultural/ethnic factors, health literacy level, socioeconomic factors, time/urgency factors, and personality/behavioral factors. Certainly, the nature and severity of the communication disorder represents an additional critical factor for those in the care of a speech-language pathologist or audiologist.

Another obvious area of safety concern for the clinician occurs when invasive procedures are necessary or certain patient risk factors are present. Examples of invasive procedures provided by speech-language pathologists include videostroboscopy, insertion and removal of laryngeal prostheses, and a number of swallowing procedures. Also, some speech-language pathologists and audiologists are involved in intraoperative monitoring during laryngeal, otologic, or neurosurgical procedures. When involved in these types of activities, clinicians should have demonstrated competence in carrying out the task, have documented institutional authorization, and should know any risks associated with the procedure. Appropriate precautions and personnel should be available in case of complications. Competency for these higher risk tasks can be established in a number of ways, including demonstration and observation over repeated opportunities, clinician testing and interviewing, simulation tasks, or written examinations. The American Speech-Language-Hearing Association provides a number of documents to assist members who are involved in performing these tasks.

It is important that those who are engaged in high-risk professional activities (or supervising others) have validated competence and that this is documented clearly. This protects the practitioner and the institution from unnecessary complications if an adverse situation arises. Most important, it protects the patient from incompetent or inexperienced practitioners, increasing the probability of a safe and satisfactory clinical outcome.

Infection Control

Clinicians in all settings should be knowledgeable experts in all aspects of infection control, ensuring that they have minimized patient (and staff) risk for exposure to infection. Appropriate procedures for cleaning or disposing of equipment and supplies that have been exposed should be established and followed. All clinicians should know procedures for isolation precaution, hand hygiene, and medical waste disposal. All hospitals require employees to be knowledgeable in this area and are required to provide necessary training. Prevention of disease transmission should be a consideration with every professional interaction. See Chapter 22, "Safety in the Workplace," for more information.

Requirements for best practice regarding safety standards are generated by a number of sources including state and local health departments, The Joint Commission (formerly JCAHO), the Occupational Safety and Health Administration (OSHA), and the Centers for Disease Control and Prevention (CDC). In most institutional settings, all providers of health care are required to demonstrate knowledge of safety requirements. In general, The Joint Commission, an accrediting body, reviews compliance with institutional safety and quality standards on a regular basis and provides recommendations for improvement when needed. ASHA has provided a website to assist practitioners to understand a variety of issues related to The Joint Commission (ASHA, n.d.). This site provides information about patient safety issues, dealing with hospital culture and diversity, and sentinel events.

OSHA (https://www. osha.gov) has as its focus protection of workers. Thus, clinicians who are exposed to risk from radiation or infectious material should be familiar with OSHA standards. The CDC is concerned with preventing and managing general health concerns in the United States. Clinicians with concerns about disease outbreaks or specific information about various conditions can find a variety of alerts and general content on the CDC website (https://www.cdc.gov).

Measuring Change, Progress, and Outcomes

General principles and specific practices associated with assessment and diagnosis in health care settings are beyond the scope of this chapter. Typically introduced in graduate curricula and practica, lifelong learning of clinical skills is the goal of every competent practitioner in SLP and audiology. These essential skills are covered comprehensively in common texts used in graduate education. A topic sometimes overlooked in disorder-specific discussions is that of measurement of change over time, which may indicate progress, deterioration, or plateauing. These observations are critical to decisions about the patient.

The benefit to the patient and the family is the centerpiece of all work in communication disorders. Benefit (or lack of it) can be measured from multiple perspectives along a continuum from short-term behavioral change to significant change in health status, participation in functional activities, or overall quality of life. In the various health care settings, early changes in communication, cognition, or swallowing can signal the very beginning of recovery. Intermediate levels of progress are seen in recovery of functional skills in listening, attention, understanding, reading and writing, and conversation. The most desired and challenging stages of communication progress are observed when patients' functional abilities are either restored or maximized so that their participation in life activities is enabled rather than disrupted by their communication, hearing, or swallowing abilities. It is worth noting that rarely are these changes attained in a simple, orderly manner. Patients may show progress in one domain of communication while experiencing little gain in another aspect. Thus, to document and measure change across the continuum of health care settings (and patient acuity), many different tools and approaches may be necessary.

Measures are critically important to everyone involved in the care process. Evidence of change and outcome are the basis for decisions related to reimbursement. They also provide guidance for the clinician as to whether treatment is beneficial and should be continued. Conversely, these measures provide support for the decision to stop treatment when minimal benefit is documented (even when ongoing assessment adjustments to the plan of treatment were made to optimize gain). Measures of change or outcome are usually based on assessments of the patient's perceived benefit, the clinician's judgment of change, or objective measures of communication performance.

Patient Self-Assessment Measures

Patients are often the best judges of the benefits of services received. Table 15–2 displays a number of tools that have been developed to help clinicians reliably quantify benefit and/or change from the patient's perspective. Most of these measures are designed to measure the patient's view of the degree of functional impairment or progress, as opposed to improving understanding of the underlying causative mechanisms. Eadie et al. (2006) provide a critical review of the psychometric adequacy of self-report mechanisms in speech-language pathology. In general, the assessment of outcomes and progress should include the patient's perspective, ensuring that the clinician and patient agree on the benefit of treatment or other interventions. At times, when a patient cannot respond to the demands of the task, a family member or other caregiver may need to assist with collection of the measurements. While this approach

compromises the validity of some assessment tools, it may provide a useful perspective from the view of the patient or the patient's proxy.

Performance-Based Measurement Tools

Numerous outcomes tools have been developed for measuring patient progress in various settings. Many of these tools are based on a classification proposed by the World Health Organization (WHO) *International Classification of Functioning, Disability, and Health (ICF)* (2001), which classified key factors associated with functioning and disability. The ICF classification is based on various categories of body functions and structures, as well as associated activity limitations, impairments, or participation restrictions. The ICF model has been adopted by the American Speech-Language-Hearing Association as foundational to scopes of practice in both audiology and speech-language pathology. In essence, the ICF model focuses on the person, their abilities, and any limitations to carrying out basic bodily functions (e.g., swallowing, breathing, hearing) and activities (e.g., talking, reading, writing, comprehending) or participating in important life activities (e.g., social relationships, work, school, community). The ICF is

Table 15–2. Sampling of Speech-Language-Hearing Patient Self-Assessment Tools Used in Health Care Settings

Focus	Instrument Title	Author (Year)
Communication	ASHA Quality of Communication Life	Paul et al. (2004)
Stroke/aphasia	Burden of Stroke Scale (BOSS)	Doyle et al. (2004)
Voice	Voice Handicap Index	Jacobson et al. (1997)
Aphasia	Aphasia Communication Outcome Measure (ACOM)	Hula et al. (2015)
Parkinsons, ALS, MS	Communication Participation Item Bank	Baylor et al. (2013)
Dysphagia	Dysphagia Handicap Index (DHI)	Silbergleit et al. (2012)
Dysphagia	Swallowing Quality of Life (Swal-QOL)	McHorney et al. (2000)
Aphasia	Assessment of Living with Aphasia	Simmons-Mackie et al. (2014)
Hearing	Hearing Handicap Inventory for Adults (HHIE)	Newman et al. (1990)

designed to encompass all aspects of human function and participation across the lifespan. It also considers the role that an individual's environment impacts health, functioning, and human performance. Thus, the ICF provides a model that allows practitioners from across various fields to consider priorities, goals, and desired outcomes for various treatment and/or rehabilitation activities. SLPs and audiologists can use the ICF as a tool to assist with clinical decision making and goal setting for their clients/patients.

One of the most widely used general measures in rehabilitation settings is the *Functional Independence Measure* (FIM) (Keith, Granger, Hamilton, & Sherwin, 1987). The FIM is a descriptive measure, completed by the clinician and designed to measure change in a number of areas including communication. Because the FIM provides a global measure of communication in the context of other areas of function (walking, eating, etc.), there has been interest in the development of communication-specific tools that provide a more detailed focus on a variety of components of speech-language and swallowing. One set of measures, *Functional Communication Measures* (ASHA, 2003), is now part of ASHA's National Outcomes Measurement System (NOMS). Use of these measures for communication and swallowing allows for assessment of the benefit of treatment services for a given patient, while also measuring the effectiveness of a particular program or service to a group of patients. Thus, the outcomes obtained from these analyses allow for a clinical service to be modified or improved based on results.

As part of their professional preparation, all professionals in speech-language pathology and audiology have been exposed to dozens of specific measurement approaches for diagnosis and assessment. Many of these tools (i.e., standardized tests of language or speech, the modified barium swallow, audiometric testing, vestibular studies, oral mechanism examination, and so on) provide a valuable window to selected functions, allowing careful description of behaviors and some underlying mechanisms as well. While these tools are essential for diagnosis and assessment, they are not always the best measures for studying patient change and progress, especially when the outcomes goal is a change in function rather than specific physiologic, cognitive, or linguistic change. Thus, it is best to use measures that are valid and integrative and include the combined perspective of the clinician and the patient to assess progress and then document it.

Documentation

SLPs or audiologists should address any questions and concerns raised by the referring specialist or primary care provider. Responses to referral sources should be clear, direct, timely, and accurate. Good guidelines for report writing and consultation can be found in a number of sources; however, only a few such sources specifically focus on writing reports and notes specifically for health settings (ASHA, 2011; Kummer, Johnson, & Zeit, 2007). Johnson and Jacobson (2007, 2016) have also written about the errors in patient care attributed to poor or incomplete documentation. Some of the errors associated with documentation are summarized in Table 15–3.

Documentation, as provided by the speech-language pathologist, serves a variety of priorities. These priorities include (1) educating and informing the referral source and other providers, (2) documenting progress toward goals and additional behavioral/clinical observations,

Table 15–3. Ten Exemplars of SLP or Audiology Communication or Documentation Errors

1. Failure to report results of high-risk or invasive procedures with accuracy or timeliness.

2. Failure to document sufficient for others to provide necessary follow-up.

3. Failure to document supervision of non-licensed (or non-certified) personnel.

4. Failure to document results from evaluations that could have diagnostic significance or could change the medical plan of care.

5. Failure to document observation of changes in patient behavior that could signal altered medical or psychological status.

6. Failure to document appropriate informed consent for any research activities that include the patient.

7. Producing diagnostic statements or interpretations outside the scope of practice or not substantiated with data or observations.

8. Failure to ensure confidentiality of patient information.

9. Failure to communicate beyond the written record (e.g., call attention to significant findings) when timing or urgency are important factors.

10. Failure to communicate clearly and appropriately with patients and their caregivers.

(3) reporting on any adverse events or outcomes, and (4) ensuring that information required for compliance or reimbursement is available.

As the first priority, documentation that educates and informs the referral source and others involved in the care of the patient is a critical component of the care process for all patients. Most important, initial speech-language-swallowing-hearing consultations should address the question of the referral source. Conley, Jordan, and Ghali (2009) reported that 25 percent of referral notes do not contain a clear question, so SLPs completing initial consultations should be sure to obtain clarity before proceeding with evaluation or treatment. Numerous publications describe good report writing guidelines, and novice speech-language pathologists should review these. In health settings, especially in hospital documentation, reports may be produced using an electronic medical records system that does not allow for the type of writing recommended in common SLP texts. Regardless of the format required, notes should be concise and clear (avoiding SLP terms that the referral source might not know) and should add information that will be helpful in subsequent decision making and patient care.

Second, when the patient is being seen for treatment beyond the initial consultation, it is important to document the goals and the response to treatment. Again, the approach to doing this will be setting dependent; however, the principles of the *SOAP* approach (subjective, objective, assessment, plan) are widely used by SLPs in clinical settings. This SOAP approach, introduced by Weed (1970), has been adapted to many clinical disciplines and is well understood within the health care enterprise. This method is familiar to colleagues in medicine, nursing, and other health fields. It allows for easy retrieval of relevant information, elimination of irrelevant observations, and clear statement of "next steps," an area that is frequently of great interest to those involved in managing hospital stays for patients. Table 15–4 offers some brief guidance for producing SOAP notes. Chapter 20 discusses documentation issues in more detail.

At the time of the writing of this chapter, the implementation of the Electronic Medical Record (EMR) is increasingly realized across the health system. As of

Table 15–4. What Are SOAP Notes?

Comment Type	Description	SLP Example
Subjective	Describe patient's emotional, physical, cognitive status; include general observations about patient's mood, appearance, attitude, or conduct.	The patient was lethargic. The patient refused to cooperate with the examination.
Objective	Summarize data related to stated goals; include measurable information. Compare data from current session to previous sessions.	The patient was able to accurately repeat 20 out of 30 multisyllabic words today; yesterday he was able to repeat 8 words. The patient was able to sustain vocalization for 12 secs.
Assessment	Interpret the data and observations that have been noted in the current session.	The patient's performance on the oral motor exam showed increased strength. The patient's scores on the test are supported by the increase in intelligibility noted in conversational speech.
Plan	Based on the assessment of what has occurred, describe the next steps. Changes in goals or recommended activities, changes in therapy scheduling or frequency, and any needed referrals might be included. Also, document any recommendations for family members.	The patient should be referred for laryngological examination. The patient should be considered for discharge from treatment. The patient's family should be encouraged to converse with the patient several times per day, focusing on current events.

2017, 96% of acute care hospitals had adopted health reporting technology (Alpert, 2016.). The inclusion of this new technology has already had a profound effect on health care delivery across settings. All providers who document in the medical record are now required to learn to enter information using these new technologies. There is minimal documentation, if any, in the literature about the specific opportunities and challenges associated with EMRs as reported by audiologists and speech-language pathologists. While detailed discussion of this trend is beyond the scope of this chapter, practitioners and academics are encouraged to become aware of specific institutional requirements and the opportunity to prepare for full utilization of information in these systems. Two points should be considered by practitioners across health settings: (1) clinical administrators should ensure that key information required for management of patients with communication disorders is included in the various templates in their particular electronic medical record system; and (2) clinicians should be sure that they highlight critical and timely communication (questions, clarifications, recommendations) so that they are clear for the rest of the health care team.

Continuing Professional Development

For the clinical practitioner in the health setting, nothing is more critical than continuous professional education and development. This concept entails going beyond the more traditional approach to continuing education as attendance at workshops and conferences or occasional reading. Every practitioner should devote a significant amount of time to learning new approaches, technologies, or delivery models that address the issues of cost-benefit to the patient and the system, improving safety for the patient, and enhancing quality of health and life. Some state licensure laws even require continuing education in specified areas such as prevention of medical errors for SLPs to maintain licensure.

Access to such professional development activities is readily available online; in some of the university-affiliated hospitals; through a number of continuing education centers and offerings; and through the American Speech-Language-Hearing Association, American Academy of Audiology, and other professional organizations.

In considering selection of a professional development program that focuses on improving one's current practice, it can be helpful to use a series of self-guided questions to direct selection of activities and information. Following are some questions for choosing health related continuing education programs in communication sciences and disorders:

1. Are there skills and knowledge that need to be developed to provide services to a specific patient population in a specific setting?

2. For the patient populations that are being served:
   a. What is the core understanding of any disease processes, common symptoms and medications, typical and atypical communication, and swallowing issues needed in order to best manage this group of patients?
   b. What are the resources available to guide "best practice" in managing this group of patients?
   c. Are there special technical procedures or skills that need to be verified before serving this patient population?
   d. What are the expected effects of treatment with this patient population and the range of outcomes that have been reported in the literature?

3. For the specific health setting (e.g., nursing home, acute care)
   a. What are the service models, regulatory issues, and reimbursement constraints that impact care in this environment?
   b. What are the documentation requirements and what technical or other skills are needed to complete documentation?
   c. What are the collaborative (interprofessional) skills required to work in this setting?
   d. What are the specific desired systematic outcomes associated with this setting? (For example, in acute care, the goals may be rapid assessment, short-term consultation and intervention, and planning for transfer. In hospice care, the goals may be comfort, nutrition, reduced communication effort, and maintaining interaction with caregivers.)

Using these basic questions, a clinician can identify those particular areas of skill and knowledge needed to function as an expert in a given health setting. By identifying these areas, the clinician can then proceed to acquire the information needed through reading, formal education, mentored "hands-on" experience in the clinical setting, and workshop/conference attendance.

As technology for content delivery has advanced, so has the number of opportunities for delivery of continuing education. While attendance at conferences continues, the number of web-based available mechanisms for continuing education is ever-increasing. In these activities, prospective attendees should use the same questions and clarifications regarding evidence, quality, and currency of the information being presented. Increasingly, information is available from providers regarding potential conflicts of interest of individuals presenting in activities based on continuing education units. Learners should always ask themselves if there is a product or service being sold and advanced. If so, the same high standards of evidence should be applied in evaluating potential benefit for patients.

Another aspect of continuing professional development focuses on the education of other professions about communication disorders. Speech-language pathologists and audiologists are always part of a team with the common goal of improving the health and function of the patient. Learning from and with these other professions is critical to good patient care. One piece of this professional exchange is to share knowledge of how individuals' communication disorder affects their progression with other members of the health care team. For example, when a patient has a hearing loss and is hospitalized, it may be necessary to give support to the staff providing care regarding use of amplification and communication strategies. A broader discussion of interprofessionalism occurs later in this chapter, and Chapter 23 of this book addresses the issue of *interprofessional practice* more comprehensively.

Supervision of Others

Speech-language pathologists and audiologists have long been involved in the supervision and mentoring of new professionals in the field. The current educational pathway typically begins in the university clinic and then extends to various practicum and internship experiences, and finally to a clinical fellowship in SLP or a fourth-year externship in audiology. Accrediting bodies and certification boards ensure that these clinical experiences are valid, rigorous, and comprehensive. There is a body of literature that addresses the topic of clinical supervision, focusing primarily on the student–clinical instructor/preceptor relationship. Examples of this body of knowledge come from the work of early leaders such as Jean Anderson (1988), who proposed a continuum/developmental model of supervision with an ongoing goal of encouraging the independence of the supervisee. McCrea and Brasseur (2003) continued Anderson's themes. Their work provides a rich discussion of the importance of the supervisory process to the development of professional competence in assistants, in new and advanced students, and in the early years of professional experience. In their book, McCrea and Brasseur encourage a change from the term *supervision* to *clinical education* and refer to the instructional role

as *clinical educator*. Moving the focus of discussion to teaching and learning is key to the ongoing development of professionals, especially as they move to levels of advanced practice.

Regardless of the terminology, professional leaders and associations acknowledge that skills and knowledge are required to deliver education to others. In particular, the American Speech-Language-Hearing Association has provided guidance in the form of consensus documents, *Knowledge and Skills for Supervisors of Speech-Language Pathology Assistants* (ASHA, 2004) and *Clinical Supervision in Speech-Language Pathology* (ASHA, 2008). These papers, along with a number of other ASHA resources, specify approaches and best practices for educating assistants, students, and clinical fellows. There are additional published articles or books that speak specifically to more advanced professional development in health settings for speech-language pathologists or audiologists. Guidance for education and professional development in these settings can be attained from two sets of resources. First, ASHA consensus documents (guidelines, technical reports, skills and knowledge statements) are available for a significant number of areas of practice, including services to patients in neonatal intensive care units (ASHA, 2004b); videofluoroscopy (ASHA, 2004a); dysphagia (ASHA, 2002b); audiologic services to infants and young children (ASHA, 2006); as well as many others.

A second set of resources that may be useful to those practicing and leading in health settings can be found in literature from other disciplines, such as physical therapy, medicine, nursing, and occupational therapy. Many disciplines have struggled with the same issues that have been challenging for those in communicative disorders, including teaching clinical problem solving and reflection, learning clinical procedures and psychomotor skills, applying evidence-based approaches, using simulation tasks and/or simulated patient scenarios, and interdisciplinary communication. It is beyond the scope of this chapter to review this literature, but a survey of current educational approaches from a number of disciplines will be enlightening and helpful to those charged with the education of others. (See Chapter 26 for a further discussion of supervision and mentoring.)

Quality and Compliance with Regulatory Processes

The ethical, legal, and other regulatory processes that impact service delivery in the health setting are extensive. In essence, all of these regulations have been put into place to protect patients and institutions, to ensure that best practices are established and used, and to reduce costs. Despite their respectable intent, these goals are, in some ways, in competition with each other and produce demands for productivity reports, paperwork, meetings, documentation, site visits by accreditation programs, and so forth. The work associated with compliance is a significant component of delivering modern health care in the United States, and those who choose to work in this setting should understand that their role includes this demanding and sometimes frustrating intrusion into clinical or research goals. Providers in hospitals, nursing homes, health care, and outpatient settings are affected by these various requirements. Administrators in these settings typically provide support for clinicians by completing required paperwork and other activities so that access to service for patients is accomplished most efficiently. ASHA (2004a) has produced a document that will be helpful to speech-language pathologists who need guidance on issues related to compliance. This document, *Knowledge and Skills in Business Practices for Speech-Language Pathologists Who Are Managers and Leaders in Health Care Organizations*, includes many resources that are useful to those trying to understand the myriad responsibilities associated with compliance.

Interprofessional Responsibilities and Competencies

Interprofessional practice and collaboration is an evolving area of discussion for the discipline. Within the national health care scene, there is widespread interest in the potential impact and professional benefit of interprofessional practice on quality of care, safety, and patient satisfaction. A recent report titled *Core Competencies for Interprofessional Collaborative Practice 2016 Update* (Interprofessional Education Collaborative, 2016) outlines an important discussion from a number of health-related professional organizations representing the disciplines of osteopathic and allopathic medicine, nursing, pharmacy, dentistry, and public health. This document presents four major domains for interprofessional practice, including: (1) values and ethics, (2) roles/responsibilities, (3) interprofessional communication, and (4) teams/teamwork. The increased prevalence of this topic in the professional literature and in the educational curricula of medical and nursing schools suggests that health professionals from a variety of disciplines, including speech-language pathology and audiology, should become familiar with the language and culture of interprofessionalism.

What are and will be the roles of those who work in the discipline of Communication Sciences Disorders (CSD) around interprofessional issues? Specifically,

within the values domain, the role of the clinician in articulating and advocating respectfully for the communication rights and independence of all patients is a key factor. Within the domain of roles and responsibilities, helping colleagues develop a realistic, respectful, and clear picture of the role of the SLP or audiologist is critical. Similarly, SLPs and audiologists need to work diligently to ensure that their understanding of the roles and contributions of other providers is clear. The last two factors—communication and teamwork—are also of critical importance to all professionals caring for a patient. Tools and strategies for effective performance on teams are widely available. These capabilities should become part of the education and practice pattern of every SLP and audiologist who anticipates a successful career in the health care environment.

Historically, speech-language pathology and audiology associations and professionals have worked to establish autonomy in their care of patients and to achieve recognition for their distinctive contribution to the health care field. Given the number of unique disciplines represented in the arena of health care, it is not surprising that others have challenged these attempts and that occasional turf wars have emerged across disciplines that have common patient interests. Despite occasional disagreements with colleagues from medical and other health disciplines, the clinical arm of speech-language pathology and audiology has flourished over the past two decades. It is common for these fields to be listed as desirable occupations with demand for speech-language pathology being projected to grow by 18% through 2026 and for audiology by 21% (Bureau of Labor Statistics, 2018). These statistical predictions for growth exceed the national averages for other occupations. Society, particularly in North America, has become familiar with the knowledge and care provided by certified and licensed speech-language pathologists and audiologists and, in turn, continues to expect expert service from these providers. The recognition and status of the professions of speech-language pathology and audiology appear to be moving in the desired direction.

The simultaneous desire for autonomy *and* interprofessional collaboration may seem incongruent. This is not the case. Autonomy in decision making about communication disorders and about the training and education needed to serve patients are essential components of good care. The SLP or audiologist has capacity to describe, measure, and prognosticate regarding the patient's communication disorder. In the interprofessional discussion, the SLP or audiologist delivers the information about the patient's communication and/or swallowing to the larger discussion of the total care, medical condition, follow-up planning, social and emotional status, and desired outcomes. The assumption is that the patient and the system will be best served when all providers bring their distinctive contribution to the discussion in a respectful manner with an open mind. Conversely, it is essential that the SLP or audiologist receive and appreciate the impact of shared information from others involved in the care of the patient, and consider the ways in which that information is beneficial in treating the patient's communication disorder. Chapter 23 addresses these issues in more detail.

Multicultural Issues and Health Disparities

SLPs and audiologists are well aware of how diverse their patients are. Educational programs require the development of knowledge and skills around multicultural issues as they affect communication and its disorders. Respect for cultural differences lies at the heart of being engaged with others in the clinical environment. Thus, skilled clinicians need the interpersonal skills to approach each situation with respect and without judgment. Additionally, differences in behavior or language that are representative of a specific culture should not be treated as abnormal or disordered. Clinicians need to learn about and use appropriate tools for assessment and intervention with an understanding of the influence of culture on communication and health practices as a prominent feature of their patient interactions. Chapter 25 in this text discusses the broad range of issues that come into play when we consider culture in clinical practice settings, and clinicians may find this review helpful as they consider their own background and knowledge in this area.

One area of concern to those who work in the health care environment is that of disparities in access and quality for certain populations. The Centers for Disease Control and Prevention describes health disparities as "preventable differences in the burden of disease, injury, violence or opportunities to achieve optimal health that are experienced by socially disadvantaged populations" (CDC, 2008). Populations at documented risk are those that are defined by race, ethnicity, income, disability, geographic location, or sexual orientation. Disparities are believed to result from poverty, environmental trends, educational inequalities, or inadequate access to health services. While the topic of disparities is a major area of concern, especially as the distribution of health care is redefined through health reform in the United States, there are specific concerns related to the practice of speech-language pathology or audiology in health settings that should be considered. See Chapter 14, "Health Care Legislation, Regulation, and Financing," for more information.

Health Literacy

Low health literacy, or the ability to find and understand health information and services, affects health outcomes. More than 50% of Americans exhibit low health literacy (Kirsch, Jungeblut, Jenkins, & Kolstad, 1993). Of particular concern to SLPs and audiologists should be the ability of their patients to comply with instructions (written or spoken) and to access the health system for needed services. Every clinician should learn how to respectfully use appropriate levels of communication and utilize feedback to ensure that the patient and/or caregiver understand necessary instructions. With the use of video, technology, picture systems, and so on, there is ample opportunity to ensure that this occurs. Also, when the SLP or audiologist suspects that the patient may be having difficulty accessing the broader health system due to communication disability or other language differences, it will be useful to assist the patient to ensure that needs are met.

Focusing on an individual patient's ability to understand and comply with health information presented by other health care professionals is not an area that the field has embraced in a serious manner. This is problematic, as it is likely that many of the tools and approaches used by SLPs and audiologists would be helpful in addressing the health literacy problem. Given that so much of health improvement requires compliance with written, oral, and digital information, there is an obvious opportunity for collaboration among the provider, the patient, and the specialist in CSD.

Communication Disorder as a Risk Factor for Reduced Health Literacy

Many people with language or other communication disorders will have difficulties with health literacy. Beyond their ability to understand and/or comply with clinical instructions regarding self-care or prescriptions, patients with communication disorders are at additional risk. Much of the access to the health care system is driven by patients' perceived health concerns and their ability to ask for assistance. When symptoms are not obvious, or if patients do not have a reliable caregiver (spokesperson), they may be unable to communicate concerns, particularly patients with aphasia, traumatic brain injury, deafness, or another major communicative disturbance that limits expression. Clinicians should advocate for the health needs of their patients when significant communication deficits are an issue. Studies are badly needed to document the occurrence of preventable illness and mental health problems, and access to preventive care for those with communication disorders. This is an area where speech-language pathologists and audiologists have a significant opportunity to influence primary care for their patients. Establishing reliable, basic communication strategies and tools for communication between patient and provider, preparing patients for visits with their primary care provider or specialty physician, and following up after appointments to ensure that patients understand and can comply with directives are roles that could add value to the scope of care provided by the clinician in communicative disorders.

Some Future Considerations

In this last section of the chapter, we consider some issues that are just emerging or are on the horizon for the practice of SLP and audiology in health settings.

Health Reform and Cost Control

In 2010, President Barack Obama introduced the Patient Protection and Affordable Care Act (ACA), with the reported intent of making health care more accessible to everyone and reducing barriers for individuals who were previously ineligible for insurance coverage (Public Law 111-148, 2010).

In the years following the implementation of the ACA, active political debate has continued regarding further expansion of health coverage. It is important to note that some political leaders are advocating reversing or eliminating this law. Conversely, there is also a strong alternative voice advocating to continue expanding health benefits for all Americans.

PL 111-148 also expands the primary care workforce by providing loan repayment programs for nurses, physicians, and physician assistants. The bill has significant focus on prevention, with particular attention to children and to senior citizens on Medicare. Additionally, there is attention to the development of new models of service to individuals on Medicare and Medicaid through a new Center for Medicare and Medicaid Innovation. Finally, the bill has provided focus on improving care for seniors, especially those at risk after they leave the hospital.

In conclusion, at the time of this writing, it appears clinicians in the health setting face two broad challenges in light of the implications of health reform and cost containment activities that are under way in the health sector. First, providers need to help referral sources, both traditional and new, to understand the link between their concerns about patient safety and effective care with the appropriate evidence-based approach to management of communicative disorders. Second, SLPs and audiologists need to constantly address the issue of treatment effi-

ciency, ensuring that costs are under control and that patients (and referral agencies) are receiving the most value. The long-term and specific implications of health care reform and its effect on service delivery, education, and reimbursement in speech-language pathology and audiology remain to be seen.

Trends in Education for Health Settings

Preparation of the next generation of practitioners is always on the minds of those who teach and those who employ new graduates. Education, especially higher education, is a dynamic process that has many stakeholders: students, the public, state and national government, employers, and, of course, the patients who will be served. A common feature among entry-level graduate programs in the health professions is that they are heavily regulated by many different agencies. All universities participate in regional accreditation, and each of the health professions is subject to specialized accreditations that specify the content and the expected outcomes for graduates.

To address the need for rapid learning and evidence-based care in an interprofessional environment, several new educational approaches are emerging in health professions education. While not readily utilized at this time in CSD programs, they hold promise for providing interesting and helpful solutions to learning integrated clinical skills. Three of these approaches—dedicated education units, clinical simulation, and standardized patients—hold promise for addressing interdisciplinary educational needs, as well as core content in the discipline, and are described below.

Dedicated (Collaborative) Education Units (DEUs)

These hospital-based units are designed with two goals in mind: excellent patient care and student-focused education. The DEU developed primarily out of the field of nursing for the purpose of changing the standard approach to nursing education. In this model, faculty members work with staff in the hospital to develop their role as clinical educators. Students are assigned in teams to the unit, in which opportunities for education, discussion, and reflection are included as part of the core operation of the unit (Moscato, Miller, Logsdon, Weinberg, & Chorpenning, 2007). Interprofessional practice that focuses on collaboration among nurses, physicians, and social workers in inpatient settings has also been described. While this model has yet to emerge with inclusion of health professionals from rehabilitation disciplines, discussions and planning are beginning at educational institutions and professional associations.

A significant goal of participation in the interdisciplinary DEU is the development of knowledge of and appreciation for the work of each participating discipline in addressing the patient's health concerns. Thus, speech-language pathology students could learn, in some detail, about the roles the nurse and physician play in using medicines to promote stabilization and recovery; could appreciate the significance of various test results; could learn from the physical therapist about safety issues in transfers and walking with patients; and could learn strategies for positioning and orientation from the occupational therapist. Evolution of this model, especially in inpatient acute care and rehabilitation settings, has the potential to change the culture of service delivery for the next generation of providers.

Clinical Simulation

The use of simulation as a tool for building clinical skills and problem-solving abilities is expanding rapidly in clinical education in the health professions. Simulation allows no-risk practice in aspects of care that previously could only be experienced with live patients (Ziv, Wolpe, Small, & Glick, 2003). The literature on use of simulation for learning procedures in surgery, emergency medicine, anesthesia, and other technically demanding areas of medicine is quite extensive (Gordon, Wilkerson, Shaffer, & Armstrong, 2001). Additional applications of simulation for situations that rely heavily on problem solving, decision making, and communication across disciplines are emerging (DeVita, Schaefer, Lutz, Wang, & Dongill, 2005). These multidisciplinary approaches rely on clinical scenarios to elicit complex problems that require communication among professionals, an application that will likely be developed to include speech-language pathologists in rehabilitation or pediatric settings. Simulation has been used successfully in audiology settings to teach technical audiology skills in assessment and in amplification (Zurek & Desloge, 2007). Additionally, in 2018 a task force of the Council of Academic Programs in Communication Sciences and Disorders (Dudding, Brown, Estis, Szymanski, & Zraick, 2018) produced a summary of best practices guiding the use of simulation in CSD. This is an area that is likely to develop in response to the demand for expanded or alternative clinical practicum experience and the need for exposure to patient populations that are sometimes inaccessible.

One area of simulation that has significant promise for the health fields is virtual reality. As the technology for this approach becomes more fluid and more "real," it is likely that virtual speech clinics and virtual patients will be readily accessible. Williams (2006) reported on a prototype project in which a virtual immersion center was developed to provide interactive simulation with students or clients in a CSD program at Case Western Reserve University. In this virtual reality setting, students could interact with patients in a 3D environment, and the instructor could control responses of the patient. This example provides a model for clinical education, though its exact replication may be limited by the need for a full room environment and considerable technology support. On the other hand, new technological advances and applications for cellphones and computers make virtual reality models for simulated clinical experiences, patient/clinician interactions, assessment and treatment scenarios, and interprofessional problem-solving activities a realistic goal for the educational environment.

Finally, a comprehensive product that uses an online approach to developing case-based skills through the use of simulation has been developed and marketed by SimuCase (Jansen, Johnson, Ondo, Pantalone, & Williams, 2015). This product provides hundreds of hours of patient examples covering a range and scope of disorders, ages, and professional settings. Clinicians are given the opportunity to develop clinical skills, practice clinical decisions and diagnostic skills, and plan interventions. Clinical scenarios are presented either via animations or through video recorded cases. At this time, many graduate programs in speech-language pathology use SimuCase as a component of their education program.

Standardized Patients

Another emerging approach to the development of patient interaction and assessment skills is the use of standardized patients (SPs). These "patients" provide a special type of simulation by serving as trained actors. Their use in medicine and nursing education programs is extensive. Several reports in the literature describe the use of SPs in speech-language pathology. Zraick, Allen, and Johnson (2003) report on the use of SPs to teach interpersonal skills to new graduate students in SLP, and English, Naeve-Velguth, Rall, Uyehara-Isono, and Pittman (2007) describe a similar application to evaluating students' abilities in counseling the parents of newly identified deaf children. Again, the use of SPs as an innovation in education is likely to continue to develop in clinical settings. Interestingly, a recent study (Baylor, Burns, Struijk, Herron, Mach, & Yorkston, 2017) has demonstrated that actors can be trained to portray aphasia and dysarthria in a believable manner.

These three emerging approaches to clinical development—DEUs, clinical simulation, and standardized patients—will need careful evaluation in the coming years. Determining the effectiveness of these approaches in preparing clinicians to face the real world will be essential. However, if it is demonstrated that valuable skills can be acquired efficiently and effectively with generalization to clinical practice, their use will be invaluable as a cost-effective measure for instruction. Additionally, students in early stages of education will be able to benefit from simulated real-world problem solving, integration of clinical and theoretical skills, and risk-free feedback on errors or alternative approaches. While these simulated environments using technology or actors may never approach real-world clinical interactions as an effective teaching modality, they do provide a potential bridging experience that new clinicians or those learning advanced skills will find beneficial.

Entry-Level and Advanced Degrees for Practice

An additional concern for the future of the disciplines is the change in requirements for the entry level to practice. Since the mid-1990s, entry requirements for audiology have evolved from a master's degree to a professional doctoral degree, the Doctor of Audiology (AuD). The profession of audiology is not alone in making these entry-level changes; professional doctorates are well established in physical therapy (Doctor of Physical Therapy, DPT), psychology (Doctor of Psychology, PsyD), and pharmacy (Doctor of Pharmacy, PharmD). In all of the disciplines mentioned, the PhD (rather than the practice degree) remains the entry-level degree for scientific/research work and academics. The field of advanced practice nursing, which includes the nurse practitioner role, has designated the DNP (Doctor of Nursing Practice) as a "practice doctorate" in nursing, and the profession of occupational therapy has identified an advanced model of education that terminates with the OTD (Occupational Therapy Doctorate). Thus, there are two major types of degree levels for practice-based professions. The predominant model, entry-level doctoral education, is required in medicine, dentistry, physical therapy, audiology, and pharmacy. The alternative, professional doctoral education after entry into the field (i.e., after basic licensure and certification requirements are established) is found in nursing and occupational therapy. It is anticipated by some that in these latter cases, "post-entry" advanced degrees will evolve to entry-level requirements, but this is speculative at this time.

In the 1960s, speech-language pathology and audiology were two of the first non-physician health professions to require a master's degree for entry-level practice

and professional certification. Two to three decades ahead of colleagues in other disciplines, communication sciences and disorders has long been a standard bearer for advancing the highest levels of education and practice. Now, with the entry level as a professional practice doctoral degree in audiology, a significant disparity exists between speech-language pathology and audiology, which are part of the same intellectual and disciplinary heritage.

There has been considerable discussion over the years regarding the role of professional doctoral education in speech-language pathology, especially in health care settings. More than 30 years ago, Aronson (1987) made a case for the "clinical PhD" as a survival mechanism for communication disorders as a health care profession. He was describing a model, similar to that seen in many clinical psychology programs, where practice is the focus. Since that time, occasional references have been made to the professional doctoral model of SLP education. Lubinski (2003) asked for the profession to reconsider its position on the issue and proposed the development of innovative models for implementing professional doctoral education in SLP. In 2015, ASHA produced Guidelines for the Clinical Doctorate in Speech Language Pathology (American Speech-Language-Hearing Association, 2015). This document provides guidance for organization of programs and highlights four domains for advanced study: depth of knowledge and advanced skill development in select areas of practice; critical thinking and problem solving; clinical education, teaching, supervision, and mentorship; and expertise in interpreting and applying clinical research.

At the time of this writing, there are eight self-identified post-professional models of professional doctoral entry in the area of speech-language pathology. These include Kean University (NJ), Loma Linda University (CA), Northwestern University (IL), Nova Southeastern University (FL), Rocky Mountain University (UT), University of Kansas (KS), University of Pittsburgh (PA), and Valdosta State University (GA).

Telehealth

Telehealth is the use of a variety of telecommunication technologies to deliver care and health education. Using media that are common in digital social interactions (i.e., Skype, Zoom, etc.) providers and patients can interact when physical distance or the patient's health condition interferes with participation in face-to-face interactions in the same location. Telehealth encompasses a broad definition of technology-enabled health care services. ASHA's 2013 membership surveys indicated that approximately 7% of audiologists and 3% of SLPs were involved in telepractice. Today, an online search provides extensive listings of therapy services and audiologic services available through a variety of organizations, hospitals, and private companies. Anecdotal evidence reveals that telepractice can be a useful approach to service delivery, but additional research is needed. Published reports document success in treatment and diagnosis of communication disorders (Duffy, Werven & Aronson, 1997; Hill, Theodoros, Russell, Cahill, Ward, & Clark, 2006). To date, there are no documented systematic clinical trials or comprehensive evaluations of this methodology. One could speculate that as technology becomes more familiar to the public and as the quality of the visual and auditory signal improves, the experience of the patient and the accuracy of the clinician would be enhanced. The potential to diminish the effect of reduced access for patients who live at a distance from the provider, for whom specialized services are needed, or for whom physical mobility is an issue are key motivators for the continued exploration of these technologies.

The implications for the advanced use of portable technology in all of the health professions are significant; however, intensive rehabilitation-oriented services that often require face-to-face interaction, such as SLP, may particularly show cost benefits from this technology. A recent online search yielded hundreds of sites that promote the use of this interactive technology with patients with both developmental and acquired communication disorders. It is clear that the marketability of this technology is high; as such, systemic evaluation of its impact on costs and benefits to patients and payers is necessary.

Summary

This chapter addresses current and future practice issues related to speech-language pathology and audiology in health settings. First, distinctive characteristics of the various health settings across the continuum of care were reviewed. Next, the critical issues of compliance, documentation, patient safety, and development of clinical skills were discussed as core to the role of the practicing clinician. Finally, exploration of several emerging topics, including health reform, evolving professional entry models, and telehealth technologies, were also considered.

The health care continuum offers a vibrant and dynamic professional setting for the skilled speech-language pathologist or audiologist. The demand for individuals to join this practice setting with a commitment to excellent patient care and innovation is evident. Advances in technology and practice offer solutions to current disparities in access and quality, and address the ever-present need for cost containment.

Critical Thinking

1. What academic and clinical preparation is needed to work effectively as a speech-language pathologist or audiologist in health care settings? What skills are needed in the various types of health care settings?

2. How can speech-language pathologists and audiologists work more collaboratively in health care settings? How does such collaboration affect our service delivery?

3. How are the current and proposed changes in health care funding likely to affect what you do as a speech-language pathologist or audiologist in a health care setting?

4. What are some nontraditional roles we might develop in health care settings? (Hint: health care literacy)

5. How does technology enhance our roles in health care settings? What technological advances might help us deliver more effective diagnostic and intervention services?

6. It is said, "If you did not write it down, you did not do it." Why is documentation critical in health care centers? How is the emerging use of the Electronic Health Record (EHR) likely to change documentation practices and trends in our fields?

7. You worked as a speech-language pathologist for seven years at a large children's hospital and are now relocating to an area where you can get a position as an SLP in a long-term care facility. Would this be an easy transfer of skills from one health care setting to another? How do the necessary skills differ across these medical settings? What would you do to prepare yourself for work in the long-term care setting?

References

Alpert, J. (2016). The medical record in 2016: Advantages and disadvantages. *Digital Medicine*, *2*(2), 48.

American Speech-Language-Hearing Association. (2002a). *Guidelines for the training, use, and supervision of speech-language pathology assistants* [Guidelines]. Available from http://www.asha.org/policy

American Speech-Language-Hearing Association. (2002b). *Knowledge and skills needed by speech-*

language pathologists providing services to individuals with swallowing and/or feeding disorders. Available from http://www.asha.org/policy

American Speech-Language-Hearing Association. (2003). *National Outcomes Measurement System (NOMS): Adult speech-language pathology user's guide.* Rockville: MD: Author.

American Speech-Language-Hearing Association. (2004a). *Knowledge and skills needed by speech-language pathologists performing videofluoroscopic swallowing studies.* Available from http://www.asha.org/policy

American Speech-Language-Hearing Association. (2004b). *Knowledge and skills needed by speech-language pathologists providing services to infants and families in the NICU environment.* Available from http://www.asha.org/policy

American Speech-Language-Hearing Association. (2006). *Roles, knowledge, and skills: audiologists providing clinical services to infants and young children birth to 5 years of age* [Knowledge and skills]. Available from http://www.asha.org/policy

American Speech-Language-Hearing Association (2008). *Clinical supervision in speech-language pathology* [Position statement]. Available from http://www.asha.org/policy

American Speech-Language-Hearing Association. (2011). *Documentation in healthcare settings.* Retrieved from http://www.asha.org/slp/healthcare/documentation.html

American Speech-Language-Hearing Association. (2013). *2013 Membership survey. CCC-A survey summary report: Number and type of responses.* Available from http://www.asha.org

American Speech-Language-Hearing Association. (2014). Where do audiologists and speech-language pathologists work? *ASHA Leader, 19*(5), 24.

American Speech-Language-Hearing Association. (2015). *Guidelines for the clinical doctorate in speech-language pathology.* https://doi.org/10.1044/policy.GL2015-00341

American Speech-Language-Hearing Association (2018). *Highlights and trends: member and affiliate counts, year end 2018.* Retrieved from https://www.asha.org/uploadedFiles/2018-Member-Counts.pdf

American Speech-Language-Hearing Association (2019). A*SHA membership profile: Highlights and trends 2019.* Retrieved May 2, 2019, from American Speech-Language-Hearing Association

website: https://www.asha.org/research/memberdata/member-counts/

American Speech-Language-Hearing Association. (n.d.). *Joint Commission resources for SLPs.* Retrieved from https://www.asha.org/SLP/healthcare/JointCommissionResources/

Anderson, J. L. (1988). *The supervisory process in speech-language pathology and audiology.* Austin, TX: Pro-Ed.

Aronson, A. E. (1987). The clinical PhD: Implications for the survival and liberation of communicative disorders as a health care profession. *ASHA, 29*(11), 35–39.

Ballard, S. L., & Dymond, S. K. (2018). Inclusive education for secondary age students with severe disabilities and complex health care needs. *Intellectual and Developmental Disabilities, 56*(6), 427–441. https://doi.org/10.1352/1934-9556-56.6.427

Baylor, C., Yorkston, K., Eadie, T., Jieseon, K., Chung, H., & Amtmann, D. (2013).The communicative participation item bank (CPIB): Item bank calibration and development of a disorder-generice short form. *Journal of Speech-Language-Hearing Resarch, 56*(4), 1190–1208.

Baylor, C., Burns, M., Struijk, J., Herron, L., Mach, H., & Yorkston, K. (2017). Assessing the believability of standardized patients trained to portray communication disorders. *American Journal of Speech-Language Pathology, 26*(3), 791–805.

Bureau of Labor Statistics, U.S. Department of Labor. (2018). *Occupational outlook handbook* (2010–11 ed.). Washington, DC: Author.

CDC (Centers for Disease Control and Prevention). (2008). *Community Health and Program Services (CHAPS): Health disparities among racial/ethnic populations.* Atlanta, GA: U.S. Department of Health and Human Services.

Center for Connected Health Policy. (2011). *What is telehealth?* Retrieved from http://connectedhealthca.org/what-is-telehealth

Conley, J., Jordan, M., & Ghali, W. A. (2009). Audit of the consultation process on general internal medicine services. *Quality and Safety in Health Care, 18*, 59–62.

Davis, R. E., Jacklin, R., Sevdalis, N., & Vincent, C. A. (2007). Patient involvement in patient safety: What factors influence patient participation and engagement? *Health Expectations, 10*(3), 259–267.

DeVita, M. A., Schaefer, J., Lutz, J., Wang, H., & Dongill, T. (2005). Improving medical emergency team (MET) performance using a novel curriculum and a computerized human patient simulator. *Quality and Safety in Health Care, 14,* 326–331.

Doyle, P., McNeil, M., Mikolic, J., Prieto, L., Hula, W., Lustig, A., . . . Elman, R. (2004). The Burden of Stroke Scale (BOSS) provides valid and reliable score estimates of functioning and well-being in stroke survivors with and without communication disorders. *Journal of Clinical Epidemiology, 57*(10), 997–1007.

Dudding, C., Brown, D., Estis, J., Szymanski, C., & Zraick, R. (2018). *Best practices in healthcare simulations in communication sciences and disorders.* Council of Academic Programs in Communication Sciences and Disorders. Available at http://www.capcsd.org

Duffy, J. R., Werven, G. W., & Aronson, A. E. (1997) Telemedicine and the diagnosis of speech and language disorders. *Mayo Clinic Proceedings, 12,* 1116–1122.

Eadie, T. L., Yorkston, K. M., Klasner, E. R., Dudgeon, B. J., Dietz, J. C., Baylor, C. R., . . . Antmann D. (2006). Measuring communicative participation: A review of self-report instruments in speech-language pathology. *American Journal of Speech-Language Pathology, 15,* 307–320.

English, K., Naeve-Velguth, S., Rall, E., Uyehara-Isono, J., & Pittman, A. (2007). Development of an instrument to evaluate audiologic counseling skills. *Journal of the American Academy of Audiology, 18*(8), 675–687.

Gordon, J, A., Wilkerson, W. M., Shaffer, D. W., & Armstrong, E. G. (2001). Practicing medicine without risk: Students' and educators' responses to high-fidelity patient simulation. *Academic Medicine, 76*(5), 469–472.

Hill, A., Theodoros, D. G., Russell, T. G., Cahill, L. M., Ward, E. C., & Clark, K. M. (2006). An Internet-based telerehabilitation system for the assessment of motor speech disorders: A pilot study. *American Journal of Speech-Language Pathology, 15,* 45–56.

Hula, W., Doyle, P., Stone, C., Hula, S., Kellough, S., Wambaugh, J., . . . St. Jacque, A. (2015). The aphasia communication outcome measure (ACOM): Dimensionality and initial validation. *Journal of Speech-Language-Hearing Resarch, 58*(3), 906–919.

Institute for Healthcare Improvement. (2011). *Making care safer.* Retrieved from http://www.healthcare.gov/center/programs/partnership/safer/transitions_.html

Interprofessional Education Collaborative. (2016). *Core competencies for interprofessional collaborative practice 2016 update.* Washington DC.

Jacobson, B. J., Johnson, A. F., Grywalksi, C., Silbergleit, A., Jacobson, G., Benninger, M. S., & Newman, C. W. (1997). The Voice Handicap Index: Development and validation. *American Journal of Speech-Language Pathology, 6*(3), 66–70.

Jansen, L., Johnson, C., Ondo, K., Pantalone, B., & Williams, S. (2015). *SimuCase User Guide 3.0: Case by case, improving skills, inspiring confidence.* Speech Pathology.com. Available at http://www.sc-media.speechpathology.com

Johnson, A. F., & Jacobson, B. H. (2007). *Medical speech-language pathology: A practitioner's guide.* New York, NY: Thieme.

Johnson, A. F., & Jacobson, B. H. (Eds.). (2016). *Medical speech-language pathology: A practitioner's guide* (3rd ed.). New York, NY: Thieme.

Keith, R. A., Granger, C. V., Hamilton, B. B., & Sherwin, F. S. (1987). The functional independence measure: A new tool for rehabilitation. *Advances in Clinical Rehabilitation, 1,* 6–18.

Kirsch, I. S., Jungeblut, A., Jenkins, L., & Kolstad, A. (1993). *Adult literacy in America: A first look at the results of the National Adult Literacy Survey (NALS).* Washington, DC: National Center for Education Statistics, U.S. Department of Education.

Kummer, A., Johnson, P., & Zeit, K. (2007). Clinical documentation in medical speech-language pathology. In A. Johnson & B. H. Jacobson (Eds.), *Medical speech-language pathology: A practitioner's guide.* New York, NY: Thieme.

Lefton-Greif, M. A., & Arvedson, J. C. (2008). Schoolchildren with dysphagia associated with medically complex conditions. *Language, Speech, and Hearing Services in Schools, 39*(2), 237–248.

Lubinski, R. (2003). Revisiting the professional doctorate in medical speech-language pathology. *Journal of Medical Speech-Language Pathology, 8*(4), li–lxii.

McCrea, E. S., & Brasseur, J. A. (2003). *The supervisory process in speech-language pathology and audiology.* Boston, MA: Allyn & Bacon.

McHorney, C., Bricker, D., Kramer, A., Rosenbek, J., Robbins, J., Chignell. K., Logemann, J., & Clarke, C. (2000). The SWAL-QOL outcomes tool for oropharyngeal dysphagia in adults: I. Conceptual foundation and item development. *Dysphagia, 15*(3), 115–218.

Moscato, S. R., Miller, J., Logsdon, K., Weinberg, S., & Chorpenning, L. (2007). Dedicated education unit: An innovative clinical partner education model. *Nursing Outlook, 55*, 31–37.

National Hospice and Palliative Care Organization. (2009). *NHPCO facts and figures: Hospice care in America.* Alexandria, VA: National Hospice and Palliative Care Organization.

Newman, C. W., Weinstein, B. E., Jacobson, G. P., & Hug, G. A. (1990). Hearing Handicap Inventory for Adults. *Ear and Hearing, 11*(6), 395–477.

Patient Protection and Affordable Care Act, 42 U.S.C. § 18001. (2010).

Paul, D., Frattali, C., Holland, A., Thompson, C., Caperton, C., & Slater, S. (2004). *Quality of Communication Life Scale.* Rockville, MD: American Speech-Language-Hearing Association.

Pollens, R. (2004). Role of the speech-language pathologist in palliative care. *Journal of Palliative Medicine, 7*(5), 694–702.

Silbergleit, A., Schultz, L., Jacobson, B., Beardsley, T., & Johnson, A. (2012). The Dysphagia Handicap Index: Development and validation. *Dysphagia, 27*, 46–52.

Simmons-Mackie, N., Kagan, A., Victor, J. C., Carling-Rowland, A., Mok, A., Hoch, J. S., . . . Streiner, D. L. (2014). The assessment for living with aphasia, *International Journal of Speech-Language Pathology, 16*(1), 82–94.

Weed, L. L. (1970). *Medical records, medical education, and patient care: The problem-oriented record as a basic tool.* Cleveland, OH: Year Book Medical.

Williams, S. (2006). *The virtual immersion center for simulation research: Interactive simulation technology for communication disorders.* Proceedings from the International Society for Presence Conference, Cleveland, OH.

Woods, M. S. (2006, August). How communication complicates the safety movement. *Hospital Safety and Health Networks.*

World Health Organization. (2001) *ICF: International Classification of Functioning, Disability, and Health.* Geneva, Switzerland.

Ziv, A., Wolpe, P. R., Small, R., & Glick, S. (2003). Simulation based medical education: An ethical imperative. *Academic Medicine, 78*, 783–788.

Zraick, R. I., Allen, R. M., & Johnson, S. B. (2003). The use of standardized patients to teach and test interpersonal and communication skills with students in speech-language pathology. *Advances in Health Sciences Education Theory and Practice, 8*(3), 237–248.

Zurek, P. M., & Desloge, J. G. (2007). Hearing loss and prosthesis simulation in audiology. *Hearing Journal, 60*, 32–38.

Education Policy and Service Delivery

Perry Flynn, MEd, Charlette M. Green, MS, and Marie Ireland, MEd

Introduction

This is an exciting time to be a school-based speech-language pathologist (SLP) or audiologist (AuD). According to the American Speech-Language-Hearing Association (ASHA), most of its members, 51.4%, work in school settings (American Speech-Language-Hearing Association, 2018). The current scope of practice provides many opportunities for these professionals to influence the lives of students in both regular and special education in positive ways on a daily basis. Today, opportunities exist for SLPs to work in regular education settings, such as a classroom, as well as in the more traditional resource settings ("pull-out") in direct and indirect ways. Many SLPs provide services for a wide variety of disorders in classrooms, on playgrounds, in cafeterias, and even off-campus vocational settings. SLP caseloads are diverse, including but not limited to students who have phonological disorders, language disorders, learning disabilities, autism, apraxia of speech, dysphagia, hearing loss, fluency disorders, and/or voice disorders. As an educational audiologist, duties likely entail hearing screenings, assessing students with hearing loss or auditory processing disorders, or providing collaborative services to students with cochlear implants. Educational audiologists may also be assessing classroom acoustics; assessing and recommending assistive technology; and counseling students, parents, and teachers. Both SLPs and audiologists participate in continuing education to maintain credentialing, but more importantly to remain abreast of the current evidence-based practices in the professions. These professionals engage in the collection of data for evidence-based practice and progress monitoring for both regular education and special education compliance purposes. Caseloads continue to reflect the growing cultural, racial, and ethnic diversity of the United States. Speech-language pathologists and audiologists are increasingly involved in school mental health initiatives as well as concussion protocols/working with individuals with traumatic brain injuries and servicing students with emotional and behavioral issues. This chapter describes the student population in the United States in preschool through twelfth grade, outlines the federal legislation that governs services to special education students, explains many of the roles and responsibilities of school-based SLPs and audiologists, and describes educational trends across the country. The information contained in the chapter is presented to share improvements in providing educational services, to examine areas of growth, and to provoke consideration of training to become a school-based SLP or audiologist.

Settings and Students: Statistics

In 2015–2016, preschool through twelfth grade students across the United States presented with specific learning disabilities (34%), speech or language impairments (20%), and only about 1% had a hearing impairment (National Center for Education Statistics, 2018b). SLPs and audiologists serve these populations as well as students who have other disabilities. Table 16–1 lists the categories and percentages of students reported to the U.S. Department of Education as part of the annual student count. Remember that students with a variety of disabilities may also have communication impairments. Historically, families often sought "special" schools for their children who had differences to avoid societal stigma. As of 2018, 95% of the students who were served under the Individuals with Disabilities Education Act (IDEA) attended regular schools, and only about 3% were enrolled in separate schools for students with disabilities (National Center for Education Statistics, 2018b). Of note, 87% of those with speech and language impairments spend most of their day in the regular classroom. This reflects a shift from a more traditional "special classroom" model to more current mainstreaming and inclusion efforts based on parent driven advocacy.

The face of education has changed tremendously in recent years. According to the National Center for Education Statistics (2018b), in 2015–2016 there were 98,280 operating public elementary and secondary schools that enrolled about 50.44 million students in the United States. Regular public schools constituted 93% of all schools in the United States with 7% of those being charter schools. The percentage of high-poverty schools, where more than 75% of the students are eligible for free or reduced-price meals, increased from 12% in 1999–2000 to 24% in 2015–2016. Many of these high-poverty schools are in urban areas, though they also exist in suburban and rural areas. Further evidence of how education has changed over the years is in the shift of the ethnic makeup of schools. In 2015, the percentage of white students was 49%. In some school districts, minority enrollment has become the majority. For example, in 7 states and the District of Columbia, white students are in the minority. In 17 states and the District of Columbia, white student enrollment has dropped below 50%. The percentage of Hispanic students is currently 25.9% and has surpassed the enrollment of black

Table 16–1. Type of Disability, Percent of Total Enrollment, and Percent of Children with Disabilities

Type of Disability	Percent Total Enrollment	Percent Children with Disabilities
All disabilities	14.0	n/a
Autism	1.1	9.0
Deaf-blindness	No statistics	No statistics
Developmental delay	0.8	6.0
Emotional disturbance	0.7	5.0
Hearing impairment	0.2	1.0
Intellectual disability	0.8	6.0
Multiple disabilities	0.3	2.0
Orthopedic impairment	0.1	1.0
Other health impairment	1.7	14.0
Specific learning disabilities	4.5	34.0
Speech-language impairment	2.6	20.0
Traumatic brain injury	0.1	1.0

Source: Based on data from the National Center for Education Statistics, 2018b.

students. Most Hispanic students are in urban or urban fringe areas. Nine-and-a-half percent of public school students are English Language Learners (ELL) equaling 4.8 million. Poverty, racial diversity, and limited English proficiency coexist in many schools. These statistics are important. Observing the percentages and trends across time enables local districts, and state and federal education agencies an opportunity to react and proactively respond to the changing climate regarding training for teachers and staff on topics such as cultural awareness and sensitivity, programming needs for ELL, interpreter services, special education supports, literacy programs, and family training and support services.

The fact that 13.2% of the total enrollment received special education services is of particular concern to SLPs and audiologists. This represented more than 6.7 million students in the 2015–2016 school year (National Center for Education Statistics, 2018b) that may have needed the services of SLPs and/or audiologists. These statistics help to identify how necessary our professions are to improve the learning outcomes of the students we serve. These students will inevitably come from a variety of racial, ethnic, and socioeconomic backgrounds. Caseloads will reflect a wide variety of types of problems and varying degrees of severity. Most students will spend the majority of their day in the regular classroom. Thus, specific skills in the area of cultural competence and educational curriculum are needed to work effectively in today's schools.

Legal Foundations Affecting Services

SLPs and audiologists will be more effective in educational settings by understanding the federal legislation that affects public education. The federal government mandates laws governing educational practices yet has given individual states power to oversee and set forth rules within its own boundaries and local communities. School-based SLPs and audiologists are expected to know and follow the laws and policies that govern their schools. As such, they have a responsibility to keep current with changes in legislation at federal, state, and local levels. The timeline shown in Figure 16–1 highlights major historical federal legislation that has affected public education. Descriptions of current laws that impact education and individuals with disabilities are discussed in greater detail further in this chapter.

Section 504 of the Rehabilitation Act of 1973

Section 504 of the Rehabilitation Act of 1973 is a national civil rights law that prohibits discrimination against individuals with disabilities that remains in effect today. Section 504 ensures that any student with a disability has equal access to an education. Any qualified student with a disability may receive accommodations and modifications under this law. Individuals who have a history of or who are regarded as having a physical or mental impairment that substantially limits a major life function are protected by Section 504. Section 504 uses the Americans with Disabilities Act definition for major life functions where caring for one's self, walking, seeing, hearing, speaking, breathing, working, performing manual tasks, or learning are impaired.

In the school setting, a 504 Plan guarantees that eligible students, who may not require the specially designed instruction that an individualized education program (IEP) affords, will be provided accommodations or modifications to the classroom environment or curriculum. These modifications and accommodations may include a copy of teacher notes, preferential seating, sound-field amplification system, or teacher training, to mention only a few of the possibilities.

Americans with Disabilities Act of 1990 and Amendments of 2008

The Americans with Disabilities Act (ADA) was enacted in 1990 to protect the civil rights of individuals with disabilities. This civil rights legislation was designed to provide those with disabilities universal access to public services, employment, transportation, and government services (Americans with Disabilities Act, 1990). Also, the ADA Amendments Act of 2008 extended the definition of disabilities to include all physical or mental impairments, even when controlled by medication, treatment, or other aids (such as contact lenses). In the public schools, there may be many students who meet the eligibility for ADA protections due to a medical diagnosis (e.g., attention deficit disorder, diabetes, vision impairment) and who require accommodations without meeting the definition of a child with a disability under IDEA—even if the condition is being successfully managed by medication.

Every Student Succeeds Act (ESSA) (2015 Reauthorization of the Elementary and Secondary Education Act of 1965)

In 2015, Congress reauthorized the Every Student Succeeds Act (ESSA). This law was originally named the Elementary and Secondary Education Act (ESEA), passed in 1965. This law has been reauthorized eight times since then and each reauthorization provided changes and updates along with a new name. It was

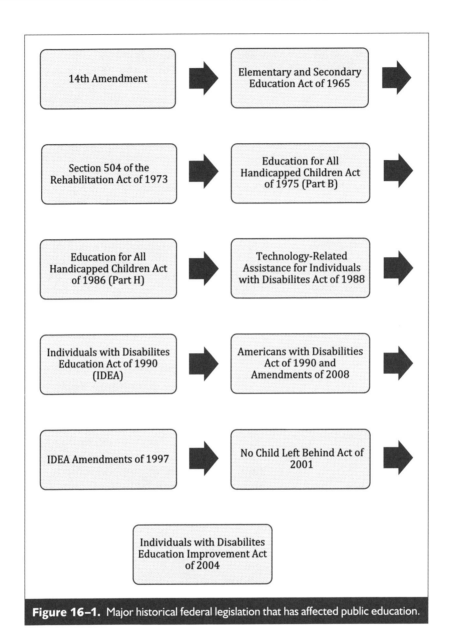

Figure 16–1. Major historical federal legislation that has affected public education.

formerly and more popularly called "No Child Left Behind," along with its other names. The ESSA provides increased accountability for education by requiring more stringent academic standards, annual student testing requirements, enforced school accountability, plans to address struggling students, and state and local report cards that are published for public viewing. Input from parents in the accountability process is a hallmark of this law, which over the years significantly raised expectations for states, school districts, and individual schools so that all students meet or exceed state standards. Previous versions of this law introduced concepts such as ensuring improved academic progress for all students, focusing on prevention versus intervention, and ensuring that special education students are first and foremost general education students as specified by providing the Least Restrictive Environment (LRE), sometimes referred to as mainstreaming or inclusion. Other improvements included requiring ratings on how all students and students within disaggregated subgroups (described below) perform on the state assessments to determine adequate yearly progress (AYP). The law required that teachers in all classrooms be highly qualified, that high academic standards were met, and those annual academic assessments aligned with state content standards. Test scores of students are then disaggregated by racial/ethnic categories, limited English proficient, economically disadvantaged, and disability subgroups. The performance of each subgroup is compared with the state target for all students who meet or exceed proficiency in academic areas to determine how well the school, school district, and state educates its students. There are a variety of consequences for schools that do not meet rigorous academic standards for their students.

Individuals with Disabilities Education Improvement Act of 2004

The Individuals with Disabilities Education Improvement Act of 2004 (IDEA) was originally enacted in 1975, entitled the Education for All Handicapped Children Act (Public Law 94-142). This law mandates a free appropriate public school education (FAPE) for children ages 3 to 21 years with disabilities. There are 14 disability categories and specific requirements that address evaluation and services for students. A FAPE includes special education and related services that are provided at public expense and are based on the student's IEP. Students with disabilities must be educated in LRE and all decisions are made by a team of individuals including teachers, administrators, related service providers, etc. Parents have the right to participate in decision making regarding evaluations and placements and provide consent in the decision-making process. An extension of IDEA 2008 addresses the birth to 3-year-old ages under Part C services, which are detailed in Chapter 17 of this book.

States are required to have a performance plan evaluating their implementation of IDEA called the Part B State Performance Plan (SPP). Each state must report annually to the U.S. Department of Education Office of Special Education and to the public on the performance of each of its school districts in a report called the Part B Annual Performance Report (APR). The law also includes provisions that help align IDEA with other education laws.

Endrew F. Supreme Court Ruling

In 2017, the Supreme Court of the United States ruled on the Endrew F. case. Endrew F. was a student with autism in Colorado. The court found that IDEA aims for "grade level advancement for children with disabilities who can be educated in the regular classroom," and therefore "de minimis progress" is not sufficient. Practically speaking, all students in special education should demonstrate "appropriately ambitious" progress. The court did not, however, define what "appropriately ambitious" progress was for students served under IDEA. This favorable ruling on behalf of a student with differences served as a catalyst to propel least restrictive and inclusion practices into regular education classrooms for core academic instruction, not only specialist type classes such as physical education, art, and music.

Education Funding

Education funding comes from federal, state, and local funds. Federal funds for education in general comprised about 3% or $102.26 billion of the 2015 federal budget, which totaled $3.8 trillion. Comparatively $1.05 trillion (27%) was spent on health care and $609.3 billion (16%) was spent on defense (National Priorities Project, 2015). Federal funding for education is provided by programs including ESSA, Title I, IDEA Part B, Improving Teacher Quality Program, 21st Century Community Learning Centers, English Language Learners Program, and Impact Aid (U.S. Department of Education [U.S. DOE], 2015). State funding is determined by the state legislature, which appropriates funds from its general fund for educational programs. Local governments receive funding from state and federal funds, but the primary source of funding at this level comes from local tax dollars. Interestingly, while the federal government gives the least percentage to education as compared with states and localities, federal laws create the largest number of requirements.

In 1975, under PL 94-142, Congress originally pledged to provide 40% of the average per-pupil costs to states educating students with disabilities. The federal contribution to date has not exceeded 18%. States may use up to 15% of their federal funds for early intervention services. The remainder of federal special education funding must be used for students who meet the definition of having a disability and are in need of specialized instruction in order to participate and progress in the curriculum of age-level peers.

Special education is expensive, and its costs are rising faster than those of regular education because of the increasing number of students enrolled. According to the National Center for Education Statistics (2018a) in 2015,

> The U.S. Department of Education provided 51 percent ($100.4 billion) of this total. Funds also came

from the U.S. Department of Health and Human Services ($27.2 billion), the U.S. Department of Agriculture ($23.9 billion), the U.S. Department of Veterans Affairs ($13.5 billion), the U.S. Department of Defense ($7 billion), the National Science Foundation ($5.8 billion), the U.S. Department of Labor ($4.8 billion), and the U.S. Department of Energy ($3.5 billion).

Medicaid in Schools

Medicaid is a program co-funded by federal and state governments in which each state develops a plan to support the elderly, disabled, and impoverished. Currently, Medicaid allows for the reimbursement of health claims for services provided to students with disabilities in the public schools and who are eligible for Medicaid. Each state creates a plan for the administration of Medicaid in School Programs and outlines the requirements for covered services, documentation and provider requirements. Audiology and speech-language pathology services that are identified in the student's IEP are reimbursable if all requirements are met. Medicaid in Schools is generally a cost-based reimbursement program that is distinctly different from the typical fee for service programs in health care. Schools receive reimbursement based on a formula that is outlined in the state plan. Understanding requirements for medical necessity, prior authorization, and provider requirements is important for SLPs and audiologists who work in schools.

Some school districts rely on Medicaid funding to supplement the costs of providing speech-language services, thereby requiring school-based SLPs to follow Medicaid billing procedures. Many ethical issues exist in the cost recovery process for Medicaid funds. Therefore, it is the responsibility of SLPs to study and adhere to the state Medicaid laws in the areas of documentation, use of graduate students for the delivery of reimbursable services, and signatures of supervising clinicians. Medicaid audits have required payback in these areas, so school districts and individual SLPs should carefully adhere to their state Medicaid laws.

Roles and Responsibilities in the Schools

The roles and responsibilities of school-based speech-language pathologists and audiologists have undergone significant changes in recent years due to changing laws and requirements in public education. The *Roles and Responsibilities of Speech-Language Pathologists in Schools* (ASHA, 2010b) states that "SLPs have integral roles in

education and are essential members of school facilities" (p. 1). The following is a discussion of the range of roles and responsibilities of SLPs within the schools. Some of these areas are also pertinent to the educational audiologist.

The Process of Working in the Schools

Range of Roles and Responsibilities

Providing services in schools offers SLPs and audiologists unique opportunities to serve a widely diverse range of children and young adults. If you choose to work in this setting, you will learn to define your roles and responsibilities in treating communication disorders related to educational performance. You will be a key player on a team within the school environment, working in partnership with educational staff and families to positively impact the lives of your students. Some SLPs serve just one building, while others serve several locations and travel from site to site.

Because school-based SLPs play a critical role in helping students meet state and district performance standards, the range of their responsibilities may be very broad and may include supporting students in both the general education and special education settings. General education is defined by the state's standard course of study. Special Education is the adaptation of methodology, content, or delivery of instruction to address the unique needs of a child identified with a disability under state eligibility criteria.

In both general and special education settings, services provided by school SLPs are based on educational relevance. Thus, a clinical or medical model of evaluation and service is not always appropriate. To be relevant, school-based SLPs need to have a thorough understanding of federal and state laws and regulations governing education requirements that must be followed. Additionally, assessment and treatment goals for students that relate to state and local educational goals will improve outcomes for both students and the school district.

Services Within General Education

Within general education, SLPs play a key role as individuals or team members, developing and implementing strategies that are specifically designed to prevent communication disorders that negatively impact student educational performance or support the needs of all students. General education systemic initiatives that support students who are not suspected of having a disability include Multi-Tiered Systems of Support (MTSS) and Response to Intervention (RTI). These school initiatives may involve school-based SLPs. Members of an MTSS or RTI team may request the input of the SLP as they discuss expected levels of student performance related to typical development. SLPs may also be asked to support the communication skills of teachers by designing strategies for improving communication and addressing differences within the classroom environment.

School SLPs may work alone to design short term programs called pre-referral interventions to address communication difficulties for students who may or may not have a speech-language disability. Typically, the SLP would design interventions that would be carried out by the classroom teacher or trained designee over a specified period of time. Analyses of collected data would then inform if the interventions were successful, if tweaking or further interventions were necessary, or if an evaluation by the SLP was indicated. Pre-referral intervention programming and/or similar types of programs help to reduce overidentification and address communication differences that do not meet the requirements of IDEA. The school SLPs' role in general education will vary according to state and local requirements and accountability initiatives.

Services Within Special Education

To meet the requirements of IDEA, school SLPs are generally involved in the assessment and treatment of students with disabilities ages 3 through 21. School-based SLPs may be asked to work with students from preschool through young adult or serve students solely in a specific age group or disability area. Children served in schools present with a wide range of communication disorders and impairments, including language/literacy, articulation, fluency, voice/resonance, auditory processing disorders, hearing impairment, feeding and swallowing, traumatic brain injury, behavioral and emotional disorders, and augmentative communication needs. The potential diversity of a school SLP's caseload requires a broad knowledge base.

Students may have multiple disability identifications under IDEA or receive SLP services because the IEP team determined those services are required to assist the child with a disability. For instance, a child identified with autism who is in a self-contained special education classroom may be receiving both speech-language therapy and occupational therapy as related services to address educational needs. Under IDEA, speech-language therapy is part of special education, either as a "stand-alone" service or as a related service. A table of some additional related services in IDEA is shown in Table 16–2.

Table 16–2. Additional Related Services in IDEA
Speech-language and audiology services
Interpreting services
Psychological services
Occupational and physical therapy
Recreation, including therapeutic recreation
Early identification and evaluation of disabilities in children
Counseling services, including rehabilitation counseling
Orientation and mobility
Medical services (but only for diagnostic or evaluation purposes, not for ongoing treatment)
School health and/or school nurse services
Social work services
Parent counseling and training

A case manager is a school staff person responsible for the coordination of supports for a student with a disability and communication with parents. When students have more than one disability identification, the case manager would typically be the child's classroom-based special education teacher. When a student's only disability is speech-language impairment, the school SLP generally serves as the case manager and is responsible for planning and leading annual meetings, mandated evaluations and re-evaluations, completing all the associated required documentation, which includes making sure that at least one other professional has had input into the IEP such as the occupational therapist, and ensuring that all sections are completed and communicated with parents within the due process mandated timelines. This will be further reviewed below.

Within the special education setting, school SLPs may conduct evaluations of identified eligible students, and provide services to those who meet qualifying criteria. Assessments may include both standardized and non-standardized instruments, including "authentic assessment" of students in their natural environment. Assessments may be for the purpose of determining eligibility for special education under IDEA or to develop academic programming. In regard to treatment, providing evidence-based interventions for students with disabilities typically comprises the bulk of the school-based SLP's day-to-day work. School-based SLPs may want to keep in mind that "speech" is not a place where children go, but a service that is provided anywhere within the school setting. Services may be provided in classrooms, in the lunchroom, on field trips, at off-campus employment sites, or wherever the IEP team and/or SLP determines the students' needs will be best met. Educationally relevant intervention may occur wherever educationally relevant communication takes place and should move away from the traditional, more restrictive "pull-out" model. It is important to remember that IDEA requires the provision of services in LRE and in as natural a setting as possible. Natural settings might include a classroom, playground, cafeteria, art room, music room, physical education gym, or even a bus parking lot.

Common strategies to manage rising caseloads and to work smarter, not harder, while being most effective include integration of the student's curriculum into therapy activities, providing special education services in the general education setting when possible, and collaborating with classroom teachers. Accommodations and modifications are written into the student's IEP. Planning meaningful lessons incorporates student interests and promotes buy-in by students. As an example, a therapy group may include students with various challenges, including fluency, articulation, and language. Students would use curriculum-based text and content, such as the weekly spelling list or a chapter from their science textbook, to further their learning while focusing on speech or language skill development.

School-based SLPs and educational audiologists need to familiarize themselves with federal, state, and local mandates related to compliance. These important activities include adhering to timelines for due process, including screenings, evaluations, and development of IEPs and IFSPs; following Medicaid billing procedures; and maintaining appropriate documentation of services. See Chapter 20, "Documentation Issues," for further details related to this most important aspect of service delivery.

Additional Responsibilities in Schools

Providing staff development, teacher training, and parent education and training are other important tasks for the school SLP and AuD. Working with administrative staff to ensure the development and maintenance of high-quality programs at the school and district levels is also a responsibility of the SLP and AuD (ASHA, 2010a). For instance, some SLPs have a specialty area, such as autism spectrum disorders (ASDs) or fluency disorders and may serve as a resource to an entire school district in meeting the needs of a specific population. These school-based SLPs with specialized interests can be supported by their SLP colleagues in collecting data for conducting research

and helping them to pursue additional professional development or continuing education opportunities to further their skills. This individual can then bring back meaningful in-service information to the department and serve as the "go-to" SLP when needs arise across the district. These additional responsibilities represent opportunities for professional and personal growth and allow the school SLP to become an integral part of the at-large school community.

Supervision of student SLPs (interns), clinical fellows (CFs), and speech-language pathology assistants is one of the roles and responsibilities of SLPs in the schools. Evidence of current knowledge of supervision practice as of 2020 is a requisite to supervising graduate students and CFs for ASHA certification (ASHA, n.d.). Many SLPs have little or no coursework during their graduate preparation in this area; however, there are many continuing education opportunities offered on the topic of supervision. By supervising graduate students and CFs, SLPs cultivate the next generation of professionals. By ensuring positive school-based experiences, SLPs also encourage graduate students and CFs to consider schools as a future work setting.

School-based SLPs may need to reach out to local universities with Communication Sciences and Disorders programs to volunteer to supervise interns. Supervisors need to make sure that their licensure and certification are current throughout the period of time they are supervising. Supervision of interns should be a mutually beneficial opportunity. Graduate students bring a wealth of current knowledge on evidence-based practices, while practicing SLPs provide the required clinical hours and fine-tuning of skills that students need to become outstanding professionals. Universities may also provide training in supervision to enhance the professional development of school-based SLPs, thus creating well-trained school-based supervisors. The role of the supervising SLP may be both challenging and rewarding and, like any supervisory relationship, is one that needs to be built on collaboration, trust, and open communication. Of note: If you are supervising a student or clinical fellow, consider joining ASHA's Special Interest Group 11, Administration and Supervision, and enroll in workshops on supervision. Both of these provide you with opportunities to learn how to work effectively with student interns and CFs as you learn more about your role as a supervisor. For more information on supervision see Chapter 26, "Supervision and Mentoring."

The school-based SLP may also be asked to supervise SLP assistants. This responsibility requires specific knowledge and skills in the area of supervision and presents with its own set of both challenges and opportunities and will be discussed later in this chapter.

Special Education Processes Under IDEA

Federal and state law governs the processes of referring and evaluating students who are suspected of having a disability and for treatment of those who are identified as eligible under IDEA. Parents have specific procedural safeguards under IDEA and the special education eligibility process must be completed within 60 days unless a state had an existing timeline in regulation.

The following sections outline the general steps in the special education process. It is important to note that state and local differences may exist. Examples of these state-specific differences include regulatory timelines, data sources, and evaluation components. SLPs should become familiar with their own state and local requirements to ensure responsible practices.

Referral. The referral for a suspicion of a disability begins the special education process. Parents, guardians, or any member of the school faculty and staff may make a referral. Whenever a referral is received by any member of the school staff, the special education process begins. A meeting may be scheduled to review the concerns and decide if the referral is appropriate. Examples of referrals that may be rejected by the team include students who exhibit developmentally appropriate articulation errors or language and reading difficulties that can be managed in regular education. If the team determines a disability is suspected, the process continues.

Review of Existing Data and Determination of Needed Data. The next step in the special education process is a team review of existing data in order to determine if any additional information is required. Examples of some existing data may include pre-referral interventions that have already been completed or that may need to be initiated to determine if a full evaluation is necessary, family reports on recent changes that may be contributing to the concerns, and/or outside reports such as a neuropsychological evaluation or physician reports. After review, the team reaches consensus on the assessment tools and measures that will be used to gather data about the student. Parent consent is required prior to beginning any new assessment or evaluation procedures.

Evaluation. Once consent is provided, school SLPs work to gather data related to the specific communication concerns shared in the referral. Additionally, they work together with teachers and parents to gather information about the educational impact of any communication impairment and need for specially designed

instruction. These data should be sufficient to answer any questions for eligibility determination, but also to develop a functional IEP should the child be found eligible with a speech-language impairment.

The evaluation must measure all suspected areas of disability and, if necessary, include a description of any non-standardized measurement tools. All evaluations must be "conducted in the student's native language or other mode of communication (unless not feasible), free from discrimination and bias, valid, and administered by trained professionals" (IDEA, 2004). For students with limited English proficiency, materials should evaluate disability and special education needs and not English language skills. The evaluation must also include a variety of tools that are tailored to measure specific areas of educational need for the individual.

An assessment is a controlled opportunity to observe and interpret behavior. Assessments are used to gather relevant, functional, and developmental information, "including information provided by the parent, and information related to enabling the child to be involved in and progress in the general curriculum" (U.S. DOE, 2004). The results of the assessment must provide relevant data that directly assist the eligibility IEP team in determining the educational needs of the child (IDEA, 2004).

This evaluation includes more than the results of standardized tests. No single procedure or tool should be the sole eligibility criterion. Evaluations that rely solely on standardized scores are merely a "snapshot" in time—a one-dimensional view of the student over a brief period of time often conducted in a separate environment, such as the "speech room" with evaluators the student has never met, using materials or questions that are unfamiliar to the student. A comprehensive evaluation includes both qualitative and quantitative data composed of standardized and non-standard assessments as well as opportunities to observe the student in multiple educational environments. Multiple observers view the student in different settings, focusing on how the impairment may be negatively affecting the student's educational performance. This observational information is required to determine the adverse effect of the impairment on the child's ability to access the general education curriculum and is required for initial evaluations. Consideration of the diagnostic accuracy of tools and tests along with attention to possible bias introduced by dialect, language learning, or poverty are critical to reducing both over- and underidentification in the school setting.

Once the SLP completes the evaluation, a report is provided to the family prior to the meeting and remains as part of the student's educational record.

Eligibility. After the evaluation is complete, a team, including the parent, meets to review the results and using state eligibility criteria, determines whether the student has a disability. This team also decides which category or categories of disability best describe the student's disability. The determination that a child is eligible for special education must be made on an individual basis by the group responsible within the child's school system for making those determinations (U.S. DOE, 2004). Students may qualify under one or more of the disability categories listed in Table 16–1. Students who meet the state eligibility criteria are determined to be eligible for special education and related services.

According to IDEA (2004), speech or language impairment includes communication disorders such as stuttering or impaired articulation, language, or voice that adversely affects a child's educational performance. In a letter to ASHA in 1980, the U.S. Department of Health, Education, and Welfare stated that "meaningful educational performance cannot be limited to showing signs of discrepancies in age/grade performance" (U.S. Department of Health, Education, and Welfare, 1980). In the letter of guidance, requested by ASHA in 2009, the U.S. DOE Office of Special Education Programs confirmed that the 1980 policy on "adverse effect" was still in effect. Further "a child's educational performance must be determined on an individual basis and should include non-academic as well as academic areas" (U.S. DOE, 2007). The term *adverse effect* is intended to encompass both academic achievement and functional performance. Keep in mind that functional performance may not always be reflected in the student's academic performance, or grade point average. For instance, a student with all A's may still have social communication deficits that have an adverse effect on overall educational (i.e., not academic) performance. The determination of adverse effect should be a data-driven one and the state or local educational agency (LEA) may have identified thresholds that help in that assertion.

Individualized Education Programs.

Once a determination is made that a child has a disability and needs special education and related services, the team develops an IEP (U.S. DOE, 2004). The team uses the results of the evaluation to write the IEP, which serves as a blueprint for services. SLPs are part of the team that writes an IEP to meet the unique needs of each individual child who is identified as having a speech-language impairment. SLPs are also part of the team when speech as a related service is being considered (see related services).

Every eligible student with a disability must have an IEP in place that is reviewed at least annually. The IEP is a written statement for each child with a disability that is developed, reviewed, and revised in a meeting that must include the parents of the child; at least one regular education teacher of the child (if the child is, or may be, participating in the regular education environment); at least one special education teacher of the child, or one special education provider of the child; and a representative of the school district who is qualified to provide or supervise the provision of instruction specially designed to meet the unique needs of children with disabilities and is knowledgeable about the general education curriculum and the availability of resources of the public agency. Other required attendees may include an individual who can interpret the instructional implications of evaluation results; other individuals who have knowledge or special expertise regarding the child, including related services personnel as appropriate and at the discretion of the parent or the agency; and whenever appropriate, the child with a disability (U.S. DOE, 2004).

Members of the IEP team can serve dual roles. For example, the speech-language pathologist may serve as the special education provider *and* the individual who can interpret the instructional implications of evaluation results.

The purpose of the IEP meeting is to consider the eligible child's strengths and areas of academic, developmental, and functional needs; concerns of the parents; and results of the initial or most recent evaluation to develop a plan for educating the student. Special factors that the team must also consider include but are not limited to behavioral factors; the language needs of the child with limited English proficiency; whether a child who is blind or visually impaired requires instruction in Braille; communication needs of the child, including opportunities for direct instruction in the child's primary language and communication mode; hearing impairments and whether the child needs assistive technology devices and services. The education plan must include measurable goals and accommodations that will allow students to access their curriculum.

Related Services.

Students with a disability are eligible to receive related services (see Table 16–2) as determined by the IEP team. These data-driven decisions should be based on the student's need for the related service in order to fully benefit from (or achieve the goals in) the primary area of eligibility. Related services may flow in and out of an IEP based on the goals determined by the team for the period of time covered by the document (usually one year). A student who is receiving multiple services and is not a "speech only" student may require a related service one year and not the next based on goals stated in the current IEP. *It is important to note that the category of speech or language impaired is the only one that can be both a primary area of special education disability and a related service.* Although the intent of IDEA

(2004) is that goals for a student be written before providers are determined and services begin in reality, providers are typically determined first and then each provider writes goals.

Service Delivery Options

School speech-language pathologists may provide services using a variety of service delivery models. Direct therapy services (individual or group sessions directly focusing on the goals identified on the IEP) to students may be used in combination with indirect services (work on behalf of the student when he or she is not present, such as programming a speech-generating device) that support a student's learning in school as well as the community. The wide range of service delivery possibilities is one of the many aspects of school-based speech-language pathology and audiology that professionals find appealing in this practice setting. Direct and indirect therapy services will be discussed in greater detail below.

Curriculum-Relevant Services

IDEA intends that all special education be connected to the curriculum. Most states have adopted the Core Content Standards (Common Core State Standards Initiative, 2010) as their curriculum. For SLPs, the intent of IDEA means that all services should be connected to the educational standards of the state. Teachers are the curriculum experts for their grade level. In whatever location students are served, SLPs should be communicating with teachers to connect special education services to the educational standards and classroom instruction. Even if SLPs are providing services using a pull-out model, they should incorporate curriculum materials provided by teachers to connect the differentiated instruction in special education to the classroom.

Direct Services

Pull-Out Services. SLPs may serve students by pulling them out of class to a separate special education environment, which is often referred to as the "speech room." This is a more restrictive environment than the classroom, but it affords the opportunity for drill and practice on concepts one-on-one or in a small group. This service delivery model may actually represent the least restrictive learning environment for some children as they may require a quieter, more focused setting for optimal learning. SLPs should tie pull-out services to the curriculum by using concepts or materials that are related to the educational standards covered in the classroom. Students often miss classroom content when they are pulled out of the classroom for these sessions.

Therefore, SLPs should consider if this service method is required for students to make progress or if services in the less restrictive environment such as a classroom or some other educationally relevant location would be more appropriate.

Classroom-Based Services. If students are determined eligible for SLP services, SLPs may provide their special education services in general education or special education classrooms, sometimes referred to as integrated inclusive, embedded, or a collaborative model. This often represents a less restrictive environment for many students, since it is their natural learning environment. Sometimes, the term "push-in" is used to describe services provided in a classroom. Keep in mind that this term may not be received in a positive way by classroom teachers whose perception is that the SLP is invading their space. This is where a conversation about the benefit of services in the natural environment and the goal of supporting services in LRE can be helpful.

Students can also be served at other locations on the school campus, including the cafeteria, playground, or gym. This model provides additional benefit to other students in the classroom setting, also called incidental benefit, which is permitted by IDEA. Reducing a student's time away from instruction and increasing educational relevance during treatment are the benefits of this service model.

Some SLPs serve students off campus at community-based vocational settings. This model often requires planning time with other professionals to best target special education goals embedded in curriculum or classroom-based routines. The goals for this type of service are often captured in the transition component of the IEP, described later in this section.

Indirect Services

Indirect services are provided on behalf of students and are delivered without the student present. These services focus on supporting the student by working with teachers, assistants, parents, other school personnel, or even other students serving as peer models or mentors. This type of service supports the learning environment for a student and may take the form of programming augmented communication devices, teaching other students how to appropriately interact with an augmented communication system user, teaching an assistant a therapy technique, or planning with a teacher to engineer a communication-rich classroom. Audiologists may also play an important role here—for example, providing support for teachers using frequency-modulated (FM) systems for hearing-impaired students, and consultation on classroom acoustics to the benefit of all students. These activities represent only a few of the possible indirect services that may be provided in a school setting. Because this type of service is provided indirectly to the student, it is important that parents have a clear understanding of this service delivery model when included in an IEP. Other terminologies such as consultation and collaboration should be used carefully, as each state or school division may define these terms differently in education and Medicaid regulations.

3:1 Model

The 3:1 model is a combination of both direct and indirect services delivered in the education setting. It is not, however, the only way to accomplish this combination in a workload approach. The 3:1 model combines 3 weeks of direct treatment sessions with 1 week for indirect treatment. This service delivery option provides direct treatment and supports other professionals and family members to improve outcomes for the student. Indirect services include those listed in the indirect services section.

Reevaluation and Continued Eligibility

According to IDEA, children with a disability must have their eligibility considered *at least* every three years to determine whether they continue to have such a disability and to assess their educational needs (IDEA, 2004). When an IEP is in place for a student, the team must review, at least every three years, existing evaluation, assessment, and other pertinent data, including current classroom-based observations and input from parents and teachers to determine whether additional evaluations are required to document the disability. Parental consent is required for any additional evaluations that are requested by the IEP team for the purpose of eligibility determination.

Transition Services

IDEA 2004 mandates that transition services be in place for special education students 16 years and older and considered for those 14 years old and above. The IEP team considers what these students will do after they leave the public schools by documenting potential interests and hobbies (leisure activities), vocational aspirations (employment), and the ability to live independently (independence). Both audiologists and SLPs have the opportunity to make insightful contributions during this discussion.

SLPs and audiologists provide services to students as they transition at all stages of their education. Many are involved in supporting the transition of students from preschool settings to kindergarten, from elementary to middle school, and middle to high school. SLPs and audiologists can directly affect the successful transition of school-age students by helping them navigate the new challenges of changing classes and interacting with many personalities in middle and high school. SLPs and audiologists can also be instrumental in facilitating successful transitions for students to work and vocational settings. Difficulties with hearing, speech, or language can serve as blocks to success for special education students at vocational sites. SLPs and audiologists are equipped with the knowledge and problem-solving skills to support students in achieving positive outcomes at job sites.

Special Issues in School Settings

Below you will find a variety of issues that arise for the school-based SLP or audiologist. These issues are impacted by state and local policy. These issues are important to school-based providers.

Evidence-Based Practice (EBP)

According to IDEA 2004, special education should be "evidence-based to the extent practicable." The treatment approaches described in the IEP should have research validation. EBP is not simply the technique; it is the convergence of researched techniques, parent and student preferences, and clinical expertise. ASHA provides a wealth of information on EBP for a variety of disorders, and Chapter 8 provides more discussion on the topic. The following case study serves to clarify the convergence of the multiple variables of EBP:

Case Study in EBP. A student has been identified as eligible for special education, and goals have been written in the area of literacy. The parents and school staff have researched the promising practices in literacy intervention and together have found three tested literacy programs they believe have research validation sufficient to provide good outcomes for the student. However, neither the school staff nor the parents have enough information about any of the programs to be able to suggest one over another. One of the programs (X) incorporates student-produced artwork, and the student in question loves to draw. In addition, the school SLP has been trained in this particular (X) method and endorses its efficacy, as it incorporates language-based learning needs such as vocabulary, concepts, problem solving, reasoning, direction following, and sequencing, which are all identified goals on this student's IEP. The team then agrees that this program (X) will be followed for the particular student. The convergence of the three areas of EBP has led the team to the best decision for this student given all considerations.

Workload Versus Caseload

For many years it has been common practice in school districts to hire SLPs and audiologists using a caseload approach that simply examines the number of students served. In more recent years, however, with the multitude of new responsibilities that SLPs perform in the schools, ASHA has endorsed a workload model that considers not only the number of students served but also many other parameters. Other work tasks include committee work, provision of indirect and consultative services on behalf of all students, collaboration with other professionals, and participation in IEP team meetings, to name a few.

Many teachers and other school professionals remain unaware of the knowledge and skills possessed by their SLP colleagues. Thus, they may not be familiar with the myriad of roles and responsibilities of the SLPs working in their facility. SLPs in the school setting may need to educate their faculty about the variety and number of the evaluation, treatment, and collaboration responsibilities that constitute the contemporary SLP workload. A faculty/administration in-service to inform school personnel on the evolving role of the SLP is a worthwhile investment of time and effort. See Resources for more information about the workload analysis approach for establishing caseload standards available on the ASHA website (ASHA, 2002a).

Scheduling

It is difficult to characterize a "typical" daily schedule for school-based SLPs or audiologists. The responsibilities of these professionals are continuously changing because of the ever-expanding scope of practice and the constantly evolving education initiatives at the federal, state, and even local levels. "Scheduling" in the context of school-based SLPs and audiologists typically refers to the provision of direct services, although numerous other responsibilities as noted in the section above also need to be factored into the overall schedule.

A variety of locations for direct service delivery are represented on the schedule of the present-day SLP or audiologist, as mentioned earlier in this chapter. Many school-based SLPs and audiologists engage in a variety of service delivery models (e.g., in the classroom, pull-out, consultation) to support the use of the LRE and to provide ecologically valid services in the "natural environment" for all students.

Designing a schedule to meet the needs of students based on their IEPs requires flexibility and collabora-tion with staff members. SLPs and audiologists need to schedule a time for observations and evaluations, consultations, planning and preparation, and, of course, lunch, or 30 minutes of unencumbered time. The master, or "bell," schedule of the individual school is the best template to use in designing a schedule for speech-language services. Once a schedule is in place, it should be shared with appropriate school personnel and, naturally, the student. The effective professional will remember that the schedule is fluid, with changes to be made as needed throughout the school year.

Some SLPs and audiologists may experience difficulty in constructing a schedule because of constraints placed on student time by teachers or administrators. When these obstacles arise, professionals may need to involve the administration of the school or district to provide input in developing a schedule that meets the needs of all students in accordance with their IEPs.

English Language Learners and Cultural Competence

Cultural and linguistic diversity in schools continues to rise and that trend will surely continue. According to recent statistics, there are approximately 5 million English-language learners in public schools today. That is twice the number from just 15 years ago, and that number was expected to double again by 2015 (National Clearinghouse for English Language Acquisition, 2007). A bilingual speech-language pathologist who is fluent in the student's native language is the most appropriate resource for assessment and treatment of English language learners with speech-language disorders. If an interpreter is needed, the public school division policy or procedure should be followed to ensure a qualified and competent interpreter is used.

Speech-language pathologists and audiologists must carefully select and train individuals who will assist in the assessment and treatment of English language learners. It is crucial that interpreters translate exactly what each party says without using nonverbal cues or rewording the phrasing of the SLP or audiologist. Interpreters should be familiar with the anticipated tasks and any assessment and intervention materials. Interpreters should take notes as needed as the session proceeds. SLPs, audiologists, and interpreters should allow time after the session to review notes, discuss responses, and address any difficulties that arise in the session. Translators may also be helpful in translating written homework and procedural forms for parents.

This population offers a unique opportunity for school teams to practice interprofessionally. English as a Second Language (ESL) teachers work together with teachers, SLPs, audiologists, and interpreters to support students in acquiring English proficiency while addressing accompanying language and/or hearing disorders, if they exist.

SLPs and audiologists will demonstrate cultural competence when working with students and families if they learn some basic words in the native language of the student. The ability to greet students in their native language creates a positive tone for face-to-face interactions. As mentioned earlier, many internet resources for translation are available; therefore, it is not difficult to initiate the meeting with a display of respect stemming from the knowledge of the student's cultural and linguistic heritage.

To the extent possible, intervention sessions should begin in the student's native language and move toward the language of educational significance, typically English. Educational performance for purposes of gauging AYP is assessed in English according to the No Child Left Behind legislation. English language learners have a two-year period of "safe harbor" from AYP testing but eventually are held accountable for mastery of academic goals, ones that are evaluated by assessments administered in English. You may find the English Learner Tool Kit (U.S. Department of Education, 2015) in the resource section very helpful. See Chapter 25 for more information on service delivery to linguistically diverse populations.

Privacy Issues

SLPs and audiologists are obligated to maintain the privacy of all students. Publicly conversing about a student, including use of social media, removing confidential files from the facility, or leaving confidential files unattended or unsecured are examples of situations that compromise the privacy of students and their families. The Family Educational Rights and Privacy Act (FERPA) (U.S. Department of Education, 2011) affords parents and students over 18 years of age certain rights with respect to educational records. School-based SLPs and audiologists have a legitimate educational interest in students' educational records, and as such, FERPA permits "disclosure without consent," allowing access to records. With this privilege comes a huge responsibility to keep all records secure, keep all discussions about a student in a private setting, and adhere to standards that respect the confidentiality and privacy of students and their families.

Increasingly, documentation and records are maintained through electronic means. This innovation provides a variety of new challenges to keep and maintain record confidentiality. Many LEAs are establishing electronic record confidentiality policies and procedures. See more about privacy issues in Chapter 20, "Documentation Issues."

Communication and Documentation

The easiest way to avoid complaints that could lead to a due process hearing is to establish professional, positive communicative relationships with the child's parents at the beginning of the special education process. Acknowledging and addressing parental concerns in a proactive way often avoids conflict. Many complaints are simply a result of a lack of timely communication from school staff. Most parental concerns can be effectively addressed through open communication, clarification, and/or active listening. If attempts to resolve parent concerns are unsuccessful, it is critical that the SLP or audiologist follow established notification procedures of the school district and inform the appropriate school and/or central office staff. The documentation of the SLP and audiologist will frequently be requested and is crucial evidence in due process proceedings.

School districts often choose to compromise or enter into a legally binding settlement agreement with parents to avoid litigation. The best protection for the SLP, audiologist, and school district is to maintain accurate documentation, including parental contacts, dates of service (including why scheduled services were not provided), session activities, and progress toward attainment of IEP goals. Additionally, it is imperative that SLPs and audiologists share IEP accommodations, such as preferential seating for a student with a hearing loss, with all the student's teachers and maintain written documentation that accommodations were provided in accordance with the IEP. Best practice dictates that the SLP and audiologist, as appropriate, communicate regularly with teachers to verify that all parts of the IEP are implemented as specified. Again, see Chapter 20, "Documentation Issues," for more in-depth discussion on this topic.

Response to Instruction/Intervention

States that permit the use of Response to Intervention have set careful guidelines for its implementation. According to the National Center on Response to Intervention (National Center on Response to Intervention, 2011), "RTI integrates assessment and intervention within a multi-level prevention system to maximize student achievement and to reduce behavior problems. With RTI, schools identify students at risk for poor learning outcomes, monitor student progress, provide evidence-based interventions, and adjust the intensity and nature of those interventions depending on a student's responsiveness, and identify students with learning disabilities or other disabilities" (p. 1). RTI has four components according to the National Center on Response to Intervention:

1. A schoolwide, multilevel instructional and behavioral system for preventing school failure

2. Screening

3. Progress monitoring

4. Data-based decision making about instruction, movement within the multilevel system, and disability identification (in accordance with state law)

School systems must consider a number of factors as they move to an RTI model. First, the school districts weigh the advantages and disadvantages of RTI over the discrepancy model (the mismatch between ability and progress in school). If they choose the RTI approach, the district must write guidelines, policies, and procedures that will govern the practice of RTI. In addition, the district must provide training to all educational personnel, choose universal screening tools to be administered to all students, and identify tiers of progression through the RTI process. A school-based team refers students experiencing failure, implements interventions, monitors student progress, and makes referral to special education if necessary.

Eligibility for special education or entitlement under RTI may occur in a variety of different ways. The "tiers" of RTI represent increasing levels of intensity of interventions. Tier 1 typically involves parent and teacher collaboration. Tier 2 typically begins with classroom-based interventions, perhaps with the involvement of the SLP, psychologist, or other identified support. At Tier 3, interventions are increased in frequency and/or intensity. In some states, Tier 3 marks the beginning of the special education process. Each progressive tier is designed to support student success in regular education and prevent the need for movement toward special education services unless the student is unresponsive to intervention. The following case study is an example of the progression through the tiers of the RTI evaluation system:

Tier 1: All the students in a kindergarten class are administered a universal screening instrument. The kindergarten teacher identifies a student who performed well below expectations on the screening tool, has exhibited learning and play skill difficulties in the classroom, and is struggling with early literacy skills. The student displays difficulty forming grapheme/phoneme relationships, as indicated by his inability to articulate and write the letters in his name. The teacher alerts the school student assistance team composed of regular education

teachers, an administrator, the SLP, and the psychologist. Following the protocol for this school, the assistance team informs the parent and asks for a meeting. The team shares its concerns with the parent and receives consent to begin interventions to support the student in learning. Because the student is minimally responsive to Tier 1 interventions that the teacher and teacher's assistant are incorporating into the classroom curriculum, the team decides to move to Tier 2.

Tier 2: The teacher again collaborates with the assistance of team members, including the SLP, learning disabilities specialist, literacy facilitator, and psychologist, to plan interventions to target the student's areas of need. The team plans the individualized interventions for the student, the setting (classroom, small group, or individual services in another room), the exact intervention(s), and the personnel who will deliver the intervention(s). The interventionists monitor progress frequently and report to the assistance team. Parents are informed at all stages throughout the process. While the student is making some limited progress, the team concludes that he/she is not responding adequately to Tier 2 intervention, so the team decides to increase the frequency and intensity with which the interventions are provided (still at Tier 2). Again, little additional progress is demonstrated on emergent literacy skills, including decoding, grapheme/phoneme relationships, and phonemic synthesis. After several weeks of intervention and progress monitoring, the assistance team with input from the parents decides to make a referral to special education.

Tier 3: Data collected from the RTI process in conjunction with psychoeducational and speech-language testing reveal that the student meets the eligibility criteria for placement in special education. IDEA procedural paperwork and an IEP are initiated, and the student is subsequently placed in special education.

Movement through the tiers of RTI may be both forward and backward depending on the level of support the student requires to be successful. RTI is a promising approach to support learning without identifying students for special education unless their areas of need cannot be met in regular education. Dynamic assessment (where skills and potential are determined) may be part of the special education process. During the RTI dynamic assessment period, a student's mild disorder or difficulties may be remediated, thereby eliminating the need to move to a special education evaluation. This approach has been viewed favorably by many families who do not want their child to be labeled as "special ed" if not absolutely necessary. Unfortunately, there is often a stigma associated with receiving special education support. Given patience and understanding, this often goes away quickly when families see their students progressing.

Literacy

One of the major functions of the school-based SLP is to serve students who exhibit or are at risk for literacy disorders. Speaking, listening, reading, and writing are activities that define literate learners. SLPs are uniquely qualified to prevent and remediate literacy disorders by focusing on prevention and remediation activities that underpin the language functions of literacy. Many SLPs engage in activities that support literate learners in both regular and special education. ASHA's Practice Portal contains much information on the SLP's role in literacy as well as many activities that target the linguistic skills to develop literate learners.

Comprehensive Assessment

IDEA requires data to document the speech and language impairment, educational impact, and need for specially designed instruction. School SLPs must maintain a broad approach to evaluation and select tools that will provide the required data for decision making and IEP development. Gathering data from academic activities, contextualized measures (state and local performance measures in general education), checklists, observations, and other non-standard measurement tools may save time and be more useful in school-based practice than standardized measures that lack sufficient specificity (Schraeder, Quinn, & Stockman, 1999). Authentic assessments are used to investigate speech and language disorders that manifest themselves in samples of classroom work and are often some of the most curriculum relevant and meaningful data that an SLP can collect (Timler, 2008). These assessment artifacts, which are used to determine how a communication disorder might impact academic achievement, can be useful in determining eligibility for special education as well as in selecting goals that will most affect academic achievement.

Working with Service Extenders

School-based SLPs may find that a speech-language pathology assistant (SLPA) has been assigned to help with day-to-day responsibilities. It is important to have a clear understanding of the delineation of the roles and responsibilities of the SLP and those of the SLPA, particularly when it comes to supervision The job description, supervision requirements, and credentialing of these paraprofessionals vary greatly from state to state, so it is important to become familiar with specific requirements within a given state. In addition, ASHA is currently in the process of developing a voluntary credential for SLPAs at the national level, described in more detail in Chapter 13.

As noted by Paul-Brown and Goldberg (2001), SLPAs are extenders of speech-language pathology services and not replacements for SLPs (p. 8). According to the Speech-Language Pathology Assistant Scope of Practice (ASHA, 2013), the tasks delegated to the SLPA by the SLP serve to increase the availability, frequency, and efficiency of services. Such tasks could include but are not limited to assisting with informal documentation, following treatment plans or protocols, documenting client performance, assisting with clerical duties, and performing checks and maintenance of equipment, all under the direction of the supervising SLP. See Chapter 13, "Support Personnel in Communication Sciences and Disorders," for detailed information.

Collaboration with Other Professionals

One of the most attractive aspects of the school setting is the opportunity to engage in interprofessional practice (IPP) by collaborating regularly with many other professionals. SLPs and audiologists work closely with occupational therapists, physical therapists, psychologists, social workers, nurses, counselors, teachers, and others to meet the needs of all students. These collaborative relationships are stimulating to all professionals, ensuring that services are provided using a "whole child" approach. Collaborative planning time between professionals is critical to interprofessional practice and may be accomplished in a variety of ways, including electronic and face-to-face meetings (Flynn, 2010).

Related to IPP is the concept of emotional intelligence. The *Harvard Business Review* has identified that professionals who are aware of their own emotional intelligence work well in interprofessional teams with exponentially improved outcomes (Goleman, 2004). See Chapter 23, "Overview of Interprofessional Practice and Interprofessional Education," for more discussion on working as part of an interprofessional team.

Dysphagia

According to ASHA (2018), SLPs play a significant role in the management of students with swallowing (dysphagia) and feeding problems in school. The 2018 ASHA Schools Survey reported that 10.5% of school-based SLP respondents have an average of 2.6 students with dysphagia on their caseload. Even so, uncertainty persists about the educational relevance of dysphagia management.

ASHA's *Guidelines for Speech-Language Pathologists Providing Swallowing and Feeding Services in Schools* provides the following reasons to explain why addressing swallowing and feeding disorders is educationally relevant and part of the school system's responsibility:

1. Students must be safe while eating in school. This includes providing appropriate personnel, food, and procedures to minimize risks for choking and for aspiration during oral feeding.

2. Students must be adequately nourished and hydrated so that they can attend to and fully access the school curriculum.

3. Students must be healthy (e.g., free from aspiration pneumonia or other illnesses related to malnutrition or dehydration) to maximize their attendance at school.

4. Students must develop skills for eating efficiently during meals and snack times so that they can complete these activities with their peers safely and in a timely manner (ASHA, 2007).

So, what is the role of the school-based SLP when it comes to a child with a swallowing and feeding disorder? SLPs in schools may be instrumental in creating dysphagia teams (Anderson & Homer, 2006) composed of SLPs, occupational therapists, child nutrition directors, and nurses. These teams problem solve to help students gain the hydration and nutrition they need to have sufficient stamina to learn in the least restrictive environment. As part of interdisciplinary decision making, it is also important for school personnel to communicate frequently with medical professionals on issues related to the consistency of food preparation and viscosity of liquid intake provided at school.

The SLP managing the student with dysphagia may need to consider and remain sensitive to cultural factors surrounding food and eating. The SLP should also be aware of legal and ethical issues when addressing feeding and swallowing disorders, including certification, licensure and scope of practice. School districts may have their own policies and procedures with which the SLP should be familiar, as well as issues pertaining to reimbursement, such as Medicaid.

Performance Appraisal

ASHA's Professional Assessment of Contributions and Effectiveness of Speech-Language Pathologists (PACE) document (ASHA, 2014) for the appraisal of the school-based SLP's performance of workload duties serves as a model for many states that now have their own evaluation instrument. Some districts are providing additional monetary incentives based on "value-added" assessments that are tied to student achievement and are another way to assess the SLP's job performance.

Each school district may have its own performance appraisal system, and personnel are typically notified of the process at the beginning of a school year or upon being hired. Performance may be evaluated annually or as part of an ongoing process throughout the school year. The evaluation may be completed by an SLP or audiologist in an administrative role, or by a school principal or other school district administrator. In any case, the evaluation process provides an opportunity to share successes, describe goals for improvement, and receive constructive feedback for professional growth. For more information on performance appraisals, see Chapter 12, "Building Your Career."

Technology

A wide range of low to high technological advances is currently available in many school settings. Document projectors, Smart Boards, whiteboards, telecommunication, computers, and a rapidly increasing number of computer software programs and applications are now available for use in the disciplines of speech-language pathology and audiology. No longer is technology just for augmented and alternative communication users.

According to the Education Superhighway (2017), 88% of public school districts have high-speed broadband internet services, which represent an increase of 30.9 million students and 2.1 million teachers since 2013. Computer labs, rather than classrooms, remain the major internet access point for students. This seems to indicate that schools have yet to fully integrate technology with teaching that takes place in the classroom, and that classroom technology may need to be upgraded, expanded, or replaced. SLPs and audiologists should have internet accessibility in their facilities, but the availability of a computer for personal use varies from district to district. SLPs and audiologists should determine whether their district is able to provide a computer, and if not, how they would be able to access one in their facility.

Telepractice

A promising technological advance in speech-language pathology is telepractice, the use of telecommunications technology to deliver speech-language pathology services at a distance (Crutchley, Dudley, & Campbell, 2010). The practice is gaining in popularity to provide services to underserved or unserved students in school settings. Many rural districts are finding it a viable means of delivering speech-language services. ASHA has developed guidelines for ethical telepractice. Chapter 27, "Technology for Student Training, Professional Practice, and Service Delivery," discusses this topic in more detail.

Audiology Services

Audiological services play a crucial role in supporting students identified for special education and those in regular education. Although these services are widely perceived to be reserved solely for students identified for special education, they should be available to all students in the form of hearing screenings and hearing conservation activities and in the engineering of classroom acoustic environments that are conducive to learning for all students. ASHA and the Educational Audiology Association provide excellent guidance for the role of audiology in schools (ASHA, 2002b). Audiologists help support a FAPE under IDEA for all students. According to ASHA (2002b), they engage in the following activities in support of FAPE:

- Identification of children with hearing loss

- Determination of the range, nature, and degree of hearing loss, including referral for medical or other professional attention for the habilitation of hearing

- Provision of habilitation activities, such as language habilitation, auditory training, speech reading (lip-reading) hearing evaluation, and speech conservation

- Creation of an administrative program to prevent hearing loss

- Counseling and guidance of children, parents, and teachers regarding hearing loss

- Determination of a child's needs for a group and or individual amplification, selecting and fitting of appropriate aid, and evaluating the effectiveness of amplification

Summary

The evolution of education reform has significantly influenced the roles and responsibilities of school-based speech-language pathologists and audiologists in recent years. Much of this legislation has enabled school-based SLPs and audiologists to have a positive impact on a varied and complex caseload of students. For those who choose to work in this dynamic environment, it is necessary to have a wide range of knowledge and skills. School settings offer the opportunity for IPP and a variety of service delivery options in the natural environment. SLPs and audiologists work with teachers, school psychologists, administrators, teacher assistants, occupational therapists, physical therapists, school nutrition workers, adapted physical education teachers, English as a Second Language teachers, and a host of others to improve outcomes for all children on their caseload.

Today's school-based SLPs and audiologists serve as consultants in the prevention of communication disorders through RTI initiatives whereby involvement in the referral process leads to evaluation and eligibility for special education and related services. As service providers, they play a key role in ensuring that due process occurs in accordance with federal and state laws. Through the demonstration of relevant service delivery incorporating core curriculum standards to enable transition across levels of education and graduation, they assist students in the ability to navigate life as independently and optimally as possible. This is no small feat, but one that comes with many rewards.

School-based SLPs and audiologists recognize the importance of evidence-based practices in their work setting. In addition to supporting students' skills in the areas of hearing, articulation, language, voice, and fluency, they gain strengths in serving students with disorders related to literacy, limited English proficiency, and dysphagia. They use technology in the delivery and documentation of services and demonstrate flexibility in scheduling services. They also understand issues related to privacy and documentation of all services provided within the setting. SLPs and audiologists may need to learn more about supervisory processes as they work with assistants, student interns, and clinical fellows. Collaboration and teaming are integral parts of the work of school-based SLPs and audiologists. The ability to share knowledge and ideas effectively in verbal and written formats is crucial to success in this setting because performance is evaluated; and accepting constructive feedback and playing a role in planning one's own professional development is also expected.

Schools provide a setting in which both the SLP and the audiologist may acquire, develop, and refine a wide range of knowledge and skills. There exists the opportunity to serve as a member of a team of professionals or as a consultant, work with family members, and provide direct services to both children and young adults. One may choose to become an expert in a specific area or a generalist in many. In either case, the challenges and the rewards are ever present, and SLPs and audiologists who choose this setting play a major role in the future of the children they serve.

Critical Thinking

1. How has federal legislation influenced the practice of speech-language pathology and audiology in the schools of the United States?

2. Discuss how speech-language pathologists and/or audiologists would explain that their services are educationally relevant.

3. Describe the factors that need to be considered by the SLP when developing a schedule for service delivery.

4. What role would the SLP play on a curriculum-planning team developed to support student performance in literacy?

5. How are Multi-Tiered Systems of Support (MTSS) and Response to Intervention (RTI) changing the role of the speech-language pathologist in a school? How do pre-referral interventions and RTI differ?

6. In what ways might telepractice change the practice of speech-language pathology and audiology in school settings?

7. What skills do you need to work effectively with students and their families from a variety of diverse backgrounds in the schools?

8. What issues might arise in the supervision of speech-language pathology assistants? How might those be different from supervisory relationships with graduate students and clinical fellows in school settings?

9. Suppose you get a professional position in an educational setting in the next year. How do you think your job will change in the next 10 years? What will you do to increase the importance of the speech-language pathologist or audiologist in the educational setting in which you work?

References

American Speech-Language-Hearing Association. (2002a). *A workload analysis approach for establishing speech-language caseload standards in the schools*. Rockville, MD: Author.

American Speech-Language-Hearing Association. (2002b). *Guidelines for audiology service provision in and for schools*. Rockville, MD: Author.

American Speech-Language-Hearing Association. (2007). *Guidelines for speech-language pathologists providing swallowing and feeding services in schools*. Rockville, MD: Author.

American Speech-Language-Hearing Association. (2010a). *Guidelines for the roles and responsibilities of the school-based speech-language pathologist*. Rockville, MD: Author.

American Speech-Language-Hearing Association. (2010b). *Roles and responsibilities of speech-language pathologists in schools*. Retrieved from http://www.asha.org/slp/schools/prof-consult/ guidelines/

American Speech-Language-Hearing Association. (2013). *Speech-language pathology assistant scope of practice*. Retrieved from https://www.asha.org/uploadedFiles/SP2013-00337.pdf

American Speech-Language-Hearing Association. (2014). *Performance assessment of contributions and effectiveness of speech-language pathologists*. Retrieved from https://www.asha.org/uploadedFiles/SLPs-Performance-Assessment-Contributions-Effectiveness.pdf

American Speech-Language-Hearing Association. (2018). *2018 Schools survey. Survey summary report: Numbers and types of responses, SLPs*. Available from http://www.asha.org

American Speech-Language-Hearing Association. (2018). *Highlights and trends: Member and affiliate counts, year-end 2018*. Retrieved from http://www.asha.org/uploadedFiles/2018-Member-Counts.pdf

American Speech-Language-Hearing Association. (n.d.). *Professional development requirements for the 2020 audiology and speech-language pathology certification standards*. Retrieved from https://www.asha.org/Certification/Prof-Dev-for-2020-Certi fication-Standards/

Americans with Disabilities Act of 1990, 42 U.S.C. § 1201 *et seq.* (1990).

Anderson, J. C., & Homer, E. M. (2006). Managing dysphagia in the schools. *ASHA Leader, 11*(13), 8–30.

Common Core State Standards Initiative. (2010). *Common standards*. Available from http://www.corestandards.org/

Crutchley, S., Dudley, W., & Campbell, M. (2010). Articulation assessment through videoconferencing: A pilot study. *Communications of Global Information Technology, 2*, 12–23.

Education Superhighway. (2017). *2016 state of the states: Education Superhighway's second annual report on the state of broadband connectivity in America's public schools*. San Francisco, CA. Retrieved from https://s3-us-west-1.amazonaws.com/esh-sots-pdfs/2016_national_report_K12_broadband.pdf

Elementary and Secondary Education Act, Pub. L. No. 89-10, 79 Stat. 27, 20 U.S.C. ch.70 (1965).

Every Student Succeeds Act, Pub. L. No. 114-95 Stat. 1177, 114th U.S.C. (2015).

Family Educational Rights and Privacy Act of 1974, 20 U.S.C. § 1232g (1974).

Flynn, P. (2010). New service delivery models: Connecting SLPs with teachers and curriculum. *ASHA Leader, 15*(10), 22.

Goleman, D. (2004). *What makes a leader.* Retrieved from https://hbr.org/2004/01/what-makes-a-leader

Individuals with Disabilities Education Act, 20 U.S.C. § 1400 (2004).

Individuals with Disabilities Education Improvement Act of 2004, Pub. L. No. 108-446, 20 U.S.C. § 1400 *et seq.* (2004).

Library of Congress. (2010, July). *Primary documents in American history: 14th Amendment to the U.S. Constitution.* Retrieved from http://www.loc.gov/rr/program/bib/ourdocs/14thamendment.html

National Center for Education Statistics. (2018a) *Digest of education statistics, 2017.* Retrieved from https://nces.ed.gov/programs/digest/d17

National Center of Education Statistics (2018b), *The condition of education 2018.* Retrieved from https://nces.ed.gov/pubs2018/2018144.pdf

National Center on Response to Intervention. (2011). *The essential components of RTI. What is RTI?* Retrieved from http://www.rti4success.org/whatisrti

National Clearing House for English Language Acquisition. (2007). *The growing numbers of English Learner Students.* Retrieved from http://www.ncela.gwu.edu/files/uploads/9/growingLEP_0708.pdf

National Priorities Project. (2015). *Federal spending: Where does the money go.* Retrieved from https://www.nationalpriorities.org/budget-basics/federal-budget-101/spending/

No Child Left Behind Act of 2001, Pub. L. 107–110 (2002).

Paul-Brown, D., & Goldberg, L. R. (2001). Current policies and new directions for speech-language pathology assistants. *Language, Speech, and Hearing Services in Schools, 32,* 4–17.

Rehabilitation Act of 1973, as amended, 29 U.S.C. § 701 (1973).

Schraeder, T., Quinn, M., & Stockman, I. (1999). Authentic assessment as an approach to pre-school speech-language pathology screening. *American Journal of Speech-Language Pathology, 8,* 195–200.

Section 504 of the Rehabilitation Act of 1973, Pub. L. No. 93-112, 87 Stat. 394, 29 U.S.C.§701 (1973).

Timler, G. (2008). Social communication: A framework for assessment and intervention. *ASHA Leader, 13*(15), 10–13.

U.S. Department of Education. (2007, March 8). Letter from Alexa Posny (Director, Office of Special Education Programs) to Catherine D. Clarke (Director, ASHA Education and Regulatory Advocacy). Retrieved from http://www.asha.org/uploadedFiles/advocacy/federal/idea/RequestClarificationLettertoPosny.pdf

U.S. Department of Education. (2011, February). *The Family Educational Rights and Privacy Act: Guidance for eligible students.* Retrieved from http:// ed.gov/policy/gen/guid/fpco/ferpa/for-eligible- students .pdf

U.S. Department of Health, Education, and Welfare. (1980, May 30*).* Letter from Edwin Martin (Acting Assistant Secretary for Special Education and Rehabilitative Services, Office of Special Education Programs) to Stan Dublinske (School Services Program American Speech-Language Hearing Association). Retrieved from http://www.asha.org/uploadedFiles/slp/schools/prof-consult/LetterPolicyInterpretation.pdf

Resources

American Speech-Language-Hearing Association. (2000). *IDEA and your caseload. A template for eligibility and dismissal criteria for students ages 3 to 21.* Available from http://www.asha.org

American Speech-Language-Hearing Association. (2002a). *A workload analysis approach for establishing speech-language caseload standards in the schools: Guidelines.* Retrieved from http://www.asha.org/ docs/html/GL2002-00066.html

American Speech-Language-Hearing Association. (2002b). *Guidelines for audiology service provision in and for schools.* Retrieved from https://www.asha.org/policy/GL2002-00005/#sec1.1

American Speech-Language-Hearing Association. (2005). *Medicaid and third party payments in the schools.* Retrieved from http://www.asha.org/practice/ reimbursement/medicaid/thirdparty-payment.htm

American Speech-Language-Hearing Association. (2006, November 2). Letter from Catherine D. Clarke (Director, ASHA Education and Regulatory Advocacy) to Alexa Posny (Director, Office of Special Education Programs). Retrieved from http://www.asha.org/uploadedFiles/advocacy/federal/idea/RequestClarificationLettertoPosny.pdf

American Speech-Language-Hearing Association. (2007). *IDEA Series: Developing educationally relevant IEPs.* Available from http://www.asha.org

American Speech-Language-Hearing Association. (2009). *Practical tools and forms for supervising speech-language pathology assistants.* Rockville, MD: Author.

American Speech-Language-Hearing Association. (2010). *Schools Survey report: SLP caseload characteristics trends 1995–2010.* Retrieved from http://www.asha.org/uploadedFiles/Schools10Caseload-Trends.pdf

American Speech-Language Hearing Association. (2011). *Literacy gateway.* Retrieved from http://www.asha.org/publications/literacy/

American Speech-Language-Hearing Association. (n.d.). *School-based service delivery in speech-language pathology.* Retrieved from: https://www.asha.org/SLP/schools/School-Based-Service-Delivery-in-Speech-Language-Pathology/

American Speech-Language-Hearing Association. (n.d.). *Tips for working with an interpreter.* Retrieved from http://www.asha.org/practice/multicultural/issues/interpret.htm

Americans with Disabilities Act of 1990, 42 U.S.C. § 1201 *et seq.* Available from http://www.ada.gov/

Common Core Standards. Available from http://www.corestandards.org/

Education Audiology Association. (2009). *School-based audiology advocacy series.* Retrieved from http://www.edaud.org/advocacy/6-advocacy-09-09.pdf

McCready, V. (2011). Generational issues in supervision and administration. *ASHA Leader, 16*(5) 12–15.

Schrag, J., & Schrag, H. (2004). *National Dispute Resolution Use and Effectiveness Study: Executive summary.* Retrieved from http://www.directionservice.org/cadre/pdf/Effectiveness%20Full%20Study.04

State Education Agencies Communication Disabilities Council. http://www.seacdc.org

U.S. Congress. (2004). Individuals with Disabilities Education Improvement Act (IDEA) of 2004. Retrieved from http://idea.ed.gov/explore/view/p/%2Croot%2Cstatute%2CI%2CA%2C602%2C3%2C

U.S. Department of Education. (1990). Americans with Disabilities Act (ADA). Retrieved from http://www.ed.gov/about/offices/list/ocr/docs/hq9805.html

U.S. Department of Education. (2004). *Federal regulations IDEA 2004.* Retrieved from http://idea.ed.gov/explore/view/p/%2Croot%2Cregs%2C

U.S. Department of Education (2010). *Elementary and secondary education, No Child Left Behind legislation and policies.* Retrieved from http://www2.ed.gov/policy/elsec/guid/states/index.html

U.S. Department of Education. (2011). *Overview: The federal role in education.* Retrieved from http://www2.ed.gov/about/overview/fed/role.html?src=ln

U.S. Department of Education. (2011). *Student placement in elementary and secondary schools and Section 504 of the Rehabilitation Act and Title II of the Americans with Disabilities Act.* Retrieved from http://www2.ed.gov/about/offices/list/ocr/docs/placpub.html

U.S. Department of Education. (2015). *English learner tool kit.* Retrieved from https://www2.ed.gov/about/offices/list/oela/english-learner-toolkit/index.html

U.S. Department of Health and Human Services Centers for Medicare and Medicaid Services. (2003). *Medicaid school-based administrative claiming guide.* Retrieved from http://www.medicaid.gov/Medicaid-CHIP-Program-Information/By-Topics/Financing-and-Reimbursement/Downloads/2003_SBS_Admin_Claiming_Guide.pdf

U.S. Department of Justice. (2010). *Highlights of the final rule to amend the Department of Justice's regulation implementing Title II of the ADA.* Retrieved from http://www.ada.gov/regs2010/factsheets/title2_factsheet.html

Zirkel, P. (1998, April). Counterpoint: National trends in education litigation: Supreme Court decisions concerning students. *Journal of Law and Education, 27*, 235.

Zirkel, P. (2007). Courtside: 'Higher' education litigation? *The Phi Delta Kappan, 88*(10), 797–799.

17

Service Delivery Issues in Early Intervention

Corey Herd Cassidy, PhD

Introduction

It is the worst nightmare of every parent or caregiver to discover that his/her child has been born with or has been diagnosed with a disability or developmental delay. Parents and caregivers often experience feelings of fear, anxiety, depression, and helplessness when they do not know where to go for services for their child or support for their family. Early intervention (EI) services are evidence-based, specialized services that are designed to meet the needs of infants and toddlers (and their families) from birth to age 3 years who have or may be at risk for developmental delays or disabilities. The primary goal of EI services is to address the identified needs of young children in order to lessen the effects of their disabilities or delays. These services are designed to decrease the family's anxiety by providing resources and supports for the child and family to ensure that the child has every opportunity to develop and learn. The Individuals with Disabilities Education Act (IDEA), is a federally mandated system originally introduced in 1975 as Public Law 94-142 called the Education for All Handicapped Children Act. It was enacted to ensure equitable educational opportunities for children aged 5 to 21 years. Over time the system has been restructured and renamed several times. As of 1997 the Act was revised to include the Program for Infants and Toddlers with Disabilities, also called Part C, to serve birth to age 3 children and their families. The most current act, the Individuals with Disabilities Education Improvement Act (IDEIA), was authorized in 2004 with additional *IDEIA Part C Final Regulations* confirmed in 2011 (IDEIA, 2011). These documents reflect empirically based practices in the arena of early intervention. This chapter presents the evidence that supports intervention in the birth to 3-year-old population as well as the most current IDEIA regulatory requirements regarding early intervention policies, procedures, and practices that impact infants and toddlers with disabilities and their families.

In 2008, the American Speech-Language-Hearing Association (ASHA) initially presented five guiding principles that reflect evidence-based best practices for speech-language pathologists and audiologists who are providing Part C early intervention services to young children and their families. Updates addressing the five principles, as well as implementation for best practice, are now also available through the ASHA Early Intervention Practice Portal (ASHA, 2019). This chapter presents each of these principles and discusses how each may be effectively implemented by speech-language pathologists (SLPs) and audiologists. The chapter discusses how SLPs and audiologists need to team with other service providers and family members within the early intervention system for the most efficacious and meaningful service delivery. Family-centered practices and the importance of considering and incorporating natural environments into the provision of early intervention services are presented and discussed. The concept of cultural competence in the early intervention arena, including the definitions and the circumstances that influence the provision of effective and appropriate family-centered services, is defined. This chapter discusses each step of the early intervention process, including considerations regarding eligibility, the creation of the Individualized Family Service Plan (IFSP), and transitioning from Part C to Part B (Special Education) or other services. In addition, the chapter presents the scopes of practice for SLPs and audiologists who work in the early intervention arena and introduces you to information on different team formats in early intervention programs. Research supporting the fact that the period from birth to age 3 is a critical time in a child's development is shared. The most current evidence regarding the foundation of and best practices in early intervention is discussed. Finally, the chapter presents general advice for providing best practices within natural environments as well as suggestions for establishing a positive and safe work environment.

What Is Early Intervention?

Before 1975, approximately one million children with disabilities were denied pertinent services and were provided only minimal education in separate facilities and institutions. Public Law (PL) 94-142, also known as the Education for All Handicapped Children Act, was passed in 1975 and is considered by many to be the most significant act in the history of education in regard to children with disabilities. This act mandated a free appropriate public education (FAPE) for all children with disabilities from 5 to 21 years of age. Through a series of reauthorizations, FAPE was extended to include children with disabilities from 3 to 21 years of age. PL 94-142 is the predecessor to both the Individuals with Disabilities Education Act (IDEA) and the Individuals with Disabilities Education Improvement Act (IDEIA). The term is often used interchangeably with IDEA and IDEIA, as it also refers to all amendments affecting the 1975 Act.

In 1986, IDEA was passed. This amendment to the original PL 94-142 provided the federal mandate for special education services in each state for children with disabilities from birth to 21 years of age. It outlined the system of funding employed for special education and related services. Provisions were put in place through Part H of IDEA to provide incentives to states to provide services to children from birth to 3 years of age. Congress established the Part H (early intervention) program of IDEA in recognition of "an urgent and substantial need" to:

- enhance the development of infants and toddlers with disabilities;

- reduce educational costs by minimizing the need for special education through early intervention;

- minimize the likelihood of institutionalization, and maximize independent living; and

- enhance the capacity of families to meet their child's needs.

IDEA Part C

In 1997, IDEA (PL 105-17) was restructured and Part H became Part C—the Program for Infants and Toddlers with Disabilities. IDEA was modified once again in 2004 as the Individuals with Disabilities Education Improvement Act (IDEIA). Federal Part C regulations now require that a statewide policy and system of early intervention services are in effect to ensure that appropriate early intervention services are available to all infants and toddlers with disabilities and/or significant developmental delay and their families. For a state to participate in the program, it must ensure that early intervention will be available to all eligible children and their families. Each state's governor must designate a lead agency to receive the funding and to administer the program. The governor must also appoint an Interagency Coordinating Council (ICC), including parents of young children with disabilities, to advise and assist the lead agency. Currently, all states and eligible territories are participating in the Part C program. Annual funding to each state is based upon census figures of the number of children birth to 3 years of age in the general population. Part C services may be extended to include children up through six years of age; however, few states have adopted this practice.

In 2011, the IDEIA Part C Final Regulations (IDEIA, 2011) were presented. The Final Regulations reflected changes made to the IDEA, as amended by the Individuals with Disabilities Education Improvement Act of 2004, and made other necessary changes needed to implement the Early Intervention Program for Infants and Toddlers with Disabilities. One of the most significant changes in these regulations provided states the discretion to extend eligibility for Part C services through age 5 years to children with disabilities who are eligible for services under Part B, Section 619 (Preschool Grants) and who previously received services under Part C.

Evidence Supporting Early Intervention

Children grow and develop differently and at their own pace. Decades of research support the fact that the period from birth to age three is a critical time in a child's development and an important time for parents to have access to accurate information and consistent support (Center on the Developing Child at Harvard University [CDCHU], 2008, 2010). Research has shown that a child's earliest experiences play a critical role in brain development. It is therefore crucial that services are provided during these early years (CDCHU, 2008). According to the CDCHU (2008, 2010), neural circuits, including those that create the foundation for learning, behavior, and health, are the most flexible during the first 3 years of life. The findings also indicate that early social/emotional development and physical health provide the foundation upon which both cognitive and language skills develop. Positive early experiences that involve stable relationships with responsive adults within safe and supportive environments and appropriate nutritional opportunities are all key elements of healthy brain development (CDCHU, 2010). According to Guralnick (2011), the earlier intervention supports and services are provided, the more likely children who have disabilities or developmental delays are to achieve successful learning outcomes related to the development of effective communication, language, and swallowing skills. Services have been shown to positively influence outcomes across developmental domains, including health, language and communication, cognition, and social/emotional well-being of infants and toddlers who have disabilities or are at risk for developmental delays (ASHA, 2008b; Branson & Demchak, 2009; CDCHU, 2010; Guralnick, 2011; Hebbeler et al., 2007; Joint Committee on Infant Hearing, 2007; Landa, Holman, O'Neill, & Stuart, 2010).

Benefits of Part C services to society also include reducing economic burden through later academic success and a decreased need for special education in the school years (Hebbeler, 2009). Therefore, intervention is likely to be more effective and less costly when it is provided earlier rather than later in life. These research findings underscore the importance of intervention in the earliest years and support the impact of IDEIA Part C services on children, families, and society as a whole.

Range of Early Intervention Services

Broadly speaking, early intervention services are specialized health, educational, and therapeutic services designed to meet the needs of infants and toddlers from birth to age 3 years who have or may be at risk for developmental delays or disabilities, and their families. The primary goal of early intervention is to decrease the effects of a disability or delay by identifying and addressing the needs of young children across five developmental areas including cognitive development, communication development, physical development (including vision and hearing), social or emotional development, and adaptive development (IDEIA, 2004). Early intervention services bring families and service providers from many aspects of the community together, including public and private agencies, child care centers, local school districts, and private providers. Supports and services are intended to work together to meet children's unique needs and those of their family in their natural environments. Early intervention services may be simple or complex depending on each child's needs. They can range from something fairly uncomplicated such as prescribing glasses for a 2-year-old to significantly more complex such as needing to develop a multi-faceted comprehensive approach with a variety of services and team members. Depending on the child's needs, early intervention services may include family training, counseling, and home visits; special instruction; speech-language pathology services; audiology services; occupational therapy; physical therapy; psychological services; medical services (for diagnostic or evaluation purposes); health services needed to enable the child to benefit from the other services; social work services; assistive technology devices and services; transportation; nutrition services; and service coordination services. Table 17–1 illustrates a sample of the coordination services that may be provided under the scope of IDEIA Part C Final Regulations.

Roles and Responsibilities of Speech-Language Pathologists and Audiologists in Early Intervention

In the early intervention arena, SLPs are qualified to provide services to families and young children who demonstrate or are at risk for developing disabilities or delays in the areas of communication, speech, language, cognition, emergent literacy, and/or feeding and

Table 17–1. Early Intervention Services Provided under IDEIA Part C Final Regulations

- Assistive technology devices and assistive technology services
- Counseling, and home visits
- Early identification, screening, and assessment services
- Family training
- Health services necessary to enable the infant or toddler to benefit from the other early intervention services
- Medical services only for diagnostic or evaluation purposes
- Occupational therapy
- Physical therapy
- Psychological services
- Service coordination services
- Sign language and cued language services
- Social work services
- Special instruction
- Speech-language pathology and audiology services
- Transportation and related costs that are necessary to enable an infant or toddler and the infant's or toddler's family to receive another service described in this paragraph
- Vision services

Source: Based on information from the Individuals with Disabilities Education Improvement Act (IDEIA) (2011).

swallowing difficulties (ASHA, 2016b). Table 17–2 presents the roles and responsibilities of SLPs in early intervention.

The knowledge, skills, and experience of audiologists who are specifically educated to provide services to young children are also needed in the EI arena. Audiology services in EI include the establishment of an accurate diagnosis of auditory and vestibular function, effective family counseling provided in conjunction with the diagnostic process, and timely service coordination for those children who require audiological services (ASHA, 2013; JCIH, 2007). Table 17–3 presents the roles and responsibilities of audiologists in EI.

SLPs and audiologists must also consider the ASHA Code of Ethics (ASHA, 2016a), which states both professions must only participate in roles that are within the professional scopes of practice. EI SLPs and audiologists must demonstrate documented high levels of competence evidenced by level of education, discipline-specific training, and experience. Additionally, the SLP and audiologist roles and responsibilities in EI are guided by both state licensure regulations and service delivery models as implemented by local agencies.

Guiding Principles of Early Intervention

Five guiding principles reflect current best practices when providing early intervention for young children and their families (ASHA, 2008a). These principles specifically note that supports and services must be (1) family centered; (2) culturally and linguistically responsive; (3) developmentally supportive and promotive of children's participation in their natural environments; (4) comprehensive, coordinated, and team based; and (5) based on the highest quality internal and external evidence that is available. Each one of these principles is discussed in greater detail throughout the chapter.

Table 17–2. Roles and Responsibilities of Speech-Language Pathologists in Early Intervention

- Demonstrate knowledge of typical norms from birth to age 5 years across developmental domains.

- Engage in prevention and early identification activities to promote healthy development and reduce risk factors that can impact a child's development.

- Understand federal, state, agency, and professional policies and procedures related to screening, evaluating, and assessing infants and toddlers with, or at risk for, disabilities

- Conduct screening, evaluation, and assessment to identify young children with, or at risk for, a delay or disorder.

- Establish eligibility for services and guide the development of an intervention program in collaboration with the family.

- Make referrals to other professionals and, with the family's consent, inform the referral source of the outcome of the eligibility process.

- Develop a plan for implementing services and supports that includes evidence-based speech-language pathology intervention approaches, methods, and settings.

- Gather and report treatment outcomes and document progress.

- Revise intervention plans and determine appropriate discharge criteria.

- Collaborate with families, caregivers, agencies, and other professionals involved on the IFSP team to support implementation of intervention strategies in everyday routines

- Support family interactions that reflect cultural beliefs, values, and priorities.

- Coordinate services (including evaluation and assessment, development of an IFSP, and access to resources) and ensure services are implemented, as agreed upon by the team.

- Participate in transition planning to ensure seamless transition and timely access to services for families moving from one program to another.

- Advocate at the local, state, and national levels regarding public policy, funding, and infrastructure for early intervention services.

- Raise awareness about the importance of early intervention by working with families and other professionals; develop and disseminate resources.

- Remain informed of current evidence-based practice in early intervention.

- Support the advancement of the knowledge base related to the nature and treatment of speech, language, cognitive-communication, and swallowing development and disorders in infants and young children.

Source: Based on information from ASHA (2019).

Family-Centered Services

The first guiding principle that reflects current best practices of SLPs and audiologists in the early intervention arena focuses on the delivery of services that are family centered (ASHA, 2008a). The principle of family-centered services is based on a family-systems model for implementing early intervention and family support assessment and intervention practices. According to Dunst and Trivette (2009), the family-systems model focuses on four evidence-based operational components. The model is implemented by first identifying the family's *concerns and priorities*. At this level, family aspirations and priorities are identified using needs-based assessment procedures and strategies to determine what the family considers important. The second step toward implementation of the family-systems model is identification of the *supports and resources* that can be used by the family to address their concerns and priorities. The family's personal social network and potential sources of information and assistance are identified, in addition to emphasizing the particular strengths of the family that increase their likelihood to utilize those resources that are needed to meet their needs. The third step in the model involves

Table 17–3. Roles and Responsibilities of Audiologists in Early Intervention

- Oversee early identification (via newborn and early childhood screening) programs and ensure that appropriate procedures are followed (Joint Committee on Infant Hearing [JCIH], 2007).

- Report results of newborn hearing screenings to state newborn hearing screening and follow-up programs (based on state-by-state regulations).

- Establish an accurate diagnosis of hearing status.

- Provide information about the child's hearing status and eligibility for Part C services to the referral source (only with the family's consent).

- Coordinate timely audiologic services.

- Evaluate infants and young children with hearing and vestibular deficits for amplification and other sensory devices, assistive technology, and vestibular rehabilitation.

- Fit and maintain amplification, other sensory devices, and assistive technology; frequently validate that the devices are providing the intended benefit.

- Provide effective family support and counseling regarding the nature of auditory and vestibular conditions and implications for language development, modes/methods of communication, communication access strategies/accommodations, and acoustic modifications.

- Advocate for a continuous process of family-focused service delivery.

- Refer families to parent-to-parent support and other consumer-based organizations.

- Educate other professionals about the needs of infants and young children with hearing and vestibular/balance deficits and the role of audiologists in diagnosing and managing them.

- Coordinate services (including evaluation and assessment, development of an IFSP, and access to resources) and ensure services are implemented, as agreed upon by the team.

- Advocate for the rights to and funding of services for infants and young children with reduced hearing, auditory disorders, and/or vestibular disorders.

- Remain informed of research in the area of early intervention to support advancement of the knowledge base related to the nature, identification, and treatment of hearing and vestibular deficits in infants and young children.

Source: Based on information from ASHA (2006, 2019).

identifying family members' existing *abilities and interests* to obtain needed supports and resources. At this point, the family's strengths and capabilities are explored and considered as a basis for promoting their abilities to obtain and mobilize their resources. The fourth and final step in implementation of the family-systems model involves coaching the family to use *help-giving practices to build their capacity*; these practices are utilized by the family to carry out actions intended to obtain supports and resources to meet their identified priorities and concerns. This final step is intended to enhance a family's ability to become more self-sustaining with respect to acquiring, recognizing, and utilizing their own competencies and skills to effectively meet their needs and achieve their goals (Dunst, 2017; Dunst & Trivette, 2009).

Effective family-centered practices involve working collaboratively with families in all aspects of service delivery. It means relating to family members as people, not "patients." A family-centered approach recognizes the importance of all family members, including brothers and sisters, grandparents, and extended family members. Furthermore, this approach involves the awareness and inclusion of the set of beliefs, values, principles, and practices that strengthen the family's capacity to enhance their child's development and learning (IDEIA, 2004). Effective family-centered practices are responsive to the unique circumstances of each family and provide families with unbiased and comprehensive information to make informed decisions (Division for Early Childhood [DEC], 2014).

IDEIA Part C requires that families are provided the opportunity to participate in all aspects of their child's services. To ensure that the family, and not just the child, receives EI services that build upon their strengths, collaboration between families and providers is the foundation of family-centered services (Crawford & Weber, 2014; DEC, 2014; Dunst, 2017; McWilliam, 2010b; Ross, 2018; Trivette & Dunst, 2007). Figure 17–1 illustrates the principles that help define collaboration and, ultimately, explain the approach and intent of early intervention. Families collaborate with providers to design and implement services that align specifically with their own preferences, resources, concerns, and priorities (IDEIA, 2011). This collaboration leads to a partnership that creates a learning environment supportive of both the child's and family's needs while achieving mutually

agreed upon outcomes and promoting family capacities (DEC, 2014; Roberts, Hensle, & Brooks, 2016). To put the components of the family-centered model and effective collaboration into practice, families and providers must form a partnership. This partnership begins by determining the definitions and roles of both the family and the SLP or audiologist. The term *family* can have many different meanings. Families define themselves by: who lives together, who makes decisions, what roles family members play, and how members support each other. Each family operates as a system, and for each child, the family system represents the group of individuals

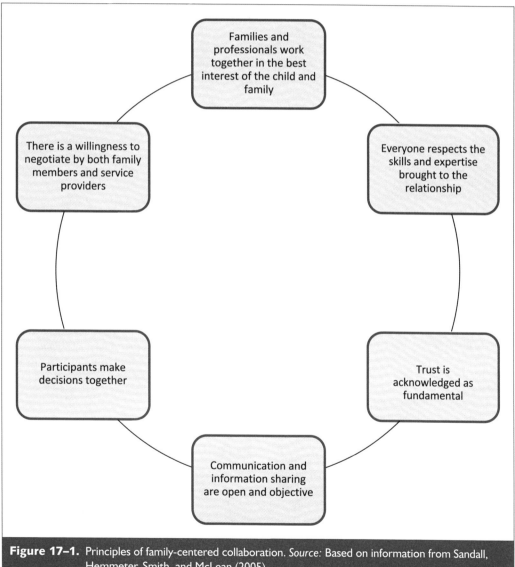

Figure 17–1. Principles of family-centered collaboration. *Source:* Based on information from Sandall, Hemmeter, Smith, and McLean (2005).

who have the most influence on that child's growth and development. Building rapport, collaborating with one another, and facilitating an individualized, supportive early intervention process are all critical components to working effectively with each family. By asking questions about routines, joining their activities, and communicating effectively, early intervention service providers learn about how each family works. Services can then be implemented that include opportunities for families and caregivers to directly participate in intervention (DEC, 2014). These steps also offer families an opportunity to see that identified family dynamic information is vitally important for individualized and meaningful services for their unique child and family (SpecialQuest Multimedia Training Library, 2007).

SLPs and audiologists must learn to adapt their knowledge and expertise to fit the needs of each child and family, ensuring that the family's needs are being addressed and learning is supported. The unique needs of each child and family determine which skills you use, how knowledge is shared, and which strategies are developed. You should combine your professional expertise and activities with the child- and family-specific expertise that the parent brings to the table. Together, you can create intervention that is focused on how the family will encourage the growth, development, and participation of their child when you are not present (McWilliam, 2004). Raver and Childress (2015) report families need to be involved and responsive to their child's needs and development to ensure intervention is effective. Engagement and involvement by families is essential to strengthen their existing knowledge and skills in order to promote the child's development of new skills and to enhance both child and family outcomes (DEC, 2014).

SLPs and audiologists who use a family-centered approach effectively collaborate with families to share information, strengthen family functioning, empower decision making, and facilitate family participation throughout the early intervention process. Establishing a positive relationship with a family is key to facilitating their participation throughout the early intervention process. You play an important role in developing the relationship and facilitating family participation. Building rapport and trust that lead to a true partnership begins with the first contact and continues through transition (Jung & Grisham-Brown, 2006). Meeting families "where they are"; practicing active listening; and helping them identify priorities, resources, strengths, and needs related to their child's development and their family lay the foundation for a supportive early intervention system.

As SLPs and audiologists, you join the parents, through your relationship, in your common concerns about their infant or toddler. You both observe the child's growth and development and offer developmen-

tally appropriate anticipatory guidance. You, therefore, need to encourage parents to take the lead in the early intervention experience. You also identify the strengths that each parent brings to the relationship with his or her child and identify and support the parent's pleasure in the child. You must take your knowledge and learn to adapt and apply it with each family in each intervention visit. Young children's development occurs within the context of their family and community (Dunst et al., 2001). It is because of the profound influences of family and community that SLPs and audiologists working in EI focus on how to support the development of infants and toddlers within these contexts. The guiding principles of Part C recognize that infant and toddler development unfolds during family routines and activities. Supports and services that focus on these routines and activities provide family members with useful, meaningful strategies that can be used daily within the context of those activities unique to each individual family (Woods, Kashinath, & Goldstein, 2004).

Establishing and Maintaining Rapport

Building rapport with a family begins with the first contact and affects the relationship throughout the process of intervention. Strong rapport takes time to establish and effort to maintain, but it can be a means of encouraging open communication and learning for everyone involved. Working from a family-centered perspective, SLPs and audiologists are able to build strong relationships with the families they serve by establishing a positive foundation. By recognizing the family's strengths and perspectives in the first stages of the early intervention process, you are able to consider the demands of intervention in relation to the benefits at each subsequent stage. Keeping an open dialogue with family members and discussing these demands and benefits on a consistent basis are key to maintaining rapport among the team members. Table 17–4 provides suggestions for building positive relationships with families.

Culturally and Linguistically Responsive Services

The second guiding principle that reflects current best practices of SLPs and audiologists in the EI arena states that families of infants and toddlers with a disability or developmental delay must have access to culturally and linguistically competent services (IDEIA, 2011). The term "culturally and linguistically diverse" refers to children and families who reside in the United States but who come from homes that speak a language other

Table 17–4. Suggestions for Building Positive Relationships with Families

- Show genuine interest in the family's life, routines, activities, interests, and in the child's needs and achievements.

- Be sensitive to each family's readiness to share information and to receive feedback.

- Facilitate a family member's participation at a level that is comfortable for him or her.

- Encourage family members to be active participants in all aspects of the early intervention process, including referral, assessment and evaluation, development of the IFPS, and intervention planning.

- Respect the family's time by being punctual for visits and offering flexible scheduling.

- Acknowledge the complexities of raising a child with developmental delays or disabilities and offering assistance as needed.

- Provide complete, unbiased information and allow family members time to make informed decisions, even when the family's decisions differ from choices you would have made.

- Respect family's rights throughout the early intervention process.

Source: Based on information from SpecialQuest Multimedia Training Library (2007) and IDEA (2011).

than English and whose cultural identity differs from mainstream U.S. culture (Puig, 2012).

Using the family systems approach, SLPs and audiologists provide early intervention services by supplying knowledge and training to families as they navigate the world of raising their children with disabilities (Dunst & Trivette, 2009). A 2007 ASHA survey of SLPs indicated that, in all settings, approximately 29% of caseloads are composed of culturally and linguistically diverse clients (ASHA, 2007). In a 2013 survey of SLPs who work in EI programs, only 7% reported being able to effectively communicate with a family without an interpreter in a language other than English; less than half thought they had received enough knowledge in their coursework to work effectively with culturally and linguistically diverse families; and only about a quarter had engaged in practical experiences with culturally and linguistically diverse families (Caesar, 2013). It is not surprising that results from the National Early Intervention Longitudinal Study indicated that families from diverse ethnic/racial backgrounds and families at lower income levels who had participated in early intervention services were less satisfied with services than Caucasian families and those families at higher income levels (Hebbeler et al., 2007; Raspa et al., 2010; Turnbull et al., 2009). To effectively support families, it is therefore necessary to develop a heightened level of sensitivity to the influences of cultural values, customs, and beliefs as well as to the strengths that cultural and linguistic identity brings to the family system (Peredo, 2016; Segal & Beyer, 2006).

SLPs and audiologists interact with families of many different cultures. Culture is defined as "people's values, religion, ideals, language, artistic expressions, patterns of

social and interpersonal relationships and ways of perceiving, behaving and thinking" (Balthrop & Coleman, 2003). Different cultural dimensions can have an influence on a family's decisions regarding EI services and supports. Cultural competence is the ability to interact effectively with all people, regardless of their culture, and to recognize how their cultural dimensions may impact a family's approach to services for their child. By becoming more culturally sensitive, you will be able to reduce your own cultural biases and recognize the cultural issues important to each family. Table 17–5 illustrates variables that should be taken into consideration with regard to differences among cultures. For additional information regarding service delivery for culturally and linguistically diverse populations, refer to Chapter 25.

Cultural competence is necessary to ensure success in every step of the process when providing early intervention supports and services. The components of the family system are strongly influenced by culture as it influences how a family defines and structures itself (Wayman & Lynch, 1991). Culture influences family functions, the family life cycle, and events that are viewed by the family as stressors. Cultural perspectives that may relate directly to services within early intervention include views of (1) children and child rearing, (2) disability and causation, (3) intervention, (4) medical treatment and healing, (5) family and family roles, and (6) language and communication styles (Hanson & Lynch, 1990; Pereda, 2016). Additionally, according to Hanson and Lynch (1990), several factors regarding the nature of early intervention itself should be considered to provide effective early intervention services to families from culturally and linguistically diverse backgrounds.

Table 17–5. Variables Regarding Cultural Differences

Personal space	In some cultures, it is common for people to stand approximately three feet apart when having a personal conversation. In other cultures, it is typical to stand much closer. Each distance may feel awkward to someone who is unfamiliar with the other style; the conversational partner may try to move closer or farther away, depending upon his/her own comfort.
Eye contact and feedback behaviors	In some cultures, individuals are encouraged to look each other directly in the eye and to participate actively in providing feedback behaviors (leaning forward, smiling, nodding, etc.). In contrast, people from other cultures may show respect or deference by not engaging in eye contact or by participating more passively in their body language and conversation.
Interruption and turn-taking behaviors	Some cultures have come to expect a conversation to progress linearly (one speaker at a time) while it may be more natural for several people to be talking at once in another culture. Listening skills that address different cultural rules regarding turn-taking in conversation must be developed when considering and accommodating multiple styles.
Gesturing	Hand and arm gesturing can vary quite a bit in different cultural backgrounds. In general, extreme gesturing should not necessarily be interpreted as excitement as it may just be an ordinary manner of communication, depending on the speaker.
Facial expressions	Variance in this form of communication is also common; it is important to not assume that someone is cold or distressed based solely on one's own cultural experience.
Silence	Americans often find it more difficult to tolerate periods of prolonged silence than do others from different cultures, and may try to fill the silence with noise.
Dominance behaviors	In some cultures prolonged eye contact, an erect posture, looking down at someone's hands or hips, looking at someone with lowered lids, and holding the head high are all examples of behavior that may be interpreted as assertive or even aggressive. The interpretation of these behaviors may vary from one culture to another.
Volume	Irritation often results when culturally different speakers consider differing levels of acceptable volume. It is important to remember that each individual may be reacting based on the rules learned in his/her own background and what may be considered normal by his/her peers.
Touching	Some cultures may perceive someone as cold and aloof if there is not much touching and/or proximity to one another. In other cultures, touching may be perceived as intrusive or rude.

Source: Based on information from Saldaña (2001).

These factors include (1) attitudes regarding intervention, (2) methods used and location of services, (3) qualifications of the service providers, and (4) styles of interaction and communication in the provision of services.

When providing services to families from diverse cultural backgrounds, SLPs and audiologists should consider those factors that affect families' perspectives as well as those considerations that may relate directly to services. By listening to the family and learning about their family system, you can better promote effective

intervention. During the initial assessment for the program planning process, you have the opportunity to ask questions and listen to the family members discuss their needs and concerns. Based on their feedback and by collaborating with family members, outcomes should be aligned with family culture, values, needs, and priorities. Additionally, using a routines-based approach to goal selection and intervention may be optimal (Kashinath, Woods, & Goldstein, 2006; Woods et al., 2004). Since intervention activities are built directly into family routines that already exist, this approach builds upon the strengths that are inherent to individual family systems while eliminating cultural mismatches. By determining optimal routines and empowering parents to incorporate opportunities into their own everyday activities, you are able to provide effective services while respecting and considering every family's culture and value system (Peña & Fiestas, 2009).

In regard to providing linguistically responsive services, you must consider both the home language(s) as well as acquisition of the language needed for the child's academic success. This consideration will look different depending on the services and supports that are being provided. IDEIA regulations define *native language* as the language typically used by an individual. In the case of a child receiving services, native language is the language typically used by the parents or caregivers (IDEIA, 2011). Unless it is not feasible to do so, prior written notice regarding early intervention services must be provided to families in their native language. Beyond the prior written notice, you will provide EI supports and services in the language(s) most likely to result in an accurate representation of the child's skills (DEC, 2014; IDEIA, 2011). You will want to teach families and caregivers how to implement strategies in their home language to maximize comprehension and carryover of both knowledge and skills (Peredo, 2016). Service providers often work with families and interpreters to support both the home language(s) and acquisition of the language needed by the child for academic success.

Ultimately, you can build strong relationships with families and address their individualized needs by recognizing that each family is a whole unit with its own unique set of values. By respecting the choices that families make in regard to child-rearing, serving the family's functional needs, and viewing the culture and the home language of the family as a strength, you can implement the principles of family-centered practice effectively to support culturally and linguistically diverse families in early intervention (Peredo, 2016).

Developmentally Supportive Services in the Natural Environment

Effective EI services meet the family where they are, at the level of their needs, and in the environments in which they find themselves. Each family exists within a system that includes the people with whom they interact, the supports and resources they have, and the places they go. The primary purpose of early intervention is

to support family efforts and to build their confidence and competence in meeting the needs of their children. With that purpose in mind, intervention visits that are provided within each family's support system and natural environment may be best suited to positive developmental outcomes for children and families (ASHA, 2008b). Furthermore, services that address family routines, concerns, and priorities through authentic experiences, active exploration, and interactions with both people and the environment that are consistent with the child's age, cognitive skills, communication skills, strengths, and interests are considered developmentally supportive (DEC, 2014).

IDEIA Part C (2004) requires that early intervention services be provided, to the maximum extent appropriate, in natural environments. According to IDEIA (2011), natural environments are defined as "settings that are natural or typical for a same-aged infant or toddler without a disability, [and] may include the home or community settings." Natural environments include the home as well as other settings in which children without delays and disabilities participate in their communities. Natural environments are not places where children go because of their disabilities, the convenience of the SLP or audiologist, or access to a special place or equipment. Natural environments are, instead, those settings and activities in which each individual child's family participates or in which they would like to participate.

When considering the provision of EI services in natural environments, SLPs and audiologists must determine not only *where* the supports are provided but also *how* they will provide them. Children learn best when they learn in context and have multiple opportunities to practice the skills and abilities throughout the day. It is much easier for infants and toddlers to generalize their newly learned skills when they have learned them during meaningful, functional activities as they happen naturally, rather than learning them in contrived situations in a clinical setting. It is your job to provide parents with this perspective.

SLPs and audiologists must learn to think beyond the traditional "home visit." You must consider the multitude of activities that occur outside of your scheduled block of time (Hanft, Rush, & Shelden, 2004). Thinking beyond the typical home visit requires a shift in how early intervention has been provided in many localities. Therefore, to help your teams move forward, you need to understand the similarities and differences between traditional "home visiting" and intervention that is provided when incorporating each family's priorities, routines, and activities. Services provided through traditional "home visits" tend to be limited to what can be accomplished during the span of time the SLP and family have allotted for the visit. Specific skills may be addressed in isolation, and activities may be discussed but not practiced because they do not coincide with the scheduled time. In contrast, supports and services that consider the concept of natural environments use that allotted "home visit" time much differently. The time is used to explore a variety of family routines and activities to find out how they can be enhanced to address IFSP outcomes, both during and between early intervention visits. Since SLPs and audiologists may join the family in those activities, the intervention visit should be scheduled in response to the activities being explored and is therefore flexible with regard to day and time.

Intervention provided in the home or other natural settings and environments gives SLPs and audiologists the opportunity to see what daily life is like for the family. Familiar everyday experiences, events, and places should be incorporated as opportunities to promote incidental teaching and natural learning throughout each day (McWilliam, 2010b; Raver & Childress, 2015; Ross, 2018; Rush & Sheldon, 2011). These interactions may include learning what goes well for each family in each scenario and determining how and what assistance the family may need. By becoming familiar with the specifics of each family's routine and activities, SLPs and audiologists can help parents develop individualized outcomes and intervention strategies based on those activities that are meaningful and useful to the family during their routine daily life.

Comprehensive, Coordinated, and Team-Based Services

The fourth of the five guiding principles of early intervention (ASHA, 2008a) states that supports and services should be "comprehensive, coordinated, and team-based." Regardless of state or local programming methods, all young children and their families follow the same basic steps as they enter into and move through the early intervention system. The process, often called the *supports and services pathway*, begins with referral for assessment and follows the child and family while they continue to receive services through the Part C program. The supports and services pathway assists in the identification of eligible families with its purpose being to maximize family and child outcomes through the delivery of EI services. It consists of seven distinct components of service delivery, including referral, intake, eligibility determination, assessment for service planning, IFSP development, implementation and reviews of the IFSP, and transition activities. Embedded in each of these processes is the legal acknowledgment of the family's and child's procedural rights and safeguards. Figure 17–2

provides the typical sequence that a family follows while involved in Part C services.

Referral

A primary referral source, such as a parent, pediatrician, or health department representative, identifies a child who may have a developmental delay or may be in need of further assessment. Referral sources often have concerns based on results of developmental screenings, observations, or a diagnosis indicating a potential developmental delay. Anyone in the community can make a referral of a child who might be eligible for Part C services as long as parent/guardian permission is secured. The referral is made to the Part C local Central Point of Entry at the lead agency. The Central Point of Entry collects the referral information and assigns a service coordinator to meet with the family. During the referral process, information regarding the local or statewide early intervention process is shared with the family, and initial information regarding the child and family is gathered. Each local lead agency develops policies and procedures in the community to ensure quick response from the Central Point of Entry and to move quickly toward the next step in the early intervention process. The IDEIA (2011) requires that providers make referrals within seven days after the infant or toddler is identified as having a possible disability or delay. Following receipt of a referral, the lead agency has 45 days to complete the intake or screening, initial evaluation, initial assessments, and initial team meeting to develop the initial IFSP for the child and the family (IDEIA, 2011).

Intake

Intake involves face-to-face and/or phone meetings with the family to continue gathering information to determine eligibility. Such information includes developmental history, medical history and medical home information, family routines, schedules, and activities of interest as well as the completion of a developmental screening, if needed. In-depth information is shared with the family regarding the Part C system including eligibility criteria, IFSP development if the child is eligible, family cost share participation, and child and family procedural rights and safeguards. At this point, the Central Point of Entry, or a service coordinator who has been assigned to the family, begins the process of eligibility determination.

Eligibility Determination

Eligibility determination is the process of determining whether a child meets the system's eligibility criteria to

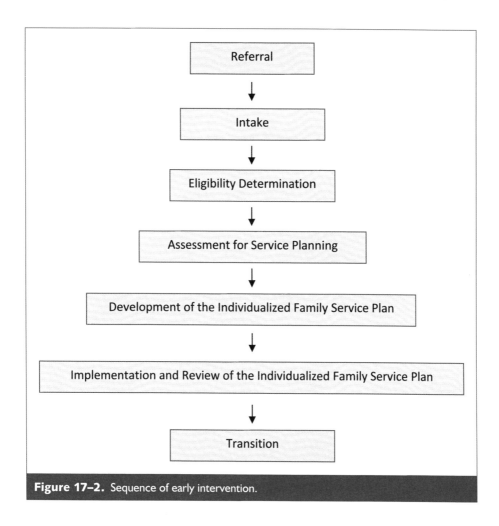

Figure 17–2. Sequence of early intervention.

receive early intervention services. This process includes the evaluation of the child's skills and needs through a review of information, including medical/developmental reports, assessment reports, observations, and parent report. According to IDEIA §303.321(a)(2)(i), evaluation is defined as "the procedures used by qualified personnel to determine a child's initial and continuing eligibility" (IDEIA, 2011). Eligibility determination is based on the child's needs within the child's natural environment, which may include the home or any community setting in which children without disabilities participate (e.g., child care centers, public playgrounds). All areas of a child's development are considered to determine whether the child has a delay and/or differences in development that might make him/her eligible for Part C services. As such, "no single procedure may be used as the sole criterion for determining a child's eligibility" (IDEIA 2011, §303.321(b)); these procedures must include administration of an evaluation instru-

ment, an interview with the parent to gather the child's history, identification of the child's level of functioning in each of the developmental areas, a gathering of information from a variety of sources to understand the full scope of the child's individual strengths and needs, and a review of the child's medical, educational, and/or other records (IDEIA, 2011). This information is reviewed by a multidisciplinary team (identified below). This team determines whether a child meets one or more of the criteria for eligibility. Part C of IDEIA 2004 states that systems must provide services to any child "under 3 years of age who needs early intervention services" (IDEIA 2004, § 632(5)(A)) because the child "(i) is experiencing developmental delays, as measured by appropriate diagnostic instruments and procedures in one or more of the areas of cognitive development, physical development, communication development, social or emotional development, and adaptive development; or (ii) has a diagnosed physical or mental condition which has a high probability of resulting in developmental delay" (IDEIA 2004, § 632[5][A]).

A state may also provide services, at its discretion, to at-risk infants and toddlers. States have some discretion in setting the criteria for each of these variables. As a result, definitions of eligibility differ significantly from state to state. Evaluation procedures used to determine developmental delay involve determining the status of the child in each of the developmental areas.

Part C of IDEIA (2011) requires a multidisciplinary composition of the team, including the parent and two or more individuals from separate disciplines or professions with one of the individuals serving as the service coordinator. The multidisciplinary evaluation team typically includes at least two early childhood professionals who are appropriately qualified in their areas of expertise (i.e., speech-language pathologist, occupational therapist, developmental specialist), at least one of whom is qualified in the primary area(s) of concern. The service coordinator works with the multidisciplinary evaluation team to facilitate the evaluations, ensuring that all of the appropriate procedures are completed and properly documented. At a minimum, a multidisciplinary evaluation team gathers information from a review of pertinent records related to a child's current health status and medical history, family report, and the results of appropriate diagnostic methods. These methods may include additional reports from other sources, criterion-referenced instruments such as developmental checklists, a developmental history, language samples, criterion-referenced or norm-referenced instruments, observation of the child, play-based evaluations, and routine-based interviews. When you are working with families for whom English is not the native language or when there is a language barrier, an interpreter must be involved. The evaluation must be completed in the native language of the family or in the language(s) most likely to result in an accurate representation of the child's skills (DEC, 2014; IDEIA, 2011).

Developmental Delay. Each state has the opportunity to determine criteria for developmental delay in its own way. Many states determine criteria quantitatively, including (1) the difference between chronological age and actual performance level expressed as a percentage of chronological age, (2) delay expressed as performance at a certain number of months below chronological age, or (3) delay as indicated by standard deviation below the mean on a norm-referenced instrument. There is wide variability in the type of quantitative criteria states use to describe developmental delay, and there also is a wide range in the level of delay states require for eligibility. Common measurements of level of delay are 25% delay or two standard deviations (SD) below the mean in one

or more developmental areas, or 20% delay or 1.5 SD in two or more areas. Traditional assessment instruments, yielding scores in standard deviations or developmental age in months, may not adequately address some developmental domains or may not be comparable across developmental domains or across age levels (Benn, 1994; Brown & Brown, 1993). For this reason, some states have included qualitative criteria for determining developmental delay. Qualitative criteria include delay indicated by atypical development or observed atypical behaviors.

Atypical Development. Children are considered to have atypical development if they demonstrate abnormal or questionable sensory-motor responses (such as abnormal muscle tone, poor quality of movement patterns, or oral-motor skills dysfunction such as feeding difficulties) or have an identified affective disorder (such as a delay in achieving expected emotional milestones, a persistent failure to initiate or respond to most social interactions, or distress that does not respond to comforting by caregivers).

Diagnosed Physical or Mental Condition. A diagnosed physical or mental condition refers to a child who has a diagnosed physical or mental condition that has a high probability of resulting in a developmental delay if early intervention services are not provided. This includes conditions such as chromosomal abnormalities; genetic or congenital disorders; severe sensory impairments; inborn errors of metabolism; disorders reflecting disturbance of the development of the nervous system; congenital infections; disorders secondary to exposure to toxic substances, including fetal alcohol syndrome; and severe attachment disorders.

At Risk. An at-risk infant or toddler is defined under Part C as "an individual under 3 years of age who would be at risk of experiencing a substantial developmental delay if early intervention services were not provided to the individual" (IDEIA 2004, § 632(1)). Although many states are interested in serving children at risk, they also fear increasing the numbers of eligible children because of escalating costs. Two categories of risk that are frequently described by states that do serve these children include conditions of biological/medical risk (e.g., repeated infections or prenatal drug exposure) and environmental risk (e.g., history of abuse or neglect). When diagnostic assessment tools do not establish eligibility, the state lead agency must ensure that informed clinical opinion is independently considered in order to establish eligibility of services for children who are considered at risk (IDEIA, 2011). States that do not serve children at risk under their guidelines for eligibility typically indicate that they will monitor the development of these children and refer them for early intervention services if and when delays are manifested.

Under Part C (IDEIA, 2004), young children who are English language learners with typical development do not qualify for early intervention services. Dual language learners who present with difficulties in developing their native language and a second language, however, may be eligible for services.

Assessment for Service Planning

Assessment, as defined by Part C of IDEIA, includes "the ongoing procedures used by qualified personnel to identify the child's unique strengths and needs and the early intervention services appropriate to meet those needs throughout the period of the child's eligibility" (IDEIA 2011, §303.321(a)(2)). This is a multistep process that includes identification of the family's resources, priorities, and concerns through family-centered assessment, multidisciplinary team observations, and assessment of eligible children. In addition to assessing the family, assessment is also an opportunity to determine the child's strengths and needs in all areas of development. The assessment process provides the IFSP team with an opportunity to identify early intervention supports and services that may be necessary to address the child's unique needs. Although assessment tools may vary, ASHA (2008b) recommends combining formal and informal assessment tools that include both standardized and non-standardized measures to provide the most comprehensive picture of the child. This combination of assessment tools provides information regarding the communication skills of the child in comparison to same-age peers. Conducting an assessment with a comprehensive battery is more conducive to encouraging family and team member participation and collaboration and to guiding the IFSP development. Some local and statewide systems have implemented specific requirements regarding the choice and use of assessment tools for the purposes of both eligibility determination and assessment for service planning.

Development of the Individualized Family Service Plan

Based on the assessment for service planning, the Individualized Family Service Plan is developed. The IFSP is a written plan for providing early intervention services to eligible children and their families. The plan is developed jointly by the family, the service coordinator, and others, such as the SLP, audiologist, physical therapist, nurse, social worker, etc., who may be providing early intervention services to the child and family. The IFSP is based on the multidisciplinary evaluation and assessment of the child and the assessment of the resources, priorities, and concerns of the child's family. The plan includes outcomes, strategies, and services that are necessary to enhance the development of the child and the capacity of the family to meet the special needs of the child (IDEIA 2004, § 303.340(2)). Part C of IDEIA mandates that the IFSP meeting must be conducted in settings and at times that are convenient to the family. The meeting and the documents must also be in the native language of the family. An interpreter must be involved if the native language of the family is not English. The SLP or audiologist must work collaboratively with the interpreter to ensure that families fully understand their rights and role in the early intervention system.

There are eight required components of the IFSP (PL 108-446, Sec. 636(d)):

1. A statement of the infant's or toddler's present levels of physical development (including fine motor, gross motor, vision, hearing, and health status), cognitive development, communication development, social or emotional development, and adaptive (self-help) development based on objective criteria. This can be listed as an age level or a range.

2. A statement (with the family's permission) of the family's resources, priorities, and concerns related to enhancing the development of the family's infant or toddler with a disability. Priorities may include the hopes and dreams of the family for their child. This statement may also include information about how the family would like its child to more fully participate in family and community activities. Resources include people in the family's life with whom they rely and interact.

3. A statement of the measurable results or outcomes expected to be achieved for the infant or toddler and the family. The statement should include emergent literacy and language skills that are developmentally appropriate for the child. The statement should also include the criteria, procedures, and time lines used to determine the degree to which progress toward achieving the results or outcomes is being made. Any modifications or revisions of the results/outcomes/services that may be necessary should be included. Outcomes are statements about what the family wants its child to learn or do. For example, an IFSP outcome may focus on the child learning to sit at the table with the family at dinner and eat with a spoon, walk around the block to the playground with the family in the evening, or say new words to tell

the family what toys the child wants. Outcomes should be individualized for each child and family. As such, they should be contextualized, functional, and discipline free. Outcomes should be relevant to the family and focused on the whole child and his or her participation in activity settings that are important to the family (Infant & Toddler Connection of Virginia, 2003).

4. A statement of specific early intervention services based on peer-reviewed research, to the extent possible, necessary to meet the unique needs of the infant or toddler and the family. The statement should include the frequency, intensity, and method of delivering services. Supports and services should be individualized. If a group of IFSPs are reviewed within a local system, the reviewer should see this individualization with varying services and supports being provided from IFSP to IFSP. Early intervention services include, but are not limited to, service coordination, speech-language therapy, physical therapy, occupational therapy, special instruction, and assistive technology. All children must receive service coordination. Additional services are dependent upon many variables and often change over the course of the child's involvement in early intervention.

5. A statement of the natural environments in which early intervention services will appropriately be provided. If the services will not be provided in a natural environment, a justification must be presented. Natural environments include locations where children live, learn, and play, and how they learn in those natural places.

6. The projected dates of initiation of services and the anticipated length, duration, and frequency of the services. Projected start dates must include the month, date, and year.

7. The identification of the service coordinator from the profession most immediately relevant to the child's or family's needs (or who is otherwise qualified to carry out all applicable responsibilities under this part). All families in early intervention have a service coordinator who is responsible for overseeing the IFSP, ensuring that all the IFSP services are provided, and that changes in the IFSP are made when necessary.

8. The steps to be taken to support the transition of the toddler with a disability to preschool or other appropriate services. This transition plan must be individualized for each child.

According to IDEIA §303.344(d)(4), when addressing the needs of children who are at least 3 years of age and receiving services through the provisions provided in the 2011 IDEIA Part C Final Regulations, the IFSP must also include "an educational component that promotes school readiness and incorporates pre-literacy, language, and numeracy skills" (IDEIA, 2011).

IFSP Implementation and Review

Implementation and review of the IFSP involves the coordination and monitoring of the delivery of IFSP supports and services. Early intervention services must begin within 30 days of the IFSP being written and agreed upon by the multidisciplinary team. Periodic reviews are held to facilitate IFSP changes as necessary. These changes may reflect the child's development and any changes, including those that may be medical in nature, that occur in regard to a family's priorities and concerns. IFSP reviews must take place at least once every six months or each time a child has either achieved a documented outcome or presents with a new area of need (IDEIA, 2004). Annual reviews must be completed within 365 days of the initial or previous annual IFSP meeting.

Transition

Transition is the entry and exit of children and families to and from early intervention services. This is an ongoing process that begins with the child and family as they enter the system and ends when they transition from the early intervention program under Part C to the next program or other appropriate services identified for the child who is no longer eligible to receive Part C or Part B services. The service coordinator tends to be the provider who is primarily responsible for assisting families through the transition process. All service providers, however, including the SLP and audiologist, should be knowledgeable about the transition process. Transition should be discussed at every IFSP meeting. As the child approaches 30 months of age, the service coordinator should increase the level of detail of these discussions in preparation for the child "aging out" of the early intervention system at the age of 3 years. Under the Final Regulations (IDEIA, 2011), notice of transition must occur no fewer than 90 days before the toddler's third birthday. Children transitioning from early intervention include those who no longer qualify for Part C supports and services prior to the age of 3 years, children who are turning 3 years and whose parents do not want to pursue Part B services (essentially preschool services), and/or children who are between 2 and 3 years of age and are preparing to transition to Part B services.

Under the Final Regulations (IDEIA, 2011), each state is provided with the opportunity to choose to extend Part C services to those children, who are eligible for preschool services, beyond the age of 3 until they enter or are eligible under state law to enter kindergarten. The state may choose to implement this option for children beyond 3 years of age until the beginning of the school year following their third, fourth, or fifth birthday. Currently, very few states are choosing this option.

Regardless of their choice, each state must include a description of the policies and procedures in place to ensure an effective and seamless transition for young children from receiving early intervention services under Part C of IDEIA to preschool or other appropriate services or for those who are exiting the Part C program altogether. Transition plans look different for each child and are dependent on the child's and family's needs. Regardless of where the child transitions, there may be an adjustment for the child and family when leaving the Part C system. You may be able to help the family with this adjustment by discussing the process and being prepared to answer any questions about the transition from Part C services to preschool services (IDEIA Part B).

Service Coordination

Under IDEIA 2004 Part C, service coordination is defined as an active, ongoing process that assists and enables families to access services and ensures their rights and procedural safeguards. Part C mandates that every family in the early intervention system receives service coordination at no cost.

In some states, the speech-language pathologist or audiologist, as a member of the IFSP team, may assume the functions of the service coordinator. When you are not responsible for the service coordination role, it is still imperative that you have an understanding of this role within the system to effectively collaborate with the service coordinator.

The service coordinator's primary function is to serve as the single point of contact for the family throughout the early intervention process. Service coordinators help the family identify and obtain needed services and assistance. Often, the service coordinator also acts as the initial point of contact and may therefore play the important role of assisting the family as they begin to understand and process the nature of their child's disability and needs. The family's first interactions with the service coordinator may have a significant influence on their level of trust and expectations of the early intervention system as a whole (Dunst, 2002).

Once a referral has been made for early intervention services, a service coordinator is assigned to the family as quickly as possible and becomes actively involved in the IFSP process. Table 17–6 illustrates the tasks that a service coordinator must accomplish efficiently and effectively.

The service coordinator supports the family members as they develop, implement, and monitor their intervention plan based on the IFSP. Service coordinators help families develop the knowledge and skills necessary to advocate for their children in the future. Service coordinators also access and coordinate resources and services for families. Ultimately, the service coordinator must ensure that the early intervention services are family centered and collaborative among the multidisciplinary team members. When service coordination is not effective, families may not have a clear understanding of their child's strengths or needs. They may be left to coordinate information and services from multiple sources on their own. In this case, intervention and transition are likely to be fragmented, and the family may be unaware of all available resources (ASHA, 2008b). All service providers must communicate regularly with assigned service coordinators to ensure cohesion between their services and the needs of the children and families.

The Team Approach

The early intervention system relies heavily on a team approach to service delivery. In addition to working closely with family members, SLPs and audiologists need to collaborate with service coordinators, specialists within other domains, physicians, and educators. Regardless of the level of severity of a child's or family's needs, services in early intervention include all types of resources or supports that the child needs and is eligible to receive (ASHA, 2008b). When team members communicate well with one another, all participants reap the benefits from the comprehensive services. Access to all necessary supports and services, the provision of skills and resources from multiple agencies, and the sharing of information and opinions across areas of expertise are just a few of the benefits of teams collaborating within the system.

The integration of services, including the coordination of the team members, is critical to the effective nature of early intervention. Additionally, they are essential elements of family-centered and best practices to support young children and their families (Early Childhood Personnel Center, 2017). Collaboration among team members provides opportunity for the development and coordination of interventions that complement one another. Team members who communicate well and collaborate across areas of expertise, including family members, benefit from joint professional development and consultation that results in enhanced knowledge and skills (Boyer & Thompson, 2014; Coufal

Table 17–6. Service Coordination Tasks

- Informing the family of their rights and procedural safeguards as well as the various timelines specified by Part C of IDEA 2004 and the final regulations implemented in 2011.
- Establishing a collaborative relationship with the family.
- Collecting information about family priorities, resources, and concerns, as well as daily routines and activities.
- Supporting the family's problem-solving skills as a course of action begins to develop.
- Planning the developmental evaluation/assessment, formulating questions that reflect the family's concerns, and addressing state eligibility standards with the family and the team members.
- Compiling and integrating information from various sources in order to develop a comprehensive developmental profile of the child.
- Facilitating communication among and between the various team members and the family in order to develop functional, meaningful outcomes based on the family and child's daily routines and activities.
- Ensuring that intervention services are provided in a timely manner and are directly related to functional outcomes and maintains communication and collaboration among team members in order to ensure that outcomes are being addressed.
- Coordinating early intervention and other services for the family (including educational, social, and medical supports and services that are not provided for diagnostic and evaluation purposes).
- Conducting referral and other activities to assist the family in identifying available providers.
- Overseeing the evaluation and review of the IFSP and subsequently monitoring the services specified in the IFSP.
- Conducting follow-up activities with the family and the team members.
- Coordinating and frequently reviewing the child's plan for transitioning from the early intervention system with the family.

Source: Based on information from ASHA (2008b) and IDEA (2011).

& Woods, 2018). As discussed earlier, the roles and responsibilities of the service coordinator are central to successful communication among the early intervention team members. Part C of IDEIA 2004 requires that members of the IFSP team coordinate their approaches, consult with one another, and recognize that the child and family outcomes are a responsibility to be shared by the entire team. Collaboration is dependent upon the type of team model that is used, the lead agency's program guidelines, and the knowledge and skills of the individual team members (ASHA, 2008b). Although collaboration among team members may vary, professional communication with the family is essential.

Part C of IDEIA 2004 uses the term *multidisciplinary* to describe the early intervention team approach, though other team models may be applied depending on the needs of the child and family. Three team models are commonly used within early intervention. In addition to multidisciplinary teams, interdisciplinary and transdisciplinary team models may be options within the local and/or state service delivery systems. Each one of these

teams is different in regard to the amount of communication and coordination required among team members (Paul-Brown & Caperton, 2001). Regardless of the model chosen, SLPs and audiologists are often integral members of early intervention teams.

Multidisciplinary Teams. In a multidisciplinary approach, service providers from different disciplines (i.e., physical therapy, occupational therapy, and audiology) assess and/or provide intervention to the family and child separately. Each provider completes an evaluation and/or assessment and makes recommendations independently of the other disciplines. Although several providers may be involved with the family, each professional works distinctly and separately in providing services. Team members therefore focus on their own disciplines and subsequent perspectives and do not tend to engage in collaborative planning or service provision. The service coordinator is typically a designated position within this type of team. Unfortunately, because collaboration among team members is often limited, cohesion of services may be affected (Paul & Roth, 2010). As stated earlier, Part C of IDEIA (2011) requires a multidisciplinary composition of the IFSP team, including the parent and two or more individuals from separate disciplines or professions with one of the individuals being the service coordinator.

Interdisciplinary Teams. Interdisciplinary teams have a greater focus on collaboration and communication. Typically, providers from various disciplines conduct the evaluation and/or assessment with the child and family individually; occasionally, an "arena" method of evaluation, in which multiple team members are present during the evaluation and/or assessment, may also be conducted. The team members then communicate with one another and integrate the findings to determine the needs, recommendations, and services for the child and his/her family (Paul & Roth, 2010).

Transdisciplinary Teams. The transdisciplinary team model involves a greater degree of collaboration among team members than the other service models. This approach is often more difficult to implement because of the need for increased collaboration and communication. It is the model, however, that is expected by IDEIA (2011) to be utilized to support the design and delivery of services for children with disabilities and delays and their families (Paul, Blosser, & Jakubowitz, 2006).

The transdisciplinary approach requires the team members to share roles and systematically cross discipline boundaries. The purpose of the approach is to pool and integrate the expertise of team members so that more efficient and comprehensive assessment and intervention services are provided. Communication among team members involves continuous give and take between all members on a consistent basis. Evaluation and assessment, as well as intervention services, are typically conducted jointly by designated members of the team assigned to the child/family; one team member will then serve as the primary service provider and will provide direct services that relate to all of the developmental disciplines for the child and family (Paul et al., 2006; Paul & Roth, 2010).

Services Based on the Highest Quality of Evidence

Part C services under IDEIA were created to enhance the development of infants and toddlers with disabilities, to minimize potential developmental delay, and to reduce educational costs to society by minimizing the need for continuing special education services as children with disabilities reach school age (IDEIA 2004, § 1400[20]).

Early intervention practices are based on the integration of the highest quality and most recent research, informed professional judgment and expertise, and family preferences and values (DEC, 2014). The foundation of support for practice includes both internal and external evidence. Internal evidence is based on policy, informed clinical opinion, values and perspectives of professionals and consumers, and professional consensus; external evidence is drawn from empirical research published in peer-reviewed journals. All of these considerations are evaluated in the delivery of early intervention services to realize positive outcomes for infants, toddlers, and their families (DEC, 2014).

Evidence Supporting Routines-Based Intervention

As stated earlier, the first guiding principle that reflects current best practices of SLPs and audiologists in early intervention addresses the delivery of family-centered services (ASHA, 2008a). This practice involves working collaboratively with families in all aspects of early intervention. A family-centered approach recognizes the importance of all family members and involves the awareness and inclusion of the beliefs, values, principles, and practices that strengthen the family's capacity to enhance their child's development and learning (IDEIA, 2004). Effective family-centered practices are responsive to the unique circumstances of each family and provide families with unbiased and comprehensive information to make informed decisions (DEC, 2014).

Routines-based intervention (RBI) is an approach that builds the capacity of the family to address the child's strengths and needs by embedding instruction within the context of a family's everyday activities and routines (Florida State University, 2011; McWilliam, 2010a). SLPs and audiologists who practice RBI collaborate with other providers, family members, caregivers, and teachers to develop child-specific strategies that are practiced within the family's natural environment (McWilliam, 2010a, 2010b, 2016; Raver & Childress, 2015). Rather than bring toys, books, and other materials into the natural environment, RBI emphasizes family-focused and family-implemented intervention using toys and objects from the family's own home or other natural environments. Implementation of this strategy encourages practice and facilitates generalization of the strategies used within treatment sessions between sessions (Crawford & Weber, 2014; Friedman, Woods, & Salisbury, 2012; Woods et al., 2004).

Audiologists and SLPs who incorporate RBI in their early intervention practice establish techniques, such as naturalistic language facilitation and/or swallowing strategies, that families can use to maximize the child's development and learning within their everyday routines and activities (Dunst, Raab, & Trivette, 2012). These techniques are based on collaboration with the parents, family, caregivers, and other providers to identify typical learning opportunities in the child's home and community; determine the child's interests, strengths, and motivation within their daily routines; and create communication and participation goals during learning opportunities (Dunst et al., 2012).

Evidence Supporting the Coaching Model

Early intervention SLPs and audiologists may often find it easier to simply "do it themselves." Effective early intervention providers, however, empower families when they coach the caregivers to support their child in their natural environments (Hanft, Rush, & Shelden, 2004; Rush & Sheldon, 2011). With the shift to family-centered services under IDEIA Part C in 2004, there has also been a shift away from direct one-to-one intervention with the child and toward implementation of an early childhood coaching model. Coaching models focus on family-implemented interventions and collaborative consultation between the service providers and the family members. Coaching in early intervention is an adult learning strategy that is intended to build the family's capacity to enhance their child's development using everyday interactions and activities. Early intervention

providers support families during visits by joining the family in their routines and activities and coaching caregivers as they practice using intervention strategies with their children (Rush & Sheldon, 2011). During the initiation of the coaching process, the door is opened to engage in a conversation regarding this approach. The SLP or audiologist and the parent develop a plan together that includes the purpose and specific outcomes of the coaching. As noted previously, the purpose within early intervention is typically to support the child's participation and development in ordinary family and community life. Following the initial discussion, the SLP or audiologist may choose to observe the parents as they use an existing strategy, try out a new skill, or demonstrate a skill that has been used between visits. The SLP or audiologist may also observe the parent engaging in an activity with the child. When the SLP or audiologist has an opportunity to see the parent and child interact, it allows them to (1) see what the parent or family member is doing well and (2) offer additional suggestions and/or modifications. Such active guidance provides an opportunity to build partnerships with families. These partnerships enhance the family members' effectiveness as they engage in everyday learning opportunities with their children (Rush & Sheldon, 2011; Shelden & Rush, 2001). Table 17–7 illustrates five research-based practice characteristics and strategies for implementation by a provider that lead to the intended outcomes of coaching in early intervention.

Table 17–7. Coaching Characteristics and the Role of the Provider	
Joint planning	At the beginning of the visit, discuss the plan and goals from the last visit with the family members. You should encourage the family to share what they have tried with their child as well as what did and did not work.
Observation	Watch the family members as they play, interact, and engage in their everyday routines and/or activities with the child. You might show them a strategy to use and encourage them to try the strategy with the child while you observe.
Action	Help the family practice new ways to help their child meet his/her goals within the context of their everyday routines and activities. Encourage the family to consider ways in which they can put into action the strategies you consider together.
Reflection	Ask questions about what the family members have already tried with their child and what is typical for their family. Listen to the family and discuss what has already worked, what has not worked, and why their efforts have or have not been successful.
Feedback	In response to the family's reflections, share information, including thoughts, ideas, and feedback that might facilitate the determination of additional strategies to best support the family as they work with their child to meet his/her goals.
Joint planning	At the end of the visit, work with the family to come up with a specific plan to address the child's goals between now and the next visit. Schedule your next visit.

Source: Based on information from Rush & Shelden (2011).

Other Considerations for Early Intervention Services in Natural Environments

When intervening with families, SLPs and audiologists must be able to establish and maintain rapport as well as professional boundaries; gather information; and handle difficult situations, including reporting suspected child abuse and neglect. These topics will be discussed next. SLPs and audiologists must also be flexible in their approaches to these activities, as each family requires a unique approach to benefit from early intervention.

General Safety

Providing best practices and quality intervention is your priority as an SLP or audiologist in early intervention. Since these best practices mean providing services primarily in families' homes and community settings, it is important for you to consider your personal safety and other issues unique to providing services outside of clinic or center-based settings. Visiting families in natural environments means that you are often on your own in unfamiliar locations. Be sure to let others know your schedule, including when you will be at specific loca-

tions. It is also a good idea to keep your cell phone with you on intervention visits for safety purposes; remember, however, to keep the ringer turned off in respect for the family that you are visiting. Visit families with another staff person when you find that you are uncomfortable on your own or as deemed appropriate. Maintaining your own safety ensures that you will have the opportunity to share your knowledge and skills with families. Table 17–8 provides additional safety tips for early intervention visits in natural environments. Additional information regarding safety in the workplace is available in Chapter 22.

Maintaining Professional Boundaries

Establishing and maintaining a relationship with families while upholding professional boundaries can be tricky for the SLP and audiologist. To build rapport, sharing some personal information can be helpful when getting to know the family. Knowing what is appropriate to share, how much, and how to handle situations when families want more information about you are important considerations when working closely with families. Another aspect of maintaining professional boundaries involves knowing how far to become involved in a family member's personal life. Parents often share a great

Table 17–8. Safety Tips for Visits in Natural Environments

- Always keep a cell phone with you on visits in natural environments.
- Keep your car keys in your pocket or on your body; do not leave them on a table or place them on the floor.
- Be aware of your clothing; avoid heels and revealing clothing and limit jewelry.
- Do not take a purse into a family's home. Put your purse or any personal belongings in the trunk of the car prior to arriving at your destination.
- Clearly document your visits, particularly if anything or anyone makes you uncomfortable or causes you concern. Discuss these concerns with your supervisor immediately.
- Visit families who live in areas where safety is a concern with another provider.
- Avoid making visits on Friday afternoons or on the first or last day of the month to areas where safety is a concern (as the arrival of paychecks or federal aid checks may cause an increase in the number of people in the area). Consider morning visits to these areas whenever possible.
- Survey the area thoroughly before leaving the car or the home; look all around for any signs of danger.
- Park on the street rather than in the driveway (in order to ensure that your car will not be blocked in by other vehicles).
- When walking to your car, have your keys available.
- Make eye contact and be friendly with people as you walk to/from a family's home; become a familiar face in the neighborhoods in which you provide services.
- Be aware of your limits and ask for help when needed. Trust your instincts; if you feel uncomfortable in a home or in a situation, excuse yourself and leave.

Source: Based on information from Partnerships for People with Disabilities (2010).

deal about their lives with the SLP or audiologist, particularly when under challenging circumstances. It is ultimately your responsibility to know when you are becoming too involved. When professional boundaries are crossed, it becomes difficult to serve the family objectively and in a manner that makes them feel empowered to help themselves.

Reporting Child Abuse and Neglect

Early intervention personnel, including SLPs and audiologists, are mandated reporters of suspected child abuse or neglect in most states. Therefore, it is important that you become familiar with how to make a report in your area, what information Child Protective Services (CPS) needs, and any documentation required when making a report. You should also be aware of internal policies within your agency for making CPS reports. Refer to Chapter 24 for additional considerations regarding child mistreatment.

Managing an Unclean Environment

Each environment in which you provide services may present a different level of cleanliness. The challenge that faces you is to maintain the balance between respect for the family and comfort for yourself while providing services in these environments. Table 17–9 provides some considerations to increase your comfort while providing family-centered services.

Summary

Early intervention is a federally mandated system that operates under the Individuals with Disabilities Education Improvement Act (IDEIA). The system, which has

been restructured multiple times since its inception in 1997, authorizes services to meet the needs of infants and toddlers and their families, from birth to age 3 years who have been or may be at risk for developmental delays or disabilities. In 2008, ASHA presented five guiding principles that continue to reflect best practices for SLPs and audiologists who are providing early intervention services to young children and their families. This chapter discussed how each of those five guiding principles may be effectively implemented by the SLP and audiologist within the early intervention system. Cultural competence, including the definitions and the considerations that influence the provision of effective and appropriate services, was addressed. This chapter defined family-centered practices, based on the family systems model, and presented the rationale for incorporating natural environments, routines, and everyday activities into the provision of early intervention services. Each step of the early intervention process, including final regulations and considerations regarding eligibility and the creation of the IFSP, was presented and discussed. The chapter outlined the team approach to early intervention, different team formats, and the basic considerations for each type of team discussed. Evidence to support the basis of early intervention and the inclusion of both routines-based intervention and coaching in service delivery were also presented. Finally, the chapter offered general advice for providing best practices within natural environments and suggestions for establishing a positive and safe work environment.

Critical Thinking

1. Discuss the five guiding principles that reflect current best practices in early intervention. How

---

Table 17–9. Considerations to Increase Comfort in an Unclean Environment

- Wear dark clothing that can be easily laundered.
- Keep a change of clothing in the car.
- Keep hand sanitizer in the car and approved disinfecting wipes in the trunk to clean any toys or materials after the visit.
- Bring a large book or small blanket to spread out on the floor on which everyone can play.
- Remember that you are in someone's home and, although it may not be as clean as your standards, it may suit the family's standards.
- Recognize that, if the unclean environment is truly a health hazard to the child (i.e., roaches in the child's bedroom or spoiled formula in the infant's bottle), you will need to communicate with the family about the issue and offer to assist in finding a solution. If the family is unable or unwilling to take action to correct the health hazard, you may need to file a report with Child Protective Services.

Source: Based on information from Partnerships for People with Disabilities (2010).

does each principle impact the role of the speech-language pathologist and the audiologist in the early intervention arena? Provide a scenario of how each one can be implemented in practice.

2. Describe a speech-language pathologist's or audiologist's role and level of involvement in regard to each of the seven components of the early intervention process.

3. The speech-language pathologist or audiologist may occasionally be responsible for coordinating an IFSP meeting. What extra duties will the speech-language pathologist or audiologist be responsible for in this situation?

4. Provide an example scenario based on the eight suggestions (other than active listening) for building positive relationships with families in the early intervention system.

5. In your own words, explain the differences between multidisciplinary, interdisciplinary, and transdisciplinary team approaches. Which one is the most effective when providing family-centered early intervention services? Explain.

6. Why do speech-language pathologists and audiologists need to be familiar with cultural competence? Provide a scenario in which a speech-language pathologist or audiologist is *not* demonstrating cultural competence with a child and family. What can the speech-language pathologist or audiologist do differently to correct the situation?

7. Speech-language pathologists and audiologists with the best intentions often have difficulty designing services that are family centered and routines based and that implement a coaching model. Read the following scenarios and answer the following questions for each one:

   a. What is missing from each of these situations? What else should be considered?

   b. How would you change these practices to make them more family centered?

   c. What would you do to ensure that these sessions are routines based?

   Scenario 1: As Joey's mom works on a few chores in the kitchen, the speech-language pathologist explains and demonstrates how Joey's sitting can be supported when he is watching television in the evenings with his family.

   Scenario 2: Jenna's father, Tony, has a neatly organized home, is systematic in accomplishing daily tasks, and is quite directive in his interaction style with Jenna. During the initial home visit, the speech-language pathologist suggests that Tony consider using more open-ended questions and arranging Jenna's toys on shelves in various rooms throughout the house to promote communication initiations from Jenna.

   Scenario 3: Candace has bilateral cochlear implants and uses both sign language and vocalizations to communicate. Her parents have requested that the audiologist visit her at home as well as at her child care center; they want both services to be coordinated to ensure that the routines and coaching strategies are consistent across the natural environments. Her child care teacher believes in a child-directed play approach and does not believe in coaching or adult direction. She wants Candace to be pulled out of her classroom to receive special education services with the audiologist and speech-language pathologist because, as she states, she "doesn't have time to work with her individually during every routine."

8. As a clinician engaging in early intervention, you are likely to go into homes that present a variety of cultural and linguistic differences in addition to varying child-rearing practices. What should you do to prepare for this experience?

9. You are likely to be working with a variety of other professionals when you provide assessment and therapy services to children and families through early intervention. Who are these other professionals? What are their roles in EI? What should you do to work effectively in a team context?

10. What ethical dilemmas might you face in working as a professional in an early intervention context? How would you resolve these?

References

American Speech-Language-Hearing Association (ASHA). (2006). *Roles, knowledge, and skills: Audiologists providing clinical services to infants and young children birth to 5 years of age* [Knowledge and skills]. Available from http://www.asha.org/policy/

American Speech-Language-Hearing Association (ASHA). (2007). *ASHA SLP Health Care Survey 2007: Caseload characteristics.* Rockville, MD:

Author. Retrieved from https://www.asha.org/uploadedFiles/research/memberdata/HC07Case loadRprt.pdf

American Speech-Language-Hearing Association (ASHA). (2008a). *Core knowledge and skills in early intervention speech-language pathology practice.* Available from http://www.asha.org/policy

American Speech-Language-Hearing Association (ASHA). (2008b). *Roles and responsibilities of speech-language pathologists in early intervention: Guidelines.* Available from http://www.asha.org/policy

American Speech-Language-Hearing Association (ASHA). (2013). *Supplement to the JCIH 2007 position statement: Principles and guidelines for early intervention following confirmation that a child is deaf or hard of hearing* [Position statement]. Available from http://www.asha.org/policy/

American Speech-Language-Hearing Association (ASHA). (2016a). *Code of ethics* [Ethics]. Available from http://www.asha.org/policy/

American Speech-Language-Hearing Association (ASHA). (2016b). *Scope of practice in speech-language pathology* [Scope of practice]. Available from http://www.asha.org/policy/

American Speech-Language-Hearing Association (ASHA). (2019) *Early intervention practice portal* [Web page]. Retrieved from https://www.asha.org/PRPSpecificTopic.aspx?-folderid=8589943999&section=Key_Issues

Balthrop, C., & Coleman, W. (2003, March). *Why is Suzy so weird? Understanding cultural differences in the classroom.* Paper presented at the meeting of the Virginia Association for Early Childhood.

Benn, R. (1994). Conceptualizing eligibility for early intervention services. In D. M. Bryant & M. A. Graham (Eds.), *Implementing early intervention* (pp. 18–45). New York, NY: Guilford Press.

Boyer, V. E., & Thompson, S. D. (2014). Transdisciplinary model and early intervention: Building collaborative relationships. *Young Exceptional Children, 17,* 19–32.

Branson, D., & Demchak, M. (2009). The use of augmentative and alternative communication methods with infants and toddlers with disabilities: A research review. *Augmentative & Alternative Communication, 25,* 274–286.

Brown, W., & Brown, C. (1993). Defining eligibility for early intervention. In W. Brown, S. K. Thurman, & F. Pearl (Eds.), *Family-centered early intervention with infants and toddlers: Innovative cross-disciplinary approaches* (pp. 21–42). Baltimore, MD: Brookes.

Caesar, L. G. (2013). Providing early intervention services to diverse populations: Are speech-language pathologists prepared? *Infants and Young Children, 26*(2), 126–146. https://doi.org/10.1097/IYC.0b013e3182848340

Center on the Developing Child at Harvard University (CDCHU). (2008). *In brief: The science of early childhood development.* Retrieved from http://developingchild.harvard.edu/download_file/-/view/64/

Center on the Developing Child at Harvard University (CDCHU). (2010). *The foundations of lifelong health are built in early childhood.* Retrieved from https://developingchild.harvard.edu/resources/the-foundations-of-lifelong-health-are-built-in-early-childhood/

Coufal, K. L., & Woods, J. J. (2018). Interprofessional collaborative practice in early intervention. *Pediatric Clinics, 65,* 143–155. https://doi.org/10.1016/j.pcl.2017.08.027

Crawford, M. J., & Weber, B. (2014). *Early intervention every day! Embedding activities in daily routines for young children and their families.* Baltimore, MD: Brookes.

Division for Early Childhood (DEC). (2014). *DEC recommended practices in early intervention/early childhood special education 2014.* Retrieved from http://www.dec-sped.org/recommendedpractices

Dunst, C. J. (2002). Family-centered practices: Birth through high school. *Journal of Special Education, 36*(3), 139–147. https://doi.org/10.1177/00224669020360030401

Dunst, C. J. (2017). Family systems early childhood intervention. In H. Sukkar, J. Kirby, & C. J. Dunst (Eds.), *Early childhood intervention: Working with families of young children with special needs* (pp. 36–58). Abingdon, Oxfordshire, UK: Routledge.

Dunst, C. J., Bruder, M. B., Trivette, C. M., Hamby, D., Raab, M., & McLean, M. (2001). Characteristics and consequences of everyday natural learning opportunities. *Topics in Early Childhood Special Education, 21*(2), 68–91. https://doi.org/10.1177/027112140102100202

Dunst, C. J., Raab, M., & Trivette, C. M. (2012). Characteristics of naturalistic language intervention strategies. *Journal of Speech-Language Pathology & Applied Behavior Analysis, 5,* 8–16. Retrieved from https://www.thefreelibrary.com/Characteristics+of+naturalistic+language+intervention+strategies.-a0299887454

Dunst, C. J., & Trivette, C. M. (2009). Capacity-building family-systems intervention practices. *Journal of Family Social Work, 12*, 119–143. https://doi.org/10.1080/10522150802713322

Early Childhood Personnel Center. (2017). *Cross-Disciplinary Personnel Competencies Alignment.* Retrieved from https://ecpcta.org/cross-disciplinary-alignment

Friedman, M., Woods, J. & Salisbury, C. (2012). Caregiver coaching strategies for early intervention providers: Moving toward operational definitions. *Infants & Young Children, 25*(1), 62–82. https://doi.org/10.1097/IYC.0b013e31823d8f12

Guralnick, M. J. (2011). Why early intervention works: A systems perspective. *Infants & Young Children, 24*, 6–28. https://doi.org/10.1097/IYC.0b013e3182002cfe

Hanft, B. E., Rush, D. D., & Shelden, M. L. (2004). *Coaching families and colleagues in early childhood.* Baltimore, MD: Brookes.

Hanson, M. J., & Lynch, E. W. (1990). Honoring the cultural diversity of families when gathering data. *Topics in Early Childhood Special Education, 10*(1), 112–132. https://doi.org/10.1177/027112149001000109

Hebbeler, K. (2009). *First five years fund briefing.* Presentation given at a congressional briefing on June 11, 2009, to discuss *Education that works: The impact of early childhood intervention on reducing the need for special education services.* Retrieved from http://www.sri.com/neils/pdfs/ FFYF_Briefing_Hebbeler_June2009_test.pdf

Hebbeler, K., Spiker, D., Bailey, D., Scarborough, A., Mallik, S., Simeonsoon, R., Singer, M., & Nelson, L. (2007). *Early intervention for infants & toddlers with disabilities and their families: Participants, services, and outcomes. Final report of the National Early Intervention Longitudinal Study (NEILS).* Retrieved from https://www.sri.com/sites/default/files/publications/neils_finalreport_200702.pdf

Individuals with Disabilities Education Improvement Act (IDEIA) (2004). Pub. L. No. 108-446, § 632, 118 Stat. 2744. Retrieved from http://idea.ed.gov/

Individuals with Disabilities Education Improvement Act (IDEIA). (2011). Part C Final Regulations. 34 C.F.R. §§ 303 (2011). Retrieved from https://www.gpo.gov/fdsys/pkg/FR-2011-09-28/pdf/2011-22783.pdf

Infant & Toddler Connection of Virginia. (2003). *Individualized Part C early intervention supports and services in everyday routines, activities and places.* Retrieved from http://www.infantva.org/documents/wkg-ITF09302003Individualized SupportsandServices.pdf

Joint Committee on Infant Hearing (JCIH). (2007). Year 2007 position statement: Principles and guidelines for early hearing detection and intervention programs. *Pediatrics, 120*(4), 898–921. Retrieved from https://pediatrics.aappublications.org/content/120/4/898

Jung, L. A., & Grisham-Brown, J. (2006). Moving from assessment information to IFSPs: Guidelines for a family-centered process. *Young Exceptional Children, 9*(2), 2–11. https://doi.org/10.1177/109625060600900201

Kashinath, S., Woods, J., & Goldstein, H. (2006). Enhancing generalized teaching strategy use in daily routines by parents of children with autism. *Journal of Speech, Language, and Hearing Research, 49*, 466–485. https://doi.org/10.1044/1092-4388 (2006/036)

Landa, R., Holman, K., O'Neill, A., & Stuart, E. (2010). Intervention targeting development of socially synchronous engagement in toddlers with autism spectrum disorder: A randomized controlled trial. *Journal of Child Psychology and Psychiatry, 52*(1), 13–21. https://doi.org/10.1111/j.1469-7610.2010.02288.x

McWilliam, R. A. (2004). Early intervention where it counts: Natural environments. *All Together Now! 10*(3), 3–6.

McWilliam, R. A. (2010a). *Routines-based early intervention: Supporting young children and their families.* Baltimore, MD: Brookes.

McWilliam, R. A. (2010b). Assessing families' needs with the routines-based interview. In R. A. McWilliam (Ed.), *Working with families of young children with special needs* (pp. 27–60). New York, NY: Guilford Press.

Partnership for People with Disabilities. (2010). *Kaleidoscope: New perspectives in service coordination* [Trainer's notebook]. Virginia Commonwealth University: Author.

Paul-Brown, D., & Caperton, C. J. (2001). Inclusive practices for preschool-aged children with specific language impairment. In M. J. Guralnick (Ed.), *Early childhood inclusion: Focus on change* (pp. 433–463). Baltimore, MD: Brookes.

Paul, D., Blosser, J., & Jakubowitz, M. (2006). Principles and challenges for forming successful literacy partnerships. *Topics in Language Disorders, 26*(1), 5–23.

Paul, D., & Roth, F. (2010). Guiding principles and clinical applications for speech-language pathology practice in early intervention [Electronic version]. *Language, Speech, and Hearing Services in Schools.* https://doi.org/10.1044/0161-1461(2010/09-0079).

Peña, E., & Fiestas, C. (2009). Talking across cultures in early intervention: Finding common ground to meet children's communication needs. *Perspectives on Communication Disorders and Sciences in Culturally and Linguistically Diverse Populations, 16*, 79–85. https://doi.org/10.1044/cds16.3.79

Peredo, T. N. (2016). Supporting culturally and linguistically diverse families in early intervention. *Perspectives of the ASHA Special Interest Groups, 1*(1), 154–167. https://doi.org/10.1044/persp1.SIG1.154

Puig, V. I. (2012). Cultural and linguistic alchemy: Mining the resources of Spanish-speaking children and families receiving early intervention services. *Journal of Research in Childhood Education, 26*(3), 325–345. https://doi.org/10.1080/02568543.2012.684421

Raspa, M., Bailey, D. B., Olmsted, M. G., Nelson, R., Robinson, N., Simpson, M. E., & Houts, R. (2010). Measuring family outcomes in early intervention: Findings from a large-scale assessment. *Exceptional Children, 76*(4), 496–510. https://doi.org/10.1177/001440291007600407

Raver, S. A., & Childress, D. C. (2015). *Family-centered early intervention: Supporting infants and toddlers in natural environments.* Baltimore, MD: Brookes.

Roberts, M. Y., Hensle, T., & Brooks, M. K. (2016). More than "Try this at home"—including parents in early intervention. *Perspectives of the ASHA Special Interest Groups, 1*(1), 130–143. https://doi.org/10.1044/persp1.SIG1.130

Ross, K. D. (2018). *Speech-language pathologists in early childhood intervention: Working with infants, toddlers, families, and other care providers.* San Diego, CA: Plural Publishing.

Rush, D. D., & Shelden, M. L. (2011). *The early childhood coaching handbook.* Baltimore, MD: Brookes.

Saldaña, D. (2001) *Cultural competency: A practical guide for mental health service providers.* Austin, TX: Hogg Foundation for Mental Health.

Sandall, S., Hemmeter, M.L., Smith B.J., & McLean, M.E. (EDs.) (2005). *DEC recommended practices: A comprehensive guide for practical application in early intervention/early childhood special education.* Missoula, MT: Division for Early Childhood.

Segal, R., & Beyer, C. (2006). Integration and application of a home treatment program: A study of parents and occupational therapists. *American Journal of Occupational Therapy, 60*, 500–510. https://doi.org/10.5014/ajot.60.5.500

Shelden, M. L., & Rush, D. D. (2001). The ten myths about providing early intervention services in natural environments. *Infants and Young Children, 14*(1), 1–13.

Shelden, M. L., & Rush, D. D. (2010). A primary-coach approach to teaming and supporting families in early childhood intervention. In R. McWilliam (Ed.), *Working with families of young children with special needs* (pp. 175–202). New York, NY: Guilford Press.

Shelden, M. L., & Rush, D. D. (2013). *The early intervention teaming handbook: The primary service provider approach.* Baltimore, MD: Brookes.

Special Quest Multimedia Training Library. (2007). *Creating bright futures: Building relationships with families* [Facilitator's guide]. Retrieved from https://eclkc.ohs.acf.hhs.gov/sites/default/files/pdf/no-search/specialquest/building-rel-bright-futures-1-worksheet.pdf

Trivette, C. M., & Dunst, C. J. (2007). Capacity-building family-centered help-giving practices. *Winterberry Research Reports, 1*, 1–10. Retrieved from http://www.puckett.org/presentations/CapacityBldg_FamilyCtr_Prac_Char_Consq_CT_Dec_2014.pdf

Turnbull, A. P., Summers, J. A., Turnbull, R., Brotherson, M. J., Winton, P., Roberts, R., & Stroup-Rentier, V. (2009). Family supports and services in early intervention: A bold vision. *Journal of Early Intervention, 29*(3), 187–206. https://doi.org/10.1177/105381510702900301

Wayman, K., & Lynch, E. W. (1991). Home-based early childhood services: Cultural sensitivity in a family systems approach. *Topics in Early Childhood Special Education, 10*(4), 56–76. https://doi.org/10.1177/027112149101000406

Woods, J., Kashinath, S., & Goldstein, H. (2004). Effects of embedding caregiver-implemented teaching strategies in daily routines on children's communication outcomes. *Journal of Early Intervention, 26*(3), 175–193. https://doi.org/10.1177/105381510402600302

18

Service Delivery Issues
in Private Practice

◇◇

Robin L. Edge, PhD

Introduction

A private practice is a business setting in which the clinician/owner independently operates the business. According to a 2018 member survey of the American Speech-Language-Hearing Association (ASHA), 21.1% of speech-language pathology members, 31.3% of audiology members, and 32.3% of dually certified members were employed in a private practice (American Speech-Language-Hearing Association [ASHA], 2019e). Of the 21.1% of speech-language pathology private practitioners, 9% worked full time in the practice and 12.1% worked part time. Of the 31.3% of private practice audiologists (AuDs), 24.1% were employed full time and 7.2% were employed part time. Of the 32.3% of dually certified members, 13.8% were employed full time and 18.5% were employed part time (ASHA, 2019e). Additional survey data showed that 42% of audiologists (ASHA, 2017) and 37% of speech-language pathologists (SLPs) (ASHA, 2015) working in a private practice were owners or co-owners of the business.

A private practice setting appeals to individuals who are typically well versed in business management and practices, and who enjoy the autonomy of working without the larger structure of a health care or school setting. This chapter discusses the basic tenets of starting a private practice including business structures, roles, and work frequency; a business plan and location; credentials and qualifications needed to start a private practice; and service rates, billing, and networking information. The information here provides an introductory overview of starting a private practice with resources cited to provide more in-depth information on each topic. It is important to note that this chapter should not be considered a substitute for consulting business and legal advice from financial and legal professionals before starting a private practice.

Advantages and Disadvantages of a Private Practice

The advantages of owning a private practice include the autonomy of creating policies and procedures for the business, being responsible for the decisions and demands of the business, and having flexible scheduling and caseload management. Although these are positive benefits of owning and operating a private practice, a significant disadvantage is that the entire business burden falls to the owner. The flexibility of one's schedule and caseload management is a desirable feature, but the downside is that revenue for a private practitioner can be inconsistent as it is dependent on patient caseload. Business revenue can be affected by the cancellation rate of patients, the availability of the therapist(s), as well as the timeliness of reimbursement by insurance or private pay. To combat this inconsistency in revenue, a private practitioner must manage finances to cover bills, taxes, and salary. Additionally, the business owner receives no paid time off for sickness, vacation, or to complete continuing education; income is decreased each day patients are not seen. Successful private practitioners must plan ahead and save for times when patients cannot be treated. Additionally, solo private practice owners do not have coverage for days off and can spend much time alone. This can be isolating and difficult for some people to manage.

Another challenge faced by private practitioners is that there are no provided benefits when owning a practice. When you start a full-time private practice, you will need to purchase health insurance individually and contribute to an individual retirement account. Purchasing independent health insurance can be costly when the business owner is not covered under another family member's plan. In addition to health insurance, established health care facilities, school systems, and other larger employee settings typically provide retirement benefits to their employees. Many employers also match employee's retirement contributions, which is income that should be considered when deciding whether or not to start a full-time private practice. As a practice owner, you would need to seriously consider providing each of these benefits for yourself and your employees.

Many of the chapters included in this text cover issues that are particularly relevant to starting a private practice, including working in health care (15), education (16), and early intervention (17), as well as professional issues (1–6), career issues (10–12), and working productively (20). These chapters should be consulted as needed as you contemplate your transition from employee at a larger agency to joining the ranks of speech-language pathology and audiology private practitioners.

Private Practice Options

Private Practice Goals

As one contemplates starting a private practice, many important decisions must be made. First, it is important to set business goals. Why does starting a private practice appeal to you? What are you looking to accomplish by starting a private practice? How do you define a successful private practice? Providing detailed answers to these questions will become the road map for the private practice planning stages. After you articulate your motivations and desired outcomes for the practice, it is important to decide how much you want to work for the business. Do you want to build a practice for full- or part-time employment for yourself or do you prefer to provide therapy services on an as needed basis? Clinicians who work full-time for their private practice do not provide therapy services outside of their practice, whereas part-time or prn private practitioners typically keep their positions at their primary place of employment and build their practice outside of their regular working hours on a part-time or as needed basis. This allows therapists to build their private practice caseload over time without the financial burden of losing their salary in the process. Before embarking on this, you should check your contract with your employer to ensure a noncompete clause is not included. A noncompete clause can be included with the contract you sign to begin work and states that you agree to not work with a rival company or start a similar business in the same area for a specified period of time (Doyle, 2018). If you signed a contract with a noncompete clause you will be unable to work in the designated geographical area until the time limit stated passes. This type of clause is one of the reasons it is always a good idea to have someone else review any contract before you sign it. As the practice grows, the SLP/AuD can transition from full-time employment at a company to full-time self-employment as it becomes financially feasible to do so. Some private practitioners provide services on a contract basis to facilities that need speech-language pathology or audiology coverage for their patients or students. This is a straightforward way to ease into private practice without the need to take on the tasks associated with third-party insurance billing.

The financial ramifications of starting a private practice should not be ignored as business trends report that it can take up to five years before a business begins to be profitable (Davidson, 2019). Although these financial implications are generalities from business research, the speed of profitability of a business is largely dependent on start-up money and overhead expenses. Obviously, the financial burden of starting a practice is lessened if the business owner can rely on income from outside sources, including family members. Having a carefully planned budget allows a practice owner to foresee the financial resources needed for a successful business while also strategically planning for long-term operating costs and potential expansion (McQuerrey, 2019). The U.S.

Small Business Administration provides resources for budget planning for a business (2019a, 2019b). A small business certified public accountant or a tax lawyer can help with the budgeting process.

Role at the Practice

The next important question to be considered when starting a private practice is what type of private practice do you want? Do you want to provide direct therapy services to patients, or do you envision hiring therapists to treat patients while you manage the practice? Some private practices are staffing companies that contract their hired SLPs/AuDs to other health care and educational agencies in need of services, rather than directly treating patients or supervising therapists. The owner of a staffing private practice focuses his or her time on recruiting therapists to work for the company as well as identifying medical and/or school settings in need of therapy services. Private practitioners can also become consultants. Rather than providing direct treatment or staffing services, consulting SLPs/AuDs are paid by other agencies to provide case review and information regarding specific patients, disorders, or treatment techniques. For example, a consulting SLP or AuD may be called as an expert witness in a trial to review the viability of treatments rendered to a patient if a family is litigating against a hospital or school system. Additionally, a clinician may consult by offering continuing education courses on an area of expertise or by offering individual counsel to therapists who may not be experienced in treating a particular disorder. The most common type of private practices in speech-language pathology and audiology are ones in which direct services are provided to patients (ASHA, 2015, 2017), with consulting only contributing a portion of most private practitioners' income.

Business Structures

Once you decide to start a private practice, the next decision to be made is the business structure of the private practice. The type of business entity desired depends on two main factors: the owner's desire to solely own the business and the liability the owner is willing to assume for the business. Liability is defined as "a comprehensive legal term that describes the condition of being actually or potentially subject to legal obligation" ("Liability," 2008). In other words, if you are liable for a business, you are obligated to pay the business debts. Based on the ownership and liability desires when starting a practice, there are four legal organization structures a private practice can have: sole proprietorship, partnership, limited liability company, or corporation (ASHA, 2011; U.S.

Small Business Administration, 2019a). A brief overview of each of these business structures will be discussed in further detail below. Please consult your local U.S. Small Business Administration and/or legal counsel for more in-depth information regarding business structures before starting a practice.

Sole Proprietorship. A sole proprietorship provides the private practice owner/operator full control over the business as the practice does not exist without the owner. Because no other individuals are involved with the practice, business decisions can be made easily when compared with business structures involving partners. Sole proprietorship is the simplest and most common business structure as there are minimal legal restrictions and no cost to start this type of business (U.S. Small Business Administration, 2019a). One difference between this structure and others is that a sole proprietorship owner reports business income and loss on his or her personal income taxes. This means the business owner is personally financially liable or responsible for any debt the business incurs. In other words, all of the owner's personal assets can be used to pay off business debt. Because only one person is responsible for the business, it can be difficult to raise capital for this business structure as the growth of the business is limited (as there is only so much one person can manage/oversee/perform).

Partnership. A partnership is the easiest business structure for two or more people to own a business together (U.S. Small Business Administration, 2019a). There are two types of partnership business structures, a limited partnership and a limited liability partnership. In a limited partnership, one partner assumes full liability for the business and pays the self-employment taxes while other partners have both limited liability and limited control of the business (U.S. Small Business Administration, 2019a). In this business structure, the partner who pays the employment taxes assumes most of the responsibility for the business and also makes the majority of the decisions for the business. In business terminology this person has unlimited liability. The remaining partners have limited liability meaning their financial responsibility for the business is limited to a fixed sum. This is contrary to the unlimited liability partner who carries unlimited responsibility for the business finances.

A limited liability partnership (LLP) is similar to the limited partnership described above with the exception that in an LLP, all owners have fixed sum limited financial liability for the business. This business structure protects all of the business partners from the debts accrued by the business, as no partner is solely personally responsible for the financial decisions made by the other business owners (U.S. Small Business Administration,

2019a). The taxation of an LLP differs from that of a limited liability company (LLC), discussed below, in that the LLP is always taxed as a partnership and an LLC has several taxation options (Murray, 2019).

Limited Liability Company. An LLC is a business structure that protects the owners' personal assets if the business faces bankruptcy or lawsuits (U.S. Small Business Administration, 2019a). An individual or group of people can own an LLC. In most cases, the business partners of an LLC's personal assets are protected should the business fall on financial trouble. Although an LLC and a limited liability partnership are similar, the main difference is that an LLC can be owned by a corporation, whereas a limited liability partnership cannot. In the partnership structure, at least one managing partner assumes liability for the partnerships action. In an LLC, all partners can have limited liability allowing benefit from the protection of the corporation structure while assuming a partnership business model (Feigenbaum, 2019). Business profits and losses go through the owner's personal income without paying corporate taxes, but self-employment taxes for Medicare and Social Security must be paid (U.S. Small Business Administration, 2019a). LLCs have lower tax rates than corporations but do provide protection of the personal assets of business owners like an LLP. This personal asset protection is the biggest benefit of this business structure. Unlike partnerships, LLCs must register with the secretary of state where the business is located (Feigenbaum, 2019).

Corporation. The final business structure is a corporation. Corporations differ from the previous business models as they are considered a legal entity separate from its owners that can be held legally responsible as a business (U.S. Small Business Administration, 2019a). This means the business owners in a corporation have no personal liability for the business decisions. The personal assets of the owners cannot be used to pay off corporation debt. Unlike the other models, corporations pay taxes on profits and are taxed again when the profits are distributed to company shareholders. They have the highest level of protection for owners/shareholders, but typically pay more taxes than the other models. Unlike other business structures, corporations can raise funds for the business through the sale of company stocks. See the U.S. Small Business Administration website for more information regarding types of corporations as well as the other business structures discussed above.

As seen in Table 18–1, each type of business structure has advantages and disadvantages. The type of business structure you choose will depend on multiple variables, including your desire to have a partner, the start-up money you may need, the personal liability coverage and tax structure you desire, and state regulations and restrictions. If you want to own the business alone, a partnership is the only business structure that will not work. If you want to own the business with others, a sole proprietorship is not appropriate. LLCs and corporations can be owned by either an individual or a group. Liability for the business owner differs with the business structures, with the sole proprietorship structure having the most personal liability for the owner and the corporation structure carrying the least personal financial liability.

Regardless of the business structure chosen, separate business accounts should be opened to keep business financials separate from the owner's personal financial information. Seeking advice from a business consultant, attorney, and/or accountant is recommended to help in this decision-making process. ASHA and the American Academy of Private Practice in Speech Language Pathology and Audiology and the American Academy of Audiology (AAA) have resources to assist with this decision as well.

Taxes

The business structure you choose will determine the tax liability of your business. If you choose any business structure besides a sole proprietorship, your private practice will need to apply for an employer ID number (EIN). An EIN is the business's federal tax ID number and is the business equivalent of an individual's Social Security number. The EIN will be used to pay taxes on income the practice makes, and in all correspondence with the Internal Revenue Service (IRS). Taxes for the sole proprietorship business structure can be filed under the owner's personal social security number. Unlike personal income tax filings, taxes for a small business are typically filed quarterly, on or around April 15, June 17, September 16, and January 15 (IRS, 2019). A certified tax accountant can work with you to estimate the amount you need to withhold for taxes based on your specific circumstances, but the standard estimate to save to cover federal taxes is 30% (Smith, 2018). In other words, only 70% of your income can be considered expendable money to run your business. Consulting a small business certified public accountant can provide much needed guidance and assistance in strategies to save for and pay taxes as well as claim exemptions on the private practice's taxes.

Financial Recordkeeping. A very important, but sometimes overlooked part of taxes for a small business is the record keeping required to claim business-related expenses on business taxes. Although the intricacies of the

Table 18–1. Advantages and Disadvantages of Business Structures

	Business Structures			
	Sole Proprietorship	**Partnership**	**Limited Liability Company**	**Corporation**
Advantages	Simple most common. Minimum legal restrictions. Owner has full control. No cost to start.	Capital easier to acquire. Support system of other owners. In LLP all owners have fixed liability.	Hybrid between partnership and corporation. Most flexibility for customization. Limited owner liability. Can be owned by individual or multiple people.	Limited liability to owners. Personal assets may not be seized. Easy to transfer ownership. Easy to expand. Funds can be raised by selling stocks.
Disadvantages	Unlimited liability for owner. Difficult to raise capital. Business growth can be limited.	In general partnership one owner has unlimited liability. Divided authority among partners. Decisions can be difficult if partners opinions differ.	More complicated structure warrants more detailed and structured agreement. Can be expensive to set up.	Most expensive to set up. Double taxation. Government regulations apply. Can only operate in state it was chartered without permission.

Source: Adapted from *Frequently Asked Questions About Business Practices.* American Speech-Language-Hearing Association, 2011. https://www.asha.org/practice/faq_business_practices_both/

specific tax laws are fluid and ever-changing (and beyond the scope of this chapter), detailed records should be kept for your business for each expense claimed on the tax return. Additionally, all business transactions (both monies made and monies spent) should be logged in a systematic and organized manner to ease the burden of filing taxes. The IRS provides resources on the web that discuss taxation for small businesses in detail (https://www.irs.gov/businesses) and it is highly recommended that a certified public accountant be consulted to assist with filing business taxes.

Stellar, clean, up-to-date record keeping is imperative for any small business, especially in the event the business is chosen for audit by the IRS. An audit is a "formal examination of an organization's or individual's accounts or financial information" ("Audit," n.d.). During an audit, all record keeping will be reviewed for accuracy, which may affect the money taxed over the audit period. If the business has worked with a certified public accountant, he or she will be able to assist with the IRS

audit. In some circumstances, the services of a tax lawyer may prove beneficial as well. Financial business records should be kept a minimum of five years after filing the tax return as audits can be conducted years after taxes are filed.

Business Plan

A business plan is the most important tool when starting a private practice. According to the U.S. Small Business Administration (2019c), before starting a business an essential first step in ensuring the business will succeed is to complete a competitive analysis to determine the market competition for the services to be provided. This competitive analysis, the precursor to the actual business plan, will help determine the need for the business based on the current market in the owner's area for speech-language pathology/audiology services. This analysis will also identify barriers that may be encountered and any indirect or secondary competitors in the area when starting a business (U.S. Small Business Administration, 2019c). The U.S. Small Business Administration website has valuable resources for completing a competitive market analysis, as does the American Speech-Language-Hearing Association (2019f).

Once the competitive market analysis is complete, it is now time to complete a business plan. A business plan is a roadmap for the proposed business that guides the owner through each stage of business development (U.S. Small Business Administration, 2019d). A detailed business plan is a necessity especially if outside funding is sought to start the business. A traditional business plan format is very detailed and typically includes an executive summary, company description, market analysis,

organization and management, services provided, marketing and patient recruiting, funding requests, financial projections, and an appendix of supporting documents including licensing, permits, and certifications (U.S. Small Business Administration, 2019d). See Table 18–2 for a summary of these sections. The business' plan should minimally include materials, space, and personnel needed, as well as detailed financial resources, revenue streams, access to patients, and marketing strategies.

Consulting various business professionals will be helpful when writing the business plan. A certified public accountant can assist with the business financials, including tax and withholding needs and establishing billing and accounts receivable procedures. An attorney who specializes in business and contract law can help

Table 18–2. Traditional Business Plan Format	
Executive summary	■ What is your company and why will it be successful? ■ Mission statement ■ Services ■ Basic information about the company's leadership, employees, and location ■ Financial information and growth plans if asking for financing
Company description	■ Specific details about services provided including consumers ■ Provide details as to what will make the business a success
Market analysis	■ Competitive research of the state of the market in your area ■ What are other businesses doing and what strengths does your business bring to the market?
Organization and management	■ Describe your business structure ■ Include who will run the business and include key information about each person
Service or product line	■ Describe your services and how they will benefit your customers
Marketing and sales	■ Describe how you will attract and retain customers ■ Describe your complete marketing and sales strategies
Funding request	■ Outline your funding requirements clearly explaining how much funding you will need and what you will use it for
Financial projections	■ Provide a prospective financial outlook for the business including income statements, balance sheets, cash flow statements, and capital expenditure budgets ■ Provide monthly projections for the first year
Appendix	■ Provide supporting documents or materials that were requested. Common items included are credit histories, resumes, product pictures, letters of reference, licenses, permits, or patents, legal documents, permits, and other contracts.

Source: Adapted from U.S. Small Business Administration (2019d). *Write your business plan.* Available from https://www.sba.gov/business-guide/plan-your-business/write-your-business-plan

throughout the business planning process and should be consulted to review all contracts and business structure decisions. The U.S. Small Business Administration website provides a business plan tool to assist in this process, and numerous online business resources are available for more direction in developing your detailed business plan (Etim, 2019; Lavinsky, 2014).

A helpful part of the business plan is calculating a revenue-to-cost ratio. A revenue-to-cost ratio compares the cost of running the business to the operating income of the business. To calculate a revenue-to-cost ratio, divide the businesses operating expenses by the operating income for the same period of time (Thompson, 2018). Operating expenses are all of the costs incurred in running the business and include fixed expenses such as rent, insurance, utilities, and taxes, as well as fluid or variable expenses such as salaries, marketing costs, and other expenses, such as licensure and certification fees, continuing education costs, equipment, technology, and testing and therapy materials. Business income or revenue includes all income produced by the business as well as interest earned on loans or savings. A revenue-to-cost ratio is a measure of how efficiently the business is running. A low revenue-to-cost ratio indicates the business is running efficiently and is not overspending to generate revenue (Thompson, 2018). A high revenue-to-cost ratio indicates a small profit margin because it takes most of the revenue made by the business to run the company. Typically, the revenue-to-cost ratio is higher upon starting the business due to the initial financial resources needed to start the business. Because of this, many businesses do not start making a major profit until up to five years after launching (Thompson, 2018; Ward, 2019). Once initial non-repeatable business start-up costs are incurred, the revenue-to-cost ratio should decrease indicating more business profits. If it does not, the business plan should be reevaluated to determine how the business can be restructured to run in a more cost-effective and financially responsible manner.

Marketing Strategy

Another integral part of the business plan is the marketing and operational strategies for outreach and advertising to attract business (ASHA, 2019d; McCoy, 2019; McCoy & Roehl, 2019; Weimann, 2003; Wetherill, 2018). Your marketing strategy addresses how you will disseminate information about your business and the services you provide. For speech-language pathology and audiology, common ways to market your services are through the ASHA, AAA, and related professional organization websites, as well as by having a strong business presence on social media, web pages and blogs, and by networking with local doctors, hospitals, rehab cen-

ters, teachers, school speech-language pathology/special education directors, support groups, personal contacts, and other private therapists for referrals. Obtaining an advanced degree or specialization certification can assist in asserting your expertise and setting yourself apart from other professionals (American Board of Audiology [ABA], 2017; ASHA, 2019g).

Location of Private Practice

Once the business structure has been determined and the business plan developed, the next decision to be made is to determine the location of the private practice. Do you want to open a clinic and have patients come to you for services or do you want to travel to them to provide services in their natural environment? Providing services in the client's home requires less start up overhead as you do not need to provide the clinic space, but travel between clients is involved. Traveling to see clients is time-consuming and lowers the number of clients that a therapist can see on a daily basis. Typically, insurance does not reimburse travel expenses or travel time, so this loss should be considered when deciding where to provide therapy services. Treating clients in a clinic space allows for more clients to be seen per day as no travel is involved but has the added expense of overhead for clinic space. Another option for treatment location is telepractice. Telepractice is using telecommunications technology to provide speech-language pathology and audiology services at a distance (ASHA, 2019o). If you plan to provide therapy via telepractice, you must be licensed in each state that your patients live. The cost effectiveness of providing services in a home health versus clinical setting should be assessed before deciding which environment to treat clients in your private practice.

Private Practice Credentials and Qualifications

Certification

Most credentials needed to start a private practice are the same as for any SLP/AuD providing services. To work in any environment, you should give serious consideration to having your CCC-SLP or CCC-A and/or ABA certification. The CCC-SLP and CCC-A are voluntary, entry-level credentials recognizing SLPs and AuDs who have met established criteria and standards of practice to deliver high quality clinical service (ASHA, 2019k).

You may also want to consider obtaining specialty certifications which can be helpful in demonstrating your expertise in an area to attract patients to your practice (ABA, 2017; ASHA, 2019g). ASHA certification requires practicing SLPs and AuDs to acquire 30 hours of continuing education every three years to remain certified. See more about specialty certifications and ASHA certification in Chapter 4. The costs for completing continuing education courses and paying association dues should be factored into the business's annual budget and cost projections, including the revenue lost by not treating patients while participating in continuing education courses.

State Licensure

No matter the work setting or state of practice location, state licensure in the state or states in which SLPs/AuDs practice must be obtained. If practicing in multiple states, such as telepractice therapy, multiple state licenses are needed and should be factored into the business' budget. ASHA provides state licensure requirements and contact information on its website (https://www.asha.org/advocacy/state/).

Liability Insurance

Medical liability insurance is a type of professional liability insurance that protects a health care provider from liability associated with "wrongful practices" that result in a client's injury, medical expenses, and property damage, in addition to the cost of defending lawsuits related to medical claims (National Association of Insurance Commissioners Center for Insurance Policy and Research, 2018). Comprehensive medical liability insurance should be purchased by each clinician working in the practice for protection in case a malpractice claim is filed by a client. There are numerous companies that provide medical liability insurance for SLPs/AuDs, with two of the most common being Healthcare Providers Service Organization (HPSO) and Proliability (formerly Mercer Consumer). ASHA and AAA members may receive a discount on professional liability insurance. Contact information is provided for each company in the resources section of this chapter.

Business Licenses

Unlike clinicians in other work settings, private practice SLPs/AuDs may be required to obtain various business licenses. State and local business licensing requirements vary from state to state and among local jurisdictions within the same state and can include multiple types of licenses and permits. These licenses and permits include a state business license, tax registration, unemployment insurance, business name registration, a local business license, and various local permits to operate the business.

A state business license is used for the state to track and monitor businesses operating in the state. Tax registration is required in states with sales tax so customers can be charged sales tax if needed. Unemployment insurance is required in some states for businesses with employees. Most states require the business name to be registered and may require local business licenses (in addition to state licenses), as well as zoning, health, building, and environmental permits (Findlaw.com, 2019). Consult local government policies and regulations and a business organization attorney to determine what type of licenses and permits the business needs as well as local zoning laws. Local zoning laws are important, especially for a home-based private practice, as some locations do not allow businesses to operate out of a residential area. It is important to note that a business license does not replace a license to practice.

Ethics

As multiple chapters in this text have highlighted, the importance of all SLPs or AuDs to conduct themselves in an ethical manner cannot be overstated (see Chapter 5 and Edge & Sirmon-Taylor, 2019). According to ASHA, the Code of Ethics "reflects what we value as professionals and establishes expectations for our scientific and clinical practice based on principles of duty, accountability, fairness, and responsibility" (ASHA, 2016, p. 2). The Code is the framework of guiding principles for SLPs and AuDs to best serve patients, research participants, and the public, and should always be adhered to (Edge, Sirmon-Taylor, & Prezas, 2016). Private practitioners should be especially careful of ethics violations, as this therapy setting requires fewer checks and balances for the owner than other settings such as medical facilities and schools. As such, accountability procedures are imperative for a private practice (Trulove & Fitch, 1998). Resources highlighting potential ethical concerns more likely to be associated with private practice should be consulted (Denton, 2009) and business policies and procedures should be developed to prevent unethical practice.

Chapter 5 discussed the ethical complaint process and risk management to decrease the possibility of committing an ethical violation. If a CCC-SLP or CCC-AuD is found to have violated the ASHA Code of Ethics, the member's full name, city, state, violated principles and rules as well as the board's decision of sanctions may be published in *The ASHA Leader* and *The ASHA Leader Online*, depending on the nature and severity of the violation. This information is then made available to the public via the *ASHA Certification and Ethics Verification* online tool on http://www.asha.org. Any public ethics violation is associated with the member for the remainder of his or her career and this negative publicity may decrease referrals to the practice and deter clients from choosing a therapist who has been found in violation of the ASHA Code of Ethics. ASHA ethics violations can also be reported to state licensure boards and would potentially impact a professional's ability to continue to practice (ASHA, 2019l).

Cultural Competence

Cultural competence is the "possession of the knowledge and skills required to manage cross-cultural relationships effectively" ("Cultural competence," n.d.). The ASHA Code of Ethics mandates an understanding and appreciation of cultural diversity (see Chapter 25) by prohibiting discrimination in the delivery of services "on the basis of race, ethnicity, sex, gender identity/gender expression, sexual orientation, age, religion, national origin, disability, culture, language, or dialect" (ASHA, 2016, p. 5). Being sensitive to the needs of culturally diverse patients and their families is not only mandated by the ASHA Code of Ethics, but also benefits any speech-language pathology/audiology practice greatly (or can harm a practice quickly if a clinician is not culturally sensitive and aware of patients' needs). It is important to be sensitive to patients' cultural diversity, as the demographics of the U.S. are becoming more and more culturally diverse. Cultural sensitivity is also important as an effort to eliminate the disparities in the health status of minorities, to provide quality services and health outcomes to patients, and to be in compliance with legislative, regulatory, and accreditation mandates (ASHA, 2019h).

ASHA's Multicultural Issues Board has developed cultural competence resources to assist its members with increasing their proficiency when working with culturally diverse patients, including a *Cultural Competence Checklist: Personal Reflection* (ASHA, 2010a) and *Cultural Competency Checklist: Service Delivery* (ASHA, 2010b). Practicing as a culturally competent clinician can provide a competitive edge in the speech-language pathology/audiology market as well as decrease the chances of liability or malpractice claims (ASHA, 2019h). Although it is important for all practicing health care providers to be culturally competent, private practitioners need to keep in mind that the success of the practice depends on a reputation of quality service provision that is culturally sensitive to its clientele.

Resources Needed for Private Practice

Start-Up Funds

The availability of financial resources is typically the most pressing need in order to start a private practice. In the business planning stage, a detailed budget projecting the financial resources needed to start the business is essential, as well as how you plan to fund the business (U.S. Small Business Administration, 2019b). It is important that the budget be realistic rather than a conservative estimate of costs in the event of unforeseen expenses. Is the funding for the business coming from savings, from a bank loan, or from a business partner? A detailed and well-developed budget is necessary for any private practice to succeed and must include obvious expenses such as space and staff, but also less obvious expenses such as marketing and reimbursement expenses. A financial business analyst can provide direction in creating a budget and potential start-up fund sources. As discussed above, depending on the type of private practice, space may or may not be needed. Regardless of space, supplies will be needed for the business such as computers, computer software, tablets, mobile apps, billing and scheduling software, and an electronic medical recording system. Relatedly, storage space will be needed, both physical and electronic, for the storage of records, in a manner compliant with the Health Insurance Portability and Accountability Act (HIPAA) (Lusis, 2008). Malpractice liability insurance will need to be purchased for the protection of both you and your clients.

Staff

Although it is possible for the private practitioner owner to be the scheduler, biller, office manager, and therapist, as the practice grows and the needs and the demands on the owner's time become more complex, staff will most likely be needed. When staff are added, you must decide which staff will best benefit the business and how they will be paid. Common private practice staff members include an office manager, a billing clerk, and other therapists. An office manager often handles the day to day management of the business, including scheduling appointments and checking people in upon arrival to the clinic. The office manager also typically inventories and orders supplies to keep the office running smoothly. The billing clerk is responsible for submitting bills for services provided and organizing the financials of the business.

Commonly, private practices hire other therapists, including SLPs/AuDs or related therapists to provide services to their patients. One important decision that must be made is how the hired therapists and staff will be paid, either by the hour or as salaried employees. Direct employees and contracted employees typically have two major differences: rate of pay and the provision of benefits. Contracted staff are typically paid more per hour than directly employed staff, as they do not receive benefits such as retirement and health insurance, and are typically only paid for the hours they provide services to patients. Direct employees, on the other hand, usually receive a lower rate of pay per hour, but are typically paid a certain amount regardless of services provided (salaried) and are often given benefits. If direct employees are salaried, typically the business provides workers compensation, unemployment, health insurance, and retirement from their employer. Seeking counsel from a business consultant will be beneficial in determining which payment method for staff that you bring into your practice is your best option.

Electronic Medical Records and Practice Management Software

Electronic medical records (EMRs) and practice management software assist clinicians with clinical documentation and scheduling, registration/insurance authorization, and billing (Krebs, 2008). ASHA provides a list of commercially available EMR and practice management software systems commonly used by SLPs and AuDs on its website, but the organization does not endorse the use of any specific software system (ASHA, 2019i, 2019j). ASHA recommends clinicians evaluate EMRs and practice management software for applicability to their practice based on the software's target use and accessibility.

Payment for Services

Private Fee-for-Service

One of the most important decisions to be made for a private practitioner is how the business will be reimbursed for services, as there are multiple payment methods. The first is only taking patients that are capable of paying for services out of pocket, known as private-fee-for-service. The major benefit of a private fee-for-service billing structure is that billing is quite simple, as insurance is not filed. The drawback of the fee-for-service payment method is that only accepting private pay may limit the practice's number of patients as some potential patients may not be able to afford paying for services out of pocket (or prefer to utilize their insurance coverage). The ability to build a full private practice caseload from patients that only privately pay without using insurance coverage may be dependent on your geographical socio-economic status, as well as your specialization and experience levels. If a full caseload cannot be achieved with only fee-for-service patients, then you will need to consider accepting insurance payments to add more patients to your caseload. Foehl (2009) provides strategies for analyzing the payer source for a private practice to maximize payer and patient mix to increase revenue in a private practice.

Insurance

The other reimbursement method for therapy services is billing patient insurance. Although the details of insurance billing are vast and ever-changing, a basic discussion of insurance billing will be presented here. There are two basic types of insurance coverage, government funded and privatized insurance. There are two major types of government funded insurance, Medicaid and Medicare and three main types of private insurance coverages, Health Maintenance Organizations, Preferred Provider Organizations, and Exclusive Provider Organizations.

Medicaid. Medicaid is a U.S. government health care program that provides insurance coverage for low-income adults, children, pregnant women, elderly adults, and people with disabilities (Medicaid.gov, 2019b). According to Medicaid.gov, 72.4 million people in the U.S. received Medicaid health benefits in January 2019. Medicaid is jointly funded by states and the federal government according to federal regulations. As such, states have autonomy as to how the program is administered, including what services are covered and specific service reimbursement rates. Although states are given great flexibility in how they structure Medicaid services for their residents, they do have to follow the broad federal guidelines. Most states provide Medicaid coverage for speech-language pathology and audiology services, but they are not required to do so by the federal government, with the exception of children birth to 21 years of age (ASHA, 2019m). Federal Medicaid policies mandate that a physician refer patients to SLPs and AuDs before services can be provided. The process of acquiring these referrals from physicians can be time and labor intensive for therapists and/or billing clerks/office managers.

Typically, health care professionals must apply to become Medicaid providers in each state in which services will be provided. The policies and procedures to become a Medicaid provider can vary greatly from state to state, with some states using Managed Care Organizations (MCOs) to provide services to patients. An MCO contracts with the state to accept a certain number of patients per month for a standard monthly payment for services, with the intent of lowering health care costs for states (Medicaid.gov, 2019a). Service providers participating in an MCO typically have little difficulty filling their caseload, but often receive lower reimbursement rates than therapists not participating in an MCO (Medicaid.gov, 2019a). This trade-off should be considered before deciding whether or not to join an MCO when starting a private practice. Each state may have multiple MCOs providing therapy services to Medicaid patients and therapists typically have to apply separately to become a provider for each MCO. This application process is often laborious and time-consuming, which should be considered when deciding whether or not to become a Medicaid provider. Each therapist in the practice has to apply for provider status individually before becoming an in-network Medicaid provider. ASHA provides resources to assist with Medicaid policies and procedures (ASHA, 2019m) and Chapter 14 of this text provides more information regarding Medicaid coverage, including International Classification of Diseases, eleventh revision (ICD-11) codes (World Health Organization, 2018). Medicaid.gov provides links to each state's Medicaid profile, with service rates typically published in each state's Medicaid provider manual (2019c).

Medicare. Medicare is the federal insurance program for people age 65 and older, some people under 65 with certain disabilities, and people with end-stage renal disease (Medicare.gov, 2019b). In 2016, the number of people receiving Medicare health care benefits was 56.8 million, with 47.8 million 65 or older and 9 million with disabilities (National Committee to Preserve Social Security & Medicare, 2019). There are different parts of Medicare that provide coverage for various services. Medicare Part A provides hospital coverage for patients under the plan. Medicare Part B covers certain doctors' services, outpatient care, medical supplies, and preventative services. Part D provides prescription drug coverage for patients, and Medicare Part C, also known as Medicare Advantage, is a bundled version of health services including Part A, Part B, and usually Part D. At the time of this writing, Medicare Part B pays for "medically necessary" outpatient speech-language pathology services at 80% of the "Medicare-approved amount" after the Part B deductible is met (Medicare.gov, 2019c, n. p.). Medicare covers hearing and balance audiology diagnostic testing, as determined by the reasons the tests were performed, but does not cover therapeutic services (Medicare.gov, 2019a). Chapter 14 of this text, ASHA, and the federal government provide resources with in depth information about Medicare coverage and billing.

Private Insurance. Privatized insurance is another potential source of revenue for a private practice. Private health insurance is provided by companies that are not part of the government, but rather are funded by the insured participants and/or the insured participants' employers. According to the Henry J Kaiser Family Foundation, 56% of Americans were covered by private health insurance in 2017, with only 9% uninsured during that same time (Henry J Kaiser Family Foundation, 2018). The remaining Americans were insured by Medicaid or Medicare in 2017. Private plans vary not only between states, but between employers in the same

state. Employers can purchase the insurance benefits they would like, so it is common for two policies from the same insurance company to have vastly different coverages and payments per service even if both businesses are located in the same city.

There are multiple types of private insurance MCOs in the U.S., including health maintenance organizations (HMOs), preferred provider organizations (PPOs), and exclusive provider organizations (EPOs). Each of these types will be discussed below, and Chapter 14 of this text provides additional information regarding private health plans. ASHA also provides resources for therapists working with private insurance companies (ASHA, 2011, 2019m).

Health Maintenance Organizations. An HMO is a health insurance plan that provides health services for patients for a fixed annual fee by acting as a liaison between health care providers and facilities and patients (health insurance.org, 2019). Medical professionals are paid the same fee regardless of the number of patients they treat. Typically, HMO plans require patients to select a primary care physician who must be seen for a referral prior to seeing other health care providers. This can slow the process of receiving the care patients need, as wait time for appointments can be long. This can also affect the time it takes patients to be referred for speech-language pathology/audiology services by their doctor. HMOs often provide preventative care, such as yearly well-check physicals or mammograms for patients, for a reduced or free copay in an effort to keep members from contracting an illness that could be prevented. Coverages may be limited or reduced, and require more out-of-pocket spending when patients see a non-HMO network provider. The insurance plan of each patient referred to the practice should be consulted for details regarding speech-language pathology/audiology service coverages and limits.

Preferred Provider Organizations. A PPO is a managed care organization of doctors, hospitals, and other health care providers that have agreements with insurance companies to provide services to insured patients for a reduced rate (healthinsurance.org, 2019). PPOs negotiate with providers to set fee schedules with the maximum amount they will reimburse for a particular service. These plans typically cost patients more in monthly premiums than HMOs but offer more flexibility for patients as they do not need to see their primary care provider for referrals to many specialist health care providers. Although they do cost the patient more than HMOs, PPOs can drastically reduce the wait time to see a specialist as a referral is not needed. Generally, PPOs cover speech-language pathology/audiology services for out-of-network providers more often than HMOs.

Again, each patient's insurance policy should be consulted for coverage rates and exclusions.

Exclusive Provider Organizations. An EPO is a health insurance plan developed as a hybrid between HMO and PPO plans. While receiving health care benefits from an EPO, patients do not have to receive a referral from a primary care physician but do have to see health care providers contracted with the EPO to be an in-network provider. Unlike the previous plans, absolutely no out-of-network providers may be used. Unlike HMOs, providers in an EPO are paid for each service rendered to a patient rather than the monthly fee given to providers in an HMO regardless of the number of patients treated. Health care providers offer reduced rates to EPOs in exchange for being a part of the network. Although the money made per therapy session is often less with an EPO versus being an out-of-network provider in a PPO, the ease of patient access by being listed as an EPO qualifying provider is often worth the decreased rate per session (ASHA, 2011).

The intricacies and details of becoming an insurance provider and billing insurance claims are beyond the scope of this chapter. Many therapists in private practice hire a billing clerk to assist with the insurance applications to become an in-network provider and with processing insurance claims. The main question regarding insurance is, should your practice join an insurance network? The advantage of being an in-network provider is that the insurance company will refer patients to your practice. The disadvantage is that you cannot bill the patient for the difference in what you actually charge for a service and what the insurance company pays you for the service (remember, they negotiate lower rates for in-network providers). With HMO and PPO private insurers, you can accept patients even if you are not a network provider. Typically, the insurance coverage for out of network providers is poor, but you can bill the patient for the difference between what you charged for the service and what you were reimbursed for the service. If you are starting a private practice and need to recruit patients, being an in-network provider will be a way to quickly fill your caseload. If you already have a full caseload, you may prefer not to join a network so you can receive higher reimbursement rates. An important caveat here is that a provider cannot charge Medicare and some private insurance companies a different rate than their normal fee for service; therefore, if you plan to accept insurance and private pay clients, the minimum amount private pay clients must be billed is the same as the standard Medicare and insurance rates (ASHA, 2019n).

The policies to become an in-network insurance provider and to bill insurance for services provided is complicated and varies by insurance companies and policies. Claims take time to be submitted to insurance companies and must be tracked to ensure payment or resubmittal after a denial. This is often a time-consuming process, so many private practitioners hire a billing clerk to submit claims for the practice. Billing clerks are trained in medical coding and billing practices and often have quicker payment times than clinicians, especially clinicians unfamiliar with ICD-11 (World Health Organization, 2018) and Diagnostic and Statistical Manual (DSM-5; American Psychiatric Association, 2013) coding systems. Most billing clerks are trained to work with government and private insurance systems and can assist with in-network provider applications as well as claims and claim management.

Rates for Services

How much should a private practitioner charge for speech, language, and or audiology services? How do beginning private practice owners know how much to charge for services? Do they call other speech-language pathology and audiology clinics in the area to verify rates and set their rates similarly? Setting rates solely based on competitors' rates alone can be considered collusion by price fixing, which may be unethical and illegal. Collusion occurs when competing companies work together to influence service pricing to create an unfair market advantage ("Collusion," n.d.). Competing businesses setting similar prices can eliminate or reduce the competition for services provided in a market. This can have a negative impact on consumers in the area and fellow business owners providing competing services.

If other health care providers in the area are not consulted on service rates, how does a new private practitioner know what fees to charge per service? Fees need to be individualized to each practice based on the priorities and needs of the business considering clinician experience, advanced training or specializations, and the cost of living in the area. Cost of living information can be found online from the U.S. Department of Labor, Bureau of Labor Statistics Occupational Employment Statistics (United States Department of Labor Bureau of Labor Statistics, 2019). Because billing fees vary by region, accessing cost of living for your area is imperative before starting a practice because it is unreasonable to charge fees that the majority of residents in the area cannot afford to pay.

After considering cost of living and clinician expertise and experience, the most important resource for setting private practice rates is the business plan. Using the business plan, factor in the costs of running the private practice including overhead and travel time. Once the rate is tentatively set, complete a cost analysis to determine how many patients you would have to see in a week to cover business expenses including salary. If the business rates are set too low, covering the overhead of the practice may be difficult and the business will fail to realize its revenue potential. If business rates are set too high, obtaining clients for the practice will be difficult and the business will not make enough money to cover expenses (Castro-Casbon, 2015). If the practice has contracts with insurance companies, these contracts should be consulted before setting private practice rates as some insurance contracts have clauses that state providers cannot bill insurance at a higher rate than uninsured patients are billed. Some insurance contracts do not allow patients to pay for services out-of-pocket and mandate that insurance must be billed for the service. If the practice plans to accept fee-for-service payments *and* insurance payments, reviewing the insurance contracts with an attorney will be invaluable to ensure you do not violate your insurance contracts or state and local policies regarding self-payments for patients.

Regardless of your fee structure for services, many private insurers, as well as Medicare and Medicaid, pay providers' fees set by Current Procedural Terminology or CPT codes. CPT codes are a set of medical codes created by the American Medical Association (2019) used to classify any medical procedure performed on a patient. Medicaid reimbursement rates by provider type and CPT code as well as information on how to become a Medicaid provider in the state can be found on each state's Department of Health website (Medicaid.gov, 2019c). ASHA publishes *Medicare Fee Schedule for Speech-Language Pathologists* (ASHA, 2019b) and *Audiologists* (ASHA, 2019a) each year. Consulting these resources will provide information on the reimbursement rates, policies, and procedures to expect when working with patients covered by Medicaid and Medicare health insurances.

Finding this information for private insurance may be more difficult, as each policy is different. Patients' insurance cards will have contact information for the company to find coverage, rate, and benefit limit information. When consulting rate information for business planning purposes, it is important to remember that this rate is not net or "take home" pay, as no taxes are taken out of the money you are paid from insurance or patients. It is your responsibility as the business owner to pay taxes on this income. Unlike being paid as an employee at a company, private practitioners must save money to pay taxes, typically on a quarterly basis. Business tax law is involved and ever-changing; therefore, the services of a certified public accountant with experience working with small businesses is recommended to help with tax planning, filing, and payment.

Billing

Billing practices for health care providers accepting third party insurance can be overwhelming and time-consuming for many clinicians. Traditionally, SLPs/AuDs are not highly trained in medical coding and billing and private practice clinicians may find billing is a difficult task. Once claims are submitted, they need to be followed with possibly more information submitted if the initial claim is denied. Many times, services must be preauthorized with the insurance company before clients are seen. The time these billing tasks take can detract from the time the business owner has to treat clients and create revenue for the business. To assist its members with learning medical coding and billing, ASHA provides six coding and reimbursement modules covering CPT codes, ICD codes, documentation (one for SLPs and one for AuDs), and application for SLPs and AuDs (ASHA, 2019c). Even with helpful resources such as these, billing third party payers can require a steep and time-consuming learning curve for many clinicians. For some, it is more cost-effective to hire a billing specialist to submit client claims. The billing clerk may be a full-time employee in the practice or may work as an independent contractor who charges a fee per claim submitted. Insurance claims for services provided should be filed in a timely manner. "Timely" may vary for each insurance provider and should be researched so you do not lose payment for claims. The difficulty navigating private insurance should not be underestimated when a clinician is considering whether or not the practice will bill third party insurance for services provided or if the services of a billing clerk or billing service will be utilized.

Outcomes Data for Private Practices

As discussed in Chapter 20 of this text, documentation of services is imperative for SLPs and AuDs regardless of employment setting (Moore, 2019). For any therapist in any setting, progress notes and clinical records should be kept in a timely and organized manner as mandated by the ASHA Code of Ethics (ASHA, 2016). The specific documentation requirements and formatting for a private practitioner will often be determined by the payer of the services. With health care costs in the U.S. increasing, justifying the need for health care services using evidence-based treatments via sound documentation is imperative to ensure insurance companies pay for services patients need (ASHA, 2004; Edge & Sirmon-Taylor, 2019; Sackett, Straus, Richardson, Rosenberg, & Haynes, 2000). Chapter 8 discusses evidence-based practice and its importance for SLPs/AuDs. Insurance companies often ask for specific types of outcomes data to ensure a high quality of care for the patients they insure. Many electronic medical records have documentation programs for various insurers built into their software formatted for specific insurance companies' requirements. In order for SLPs and AuDs to justify the value of the services provided, they must use reliable data collection methods. Formatting requirements may change based on insurance policies and procedures, but the underlying tenet of assessing patient gains hopefully, at least in part, due to your treatment, remains constant.

Networking

When starting a private practice, building a network of collaborators will be extremely beneficial (Schwab, 2016). Examples of helpful collaborators are SLPs/AuDs who specialize in areas you do not, or medical doctors, psychologists, and physical and occupational therapists to whom you can make (and hopefully from whom you will also receive) referrals. This networking can happen through professional networking events in your community. You can also use these events as a marketing strategy for your business. Joining local civic organizations in your area such as the chamber of commerce or community service organizations such as the Rotary Club are other ways to create a network for your business. One of the easiest referral sources is by word of mouth, so getting out to get the word out about your business is key. Joining online business meetup groups and having a strong web presence are other ways to broaden your network. Attending continuing education events or health care symposiums in the local area is another way to meet fellow health care providers and broaden your network. Chapter 12 of this text provides more information on professional networking to successfully advance your career.

Summary

This chapter presented issues related to individuals wishing to pursue a speech-language pathology or audiology private practice. Although one can work as a private practitioner on a part-time or "as needed" basis, this chapter was written from the perspective of a clinician going into private practice as a full-time practitioner/owner. The benefits of owning a private practice were discussed, including the flexibility of scheduling and the autonomy of creating the policies and procedures for the practice. The biggest drawback of a private practice is that it is extraordinarily hard work, as the entire business burden falls to you and you MUST manage

finances well to cover all of the direct and indirect costs of running a practice. Income as a private practice owner may be inconsistent as it depends on client availability, payment methods, and timing of payments from payers. The expense of paying for one's own benefits and taking time off for illness and vacation should not be underestimated. It is common for new businesses to make minimal profit for the first few years, which should be considered before deciding to pursue a practice full-time. The learning curve for a new private practitioner is steep, as 66.65% of owners surveyed reported it took between one and three years to adjust to working in a private practice, with 42.85% reporting it took two or three years to adjust to the business (Fortson, 2014). As seen in Table 18–3, clinicians reported a variety of issues

Table 18–3. Private Practitioners Report of the Hardest Part of a Private Practice

Challenge	Percent Practitioners Reporting
Insurance billing	25
Regulations	16.67
Recruiting clients	12.5
Personal record keeping for tax purposes	8.3
Scheduling	8.3
Cancellations	4.1
Running a small business with no business background	4.1
Dealing with parents who are not responsible	4.1
Staff management	4.1
Different insurance policies for each client	4.1
Responsibility	4.1
Hiring staff for rural areas	4.1

Source: Adapted from Fortson, M. K. (2014). Private practice in speech-language pathology and audiology: Experience, preparation, and confidence levels of practicing professionals. *Rehabilitation, Human Resources and Communication Disorders Undergraduate Theses, 28.* Available from https://core.ac.uk/download/pdf/72840169.pdf

as the most challenging aspect of owning a private practice. Private practice options were also discussed including working full- or part-time in the business, the role of the owner in the business, business structures, and the importance of a business plan. The location of the practice, credentials, qualifications, resources needed to start a practice, along with the importance of ethics and cultural competence, and billing issues were also discussed.

Owning and operating a private practice can be very invigorating and rewarding, but the glamorous thought of owning a practice should not downplay the difficult work involved in developing and maintaining a successful private practice. SLPs and AuDs need experience in the field before deciding to start a practice, as this work experience is invaluable in providing quality patient care without the support system of fellow service providers and colleagues often received when working at a larger company. When private practitioners were asked what best prepared them to run a practice, 95.8% said experience in other therapy settings (Fortson, 2014), highlighting the value of gaining experience before trying to build a practice. Working at a private practice can feel isolating and lonely, so it is extremely important for clinicians to reach out to other private practitioners for support. Members of the American Academy of Private Practice in Speech Pathology and Audiology may be a beneficial support group as well as the resources provided by the American Speech-Language-Hearing Association (ASHA, 2011; Dougherty, 2014) and the American Academy of Audiology (2008).

Critical Thinking

1. What are the advantages and disadvantages of owning a private practice?

2. Describe the process you will take to determine if a private practice is appropriate for you.

3. What are the different ways private practitioners are paid for the services they provide?

4. Compare and contrast the business structures discussed in the chapter. Which one is the simplest? Most complicated? Which is the easiest to acquire start-up funds? Which business structures are appropriate for a single business owner? Which are appropriate for a group of business owners?

5. You have decided to open a private practice and head to the bank for a small business loan. The banker asks you for a detailed business plan. Discuss the items you will include in your business plan.

6. What credentials and qualifications do you need to start a private practice?

7. Why is having cultural competence important for a private practitioner?

8. List all of the resources you would need to start a private practice.

9. How will you determine the rates you will charge for services at your private practice?

References

American Academy of Audiology. (2008). *Private practice checklist.* Retrieved from https://www.audiology.org/sites/default/files/PracticeManagement/BEST_PrivatePracticeChecklist.pdf

American Board of Audiology. (2017). *ABA board and specialty certification.* Available from https://www.boardofaudiology.org/

American Medical Association. (2019). *CPT (current procedural terminology).* Retrieved from https://www.ama-assn.org/amaone/cpt-current-procedural-terminology

American Psychiatric Association. (2013). *Diagnostic and statistical manual of mental disorders* (5th ed.). Arlington, VA: Author.

American Speech-Language-Hearing Association. (2004). *Evidence-based practice in communication disorders: An introduction* [Technical report]. Retrieved from https://www.asha.org/policy/tr2004-00001/

American Speech-Language-Hearing Association. (2010a). *Cultural Competence Checklist: Personal reflection.* Retrieved from https://www.asha.org/uploadedFiles/Cultural-Competence-Checklist-Personal-Reflection.pdf

American Speech-Language-Hearing Association. (2010b). *Cultural Competence Checklist: Service delivery.* Retrieved from https://www.asha.org/uploadedFiles/Cultural-Competence-Checklist-Service-Delivery.pdf

American Speech-Language-Hearing Association. (2011). *Frequently asked questions about business practices.* Retrieved from https://www.asha.org/practice/faq_business_practices_both/

American Speech-Language-Hearing Association. (2015). *SLP health care survey 2015: Private practice owners and co-owners.* Retrieved from https://

www.asha.org/uploadedFiles/2015-SLP-Health-Care-Survey-Private-Practice.pdf

American Speech-Language-Hearing Association. (2016). *Code of ethics* [Ethics]. Available from http://www.asha.org/policy

American Speech-Language-Hearing Association. (2017). *2016 Audiology survey report: Private Practice.* Retrieved from https://www.asha.org/uploadedFiles/2016-Audiology-Survey-Private-Practice.pdf

American Speech-Language-Hearing Association. (2019a). *2019 Medicare fee schedule for audiologists.* Retrieved from https://www.asha.org/uploadedFiles/2019-Medicare-Fee-Schedule-for-Audiologists.pdf

American Speech-Language-Hearing Association. (2019b). *2019 Medicare fee schedule for speech-language pathologists.* Retrieved from https://www.asha.org/uploadedFiles/2019-Medicare-Fee-Schedule-for-Speech-Language-Pathologists.pdf

American Speech-Language-Hearing Association. (2019c). *ASHA's coding, reimbursement, and advocacy modules.* Retrieved from https://www.asha.org/Practice/reimbursement/modules/

American Speech-Language-Hearing Association. (2019d). *ASHA marketing solutions: Private practice.* Retrieved from https://marketing.asha.org/work-settings/private-practice/

American Speech-Language-Hearing Association. (2019e). *ASHA summary membership and affiliation counts, year-end 2018.* Retrieved from https://www.asha.org/uploadedFiles/2018-Member-Counts.pdf

American Speech-Language-Hearing Association. (2019f). *Business plan market analysis: Describe the industry and your competition.* Retrieved from https://www.asha.org/practice/marketanalysis.htm

American Speech-Language-Hearing Association. (2019g). *Clinical specialty certification.* Retrieved from: https://www.asha.org/certification/specialty/

American Speech-Language-Hearing Association. (2019h). *Cultural competence.* Retrieved from https://www.asha.org/Practice-Portal/Professional-Issues/Cultural-Competence/

American Speech-Language-Hearing Association. (2019i). *Electronic medical records (EMR) and practice management software for audiologists.* Retrieved from https://www.asha.org/Practice/EMRs-and-Practice-Management-Software-for-Audiologists/

American Speech-Language-Hearing Association. (2019j). *Electronic medical records (EMR) and practice management software for speech-language pathologists.* Retrieved from https://www.asha.org/Practice/EMR-and-Practice-Management-Software-for-SLPs/

American Speech-Language-Hearing Association. (2019k). *General information about ASHA certification.* Retrieved from https://www.asha.org/Certification/AboutCertificationGenInfo/

American Speech-Language-Hearing Association. (2019l). *How ASHA's Board of Ethics sanctions individuals found in violation of the Code of Ethics.* Retrieved from https://www.asha.org/Practice/ethics/sanctions/

American Speech-Language-Hearing Association. (2019m). *Introduction to Medicaid.* Retrieved from https://www.asha.org/practice/reimbursement/medicaid/medicaid_intro/#federal

American Speech-Language-Hearing Association. (2019n). *Private health plans frequently asked questions: Speech-language pathology.* Retrieved from https://www.asha.org/practice/reimbursement/private-plans/php_faqs_slp/

American Speech-Language-Hearing Association. (2019o). *Telepractice.* Retrieved from https://www.asha.org/PRPSpecificTopic.aspx?folderid=8589934956&section=References

Audit. (n.d.). In *Merriam-Webster's online dictionary.* Retrieved from https://www.merriam-webster.com/dictionary/audit

Castro-Casbon, J. H. (2015). *Why the "going rate" for private therapy services doesn't matter.* Retrieved from https://www.independentclinician.com/blog/why-the-going-rate-for-private-therapy-services-doesnt-matter

Collusion. (n.d.). In *Cambridge dictionary.* Retrieved from https://dictionary.cambridge.org/us/dictionary/english/collusion

Cultural competence. (n.d.). In *Medical dictionary for the health professions and nursing.* Retrieved from https://medical-dictionary.thefreedictionary.com/cultural+competence

Davidson, E. (2019, April 9). *The average time to reach profitability in a startup company.* Retrieved from https://smallbusiness.chron.com/average-time-reach-profitability-start-up-company-2318.html

Denton, D. R. (2009). Watch out for these ethical traps in private practice. *ASHA Leader, 14*(10).

Dougherty, D. (2014). 8 deadly private practice don'ts. *ASHA Leader, 19*(1). Retrieved from https://leader.pubs.asha.org/doi/full/10.1044/leader.FTR4.19012014.np

Doyle, A. (2018). *What is a noncompete agreement?* Retrieved from https://www.thebalancecareers.com/what-is-a-non-compete-agreement-2062045

Edge, R. L., & Sirmon-Taylor, B. (2019). Using ethics in evidence-based practice: A clinical paradigm. *eHearsay, 9*(1).

Edge, R. L., Sirmon-Taylor, B., & Prezas, R. (2016). A comprehensive review of the 2016 ASHA Code of Ethics. *Journal of Human Services Training, Research, and Practice, 1*(2), Article 5.

Etim, U. (2019). *How to write a professional business plan.* Retrieved from https://utibeetim.com/how-to-write-a-professional-business-plan/

Feigenbaum, E. (2019, February 5). *Limited liability partnership vs. limited liability company.* Retrieved from https://smallbusiness.chron.com/limited-liability-partnership-vs-limited-liability-company-3736.html

Findlaw.com. (2019). *State and local small business licenses for start-ups.* Retrieved from https://smallbusiness.findlaw.com/starting-a-business/state-and-local-small-business-licenses-for-start-ups.html

Foehl, A. (2009). Payer and patient mix: Keys to a healthy private practice. *ASHA Leader, 10.*

Fortson, M. K. (2014). Private practice in speech-language pathology and audiology: Experience, preparation, and confidence levels of practicing professionals. *Rehabilitation, Human Resources and Communication Disorders Undergraduate Theses, 28.* Retrieved from https://core.ac.uk/download/pdf/72840169.pdf

Healthinsurance.org. (2019). *Glossary.* Retrieved from https://www.healthinsurance.org/glossary/

Henry J Kaiser Family Foundation. (2018). *Health insurance coverage of the total population: 2017.* Retrieved from https://www.kff.org/other/state-indicator/total-population/?currentTimeframe=0&sortModel=%7B%22colId%22:%22Location%22,%22sort%22:%22asc%22%7D

Internal Revenue Service. (2019). *Employment tax due dates.* Retrieved from https://www.irs.gov/businesses/small-businesses-self-employed/employment-tax-due-dates

Krebs, J. M. (2008). Paper, paper everywhere? How to go paperless in your private practice. *ASHA Leader, 13,* 20–22.

Lavinsky, D. (2014). *How to write a business plan.* Retrieved from https://www.forbes.com/sites/davelavinsky/2014/01/30/how-to-write-a-business-plan/#7944eb147d04

Liability. (2008). *West's encyclopedia of American law* (2nd ed.). Retrieved from https://legal-dictionary.thefreedictionary.com/liability

Lusis, I. (2008). Private practice and HIPAA. *ASHA Leader, 13.*

McCoy, Y. (2019). Finding the right market for your private practice, Part 1. *ASHA Leader Live.* Retrieved from https://blog.asha.org/2019/01/16/finding-the-right-market-for-your-private-practice-part-1/

McCoy, Y., & Roehl, T. (2019). Ways to grow your private practice client base. *ASHA Leader Live.* Retrieved from https://blog.asha.org/2019/03/04/ways-to-grow-your-private-practice-client-base/

McQuerrey, L. (2019). *Why is it important for a business to budget?* Retrieved from https://smallbusiness.chron.com/important-business-budget-385.html

Medicaid.gov. (2019a, April 28). *Managed care.* Retrieved from https://www.medicaid.gov/medicaid/managed-care/index.html

Medicaid.gov. (2019b, April 28). *Medicaid.* Retrieved from https://www.medicaid.gov/medicaid/index.html

Medicaid.gov. (2019c April 28). *State overviews.* Retrieved from https://www.medicaid.gov/state-overviews/index.html

Medicare.gov. (2019a April 28). *Audiology services.* Retrieved from https://www.cms.gov/Medicare/Medicare-Fee-for-Service-Payment/PhysicianFeeSched/Audiology.html

Medicare.gov (2019b). *The official U.S. Government site for Medicare.* Retrieved from https://www.medicare.gov/

Medicare.gov. (2019c, April 28). *Speech-language pathology services.* Retrieved from https://www.medicare.gov/coverage/speech-language-pathology-services

Moore, B. (2019). Documentation issues. In M. W. Hudson & M. DeRuiter (Eds.), *Professional issues in speech-language pathology and audiology* (5th ed.). Clifton Park, NY: Delmar Cengage Learning.

Murray, J. (2019, January 30). *How to form a limited liability partnership: How an LLP differs from other partnership types*. Retrieved from: https://www.thebalancesmb.com/how-to-form-a-limited-liability-partnership-398325

National Association of Insurance Commissioners Center for Insurance Policy and Research. (2018, May 31). *Medical professional liability insurance*. Retrieved from https://www.naic.org/cipr_topics/topic_med_mal.htm

National Committee to Preserve Social Security & Medicare. (2019). *Medicare*. Retrieved from https://www.ncpssm.org/our-issues/medicare/medicare-fast-facts/

Sackett, D. L., Straus, S. E., Richardson, W. S., Rosenberg, W., & Haynes, R. B. (2000). *Evidence-based medicine: How to practice and teach EBM* (2nd ed.). New York, NY: Churchhill Livingstone.

Schwab, E. F. (2016). Surviving and thriving your first year in private practice. *Seminars in Hearing, 37*(4), 293–300.

Smith, R. (2018). *How much to set aside for small business taxes*. Retrieved from https://bench.co/blog/tax-tips/how-to-set-aside-business-taxes/

Thompson, J. (2018). *How to calculate a cost-to-income ratio*. Retrieved from https://bizfluent.com/how-6398870-calculate-cost-to-income-ratio.html

Trulove, B. B., & Fitch, J. L. (1998). Accountability measures employed by speech-language pathologists in private practice. *American Journal of Speech-Language Pathology, 7*, 75–80.

United States Department of Labor Bureau of Labor Statistics. (2019). *Occupational employment statistics*. Retrieved from https://www.bls.gov/oes/tables.htm

U.S. Small Business Administration. (2019a). *Choosing a business structure*. Retrieved from https://www.sba.gov/business-guide/launch-your-business/choose-business-structure

U.S. Small Business Administration. (2019b). *Fund your business*. Retrieved from https://www.sba.gov/business-guide/plan-your-business/fund-your-business

U.S. Small Business Administration. (2019c). *Market research and competitive analysis*. Retrieved from https://www.sba.gov/business-guide/plan-your-business/market-research-competitive-analysis

U.S. Small Business Administration. (2019d). *Write your business plan*. Retrieved from https://www.sba.gov/business-guide/plan-your-business/write-your-business-plan

Ward, S. (2019). *How to get your new small business to make money*. Retrieved from https://www.thebalancesmb.com/the-two-main-problems-of-starting-a-small-business-2948554

Weimann, G. (2003). Where to start marketing? Develop a plan! *ASHA Leader, 8*(2), 10–11.

Wetherill, A. (2018). Steps to a successful business plan. *ASHA Leader, 23*(7), 40–41.

World Health Organization. (2018). *International statistical classification of diseases and related health problems* (11th rev.). Retrieved from https://icd.who.int/browse11/l- m/en

Resources

American Academy of Audiology
11480 Commerce Park Drive, Suite 220
Reston, VA 20191
Telephone: 703-790-8466
Website: https://www.audiology.org

American Academy of Private Practice in Speech
Pathology and Audiology
PO Box 252 Granville, NY 12832
Email: office@aappspa.org
Website: https://www.aappspa.org

American Speech-Language-Hearing Association
2200 Research Blvd.
Rockville, MD 20850-3289
Telephone: 301-296-5700
Website: https://www.asha.org

For ASHA's Coding, Reimbursement, and Advocacy Modules, see https://www.asha.org/Practice/reimbursement/modules/

For ASHA's Cultural Competence Resources, see https://www.asha.org/Practice-Portal/Professional-Issues/Cultural-Competence/

For ASHA's Ethics Resources, see https://www.asha.org/practice/ethics/

For ASHA's Marketing information, see https://www.asha.org/practice/marketing/

For ASHA's overview of Medicaid Coverage, see https://www.asha.org/practice/reimbursement/medicaid/

For ASHA's overview of Medicare Coverage, see https://www.asha.org/practice/reimbursement/medicare/medicare_intro/

For ASHA's Multicultural Affairs and Resources, see https://www.asha.org/practice/multicultural/

For ASHA's Resource Guide for Audiologists in Private Practice, see https://www.asha.org/aud/private/

For ASHA's Resource Guide for Speech-Language Pathologists in Private Practice, see https://www.asha.org/slp/ppresources/

For ASHA's state licensure information, see https://www.asha.org/advocacy/state/

HPSO
    1100 Virginia Drive, Suite 250
    Fort Washington, PA 19034
    Phone: 1-800-982-9491
    Website: https://www.hpso.com

Internal Revenue Service
    See local white pages or website for address and telephone number of local office.
    Website: https://www.irs.gov/

Mercer Consumer/Proliability
    12421 Meredith Dr.
    Urbandale, IA 50398
    Phone: 1-866-795-9340
    Website: https://www.proliability.com

U.S. Small Business Administration
    409 3rd St. SW
    Washington, DC 20416
    Website: https://www.sba.gov/

19

Strategically Promoting Access to Speech-Language Pathology and Audiology Services

Brooke Hallowell, PhD

Introduction

Access to quality speech-language pathology and audiology services for people who need them is limited in myriad ways, even though the number of people throughout the age range needing such services is steadily increasing. To best position ourselves to counteract strategically the forces that threaten access to us as professionals, we must have a clear understanding of the barriers to access and a sound rationale for the need for speech-language pathology and audiology services. In this chapter, we discuss the factors that impede access despite a dire and growing need for services. We then discuss strategic means of enhancing access by optimizing reimbursement for clinical services, finding alternative ways to fund clinical services, pursuing legislative channels to enhance access, engaging in advocacy, using care extenders, taking advantage of technology, educating the public, and modifying our service-providing environments.

Identifying Barriers to Access

A first step in considering how we may strategically promote access to the services of audiologists and speech-language pathologists (SLPs) is to examine why it is that many of the people who need these services cannot or do not obtain them. Identifying challenges to access helps us then consider opportunities for enhancing access by strategically addressing those challenges. Here, we will consider barriers to access that relate to infrastructure, funding, cultural complexities, and navigation through the health care systems.

Addressing Challenges with Infrastructure

Despite wonderful progress in expanding our professions throughout the world over recent decades, many countries still lack formal programs to educate SLPs and audiologists, and recognition by governments and health care systems of our professions. In some regions of the world, our professions are in their infancy. Even where the professions exist, there are commonly insufficient numbers of clinicians to meet local and national needs. Additionally, people living in rural areas throughout the world tend to have poorer access to services than those living in more urban areas (Jones, McAllister, & Lyle, 2017). Thus, simply in terms of geographic limitations, much of the world's population does not have access to our services. Needs for transportation, facilities, and workforce are best addressed through collaborative efforts of government agencies, colleges and universities, professional organizations, not-for-profit entities, and passionate professionals representing our professions.

Examining Funding Challenges

In much of the world, reimbursement and funding problems constitute the greatest barriers for access to audiology and speech-language pathology services. In higher-resourced countries where the professions of speech-language pathology and audiology are well established, an emphasis on cost containment in all areas of health care delivery is at the root of many of barriers to access. Children and adults with disabilities face unique difficulties as they attempt to obtain services through progressively more unwieldy health care systems (Braithwaite, 2018). Overall, access to our services is being reduced by the coverage and reimbursement limitations imposed by third-party payers and ever-changing means of determining how our services are to be reimbursed.

In the United States, physician referrals are decreasing, authorizations for evaluations and treatment are slow in coming, denials are increasing, and the appeals process can be cumbersome and lengthy. Additionally, public and private health insurance carriers' reimbursement rates are commonly well below the actual cost of providing services (Lim, McManus, Fox, White, & Forsman, 2010; McManus et al., 2010). As a result, some health care employers are eliminating positions or are placing clinicians on as-needed schedules, actions that further jeopardize access to services. Primary care physicians are more aggressively guarding scarcer financial resources to ensure the availability of basic health care for their patients. Many physicians see audiology and speech-language pathology services as a low priority or a service that should be paid for by other entities, such as school districts, public service organizations, or clients themselves. Insurance companies are following suit.

Identifying Cultural Barriers to Access

Given increased diversity through worldwide migration and immigration and increasing acceptance and empowerment of marginalized groups, clinicians everywhere are more and more likely to be working with people who are diverse in multiple respects. To ensure access, service-providing agencies must demonstrate understanding of concerns and needs of people who are diverse in terms of race, ethnicity, religion, education, sex, sexual orientation, gender identity, income, and languages spoken. If they do not, large populations of people will not gain access in the first place or will be alienated from services they need. Our cultural competence as clinicians is vital to engaging diverse people to benefit from our services and helping them to retain access to us.

When expanding services for specific populations, it is important that cultural beliefs, such as those regarding health care and the nature of disabilities, be considered. Hospital-based services may not attract people who would more likely gravitate to community-based and non-medicalized models of care. Not having proficient speakers of a client's language available to provide services severely limits what we can offer. Disregard for cultural and religious beliefs leads to stunted opportunities for access to care. For example, consider the consequences of the following assumptions on a person's willingness to engage in our services:

- that a person is comfortable with the diagnostic process of labeling a disability despite a strong sense of stigma associated with disability, or a desire to protect a loved one from being labeled as having a problem

- that a person will not see his or her engagement in rehabilitation as a refusal to accept a disability that was bestowed on him or her by a higher power

- that the foci of our interventions are on individuals rather than on their families and support systems.

Recognizing the Burdens of Navigating Health Care Systems

Understanding today's medical literature and health insurance materials can be a daunting challenge for even the most sophisticated person. For those with literacy problems, difficulties are substantial and, as a result, differentially impact access and related needs for patient support and advocacy.

Ensuring that Others Understand the Need for Our Services

Why is it critical that an individual obtain services for communication disorders? What are the consequences for a child or adult with communication challenges when services are inaccessible or non-existent? The answers to these questions must be addressed and elaborated upon continuously by members of our professions if we are to substantiate the need for our services to consumers, third-party payers, legislators, and other professionals in health care and education. Likewise, the effectiveness of our interventions must be demonstrated and promoted continuously.

The need for services provided by audiologists is expected to increase by 21% from 2016 to 2026; the need for speech-language pathologists is expected to increase by 18% during the same time period (U.S. Department of Labor, 2019). There are several reasons for this growing need:

- The aging population is expanding, with corresponding increases in hearing loss, balance challenges, and neurologically based challenges to speech, language, cognition, and swallowing (U.S. Department of Labor, 2019).

- Advances in medical technology are saving lives and increasing the life span (U.S. Department of Labor, 2019).

- Bilingual/multilingual populations, which have proportionately greater needs for speech and language diagnostic and intervention services, are expanding (Centeno & Kohnert, 2009; National Center for Education Statistics, 2015).

- There is a greater emphasis on early identification and diagnosis, as well as increased referrals of students to professionals (U.S. Department of Labor, 2019).

- There is a greater emphasis on health promotion and disease prevention (Novelli, 2008; Pelletier, 2009).

- While enrollments in elementary and secondary schools have fluctuated in recent years, enrollments in special education for specific learning disabilities, which ideally benefit from speech-language pathology and audiology services, continue to increase (National Center for Education Statistics, 2018).

Another factor affecting the need for services for people with communication disorders is the accelerating worldwide dependence on information technology, requiring people to have ever more effective communication abilities. On a daily basis, we are required to manage greater amounts of complex language-based information. Those who have untreated communication challenges risk becoming marginal participants in our society, observers standing on the sidelines. In the United States, literacy data are not promising, especially in lower-income areas. Only about one third of elementary students in the United States are proficient in reading and math, as assessed by the National Assessment of Educational Progress (National Center for Education Statistics, 2018). Many of the parents and guardians of children with low literacy levels, especially those with low income, are unable to provide basic reading support due to their own low education levels. Children who are poor readers, particularly those raised in poverty, have a greater likelihood than good readers to experience academic failure and to enter adulthood in poverty, with a greater likelihood of teenage parenthood and criminal behavior (Maughan et al., 2009; McNeilly, 2016; Snow & Powell, 2008).

The prevalence of language learning disabilities and illiteracy in state prisons provides dramatic evidence of the cost of not providing speech-language pathology and audiology services. Up to 75% of individuals remanded to adult correctional facilities have significant communication disorders, which are vitally linked to literacy (Shippen, Houchins, Crites, Derzis, & Dashaunda, 2010; Sondenaa, Wansholm, & Roos, 2016). Likewise, teenage parents raised in poverty have a high prevalence of speech-language and literacy problems. Such problems may affect not only their own economic and social futures but also those of their children, who may not benefit from literate environments or from competent speech-language models (Noria, Borkowski, & Whitman, 2009). Additionally, in high-technology industries, employers report difficulty recruiting candidates with even minimal literacy and mathematical abilities (Rainee & Anderson, 2017). For many individuals, access to our services is crucial for establishing the communication skills necessary for success in education, employment, and social interaction.

The social consequences of communication disorders remain fundamentally challenging, too. Despite worldwide efforts to improve the ways people with disabilities are treated and regarded, many individuals with communication disorders face stigmatization, low self-esteem, and social exclusion.

Optimizing Reimbursement for Clinical Services

Unless the financial viability of service providers and their institutions is ensured, there will be limited or no access to speech-language pathology and audiology services. The primary means by which financial viability can be maintained is through the enhancement of clinical revenues, that is, earned income. In today's health care environment, multiple sources of reimbursement for evaluations, treatment, and consultation must be identified and developed. Contractual agreements with third-party payers (insurance companies) can be carefully negotiated to ensure clinical revenues and minimize financial risk. One must know in detail the policies and procedures of multiple payers and stay abreast of changes in policies and procedures of each payer. This requires dedication to ongoing communication with payers and follow-up to those communications by the provider.

One especially effective approach to optimizing an organization's payer reimbursements is to identify the most common reasons for authorization and/or treatment denials an organization experiences and then develop action plans that address each reason. Generally, the most common reasons for denials in the United States include the following:

- There is insufficient documentation.

- An appropriate physician referral was not obtained.

- The service provided was not covered by the client's health insurance plan.

- The service was deemed "not medically necessary."

- The authorization period had lapsed.

- The patient was no longer improving.

Given that these causes typically make up 80% to 90% of the reasons for denial by public and private insurance companies, clinical professionals and administrators may best use their time and resources by proactively addressing the causes of each of these problems. By implementing careful documentation strategies, along with ongoing verification procedures to ensure attention to each of these potential pitfalls, service providers may greatly reduce the percentage of reimbursement claims that are denied. Many service providing organizations have implemented automated denial management processes for a systematic approach for analyzing claim problems, tracking denials and appeals, and preventing future denials.

Also essential to predictable clinical revenue flow is a sound understanding of the diagnosis and treatment classification coding systems that are the basis for reimbursement in the United States—that is, the International Classification of Diseases (ICD) and Common Procedural Terminology (CPT) codes, as they relate to speech-language pathology and audiology services. Failure to keep abreast of variations in coding and billing procedures from one insurance carrier to another and to use current ICD and CPT coding can be costly (McManus et al., 2010; White, 2008). The American Speech-Language-Hearing Association (ASHA) provides substantial resources to members seeking guidance in billing, coding, and reimbursement best practices (cf. American Speech-Language-Hearing Association, n.d.).

Fortunately, compliance with the Health Insurance Portability and Accountability Act (HIPAA) helps reduce problems of inconsistency in billing codes accepted by various payers through required use of uniform coding processes. Medicare administrative contractors, such as National Government Services, are required to meet regularly with providers to identify coding, billing, and documentation problems that bring about denials. Working with providers, such entities strive to eliminate these problems, thus saving resources for providers and payers. Educating administrators, payers, and physicians about possible health care cost savings associated with speech, language, swallowing, and hearing services is an additional means of enhancing access to these services.

Another approach to enhancing clinical revenues is offering services for which clients or their employers pay directly. Direct payment is the usual form of reimbursement for some services, such as accent modification and individualized coaching for professional speakers. Patients and clients may also pay out-of-pocket for most clinical services. Emphasizing the possibility of direct payment to those who can afford it is an alternative route to accessing care that is not dependent on insurance coverage and helps to enhance providers' clinical revenues. Some SLPs have enhanced communication access greatly by developing centers where intervention, activity, and support groups are emphasized over one-on-one sessions, and where insurance coverage may not even be relevant. Given the numbers of people helping to cover costs of group meetings, costs are lower than for individual sessions. In addition, by working outside the confines of insurance regulations, clinicians may be more creative in expanding programming options. Wonderful examples of such centers are touted by Aphasia Access (https://www.aphasiaaccess.org), a collaborative group of clinicians, researchers, educators, people with aphasia, and care partners. Aphasia Access is dedicated to expanding opportunities for people with aphasia to enhance life participation through meaningful communication, well beyond the typical brief periods for which they are eligible for services through their insurance carriers.

Rebutting Denials Based on "Medical Necessity"

As health care organizations attempt to rein in health care costs, the loosely defined and yet broadly and inconsistently applied concept of medical necessity is frequently used to deny authorizations or reauthorizations for care. Strictly defined, medical necessity relates to treating conditions that result from illness, injury, or disease. First-level claims reviewers, whose purpose it is to protect health insurance company funds, typically apply this restricted definition, leading to denied claims for audiology and speech-language pathology services.

In most instances, claims reviewers have minimal to no understanding of speech-language pathology or audiology and thus are poorly prepared to render informed decisions concerning the medical necessity of our services. Because of their inexperience with our professions, third-party payers are often more easily convinced of the necessity for the treatment of physical disabilities than they are of the need to treat problems associated with cognitive and communication disorders. Further, reviewers in commercial insurance companies tend to implement medical necessity requirements based on cost, predictable outcomes, and the medical nature of conditions being treated, not on knowledge specific to audiology and speech-language pathology (Fox & McManus, 2001). Clinicians must be able to provide substantive arguments demonstrating how most of our services do, in fact, meet definitions and criteria of medical necessity.

The term "medical necessity" does not have one standardized definition that is agreed upon across health plans and government entities. Thus, each third-party payer has considerable discretion for determining the type, scope, and duration of covered benefits as they relate to the construct in contract language. Overall, the criterion of medical necessity requires that the service we are providing is:

- appropriate, given the person's age, health status, and diagnosis

- based on published evidence that the service will elucidate, prevent, or improve the person's condition

- likely to lead to greater quality of life and better functioning in whatever ability has been impaired.

When documenting medical necessity, clinicians typically include details about aspects of medical history that have influenced the individual's status, a diagnosis related to the clinician's scope of practice (e.g., aphasia, sensorineural hearing loss), date of onset, an evidence based treatment plan, and progress notes that refer to the medical necessity.

Emphasize Evidence-Based Practice

Evidence-based practice (EBP) is a concept applied increasingly by many payers to further restrict access and reduce care and, thus, their payments. This topic is discussed in depth in Chapter 8. Simply stated, health insurance companies tend to permit authorizations and reimbursements only for those interventions for which efficacy and effectiveness are supported by published research. While laudable in principle, implementation of strict EBP rules reduces access to all health care disciplines for minorities and underrepresented groups (women, children and adolescents, people of color, and older people) who generally are disproportionately excluded from clinical effectiveness studies (Epstein, 2008; Kneipp, Lutz, & Means, 2009; Nolan & Bradley, 2008). As a result, these groups suffer disproportionately when an insurance company's coverage is dependent on published evidence of a treatment's effectiveness.

Despite concerted efforts to address treatment efficacy and outcomes research in communication sciences and disorders, work to develop a solid foundation in EBP through our own disciplines lags behind the implementation of EBP requirements imposed by the insurance industry and by government policymakers. ASHA and members of several of its affiliated special interest divisions, as well as the Academy of Neurologic Communication Disorders and Sciences (ANCDS; ancds.org), have prepared extensive bibliographies summarizing treatment efficacy in a wide range of clinical areas such as stuttering, cognitive and communicative problems associated with traumatic brain injury, feeding and swallowing disorders, hearing loss, hearing aids, audiological rehabilitation, aphasia, child language disorders, autistic spectrum disorders, phonological disorders, and dysphagia. ASHA offers a free, searchable collection of "evidence maps" on its website (http://www.asha.org). A rich resource of EBP guidance across the speech-language pathology scope of practice is SpeechBite (speechbite.com), an online searchable database that provides intervention studies and ratings of the research quality of each.

This information helps support claims of effectiveness and to reverse denials based on the concepts of medical necessity and evidence-based medical necessity. It may also be used advantageously when negotiating contracts with insurance companies.

Ensuring Alternative Funding Approaches

In the face of dramatic cuts in reimbursement rates, organizations typically must enhance access to services by systematically developing funding alternatives that supplement clinical revenues. These alternatives have long been central to the operation of most not-for-profit organizations, which are commonly required to provide services to clients regardless of their ability to pay. In the midst of grave reductions in clinical revenues in the current service delivery arena, alternative funding sources are now more critical than ever. Even for-profit agencies are developing their own not-for-profit foundations or are partnering with extant foundations that will help support the provision of services to clients whose access might otherwise be curtailed.

Service-providing agencies can best support their nonclinical revenue base by strategically developing a funding plan consisting of several possible revenue sources (Henri & Hallowell, 1999a). Essential components include the following:

- Ensuring a fundraising-oriented board of directors and chief executive officer or executive director, an experienced development professional, staff, volunteers, and any additional "friends" of the organization.

- Developing a case statement that describes the agency's mission and vision and details of why donors should invest their resources in its programs and services.

- Establishing a resource development or fundraising team, including members of the organization's donor base of individuals, patients/clients, foundations, and corporations that support programs and services for people with communication disorders. The donor base may include, but should not rely solely on, federated donor bases, such as United Way, United Black Fund, or Easter Seals Society.

- Engaging in specific fundraising activities. These may include the following:
  - An annual fund campaign—This is typically conducted during the last quarter of a calendar year to take advantage of contributions that individuals and corporations make to reduce their income tax liability.
  - Special events—Examples are benefit concerts, special recognition dinners, golf outings, fashion shows, marathons, and evenings at the theater. In addition to raising operating revenue for the organization, these events generate publicity, media attention, and community goodwill. They also introduce potential donors to the organization and its mission.
  - Online fundraising—Most organizations' websites now have links on their home pages to guide potential donors on how to support the organization.
  - Planned and deferred giving programs—These long-range funding programs typically yield benefits in an average of five to seven years. They include bequests, gift annuities, charitable remainder annuity trusts, charitable remainder unitrusts, pooled income funds, charitable life insurance, and gifts of real estate and goods (e.g., works of art). Guidance from professionals with expertise in planned giving, estate planning, law, and accounting is essential to successful planned and deferred giving programs.
  - Corporate partnerships—Partnerships between corporations and not-for-profit organizations serving people with communication disorders may help to augment client access through agencies' improved fiscal stability. Corporations are most likely to "adopt" a charity or one of its programs in communities where corporations have a significant presence (e.g., in areas where their corporate headquarters are located).
  - Fraternal organizations and sororities—In the United States, community fraternal organizations such as the Eagles, Elks, Junior League, Kiwanis, Lions, and Rotary are all sources of usually client- or program-specific funding. SERTOMA and Scottish Rite, though present in only certain regions of the United States, are also fraternal organizations with long-standing histories of support for audiology and speech-language pathology services. Delta Zeta sorority has historically supported programs that serve people who are deaf or hard-of-hearing. Most of these entities entertain proposals to fund services,

equipment, or materials needed by individuals unable to afford these.

☐ Research funding to support clinical services —Clinical research funding from local, regional, state, and federal agencies may strengthen a service-providing agency's fiscal stability. Often, research instrumentation and materials purchased through grant funds (e.g., diagnostic equipment, published tests, treatment materials, computers, and software) enrich not only the research environment but the organization's clinical environment as well. Also, indirect cost or "overhead" monies provided by funding agencies can be used to support an organization's general operational costs, thus enhancing clinical access.

Agencies that do not have in-house development expertise can contract with fundraising consultants for specific resource development projects and/or long-range planning. In many instances, these arrangements are more cost-effective and further allow the organization's staff to concentrate on more profitable activities, such as acquiring major gifts.

Advancing Legislation to Improve Access

In the United States, several pieces of federal and state legislation have been passed to ensure that children and adults with special conditions have access to adequate and appropriate levels of service. Knowledge of federal laws, their state equivalents, and the rules and regulations that guarantee access to special services, including speech-language pathology and audiology, is essential. The Social Security Act, for example, contains several "titles," that is, chapters or subsections, that ensure reimbursement for speech-language pathology and audiology services, including the following:

■ Title 5, which supports the Maternal Child Health Bureau's programming for children with special needs and includes newborn hearing screenings

■ Title 18, Medicare, which provides for speech-language pathology and audiology coverage (Medicare coverage is also available for those under the age of 65 who have disabilities lasting longer than two years, such as chronic neurological conditions)

■ Title 19, Medicaid, which addresses health care and long-term care of people who meet low income and asset guidelines

■ Title 20, the Social Services Subsidy, which in some instances supports social work services and, in turn, can help families access speech-language pathology and audiology services

■ Title 21, Children's Health Insurance Program (CHIP), a funding source for speech-language pathology and audiology services, usually administered by a state's Department of Human Services, Medicaid Division

■ Individuals with Disabilities Education Improvement Act (IDEA), the primary funding vehicle for states' preschool early intervention, elementary, and secondary special education programs

■ Rehabilitation Act, which funds rehabilitation services, including audiology and speech-language pathology, for individuals ranging in age from 16 and up

Many of these reimbursement mechanisms have mixed histories in terms of their effectiveness in supporting services for populations with special chronic or degenerative conditions.

Several other pieces of federal legislation indirectly support our services in the United States. The Americans with Disabilities Act (ADA), for example, does not ensure funding per se but may require employers to make available certain resources in cases in which communication disorders have a demonstrated impact on an individual's ability to perform job duties. Likewise, the Rehabilitation Act is a national law that prohibits discrimination against qualified people with disabilities for employment in the federal sector. Additionally, the Every Student Succeeds Act (ESSA) is intended to support education of all children, including those with disabilities, in the public schools, through high standards, an emphasis on school and teacher accountability, and selective funding programs.

Advocating for Our Professions

The goals of improved access and quality of care of most current health insurance companies are often in direct conflict with their goals of cost containment (Henri & Hallowell, 1999b). Improving access for speech-language pathology and audiology services requires that action plans for advocacy be thoughtfully developed and executed at various levels of governmental bureaucracies, in the public and private reimbursement arenas (Hallowell, 2017; Henri, Hallowell, & Johnson, 1997; White, 2008).

People coping with communication disorders are often at a disadvantage when the need arises for personal advocacy concerning access or reimbursement.

Many individuals with communication disorders have difficulty advocating vigorously for their own needs. This problem may be further compounded by difficulties related to communication infrastructure, travel, distance from legislators in rural areas, and literacy. Furthermore, individuals who would benefit from our services often do not have the knowledge necessary to confront a complex bureaucratic system to obtain coverage for needed services. Audiologists and SLPs thus have numerous opportunities to initiate or support consumers' advocacy efforts. These opportunities require that we professionals be knowledgeable about the content and the process required for an effective advocacy effort (Hallowell, 2017; Henri, 2010).

Historically, most audiologists and SLPs have had little experience, and often little inclination, to participate in the arena of public policy development, political advocacy, and lobbying. Given the ongoing dramatic challenges to consumer access and the consequent fiscal instability of service-providing agencies, though, it is no longer possible for clinicians, administrators, educators, and consumers to remain passive, adopting a "let someone else do it" attitude. Together, professionals and consumers must participate in coordinated efforts aimed at educating and influencing decision makers about the value of audiology and speech-language pathology services and especially about the societal consequences of not providing these services. Information related to access issues must be disseminated and used as a basis for action. Specific actions for advocacy are described here and are outlined in Table 19–1. Given the regional and national variations in how such actions may be carried out, many of the actions described here are couched in terms that are primarily appreciable in the United States; all are modifiable for actions in other regions and countries.

Actions for Advocacy and Professional Assertiveness

Advocacy Among Clinicians and Clinical Administrators. Specific action steps in which clinicians and clinical administrators may make solid contributions to advocacy efforts to improve consumer access are summarized here.

Continuing Education. Clinicians who consistently and attentively read current publications and participate in

Table 19–1. Actions for Advocacy and Professional Assertiveness	
Advocacy among clinicians and clinical administrators	■ Continuing education ■ Consumer education and mobilization ■ Addressing literacy and non-native speaker challenges ■ Marketing to and education of referral sources ■ Appealing denials of treatment authorization and reimbursement ■ Promoting access to people with geographic and transportation challenges ■ Financial support ■ Active writing to legislators ■ Inviting legislators to work settings ■ Visiting legislators in their local offices or on Capitol Hill ■ Engaging in quality assurance
Advocacy among consumers and their significant others	■ Active pursuit of coverage for speech-language pathology and audiology services ■ Reporting of health care policy coverage inconsistencies ■ Education of employers ■ Mobilization of consumer groups
Advocacy among educators and students	■ Continuing education concerning modes of service delivery and health policy and about the effects on people with communication and swallowing disorders ■ Curricular revision ■ Education of medical students and their professors ■ Engagement in concerted legislative advocacy

seminars and workshops to improve their knowledge concerning managed care and its impact upon our services will be most effective as advocates. ASHA and the American Academy of Audiology (AAA) offer resources to assist members in their efforts to stay attuned to heath care policy changes and maintain current understanding of coding and billing procedures. The reader is encouraged to visit the ASHA and AAA websites regularly and read reimbursement-related articles that routinely appear in *The ASHA Leader*, an online ASHA publication. State associations may also be excellent resources for continuing education related to enhancing consumer access.

Consumer Education and Mobilization. Clinicians must take advantage of the direct access they have to consumers to provide counseling and education that will motivate consumers and their families to appreciate:

■ the complex relationships between an individual's communication abilities and the success one experiences in other life arenas, such as progress in school or independent living;

■ any restrictions consumers' insurance companies place on the treatment of communication and/ or swallowing disorders; and

■ specific means by which consumers may become more involved in advocacy.

Addressing Literacy and Non-Native Speaker Challenges. Case managers, volunteers (e.g., retired insurance specialists, law students), and community members with shared cultural and linguistic backgrounds may be enlisted to help those with literacy problems to navigate and understand health care and health insurance information. All written materials should be written in what the Institute of Medicine calls plain language. This includes organizing the most important action-focused information first, breaking information into understandable units, avoiding jargon, and making the pages easy to read. Also, ensuring that materials are translated and published in multiple languages is important for those who are less proficient in English than another language.

Education of and Marketing to Third-Party Payers. Providers must convince insurance representatives of the need to include speech-language pathology and audiology services in health care plans. We must also convince physicians of the necessity of our services.

Marketing to and Education of Referral Sources. Many of the decision makers who have the greatest potential for making an impact on patient access are often unaware of the issues faced by people with communication and swallowing problems and of the vital role that SLPs and audiologists play. It is important that decision makers such as physicians, discharge planners, and directors of student services and special education programs be educated about the link between communication abilities and one's success in life.

Appealing Denials of Treatment Authorization and Reimbursement. Providers must work with their clients to appeal vigorously all decisions denying coverage of services. A concerted appeals process in a service providing agency helps improve access to services in that agency, as success rates for concerted appeals are high. To support these efforts, ASHA provides guidance on appealing denials on its website (https://www.asha.org), including model letters that can be sent to health insurance companies to reverse authorization and reimbursement denials as well as treatment efficacy statements that can be appended to an appeal letter as a supporting document. The AAA also provides guidance to its membership on issues related to reimbursement.

Promoting Access to People with Geographic and Transportation Challenges. It is important that service providers develop and promote telehealth services to enhance access for those who have limited access to on-site services. Clinical agencies should also provide their clientele with information on how to access public transportation, and the option of home health care if possible.

Financial Support. Contributions to Political Action Committees help to advance concerted professional advocacy efforts at state and federal levels. ASHA and AAA each support a political action committee and hosts online content to assist members in advocating for services.

Writing to Legislators. As they want to remain in office and be reelected, legislators have a vested interest in knowing their constituents' concerns. Without the strong voice of professionals who understand the impact of policy decisions on consumers, legislators are unlikely to be sensitive to and knowledgeable about critical issues important to informed decision making. Professionals do not need to be sophisticated about legislative processes to join in legislative campaigns to address the numerous challenges to patient access. National, state, and local organizations offer ample guidance.

Taking advantage of ASHA's grassroots advocacy resources, free of charge, allows professionals to read concise descriptions of issues that need to be addressed and specific actions professionals may take. These actions almost always involve calling, writing, or emailing legislators. At annual ASHA and AAA conventions, congressional affairs staff members offer hands-on help with letter writing and related advocacy projects. Further assistance is available through the "Professionals" segments of ASHA's website and the "Practice Management" section of the AAA website.

Inviting Legislators to Work Settings. Hosting a member of Congress in the clinical environment allows clinicians to directly discuss and demonstrate problems of access, the need for access, and the ways in which speech-language pathology and audiology services improve the quality of life of legislators' constituents.

Visiting Legislators in Their Local Offices or on Capitol Hill. The Government Relations staff of ASHA arranges appointments for professionals visiting Washington, DC, and provides in-person briefings and other materials. Because legislators have temporary terms, it is a good idea to visit and write to elected officials on a yearly basis to keep them informed about critical access and service delivery issues confronting children and adults in their districts. See Chapter 30 for further discussion of legislative advocacy.

Participating in Clinical Research. Given the dire need for empirical research to support EBP, clinicians' roles in research are more important than ever. For those not having skills, time, training, or resources to initiate or oversee research programs, there are ample possibilities for collaboration with university-based researchers. The American Speech-Language-Hearing Foundation offers special funding opportunities for clinicians collaborating with researchers in clinical research.

Engaging in Quality Improvement. By maintaining ongoing quality improvement programs, providers continue to demonstrate cost-effective, functional treatment outcomes, which are essential to local, state, and national advocacy efforts. ASHA and AAA have developed resources to assist their membership in developing and maintaining quality improvement programs.

Advocacy Among Consumers and Their Significant Others. Consumers and their significant others are among the most powerful and credible advocates in improving access to audiology and speech-language pathology services. As there are often limitations due to consumers' communication disorders, support from family and from clinicians in encouraging consumer advocacy is essential. Specific ways in which consumers and their significant others may make solid contributions to advocacy efforts to improve access to services include active writing to legislators and visiting legislators in their local or Capitol Hill offices, as described previously under "Advocacy among Clinicians and Clinical Administrators." Backing by the speech-language pathologist or audiologist in each of these efforts may be helpful, as may be the support of the consumer's primary care physician.

Active Pursuit of Coverage for Speech-Language Pathology and Audiology Services. It is important that consumers pursue adequate coverage by health insurance companies. Consumers often are unaware of the coverage provided by their health care policies and restrictions that many place on speech-language pathology and audiology services. Careful study of a health plan's coverage and policies is a first step toward proactively seeking greater access to services. For those covered by employer-sponsored plans, staff members of the employer's human resources department may offer assistance in checking on specific coverage issues. Referring an insurance case (or "utilization") reviewer to a particular policy document may easily resolve some coverage issues. In cases in which needed services are not covered, consumer appeals to third-party payers regarding the need for services to enhance independence, educational status, medical management, and/or overall quality of life may help to shape future policy modifications.

Reporting of Health Care Policy Coverage Inconsistencies. When there are discrepancies between what an insurance company purports to cover, through its promotional materials and policy documentation, and its actual practice in terms of authorizing and/or reimbursing for services, appeals brought by consumers are critical. Discrepancies can be reported at a variety of levels. Working through a hierarchy of contacts is recommended, beginning with insurance case reviewers, thereon to consumer liaisons, and up to CEOs. If necessary, state insurance commissioners may be contacted. If reporting at each of these levels fails, contacting your United States congressperson or senator often helps. Other avenues for advocacy in the face of restricted services include letters to the editor in newspapers and professional journals and carefully constructed press releases that may lead to newspaper, radio, and/or television coverage of access problems. If aired constructively, such media coverage may help to foster public education about access issues while exerting due pressure on insurance companies.

Education of Employers. Organizations that pay for insurance coverage for their employees should be urged to reconsider contracts with companies that have a pattern of limiting or violating their coverage policies or of not covering critically needed services. Consumer feedback to employers' human resources departments helps raise awareness of a plan's effectiveness and worth and has been found to be especially effective.

Mobilization of Consumer Groups. The advocacy power of individual consumers may be compounded exponentially through consumer groups. Personal and political advocacy efforts among members of local, state, and national organizations for people with specific communication disorders may be especially effective in the retention and expansion of access to services.

Advocacy Among Educators and Students. Before they enter the clinical workforce, it is important that students gain awareness and knowledge of professional practice issues and how they may work to foster positive changes within their profession. Such preparation is especially essential in medical, rehabilitation, and skilled nursing contexts, where supervisors and other experienced practitioners are increasingly called to engage in billable clinical service as opposed to training and supervisory activity related to issues of insurance coverage (i.e., coding, authorizations, documentation, billing, appeals, and marketing). Graduates who are savvy about these issues and about productive actions for advocacy will have a distinct advantage over others in the job market and in their initial stages of clinical practice. An additional advantage to having students get involved in professional practice issues is that students can achieve significant advocacy work while they are still in school.

Specific actions in which faculty members and students may engage to advance advocacy for clinical access are addressed here.

Continuing Education Concerning Modes of Service Delivery and Health Policy and About the Effects on People with Communication and Swallowing Disorders. It is essential that all faculty members in clinical programs obtain an understanding of health care reimbursement principles and their ramifications for practice in speech-language pathology and audiology. Such an understanding, in turn, helps foster students' potential for strategic advocacy as well as effective future professional practice (Hallowell & Henri, 1996). Continuing education is available through current publications, internet resources, conferences, seminars, and workshops. Three methods of advocacy by educators and students are curricular revision, education of medical students, and engagement in concerted legislative advocacy.

Curricular Revision. Coursework emphasizing the interconnections among functional clinical outcomes, cost-effectiveness of intervention, reimbursement, and consumer access will help to foster professional advocacy for years to come. Infusing such concepts throughout the curriculum will help students to see the import of such concepts in their current and future professional roles.

Interprofessional Education. Opportunities to engage students from varied health-related professions in preceptorships related to our field, and clinical observation of audiology and speech-language services, enhance appreciation of our services among future clinician across disciplines. Likewise, presenting lectures or workshops to students and professors in other fields helps elevate the community's understanding of the impact of communication disorders upon a person's life trajectory and how these conditions may be beneficially addressed.

Engagement in Concerted Legislative Advocacy. Students and faculty have clout as political constituents whose voice may have an impact on legislators. It is important that faculty and students be encouraged to participate in advocacy efforts sponsored by ASHA, the National Student Speech Language Hearing Association (NSSLHA), AAA, the Student Academy of Audiology (SAA), and state and local student and consumer groups. Academic classes or student groups may organize letter-writing campaigns involving significant numbers of participants.

Care Extenders

One way to cope with limitations in access to professional specialized care that people with communication and swallowing disorders are facing is to expand the reservoir of individuals who may provide needed care. "Care extenders" consist of individuals who are not certified or licensed SLPs or audiologists, but who nevertheless are involved in helping to further the development or rehabilitation of communication and swallowing skills. Ideally, they are trained and monitored by a fully certified clinician. They may be "support personnel" (aides, technicians, or assistants), clinicians in training, family members, or community volunteers.

Support Personnel

Many SLPs and audiologists find the use of professional aides, technicians, and assistants to be essential for ensuring clients' access to care. Support personnel may help in the handling of large caseloads, such that more clients are treated and/or more treatment time per client is offered than would otherwise be possible). They may also allow fully credentialed clinicians more time to treat individuals with severe and complex communication disorders, thus improving overall quality of care. An additional advantage is that the level of care needed by an individual may be more closely matched with the level of training and experience of an aide or assistant.

Services once thought to be within the sole domain of the speech-language pathologist or audiologist, but that do not require the skills and expertise of professionals with all the training and experience required for clinical certification, may be offered by people whose services are far less costly. Support personnel vary widely in their level of academic and on-the-job training. Speech-language pathology aides, for example, generally have training in specific areas of practice and have more limited responsibilities than assistants. The increase of support personnel in speech-language pathology and audiology has led to further proliferation of regulations and standards. Within the United States, states vary in the use of terms used to refer to the various levels of training and/or licensure required of support personnel. State laws also vary in terms of the tasks in which support personnel are permitted to engage.

Examples of tasks that speech-language pathology assistants may perform under the supervision of an SLP, according to ASHA's Speech-Language Pathology Assistant Scope of Practice (ASHA, 2013), include conducting speech-language screenings and participating in treatment plans or protocols that have been established by a certified speech-language pathologist. Examples of tasks that audiology technicians may perform under the supervision of an audiologist include conducting hearing screenings, application of electrodes for electronystagmography testing, and calibration checks for audiological equipment. Support personnel may perform clerical duties, document test results and patient/client progress, prepare diagnostic and treatment materials, schedule diagnostic and treatment activities, and participate in research projects, in-service training, and public relations programs. Examples of tasks that support personnel are generally not permitted to perform include diagnostic testing or interpretation of test results, hearing aid fitting, patient/client or family counseling, development or modification of a patient's/client's individualized treatment plan, and discharging a patient/client from services. Regardless of specific duties performed, an ongoing supervisor relationship by a fully licensed and certified speech-language pathologist or audiologist is critical.

Despite the advantages mentioned, the use of support personnel has not been fully embraced in our discipline. Those opposing support personnel maintain that the quality of care rendered to patients is diminished, that time savings through services provided do not merit the increased time demands for supervision, and that the job security of licensed professionals is threatened (McCartney et al., 2005). There is also concern that cost-minded health care and educational administrators will abuse the use of support personnel by compelling them to provide services outside their scope of practice and by implementing cost-saving hiring practices in which ideal supervisor-to-support staff ratios are exceeded. An additional disadvantage is that many health insurance companies still do not recognize support personnel as qualified service providers and therefore do not pay for treatment delivered by these people. See Chapter 13 for more discussion of this topic.

Graduate Students

The provision of supervised evaluation and treatment services by graduate students in speech-language pathology and audiology has long been a source for extending care to clients/patients. In many university clinics, ample free and low-cost services are made available to surrounding communities while providing diverse clinical learning opportunities to student clinicians. Additionally, networks of student volunteers may be helpful in extending services beyond clinical and diagnostic treatment sessions. Examples are students serving as communication partners (Lyon, 1992), in-home respite caregivers (Hallowell, 2000), or volunteers in a wide array of clinical educational contexts.

Trained Volunteers

Trained volunteers can be effective care extenders. As no compensation is involved, and as these individuals are clearly identified to clients/patients as volunteers, there are fewer legal and licensure-related problems than in the use of multiskilled professionals. Volunteers provide additional opportunities to practice and maintain developing communication skills. Before their direct involvement with patients or clients, volunteers may be required to observe treatment sessions and then may be guided by the clinician in the provision of treatment-reinforcing activities such as repetitive drills. Volunteers may also be trained to handle other tasks, such as clerical work, scheduling, and equipment maintenance, allowing skilled clinicians more time to spend with clients/patients.

Family Members and Other Caregivers

Engaging family members and other people who play important roles in the lives of people with communication challenges has always been essential to the effectiveness of our work. Given the current health care service delivery climate, such people are often required to assume greater responsibilities in caring for their significant others. As with trained volunteers, coaching and training by the skilled clinician are essential. Treatment-complementing activities provided by a properly guided caregiver can be highly effective; in fact, they are essential for enhancing the life participation goals of the people we serve.

Expanding Access Through Technology

Advances in technology improve and augment the clinical services of SLPs and audiologists. For many individuals, these advances improve access to services, particularly for those with limited physical accessibility to evaluations or intervention. Technology also may be a cost-effective support for clinicians wishing to access current information to improve their clinical skills. See Chapter 27 for continued discussion of technology as a professional issue.

Telehealth

Telehealth is the use of electronic information and communications technologies to provide and support health care services when there is a distance between participants. The term *telehealth* is sometimes used interchangeably with *telemedicine*, although many authors and practitioners in health professions prefer the connotation of the former term, as it is more inclusive of professions outside of primary medical practice. The term *telerehabilitation* is also used by some. Some clinicians working in schools and in other non-medical contexts prefer the term *telepractice*. Audio, visual, and text media are generally combined in telehealth applications. From its inception, one of the most promising aspects of telehealth has been the improvement of access to care in remote areas where skilled service providers are scarce or absent (Swanepoel et al., 2010). In addition to the lack of geographic access to service providers, other barriers to care might be alleviated by telehealth. These barriers include the following:

■ Distance from services

■ Transportation challenges

■ Limited financial resources, including insurance coverage and subsidized services

■ Family, educational, and cultural factors

■ Health care delivery characteristics, including poor care coordination, long waiting times for appointments, shortages of specialists, and bureaucratic obstacles to services (Theodoros, 2012; Theodoros & Russell, 2008).

In addition to expanding access for disadvantaged populations and patients in rural areas, opportunities have expanded for home health services through technology. As home health care remains an important form of service delivery, it is essential that clinicians stay abreast of telehealth mechanisms that may allow replacing some home visits with video visits, checking up on carryover of treatment activities, and furthering patient and family education in naturalistic environments rather than in unfamiliar clinic spaces. An additional advantage of providing care through distance technology is that it may expand clinicians' availability to people who live in areas that are considered unsafe, such as some urban neighborhoods, correctional facilities, and even within active international war zones (Doolittle, Otto, & Clemens, 1998; Hart, 2010; Khazei, Jarvis-Sellinger, Ho, & Lee, 2005).

In conjunction with the expansion of digital technology, enabling image capturing, compression, transmission, and interpretation, interest in telehealth is expanding rapidly across a vast array of health care professions. High-speed, high-bandwidth telecommunication systems are expanding globally. In addition to improved access, advantages reported by evaluators of some rural telemedicine programs include reduction of duplicative diagnostic services, improved consumer confidence in local medical personnel and facilities, reduced need for referral to service providers outside the local area, improved recruitment and retention of health care personnel, improved productivity and workload management, and improved continuing education for service providers (Boisvert & Hall, 2019; Brown, 2005). Clinical applications in telehealth are found in virtually every health specialty.

A growing number of published empirical studies directly address the effectiveness of telehealth delivery in audiology and speech-language pathology. Studies involving comparisons of face-to-face and telehealth assessments support the feasibility, reliability, and acceptability of telehealth evaluations of acquired speech and language disorders (Theodoros, 2012; Wales, Skinner, & Hayman, 2017).

New developments in technological access to care will be shaped by ongoing developments in health policy as it affects telehealth. The following factors will be most influential in continuing efforts to expand service delivery options for professionals in our disciplines:

■ Licensure issues, especially for services provided among states

■ Training in the use of telehealth technology

■ Establishment of standards

■ Reimbursement issues

■ Patient confidentiality issues

■ Attitudes of providers and patients

■ Means of ensuring quality of clinician–patient relationships

■ Potential cost savings

■ Demonstration of clinical outcomes

■ Telecommunications infrastructure and cost (Theodoros, 2012; Yoo et al., 2004)

Information Technology

Given that access to care involves more than direct contact with a skilled clinician, the notion of technological access also includes the use of telecommunications and information technology to improve access to information that may allow consumers and potential consumers to learn about communication problems, diagnostic and treatment options, and prevention strategies. For those who remain without computers and connection to the internet and/or telephones, access to information resources is tenuous. Funding for technology through regional clinics and public facilities, such as libraries, is highly variable across the country, and is often subject to changes in tax or grant allocations and annual budgets. Deficits in language and literacy skills may impose further obstacles to care for disadvantaged populations. Gaps in access may actually widen if information services are improved only for those with the means, education, and skills to pursue those services. See Chapter 27 for more information on telepractice and technology in the professions.

Educating the Public

Most individuals take communication for granted and are frequently unaware of the link between one's communication abilities and one's success in life. To improve access to speech-language pathology, audiology, and swallowing services, it is increasingly more critical to improve the general public's and consumers' awareness and knowledge about speech-language pathology and audiology services. Examples of awareness campaign content and methods and tips for expanding awareness through social media and professional networking sites may be found through ASHA, NSSLHA, and AAA websites. Ideas for celebrating Better Hearing and Speech Month (in May of each year) are readily shared through ASHA and NSSLHA websites and social media platforms. Likewise, the AAA website offers ample information about how to reach out to media, consumers, and health care providers, plus ideas for getting involved in World Hearing Day and Better Hearing Month (also in May).

Adjusting Service-Providing Environments

Certain environmental and operational adjustments must be made to improve client access to speech-language pathology and audiology services. Flextime and compressed workweeks are becoming the norm. Recognizing the value of schedules that are more convenient for their consumers, organizations are expanding their daily work hours and days of operation and, as a result, improving their revenues. Speech-language pathology

and audiology providers are following suit. In environments where traditional appointment schedule models create significant hardships for the people we serve, creative, nontraditional scheduling approaches have been found helpful. Another tactic being used to improve access and attendance is the development of interagency collaborations in which several agencies contribute to fund a minibus to bring clients to their locations. To improve geographic access, satellite offices (leased, shared, or donated space) may be considered.

Summary

In this chapter, we identified significant barriers that influence access to audiology and speech-language pathology services and stressed the broad and serious consequences of current service delivery trends on our field. We also emphasized the growing need for our services throughout the age continuum. Access to audiology and speech-language pathology services can be significantly enhanced through comprehensive, focused strategies that remove or minimize barriers and maximize the use and impact of health care and educational resources, both financial and human. With this in mind, we described effective strategies to improve revenues, decrease costs, and increase clinical outcomes. To subsidize diminishing reimbursements, strategies to create alternative funding sources were presented. More than ever, it is today the responsibility of all audiologists and speech-language pathologists to ensure that barriers are eliminated and resources are maximized. To accomplish these goals, our roles in educating the public and in advocacy were described.

Critical Thinking

1. What are the key factors that have led to a growing need for services in speech-language pathology? What are the key factors that have led to decreased access to those services?

2. Imagine that you are the chief executive officer of a not-for-profit center for the treatment of communication disorders. What are the key steps that you would take to maximize your center's (a) clinical revenues and (b) nonclinical revenues?

3. When justifying your services to a third-party payer, how would you defend the treatment for each of the conditions listed below as "medically necessary"?

   a. Adult dysphagia

   b. Infant dysphagia

c. Adult aphasia

d. Adult acquired neurogenic motor speech disorders

e. Child language delay

f. Child articulation disorder

g. Child hearing impairment

h. Adult hearing impairment

i. Child central auditory processing disorder

In addition to your own descriptions of medical necessity, what other information and references might you include in your documentation to third-party payers regarding the medical necessity of your services?

4. In what specific actions for advocacy might you engage in your current educational or work context to enhance access to speech-language pathology and audiology services for people who need them? Write an action plan for achieving one or two of those actions within the next month, either alone or with students or professional colleagues. Include specific dates for each activity in which you would need to engage to achieve that action.

5. What is the role of local, state, and national professional organizations in improving access to audiology or speech-language pathology services?

6. Suppose you have a client who needs a hearing aid but has no health insurance or financial means to purchase the device. Do you have a responsibility to help the client find financial support? What sources might help in this situation?

7. Consider possible options for delivering audiology and speech-language pathology services to people who are financially, geographically, or otherwise limited in access. Choose one example of such means and describe a hypothetical scenario in which an individual would be best served through that mode of service delivery. Include details about the geographic region, socioeconomic context, and the individual's clinical profile (age, diagnosis, symptoms, services needed, etc.) as well as details about how the individual would benefit in terms of enhanced access to care.

8. Imagine that you are employed at a large university hospital and have been asked by a medical school professor to give a workshop on either speech-language pathology or audiology to the medical students. What would be your goals in this workshop? How would you get the students meaningfully engaged in the content

such that they would be likely to retain and use the information?

9. Imagine that you are director of a large urban center for the treatment of communication disorders that serves clients across the age span, and you just heard that one of your federal legislators will be visiting your agency for a two-hour morning visit. What would you want to accomplish on this visit? What aspects of your program would you want to showcase? What topics would you want to prioritize for the content of your conversations?

Acknowledgment

Recognition is extended to Dr. Bernard P. Henri for his strong contributions to earlier versions of this chapter.

References

American Speech-Language-Hearing Association. (2013). *Speech-language pathology assistant scope of practice*. Retrieved from https://www.asha.org/uploadedFiles/SP2013-00337.pdf

American Speech-Language-Hearing Association. (n.d.). *Billing and reimbursement*. Retrieved from https://www.asha.org/practice/reimbursement/

Boisvert, M. K. & Hall, N. (2019). *Telepractice for school-based speech and language services: A workload management strategy*. Perspectives of the ASHA Special Interest Groups, 4(1). https://doi.org/10.1044/2018_PERS-SIG18-2018-0004

Braithwaite, J. (2018). Changing how we think about healthcare improvement. *British Medical Journal*. https://doi.org/10.1136/bmj.k2014

Brown, N. A. (2005). Information on telemedicine. *Journal of Telemedicine and Telecare, 11*, 117–126.

Centeno, J., & Kohnert, K. (2009). Serving linguistically and culturally diverse adults with communication disorders: Multidisciplinary perspectives and evidence. *Seminars in Speech and Language, 30*(3), 137–138.

Doolittle, G. C., Otto, F., & Clemens, C. (1998). Hospice care using home-based telemedicine systems. *Journal of Telemedicine and Telecare, 4*, 58–59.

Epstein, S. (2008). The rise of "recruitmentology": Clinical research. Racial knowledge, and the politics of inclusion and difference. *Social Studies of Science, 38*(5), 801–832.

Fox, H. B., & McManus, M. A. (2001). A national study of commercial health insurance and Medicaid definitions of medical necessity: What do they mean for children? *Ambulatory Pediatrics, 1*(1), 16–22.

Hallowell, B. (2000). A student-run respite network for caregivers of persons with dementing illness. *Communication Connection, 14*(1), 10.

Hallowell, B. (2017). *Aphasia and other acquired neurogenic language disorders: A guide for clinical excellence.* San Diego, CA: Plural Publishing.

Hart, J. (2010). Medical connectivity: Expanding access to telespeech in clinical settings: Inroads & challenges. *Telemedicine Journal and E-Health, 16*(9), 922–924.

Henri, B. P. (2010). Business: At the table or on the table: It's our choice. *American Speech-Language Hearing Association Special Interest Division 11 Perspectives on Administration and Supervision, 21*, 3–8.

Henri, B. P., & Hallowell, B. (1999a). Funding alternatives to offset the reimbursement impacts of managed care. *Newsletter of Special Interest Division 2, Neurophysiology and Neurogenic Speech and Language Disorders.* Rockville, MD: American Speech-Language-Hearing Association.

Henri, B. P., & Hallowell, B. (1999b). Relating managed care to managing care. In B. S. Cornett (Ed.), *Clinical practice management in speech-language pathology: Principles and practicalities.* Gaithersburg, MD: Aspen.

Henri, B. P., Hallowell, B., & Johnson, C. (1997). Advocacy and marketing to support clinical services. In R. Kreb (Ed.), *A practical guide to treatment outcomes and cost effectiveness* (pp. 39–48). Rockville, MD: American Speech-Language-Hearing Association Task Force on Treatment Outcomes and Cost Effectiveness.

Jones, D. M., McAllister, L., & Lyle, D. M. (2017). Rural and remote speech-language pathology inequities: An Australian human rights dilemma. *International Journal of Speech-Language Pathology, 20*(1), 98–101.

Khazei, A., Jarvis-Selinger, S., Ho, K., & Lee, A. (2005). An assessment of the telehealth needs and health-care priorities of Tanna Island: A remote, under-served and vulnerable population. *Journal of Telemedicine and Telecare, 11*, 35–40.

Kneipp, S. M., Lutz, B. J., & Means, S. (2009). Reasons for enrollment, the informed consent process, and trust among low-income women participating in a community-based participatory research study. *Public Health Nursing, 26*(4), 362–369.

Lim, S., McManus, M., Fox H., White, K., & Forsman, I. (2010). Ensuring financial access to hearing aids for infants and young children. *Pediatrics. 126*(1), S43–S51.

Lyon, J. G. (1992). Communication use and participation for adults with aphasia in natural settings: The scope of the problem. *American Journal of Speech-Language Pathology, 1*, 7–14.

Maughan, B., Messer, J., Collishaw, S., Pickles, A., Snowling, M., Yule, W., & Rutter, M. (2009). Persistence of literacy problems: Spelling in adolescence and at mid-life. *Journal of Child Psychology and Psychiatry, 50*(8), 893–901.

McCartney, E., Boyle, J., Bannatyne, S., Jessiman, E., Campbell, C., Kelsey, C., . . . Ohare, A. (2005). 'Thinking for two': A case study of speech and language therapists working through assistants. *International Journal of Language and Communication Disorders, 40*(2), 221–235.

McManus, M. A., Levtov, R., White, K. R., Forsman, I., Foust, T., & Thompson, M. (2010). Medicaid reimbursement of hearing services for infants and young children. *Pediatrics, 126*, S34–S42.

McNeilly, L. (2016). Rise in speech-language disorders in SSI-supported children reflects national trends. *ASHA Leader, 21*(3). https://doi.org/10.1044/leader.PA2.21032016.np

National Center for Education Statistics. (2015). Elementary and secondary education. *Digest of Education Statistics.* Retrieved from https://nces.ed.gov/pubs2016/2016014_2.pdf

National Center for Education Statistics. (2018). *Children and youth with disabilities.* Retrieved from https://nces.ed.gov/programs/coe/indicator_cgg.asp

Nolan, P., & Bradley, E. (2008). Evidence-based practice: Implications and concerns. *Journal of Nursing Management, 16*(4), 388–393.

Noria, C. W., Borkowski, J. G., & Whitman, T. L. (2009). Parental influences on self-regulation and achievement in children with adolescent mothers. *European Journal of Development Psychology, 6*(6), 722–745.

Novelli, W. (2008). Transforming the healthcare system: A focus on prevention. *Healthcare Financial Management*, 62(4), 94–99.

Pelletier, K. (2009). A review and analysis of the clinical and cost-effectiveness studies of comprehensive health promotion and disease management programs at the worksite: Update VII 2004–2008. *Journal of Occupational and Environmental Medicine*, 51(5), 822–837.

Rainee, L., & Anderson, J. (2017). *The future of jobs and job training*. Pew Research Center. Retrieved from https://www.pewinternet.org/wp-content/uploads/sites/9/2017/05/PI_2017.05.03_Future-of-Job-Skills_FINAL.pdf

Shippen, M. E., Houchins, D. E., Crites, S. A., Derzis, M. C., & Dashaunda, P. (2010). An examination of the basic reading skills of incarcerated males. *Adult Learning*, 21(3/4), 4–12.

Snow, P. C., & Powell, M. B. (2008). Oral language competence, social skills and high-risk boys: What are juvenile offenders trying to tell us? *Children & Society*, 22(1), 16–28.

Sondenaa, E., Wansholm, M., & Roos. E. (2016). Case characteristics of prisoners with communication problems. *Open Journal of Social Sciences*, 4(4). Retrieved from https://file.scirp.org/Html/5-1760857_65496.htm

Swanepoel, D., Clark, J., Koekemoer, D., Hall, J. W., III, Krumm, M., Ferrari, D. V., . . . Barajas, J. J. (2010). Telehealth in audiology: The need and potential to reach underserved communities. *International Journal of Audiology*, 49(3), 195–202.

Theodoros, D. (2012). A new era in speech-language pathology practice: Innovation and diversification. *International Journal of Speech-Language Pathology*, 14, 189–199.

Theodoros, D., & Russell, T. (2008). Telerehabilitation: Current perspectives. In R. Latifi (Ed.), *Current principles and practices of telemedicine and e-health* (pp. 191–209). Amsterdam, Netherlands: IOS Press.

U.S. Department of Labor. (2019). *Occupational outlook handbook*. Retrieved from https://www.bls.gov/ooh/healthcare/

Wales, D., Skinner, L., & Hayman, M. (2017). The efficacy of telehealth-delivered speech and language intervention for primary school-age children: A systematic review. *International Journal of Telerehabilitation*, 9(1), 55–70.

White, S. (2008). Bottom line. Coding and reimbursement for auditory rehabilitation. *ASHA Leader*, 13(16), 3.

Yoo, S. K., Kim, D. K., Jung, S. M., Kim, E., Lim, J. S., & Kim, J. H. (2004). Performance of a web-based, real-time, tele-ultrasound consultation system over high-speed commercial telecommunication lines. *Journal of Telemedicine and Telecare*, 10, 175–179.

SECTION IV

Working Productively

20

Documentation Issues

◇◇

Barbara J. Moore, EdD

Introduction

No matter the profession, complaints about paperwork are part of the common culture. A necessary evil of our times, paperwork creates the evidence, the record that shows we have followed the law and completed our work in accordance with requirements set forth by government, associations, and other regulatory agencies. Through documentation, we prove compliance, design plans, present a rationale, justify recommendations, and submit financial remuneration requests. This chapter outlines the various types of documentation common to speech-language pathologists and audiologists in the variety of work settings in which we practice, including schools, private practice, and medical settings. As this chapter shows, accurate completion of documentation is essential for speech-language pathologists and audiologists, regardless of the setting, because "if it's not documented, it didn't happen" (Hapner, 2008; Moore, 2010b).

General Principles of Documentation

Speech-language pathologists and audiologists provide services in a variety of settings: schools, hospitals, clinics, universities, private practice offices, telepractice, and possibly others. With the exception of fee-for-service arrangements in private practice, where a client pays directly for the service rendered, the vast majority of our professional services are funded through third-party payers, generally either government funding or insurance. As a result, there are requirements for documentation to demonstrate that requirements are met. The ASHA Code of Ethics (American Speech-Language-Hearing Association [ASHA], 2016), Principle I, Rule O requires that "individuals shall protect the confidentiality and security of records of professional services provided, research and scholarly activities conducted, and products dispensed. Access to these records shall be allowed only when doing so is necessary to protect the welfare of the person or of the community, is legally authorized, or is otherwise required by law" (pp. 5–6). This requirement, then, applies to all work settings.

Third-party payers set forth eligibility requirements for services. The laws for education and the requirements for insurance, including Medicaid and Medicare, establish the foundation on which documentation requirements are built. The professional community of communication sciences and disorders establishes the expectations within the discipline that will form the content of what is documented. Clear documentation is critical regardless of the work setting, as it establishes justification and rationale for treatment, reveals the progress that did or did not happen, and creates a legal record of what has happened.

In graduate school, you may think that report writing is the biggest part of documentation in the work world. In fact, it is far more. Learning to document correctly and adequately is a skill that is necessary and must be practiced, just like clinical skills. Speech-language pathologists and audiologists should always be attentive to their own documentation, as well as learning procedures from other clinicians. Throughout a career, you should actively seek information about documentation practice. For example, before you submit a report, you might consult writing manuals, review other approved reports, select appropriate procedural terminology, use a spell-checker, and ask others to review your completed work.

Regardless of the work setting, you will be expected to use a formal writing style in your documentation, which means the use of Standard American English as well as the formal conventions of written language. Certainly, abbreviations and codes will be used, as appropriate to the type of documentation. Keeping to the standards of the field is vital not only because the documentation drives the actions of the reader but also because it is a reflection on you, the writer, and on your program.

Although schools and medical settings are funded by different sources, the basics of clinical documentation remain the same. Clinicians in any setting must remember Hapner's (2008) warning: "If the record is not clear, concise, and comprehensive, then the therapeutic process is at risk" (p. 33). Many individuals who are lax in their paperwork justify their transgressions by stating that the burden of paperwork is "too much" or that "it doesn't matter." In fact, the documentation is the record on which decisions about eligibility and services are made. The documentation guides teams, other professionals, and funding decision makers about how to do their jobs in relation to the student, client, or patient. Poor documentation can lead to funding denials, eligibility uncertainty, and inappropriate diagnosis and treatment. It also can lead to professional consequences, when colleagues and others question why inappropriate documentation was completed and/or are challenged to make service and placement decisions based on inadequate documentation. This can not only reflect on a clinician's professional reputation but also result in incorrect clinical and service decisions.

To ensure that paperwork is completed correctly, it is helpful to understand the funding source and reasons for the documentation requirements. In both medical and educational settings, the "how to" of documentation may change periodically. It is an expectation that the clinician will keep up with such requirements to avoid denials, delays, or legal action.

Documentation in Educational Settings

School-based speech-language pathology and audiology services are generally provided under the authorization of the Individuals with Disabilities Education Improvement Act (IDEA, 2004), which is the federal law that authorizes special education in the United States. While most of the paperwork required in schools must comply with IDEA requirements, the IDEA is not the only law that governs or guides what is required, how processes should proceed in school settings, and what documentation is required. Federal laws are identified as public laws (PLs), which outline major components of the law. Regulations that implement the laws are set forth in the Code of Federal Regulations (CFR). States are required to enact legislation that aligns state law with federal laws. States can exceed federal law, but they cannot have laws with lower mandates than what exists in federal legislation. State interpretations and provisions may be different from state to state. Additionally, local school board policy and local practice may have specific procedures that are not found in federal or state law but are required for local implementation of state and federal requirements. Parents and staff often become confused about which requirements are federal or state laws, or local practice. Most typically, forms and required paperwork will be designed to comply with legal requirements. Following are the major laws, or "big laws" that pertain to school services and records:

- Family Educational Rights and Privacy Act (FERPA)

- Health Insurance Portability and Accountability Act (HIPAA)

- Individuals with Disabilities Education Improvement Act (IDEA 2004)

- Rehabilitation Act of 1973 and Section 504

- Elementary and Secondary Education Act (ESEA)/Every Student Succeeds Act (ESSA)

- Americans with Disabilities Act (ADA)

This chapter reviews each of these laws and their application to speech-language and hearing services in schools. A summary of these laws, their purpose, and the types of documentation required are provided in Table 20–1.

continues

Table 20–1. Summary of Federal Laws Pertaining to Documentation in Schools

Federal Law	Original Enactment	Most Recent Authorization	Legal Foundations	Documentation
Individuals with Disabilities Education Improvement Act (IDEA 2004)	November 26, 1975, originally passed as PL 94-142, the Education for All Handicapped Children Act	December 3, 2004	IDEA 2004 requires the provision of special education and related services for students identified as children with disabilities. When students are identified as having a disability, they become members of a protected class; therefore, they secure procedural safeguards, which are realized in the procedural requirements of special education. The following are foundational concepts in special education: ■ Free appropriate public education ■ Least restrictive environment ■ Zero reject ■ Due process of law for families and children: timelines, consent, appeal procedures	**Purposes** To show that legal requirements were met, including timelines and regulations To demonstrate that parents were included in the decision making **Typical documents** ■ Individualized Education Program (IEP) ■ Assessment reports ■ Parent rights ■ Consent forms
Rehabilitation Act of 1973; Section 504	September 26, 1973	December 2008	Section 504 of the Rehabilitation Act of 1973 is a federal civil rights law that prohibits discrimination against individuals with disabilities in programs and activities that receive federal financial assistance. Section 504 is intended to prohibit discrimination on the basis of disability.	**Purpose** To ensure that the process is documented. (Section 504 has regulations but not the tight timelines and definitive criteria that special education has.) **Typical documents** ■ Section 504 accommodation plan ■ Reports ■ Consent for data collection

Table 20–1. *continued*

Federal Law	Original Enactment	Most Recent Authorization	Legal Foundations	Documentation
Rehabilitation Act of 1973; Section 504 *continued*			All IDEA students are also covered by Section 504, but not all 504 students are eligible for services under IDEA. It is not necessary for IDEA-eligible students to have a 504 plan.	
Family Educational Rights and Privacy Act (FERPA)	August 21, 1974, as part of the reauthorization of the Elementary and Secondary Education Act (ESEA), the Education Amendments of 1974	October 26, 2001, as part of the USA Patriot Act of 2001	FERPA provides students' parents the right to access educational records and also the right to protect transferability of records without their consent.	**Purpose** To provide regulations regarding sharing of student records to ensure the protection of privacy rights **Typical documents** School records as defined under the law
Elementary and Secondary Education Act (ESEA)/Every Child Succeeds Act (ESSA)	April 11, 1965	ESSA was the reauthorization of ESEA (e.g., Title I), signed into law December 10, 2015.	ESEA/ESSA intends to ensure that all children reach proficiency on state content standards and state assessments, to close the achievement gap between high- and low-performing students and between advantaged and disadvantaged students, and to ensure that all students are college and career ready.	**Purpose** To ensure the academic achievement of all students, including students with disabilities, English Learners, students from low socioeconomic homes, and minority students **Typical documents** ■ Testing results ■ Data ■ Accountability reports
Health Insurance Portability and Accountability Act (HIPAA)	August 21, 1996	April 14, 2003	HIPAA sets forth simplified health insurance administration by establishing standards and requirements for the electronic transmission of certain health information.	**Purpose** Privacy of PHI

Federal Law	Original Enactment	Most Recent Authorization	Legal Foundations	Documentation
Health Insurance Portability and Accountability Act (HIPAA) *continued*			It specifically addresses protected health information (PHI), which includes any physical or mental health information. Education records subject to the protections of FERPA are excluded from HIPAA. The HIPAA privacy rule mandates that a "covered entity" may not use or disclose PHI except as permitted by the rule. A school district is considered the "covered entity." The PHI is germane, in most cases, to conducting evaluation and development of the IEP and/or Section 504. The intent of both HIPAA and FERPA is confidentiality. Some of the agencies (i.e., medical) that work with school districts and want records must abide by HIPAA's PHI rules, so there must be consent to exchange information.	**Typical documents** Most school records are covered under FERPA and excluded from HIPAA, including IEPs, evaluations, IEP meeting tapes, Medicaid reimbursement claims, student health records, and personal notes, when the personal note has become a school record (Shorter, 2004).
Americans with Disabilities Act (ADA)	July 26, 1990	September 26, 2008	ADA (1990) deals with accessibility to public domains (including communication access) and "prohibits discrimination on the basis of disability in employment, programs, and services provided by state and local governments, goods and services provided by private companies, and in commercial facilities" (U.S. Department of Justice, 1999, in Moore & Montgomery, 2008).	**Purpose** Prohibits discrimination against people with disabilities; intended to give broad protections by providing physical and communication access **Typical documents** ■ Employment records ■ Facilities records ■ Some school records ■ Other records that document provision of accessibility for the public

Laws Regulating Student Records: FERPA and HIPAA

Laws in education are centrally concerned with protecting student confidentiality, specifically related to students with disabilities. These students are considered a protected class of individuals. The Family Educational Rights and Privacy Act (FERPA) is the federal law that addresses student records, including who can access student education records. The discussion here pertains to K–12 education, although the law does apply to higher education. When students are over 18, all rights given to the parents are assumed by the adult student. This law ensures that parents have an opportunity to have the records amended and provides families some control over the disclosure of information from the records. According to FERPA, educational records are records that are related to the student and maintained by an educational agency or institution or by a party acting for the agency or institution (20 USC 1232g[a][4][A]) (FERPA) (U.S. Department of Education, n.d.). The legislation provides clarification on parents' access to student records, in addition to limiting the transfer of records by requiring consent for record transfers.

An overview of the requirements for access to school records is outlined in Table 20–2 (U.S. Department of Education, 2011). These requirements pertain to all student records, but they set forth the foundation for

---

Table 20–2. FERPA Requirements for Access to School Records

FERPA Requires Schools to:

- Provide student with an opportunity to inspect and review his or her education records within 45 days of the receipt of a request;
- Provide a student with copies of education records or otherwise make the records available to the student if the student, for instance, lives outside of commuting distance of the school;
- Redact the names and other personally identifiable information about other students that may be included in the student's education records.

FERPA Does Not Require Schools to:

- Create or maintain education records;
- Provide students with calendars, notices, or other information that does not generally contain information directly related to the student;
- Respond to questions about a student.

Under FERPA a School Must:

- Consider a request from a student to amend inaccurate or misleading information in the student's education records;
- Offer a student a hearing on the matter if it decides not to amend the records in accordance with the request;
- Offer a student a right to place a statement to be kept and disclosed with the record, if as a result of the hearing the school still decides not to amend the record.

A School Is Not Required to Consider Requests for Amendment under FERPA that:

- Seeks to change a grade or disciplinary decision;
- Seeks to change the opinions or reflections of a school official or other person reflected in an education record.

A School Must:

- Have a student's consent prior to the disclosure of education records;
- Ensure that the consent is signed, dated, and states the purpose of the disclosure.
- Ensure the information disclosed has been appropriately designated as directory information by the school.

Source: ≈ Adapted from U.S. Department of Education (2011).

confidentiality of student records and student information under IDEA. Speech-language pathologists, audiologists, and other educators, including administrators, can sometimes be confused about requests for student records. What if the parents are divorced and do not get along? What if we need to talk to the doctor, but the parent does not agree to the contact? What if the grandmother who takes care of the student is asserting that the student's parents are not making the best choices, and she needs to see the student records? There are a variety of circumstances of records requests or informational releases that might seem in the student's best interest but do not fall within the parameters of allowable provisions. The best advice to school personnel is to always check with administration or legal counsel if you have a question. However, here are some good, quick rules to live by:

- Do not generate letters or records that do not otherwise exist in the student records. This situation may apply if a parent or attorney for the student requests that you generate an opinion regarding which parent is better suited for custody, or if a child's family should be deported when access to services may not be available in another country. Generating documents that render opinions about such issues can pull you into legal battles in which you have no business.

- Be extraordinarily cautious about student information that you put in email or other electronic methods. Increasingly, email may be considered a student record and subject to subpoena.

- Thorough documentation about phone calls, attempts to schedule meetings, and therapy notes are all necessary and important. Some of these documents can be considered student records, so cautious about ensuring that documentation is professional.

Under FERPA, all schools are required to provide an annual notification to parents and the community regarding the rules for access to student records. The means of notification can include student newspaper, calendar, student programs guide, rules handbook, or other means likely to inform students. The notification does not have to be made individually to students (U.S. Department of Education, 2011). This annual notification spells out the rights of parents and specifies the information that must be provided by the school. Parents have the right to:

- Inspect and review records

- Seek amendment of inaccurate or misleading information in their education records

- Consent to most disclosures of personally identifiable information from education records

This chapter emphasizes the critical importance of documentation. In schools, the rules pertaining to student records lay the foundation for what information should be documented in addition to the rules for who has access to these records. School personnel should assume that anything that is written has the potential for being accessed or reviewed by the parents and/or their counsel. Further information about assessment reports and Individualized Education Program (IEP) requirements follows later in this chapter.

One final consideration about student records is the requirement for maintaining or destroying these records. Record retention requirements are determined by the type of pupil record it is. School-based practitioners should check with their local district to determine what the policies and procedures are for maintaining and destroying records. Following is a list of three major types of pupil records: mandatory permanent, mandatory interim, and permitted student records.

- *Mandatory permanent pupil records* are required by state law and usually include identifying information about the pupil; when the student attended the schools in the district; and records of subjects taken, grades, immunizations, and date of graduation or exit.

- *Mandatory interim pupil records* are held for a stipulated period of time and include health information, special education information, language training records, progress reports, parental restrictions, parent/pupil challenges to records, parent authorizations/prohibitions for student participation in certain programs, and results of standardized tests.

- *Permitted pupil records* include counselor/ teacher rating scales, standardized tests older than three years, routine discipline, behavioral reports, discipline notices, and attendance records (ASHA, n.d.-a; Moore, 2018).

The Health Insurance Portability and Accountability Act (HIPAA) is the law that pertains to protected health information (PHI). Originally enacted in 1996, the 2003 amendments addressed electronic transmission of records and increased restrictions on accessibility to health records. Because school personnel are often seeking information from health care providers, there is periodically confusion and questions regarding which HIPAA requirements apply in school settings. The answer is that education records are subject to the protections of FERPA and are excluded from HIPAA. The HIPAA privacy rule mandates that a "covered entity" may not use or disclose PHI except as permitted by the rule. A school district is considered the "covered entity." The PHI is germane, in most cases, to conducting evaluation and development of the IEP and/or 504 plan. Again, the intent of both HIPAA and FERPA is confidentiality. Speech-language pathologists and audiologists practicing in health care settings will have greater awareness of the influence of HIPAA in their work settings than professionals working in schools. Most school records are covered under FERPA and excluded from HIPAA, including IEPs, evaluations, IEP meeting recordings, Medicaid reimbursement claims, student health records, and personal notes, when the personal note has become a school record (ASHA, n.d-a.; Moore, 2018; Moore & Montgomery, 2018).

IDEA 2004 Documentation Requirements

The Individuals with Disabilities Education Improvement Act (IDEA, 2004) is the law that authorizes special education in the United States. The IDEA was originally enacted as the Education for All Handicapped Children Act, PL 94-142, in 1975. The foundation of this law is rooted in civil rights, taking its influence of "separate but equal is not equal" from the Supreme Court decision *Brown v. Board of Education* in 1954 (Moore & Montgomery, 2018). Because of these roots in civil rights, students who are identified as children with disabilities (CWD) are considered members of a protected class in this country. Consequently, they engender procedural rights and protections in order to ensure these civil rights. It is for this reason that documentation under IDEA is critical, as it is the proof that school districts and service providers have followed the foundational components of the rights provided under the law.

Attorneys and school district administrators often tell staff that their work needs to be "legally defensible." Documentation is the vehicle through which personnel create the "legally defensible" record, which, in essence, shows that the process was followed and that the district's IEP team created a program that met the requirements of the law. In special education, processes are extraordinarily important. School-based personnel will participate as members of teams that create documentation that serves to verify that the processes were followed. Records should be able to stand on their own. Through the records created, the story of the student's experience should be told, and the reader should be able to "thread the needle," connecting all components of the student's history. If and when the school district is challenged in a due process hearing, it is the documentation that will provide the evidence that "something took place" (i.e., logs, postal receipts, fax confirmations,

and so on). The documentation serves as the historical record, but if we think of it as telling the child's story, we are more inclined to ensure that we are doing our part in demonstrating the reasons why decisions were made and actions were taken.

Special education eligibility is determined through a multidisciplinary assessment. The speech-language pathologist and/or audiologist will need to complete a report documenting the findings of the assessment. Assessment reports and pre-referral/response-to-intervention and multi-tiered systems of support (MTSS) processes and documentation are discussed in another section. The eligibility determination and IEP meeting process are outlined in Table 20–3.

The main document under IDEA is the IEP. The IEP is to be developed either following an assessment or for an annual review. Most IEPs are now electronic or web based. In many electronic systems, the IEP form reflects all of the federal requirements, designed to ensure that IEP teams meet the required elements. The benefit of electronic systems is that they are developed so that no portion of the IEP can be left blank. However, there is some criticism that electronic systems lend themselves to looking like they are not individualized, specific with goal development, and/or that they do not allow for parent input. Ensuring and documenting parent input is critical, especially with an electronic system. One of the best ways to do this is within the notes section of the IEP (Table 20–4).

While electronic IEPs may seem to make documentation easier, it is the IEP process that is critical. Table 20–4 illustrates how the IEP process should occur. The IEP document itself should include meaningful interpretation of data by building a bridge, or "threading the needle" between the student's performance (i.e., assessment or other data, student classroom performance, student grades, observational information, input from other teachers and specialists) and the proposed goals. Other texts (Moore & Montgomery, 2018) describe the components of the IEP, and that is not the intention of this chapter. What is important for this chapter is the content of the documents developed, in order to ensure compliance, accuracy, and legal defensibility. The following sections highlight key areas for documentation in the special education process.

Report Writing

The most typical report completed in a school setting is an assessment report. The assessment process is laid out in the law to include evaluation processes which will lead to a determination of eligibility as well as informing the IEP team as to the student's needs. The terms "assessment" and "evaluation" may be used interchangeably,

Table 20–3. Special Education Identification Process
Multi-Tiered Systems of Support
Pre-referral processes/Response to Intervention (RtI)/Multi-Tiered Systems of Support (MTSS) ↓
Referral for assessment from an Instructional Support Team (IST)/Problem Solving Team/Parent ↓
Multidisciplinary Assessment ↓
Eligibility Determination during IEP meeting ↓
Identification of Areas of Need (if eligible) ↓
IEP Goal Development (based on areas of need) ↓
Determination of Program, Placement, and Services (needed to address goals; no service without a goal)

Table 20–4. IEP Meeting Process
Determination of Present Levels of Educational Achievement ■ Review evaluation data ■ Review classroom performance ■ Review other related information ■ Consider input from parents, teachers, and specialists
Determination of Goals and Short-Term Objectives or Benchmarks ■ Based on identified areas of need ■ Designed to enable the child to progress in the general education curriculum ■ Must be measurable
Determination of Program, Placement, and Services ■ Includes services needed in order for goals to be achieved ■ Designed to confer meaningful educational benefit

Source: From *Speech-Language Pathologists in Public Schools: Making a Difference for America's Children* (3rd ed., p. 163), by B. J. Moore and J. K. Montgomery, 2018, Austin, TX: Pro-Ed. Copyright 2018 by Pro-Ed. Reprinted with permission.

but have specific meaning in law, special education, and communication disorders. Assessment refers to the process of gathering diagnostic information, and evaluation refers to the decision-making processes which will determine if a student qualifies as CWD and the extent to which his/her needs require special education and related services (Moore & Montgomery, 2018; 20 U.S.C. § 300.315) Some school districts require an annual report of student progress, but such reports typically follow a format laid out by the local education agency (LEA). Such a report would be different than the annual IEP, which does require an update of the student's present levels of performance and academic achievement. Annual speech or audiology reports are not required under federal law, but updating performance on the IEP is.

An assessment report is required whenever an evaluation occurs. It must document suspected areas of need; connect to findings in other reports, including both prior speech and language reports, as well as reports from other service providers; document current areas of concern; and be written in a professional manner, using professional terminology. In some school districts, the multidisciplinary assessment team (MDAT) will write one comprehensive report to ensure that the connection between the findings of the professionals is obvious in the report. While this is a highly recommended practice, it may not be the practice in every district.

Assessment reports generally conform to the following format (Moore, 2010a, 2010b, 2018):

- Reason for assessment
- Background information
- Assessments:
  - ☐ Standardized instruments or tests
  - ☐ Observation in natural setting
  - ☐ Non-standardized measures or methods
  - ☐ Activities within natural setting
- Behaviors observed during assessment
- Information on progress in academic or curricular areas
- Information on classroom assessments and statewide assessments
- Information from others (teacher, parent, aide, other MDAT members)
- Input from the student on his/her disabling condition, thoughts, desires, and wishes
- Impressions

- Summary/conclusions
- Recommendations

Pitfalls in assessment reports occur when school personnel do not connect their assessment results to the actual daily classroom work and functioning in school. Assessment reports that only provide test results and discussion of clinical results and do not connect these results to classroom performance do not meet the premise of "threading the needle" among assessments, IEP development, academic achievement, and functional performance.

The same is true for audiology reports. An audiogram placed in the student file without interpretation connected to the classroom or in relation to findings from other MDAT members does not serve the student well, nor does it provide necessary information to parents and other service providers. Both speech-language pathologists and audiologists in schools can assume that their clinical impressions must be directly and overtly connected to the student's classroom performance. Not only is this good practice, it is required by law and is good for the student.

Therapy Notes, Progress Monitoring, Personal Notes, and Email

During training in communication sciences and disorders, speech-language pathologists and audiologists are drilled in the requirements of documenting client performance during therapy. Swigert (2018) observes: "Many times, the speech-language pathologist feels as if she spends more time documenting than doing. Therefore, it is important to learn not only how to document, but how to do so efficiently" (Introduction). Although this skill is emphasized in training programs, when working in educational settings, these habits are prone to slippage. Keeping therapy notes for therapeutic sessions is an expectation in a school setting, just as in any other setting.

Progress during treatment sessions should be charted for each session. These notes are considered part of the student record and can and will be requested by parents and attorneys as evidence that the session occurred, as well as how progress is being attained. Progress monitoring is critical in school settings, both within special education as well as in pre-referral interventions (See Response-to-Intervention and Multi-Tiered Systems of Support). Speech-language pathologists and audiologists are trained in these methods and may serve as a resource to educational personnel. Charting and progress monitoring are expectations of our professional work and are required in all work settings for clinical practice, including schools. IEP goals are written with measurable targets. To track phonological production, fluency counts, or grammatical units, charting or progress monitoring will occur and should be part of the therapy notes.

Although it is not a requirement in schools, following a SOAP note format is useful for therapy note documentation in schools as well as medical and private practice settings (Table 20–5).

Writing a SOAP note for school settings may seem onerous to school-based clinicians, but this type of documentation will pay off for both Medicaid billing and for any legal challenges. In fact, the therapy note does not have to be onerous. Consider the following example for an in-class session:

S— Student chatting with friends before class began. Attentive to teacher instructions.

O— Applied vocabulary strategies for verbal rehearsal during class activity. Student observed three times using strategy appropriately with history terms *tariff*, *taxation without representation*, and *revolution*.

A— First application of strategy without prompting.

P— Continue per IEP.

Keeping this type of a note is neither difficult nor particularly time-consuming. Do remember, however, to initial and date each note so that authentication of the author of the note is provided. Writing the note at the end of the session or right after the session is completed ensures both accuracy and completion of the requirement. Many school (and medical/clinic) sites are now having clinicians document in real time, during the session as it occurs to reduce inefficiencies and increase productive face-face billable time.

Keeping therapy notes is important for many purposes. In addition to therapeutic interactions, school-based practitioners are encouraged and reminded about keeping documentation of all interactions with parents and all issues pertinent to the case. Particularly in challenging or "high-profile" cases, school-based practitioners may feel a need to keep "personal notes" or a "personal file." Sometimes, these notes pertain to challenging interactions with parents or other agencies. Although courts and legislatures have protected the use of personal notes, especially if used for the purpose of serving as a memory aid or reminder of a situation, a personal file may still be subpoenaed. Special education or school personnel may sometimes feel threatened or that they need to document situations for their own personal reasons, separate from the requirements of the law or professional responsibilities. Thus, always be cognizant that someone else may read that file.

School personnel also need to be cautious regarding email. Email can be subpoenaed. In most work settings, email is widely used. Email can be problematic because it is easily forwarded; it can also end up in a student file, making it part of the student record and, as such, available to the parent. You may, in fact, wish to print and save some email, but do so with the knowledge that it may be considered a student record. In some cases, this may be appropriate. Practitioners should be very careful with what to put in email. This includes both your personal email as well as your work email. The author recently participated in a due process hearing where emails made up a significant amount of the evidence. As a general rule, if you don't want the child's parent, your boss, your mother, or a judge reading the email, don't send it! (Moore, 2010a, 2010b, 2018).

One other caution about electronic communication involves social networking. Facebook, Twitter, YouTube, and the ever-emerging world of social networking are

Table 20–5. SOAP Notes
Subjective—Write your opinion or impressions regarding relevant student or client behavior status in a brief statement.
Objective—Record measurable information or progress monitoring data collected for each task during the therapy session.
Assessment—Describe your analysis and/or interpret data for current session and compare with student's or client's previous level of performance.
Plan—Identify proposed therapy targets for the next session.

widely accessed. Within these domains, individuals typically feel free to share widely their daily experiences, including their feelings about bosses, coworkers, and other situations in their lives, including, in the case of educators, information about children. Children should be protected at all times, especially by those who are responsible for their well-being. Remember, too, that FERPA and IDEA have confidentiality protections that are easily violated when personally identifiable information is shared. This is true in the lunchroom, the faculty lounge, and on social networking sites, where anyone can access information. Again, be careful and cognizant of the problems this can present.

Some systems for electronic billing of Medicaid also have electronic systems for note taking. Both IDEA and Medicaid require that school districts maintain records for at least three years after the student separates from the educational system. Storing of files is often an inefficient system in many school districts, so electronic storage is simple. Additionally, this method ensures that records are not lost.

One final comment on therapy notes and documentation: As recommended throughout this chapter, in addition to maintaining therapy notes, you should develop the habit of documenting all communications with parents, teachers, and issues pertaining to a student. Many school-based practitioners find it easy to keep all documentation in one file. Many clinicians just keep individual files on each student, maintaining therapy notes on one side and other documentation on the other side of the file. The advent of electronic records has created increased issues in this area. Be sure to know your state and district's policy for record retention and maintaining documentation. Most LEAs have a procedure for keeping such records as well as how these records are to be disposed of at the appropriate time.

The following tips summarize this section:

- Yes, it's true: *if it's not documented, it didn't happen!*

- Develop the habit of documenting everything, including conversations with parents, phone calls, intervention notes, and anything else.

- Do not rely on your memory. It will fail you, and it will not be the same as someone else's, especially that of a parent.

- Lack of documentation is lethal. Poor documentation is worse (Moore, 2010a, 2010b).

IEP and IFSP Components

The IEP and the Individualized Family Service Plan (IFSP), developed for infants and toddlers receiving services under Part C of IDEA, are the cornerstones of documentation in special education. The documentation requirements provide the foundation for ensuring that the LEA has designed a plan that is individualized to a given child's unique needs. Through the IEP process (see Table 20–4), a document is developed that, in essence, serves as the contract whereby the responsible parties develop a program intended to confer educational benefit to the student (Moore & Montgomery, 2018). These are more than words. The IEP process, a federally mandated requirement, results in a document that is legally binding and portable, meaning that the family can take this document to any school district in the United States and that district will be required to provide the services identified in the IEP without delay. If you have ever been confused by the lack of clarity in an incoming IEP document, you understand why clear documentation on the IEP is so important for the student. Sometimes this happens even within one's own district. Remember too that there are variations in the processes for students who move into a district, as policies, practices, and procedures for 30-day placements may vary from state to state and district to district. See Chapter 16 for discussion of policies and procedures in educational settings.

IFSPs are developed with a different focus than the IEP. Services to infants and toddlers occur primarily in the home, and issues related to infants and toddlers are addressed through family system support and through direct services to the child. IFSPs are outcome driven, and the documentation of an IFSP is designed accordingly. Providing services in a natural environment, and combining resources of educational and other state and local agencies, is a common way of dealing with these needs of the children and families. Programming for infants and toddlers is very different from state to state and is not addressed here. Early intervention (EI) is a growing area of service under IDEA due to technological advances and increasing awareness of the importance of providing services to children and families as early as possible. The specialization of documentation requirements is highly dependent on state and local regulations. See Chapter 17 for in-depth discussion of early intervention.

Present Levels of Academic Achievement

Special education requirements have ensured monitoring of student progress in the general curriculum since the inception of the federal law in 1975. The mandates for accountability within IDEA 2004 interface with the requirements of the Elementary and Secondary Education Act (ESEA), reauthorized in 2015 as the Every Student Succeeds Act (ESSA). The requirements mandate that school districts demonstrate academic growth in various subgroups, including students with disabilities. These mandates have led to heightened awareness of the need for speech-language pathologists to be familiar with core standards and curriculum requirements. (Moore & Montgomery, 2018; Wallach, 2008).

The ESSA represents the system mandates for accountability in academic achievement for students with disabilities as one of the subgroups to be reported. An individual mandate is required under IDEA 2004, where the IEP team must identify the student's present levels of academic achievement and/or functional performance (IDEA §§ 614[d][A][i][I]). Statements about students' performance should always be positive, never using negative language (Moore & Montgomery, 2018). Information must include how the child's disability affects involvement and progress in the general curriculum (i.e., the same curriculum as for nondisabled children). For preschool children, as appropriate, documentation should focus on how the disability affects the child's participation in appropriate activities (34 CFR § 300.320).

The IDEA 2004 requirement ensures that the IEP team is considering the student's needs in relation to academic achievement. Table 20–4 illustrates the redundancy that is built into the process. The multidisciplinary assessment team assesses all areas of suspected disability and then identifies the areas of academic need that result from the deficits identified in the assessment. If the IEP meeting is not a review of an initial or triennial assessment, then there will be no assessment upon which to base the present levels. However, this does not mean that the IEP team should rely on old reports. This means that other documentation should be brought to the IEP meeting and be considered when developing present levels that indicate areas needing goals. According to Moore and Montgomery (2018, p. 129):

Depending on the type of meeting being held, present levels of educational performance are considered by any and all of the following methods:

- Reviewing evaluations, assessment(s), including statewide, school-wide or classroom, as well as specialist or psycho-educational assessments

- Reviewing classroom work

- Reviewing grade reports

- Reviewing teacher or specialist report (oral or written)

- Considering parent and student information and interests

- Reviewing the previous year's goals and the progress made

- Considering new information brought forth by any member of the team

- Considering reports on student progress and behavior by service providers

- Reviewing discipline and behavioral information

The question for the IEP team, including the speech-language pathologist and/or audiologist, is how the communication disorder affects a student's ability to progress in the curriculum. To know this information, all personnel must be in communication, be familiar with the curricular requirements of the student's grade level and/or program, and address how the student's disability impacts his/her ability to progress in the curriculum. For students with more significant disabilities, functional performance is documented in this area of the IEP.

As a result of this shift in thinking and requirements, the present levels of academic achievement should not include simply rewriting individualized standard test scores or information from previous IEPs. Instead, the link between the areas of need and goals should be evident. For example: "Sara's difficulties in word retrieval and rapid naming adversely affect her reading comprehension abilities. She is able to participate in the classroom activities utilizing the core text with support provided through the Learning Lab program. Her independent reading level is 2.0 according to the Accelerated Reader assessment given on March 3, 2019."

Some students who receive speech and language services for articulation, fluency, voice, or even language related issues may not have deficits in core academics. In these cases, it is important that their grade-level performance be documented on the IEP. Sometimes, practitioners are tempted to leave blank areas where the student has no needs, but this is not the correct procedure. Another rule of documentation is "Leave nothing blank." On the other hand, functional performance related to the student's communication needs, such as phonology, fluency, or voice, should be documented in the IEP. For example: "Bobby's speech is characterized by multiple disfluencies, most often sound repetitions and prolongations. These disfluencies affect his ability to participate in classroom activities such as read-alouds and group discussions as well as general school activities such as lunch and 'clubs' as he tends to stay quiet and not offer his valuable thoughts and ideas and/or is not socially accepted as others pay attention to how he speaks versus the content of his message. Therefore, the focus of his current IEP is learning to utilize fluency shaping techniques across the school environment."

Goals, Objectives, and Benchmarks

IEP goals must be measurable and should be based on common core standards. Electronically based IEP systems often have an expanded base of prewritten goals from which to pick. The ASHA website (ASHA, n.d.-b) also has resources for development of IEP goals. A quick guide to writing IEP goals is provided by the Association of California School Administrators (2006):

Who:	the student
Does what:	observable behavior
When:	by reporting date
Given what:	conditions
How much:	mastery or criteria
How will it be measured:	performance data

Benchmarks are not required for annual academic goals, but some LEAs still prefer these to be written. What is required are reports to parents on the progress toward the goal. This reporting must occur on the same schedule as general education updates on the students' progress. Again, most districts have processes for such reporting, but frequently these, often quarterly, reports are not included in the IEP file, which means there is no evidence that the requirement was followed. The IEP must describe how progress of the pupil toward meeting the annual goals will be measured. Additionally, the IEP must include when the periodic reports will be made. The record needs to reflect that goals have been reported to the parents at the required intervals (34C.F.R. SS 300.320[a][3]).

Under the ESSA, states are required to have state standards which are used for IEP development. As of the writing of this chapter, 41 states have adopted the Common Core State Standards, a joint initiative of the National Governors Association Center for Best Practices and the Council of Chief State School Officers (National Governors Association Center for Best Practices, Council of Chief State School Officers, 2010). Speech-language pathologists must know the core standards that are adopted in their state, and how these are utilized to develop IEP goals.

If a student is failing to make progress on the agreed upon IEP goals, the service provider's responsibility is to reconvene the IEP team to discuss the reasons for the lack of progress. Failure to make progress on IEP goals can be seen as a denial of the student's free appropriate public education (FAPE). An IEP meeting should be held whenever students are not making progress, which is both recommended and required in order to address the issue (i.e., document it), and to adjust the IEP accordingly. Failure to do this can lead to legal and compliance issues. Examples of adjustments include changing or dropping a goal or service. Do not let lack of student progress go undocumented. Lack of progress needs to be addressed for all concerned.

IEP Meeting Notes

Whether to keep IEP meeting notes is often a local district or LEA decision, and some administrators have very strong opinions about how they want the special education personnel in the district to operate. This author is one of those special education directors who has strong opinions about meeting notes and highly recommends the use of meeting notes for several reasons. Meeting notes should document (1) the purpose of the meeting; (2) the offer of parent rights and procedural safeguards; (3) that the IEP team followed the IEP process (see Table 20–4); (4) parental participation, including questions and issues raised by the parent and how those issues were addressed; (5) recommendation of goals and adjustments made, if applicable; (6) discussion of the consideration of continuum of services; and (7) the district's offer of FAPE. Be sure to decide as a team at the school who will take the meeting notes. It is very difficult for the case manager to report at the meeting, run the meeting, and take the meeting notes. Before any meetings take place, members of the team should identify what roles each member will serve. In other words, figure out what needs to be done and who will do it. Taking meeting notes is a developed skill that is important to the district's evidence and documentation.

Multi-Tiered System of Support/Response-to-Intervention

The development of Multi-Tiered Systems of Support (MTSS) across the nation reflects systematic development of interventions designed to coordinate efforts to support students with academic, behavioral, social-emotional and mental health issues. Such systems are both state and school specific. Speech-language pathologists, audiologist and other special education staff will likely have some role within these models of prevention, which strive to keep students from needing to be identified as a student with a disability in order to get help or support. Within the MTSS may be Response-to-Intervention (RtI) models that have been developed in the general education program. Again, these models are widely variable across all school districts.

The push to provide interventions within general education and before a referral for special education assessment led to the development of intervention programs within an RtI framework. In this model, interventions were provided for either academic or behavioral needs within general education. Subsequently, a larger framework, MTSS, integrated RtI along with other models of Positive Behavior Interventions and Supports (PBIS), Title I, and even special education to provide a larger framework for building tiers of intervention that span universal teaching practices to more individualized and more intense interventions for students with greater needs. All of this is designed within the general education program.

In many cases, speech-language pathologists and audiologists have been involved with the development of the model at their school. In other cases, speech-language pathologists and audiologists are not involved in RtI services at their schools. At the heart of MTSS/RtI is the belief that early and systematic approaches to assist students who are having academic and behavioral challenges can prevent students from ultimately requiring special education. Many processes are involved in these models of intervention. A problem-solving team analyzes universal screening and progress monitoring data and makes determinations about what will happen if a student does not respond to the intervention program. In consideration of documentation for MTSS/RtI programs and the participation of speech-language pathologists and audiologists, a key is to look to the processes and programs in existence at a school site or district.

Speech-language pathologists and audiologists may be involved in many different aspects of MTSS/RtI, including planning and providing services in any of the three tiers of intervention (Moore & Montgomery, 2018). At the core of MTSS/RtI operations is progress monitoring and data-driven decision making. Rudebusch (2008) provides numerous examples of tracking systems, worksheets, and progress monitoring systems that can be used by clinicians participating in RtI. Increasingly, there are more resources that can help school-based personnel participate and document their involvement in RtI/MTSS.

Documentation Under Other Educational Laws: ESEA and Section 504

Data and documentation are also required in the school setting under the Elementary and Secondary Education Act (ESEA) and Section 504. Although these laws may seem unrelated, both strive to ensure access to equal opportunities in educational programs. Just like IDEA, these laws also address the participation of students with some sort of disadvantage who otherwise may be denied or have limited access to resources designed to support their successful participation in school.

The Elementary and Secondary Education Act (ESEA)

ESEA was enacted in 1965 during the civil rights era, under the administration of Lyndon Baines Johnson. ESEA authorized Title I, which provides local school districts with financial assistance for the education of low-income children. In 2015, the ESEA was reauthorized as the Every Student Succeeds Act (2015). This law continued the accountability focus of its predecessor (No Child Left Behind, 2002) but moved the accountability mandates to reflect an understanding that children are more than just test scores. Notably, ESSA requires that all states must have challenging academic achievement standards (e.g., previously mentioned for developing goals in IEPs), focus on college and careers, including mandates for alternate achievement standards and alternate achievement testing for students with significant cognitive disabilities, and disaggregation of accountability data by subgroups, including students with disabilities. The design for accountability is given to states, but the reporting system must include indicators for student engagement, English-language proficiency, academic proficiency in English-language arts and math, college and career readiness, graduation rate and school climate. States can add what they think is important. Focus on English learners and students with disabilities is evident.

From these requirements, speech-language pathologists should realize the importance for knowing and understanding the state testing system in their state, accountability metrics, and all of the intervention programs that may be accessible to these students. A key point under these requirements has been an increased understanding of intersectionality. This means that students may be identified as children of poverty (i.e., low income), English learners and students with disabilities. They might also be a foster youth. Each of these conditions impacts their learning. When students have needs in multiple areas, it is critical for staff to coordinate their services in order to address all needs and options to support the student and their family. What this means is that the speech-language pathologist cannot operate in a silo; we must operate as a member of a larger community garnering resources to support students as needed. Documentation within these programs may be redundant, but will also vary from state to state, since these provisions are part of the state plan approved under the federal program.

Section 504 and the Americans with Disabilities Act (ADA)

Section 504 of the Rehabilitation Act of 1973 (Rehabilitation Act of 1973) is a federal civil rights law that prohibits discrimination against individuals with disabilities in programs and activities that receive federal assistance. The interpretation of who is disabled under Section 504 is broader than under IDEA. Most recently reauthorized in 2008, the provisions of 504 have actually been broadened. According to the Code of Federal Regulations, students are deemed eligible as students with a disability under Section 504 if the student is determined to be an individual who:

> Has a physical or mental impairment that substantially limits one or more major life activities, including caring for one's self, performing manual tasks, walking, seeing, hearing, speaking, breathing, sleeping, learning, reading, concentrating, thinking, communicating, and working. (34 CFR 504.3)

Students are found to be eligible following a data collection process or assessment. If a student is eligible, a 504 Accommodation Plan will be developed. While 504 does not have the same time lines as IDEA, there are procedural safeguards, rights, and protections provided under this law. Students who are eligible under 504 may be entitled to receive services available through special education to address their needs, but each state varies on how broad the continuum of services is for students under 504. An example of this could be a student who is hearing impaired and requires support with audiological equipment, but does not require specialized academic instruction. In such a case, the audiologist or speech-language pathologist may provide such services and support. It is always necessary to document how assessment and plan development follow prescribed 504 processes. The process often feels unfamiliar to special and general education personnel because of the lack of specific requirements. A good rule of thumb is to follow the well-established time lines of special education.

The Americans with Disabilities Act (1990) is not an education law but, like 504, is a law that applies to educational settings due to the fact that education institutions receive federal funds. ADA is a law that requires access in public domains, including both physical access to buildings, as well as communication access for individuals with hearing loss and other communication limitations. Through the ADA, physical modifications to public buildings have been realized. These structural changes include creating accessible restrooms, providing accessible audio systems, and putting in ramps so that individuals with mobility challenges are not limited with movement in and around a building. Issues relating to documentation of accessibility can and do still arise in IEP meetings. Special education generally needs to work with the facilities and transportation departments of the district to ensure accessibility to students. Special education personnel may also get involved when members of the public need access, even though the issue is not student related.

Special Issues with Documentation in Schools

Documentation requirements in schools are cumbersome, and failure to comply can bring about liability for the school district. Worse, at times failure to comply can bring about hard feelings between school professionals and parents. In concluding this section on documentation in schools, we consider some special issues.

Request for Records. When parents or their representatives request records, all educational records need to be provided. This means health records, cumulative records, discipline reports, teacher records, and the special education file. Be sure to share any request for records with your principal or special education office administrator immediately, as time lines apply. A request for records often indicates that the family is unhappy with some aspect of their child's program. In a time of electronic record keeping, it is necessary to ensure that all records that should have been uploaded are also in the hard copy file. The separation of electronic documents and recordings, if any exist, can create challenges if these are not put in the hard copy record, as this is still considered the official record.

Request for Copies of Protocols. Speech-language pathologists and audiologists are sometimes confused about providing copies of protocols to parents when requested. The confusion comes because we are told that it violates copyright laws to copy protocols. Copying protocols is a violation of copyright laws if an individual copies a blank protocol in order to avoid spending the money to purchase new protocols. Once a protocol has been used during an assessment, the protocol becomes a student record and is permitted to be copied. When this record is copied, be sure to copy all pages of the protocol, including the blank pages.

Providing Parents Copies of Records in Their Primary Language. Parent participation is a cornerstone of special education. School districts have a responsibility to ensure that parents can fully participate in the IEP process. Having oral interpretation at an IEP or other school meeting is commonly understood, but parents whose primary language is other than English also have the right to have copies of IEPs and assessment reports provided to them in their primary language. The LEA will have procedures to complete such requests.

Legal Considerations. First and foremost, the legal documentation required in special education gives assurance that the required procedures have been followed. In a due process hearing, when a parent's testimony, or the testimony of a witness, contradicts the testimony of the district's witnesses, credence will be given to any documentation the district can provide to support the witness's testimony. In a legal battle, the judge will look for both substantive and procedural violations. The procedural requirements are those that involve the procedures: time lines, notices, IEP meeting documentation, and so on. The question will be "Did the district fail to comply with the procedures mandated under IDEA, and, if so, did the procedural violation rise to the level of a denial of the child's right to a free appropriate public education (FAPE)?" The substantive component of the IEP is the essence of the program. Based on what was delivered, did the student receive an educational benefit? Again, the standard the judge will consider is whether the student received FAPE. IDEA does not allow judges to determine that FAPE was denied simply because some procedural violations occurred. However, if the procedural violation led to a denial of FAPE, the district will lose the case.

A request for a test protocol, like a request for records, can be an indicator that the family is unhappy or feels the need to share the records with someone, such as a legal representative. If the family or representative requests a copy of a test protocol, it may be that person's intention to have someone check the scoring (Moore, 2010a). If someone is launching a challenge to the results and recommendations, a natural place to start for that person could be the test protocol to find any possible scoring error. Such an error might tumble the foundation upon which the recommendations were based. The lesson is to be very careful when scoring assessments. We all make mistakes, but big problems can occur if scoring errors were made and if the incorrect score was relied upon for making recommendations for goals, service, or placement recommendations. The moral of this story is that documentation is not only writing things down but also being careful in ensuring accurate administration and scoring. Legally defensible documentation relies on linking to evidence-based practice and threading the needle between assessment, identification of needs, and IEP goal development.

Documentation in Health Care Settings

While services in school settings are authorized under the requirements of federal education laws, services in health care settings are authorized under insurance requirements, which primarily are based on the requirements of Medicare. As mentioned earlier in this chapter, unless a client is paying directly for services (e.g., private pay) in a private practice setting, all other speech, language, and audiology services are paid for through third-party payers, all of whom have specific regulations. Health care settings include hospitals, rehabilitation centers, home health care, skilled nursing facilities, or other long-term care settings. In some cases, private practice and university clinic settings may also accept and bill Medicare and other health insurance.

Documentation in health care settings is all about reimbursement and may require a "shift in thinking" for speech-language pathologists and audiologists, who may believe documentation should focus on procedures and performance (Coleman, Majerus, Meska, & Goulding, 2008). According to Hapner (2008), increased scrutiny on the need for skilled services and therapy caps increases the attention that speech-language pathologists and audiologists need to pay to documentation. Additionally, remember that the individuals who are reviewing claims are typically not speech-language pathologists or audiologists. Consequently, clinicians in these settings need to be sure they not only know the requirements but also document so someone outside of the profession can understand the notes (Coleman et al., 2008; Hapner, 2008; Sutherland Cornett, 2006; Swigert, 2003). Reviewers need to be able to determine easily if the services are medically necessary and that criteria are met (Coleman et al., 2008).

Swigert's (2018) guidance is to consider the many reasons for documentation, including: client management, sharing information with others, basis for review of records, serving as a business document, and serving as a legal document. Hapner (2008) warns, "Poor record keeping poses a threat to evaluation and follow-through with therapy, to insurance reimbursement, and to the development of a clinical record that meets legal standards" (p. 33).

Medicare provides health insurance for individuals who are over 65 years of age and for individuals with certain disabling conditions. Medicare is divided into two programs: Medicare Part A and Medicare Part B. Part A is hospital insurance and covers services provided in hospitals, skilled nursing facilities, home health care services, and hospice. Part B services cover physician services, audiology testing services, outpatient services, and rehabilitation services (ASHA, n.d.-d). Telepractice is also an acceptable way to deliver speech-language and audiology services under Medicare (ASHA, n.d.-h). Documentation requirements are the same.

Billing and documentation under Medicare are extremely complex. This chapter provides general information about documentation issues under the Medicare system; however, specifics about codes, fees, and other related issues are not addressed here. ASHA's website and the website for the Centers for Medicare & Medicaid Services (CMS) have information that is particularly helpful.

Clinical notes are required under Medicare for purposes of billing and documenting services. The documents include evaluation notes, treatment encounter notes, progress notes, and discharge notes. An important part of documentation in health care settings is the billing codes. There are three types of codes: CPT codes, HCPCS codes, and ICD-10-CM codes (Table 20–6). The system of codes is regulated by the CMS, which has established recognized codes under HIPAA (ASHA, n.d.-b).

Although billing codes, their updates, and changes often dominate discussions about documentation in health care settings, Hapner (2008) clarifies the importance of clinical note writing:

- allows documentation of events, findings, and clinical impressions during encounters with patients;

- enhances clinical follow-through with the transfer of information from evaluation to intervention, or from session-to-session to ensure the progression of therapy;

- is used to transfer information from speech-language pathologist to physician; or

- is used to transfer information from one speech-language pathologist to another to

- continue the clinical process (p. 34).

Medicare requires that services provided need to be "reasonable and necessary." The ASHA document *Speech-Language Pathology Medical Review Guidelines* (ASHA, 2015) identifies the documentation required to establish the basic elements of coverage:

- The services must be consistent with the standards found in the Medicare manuals, Local Coverage Determinations, and guidelines and literature from the professions.

- The services can only be safely and effectively performed by a skilled speech-language pathologist due to the level of intricacy of the service or the clinical complexity of the patient.

- The patient's diagnosis may not be the only factor in determining reasonable or necessary. The patient's need for skilled services must be evident in the documentation.

- The amount, frequency, and duration of therapy must be accepted standards of care as documented by professional guidelines and literature (p. 8).

Types of Clinical Documentation

Creation of a clinical record provides "an overall indicator of clinical service and quality, and serves as a basis for planning care and for service continuity" (Sutherland Cornett, 2006, p. 3). Each of the different types of notes has specific requirements, depending on the purpose of the note.

Evaluation notes require the following:

- Documentation of diagnosis, description of problem, date of onset, current functional status

- Use of standardized measures for objective testing to document patient status

- Statement of prognosis and time frame for therapy

Table 20–6. Billing Code Systems

Code System	Abbreviation	Services Covered	Administrator
Current Procedural Terminology	CPT	Procedures or services	American Medical Association (AMA)
Healthcare Common Procedures Coding System	HCPCS	Devices, supplies, equipment	Centers for Medicare and Medicaid Services (CMS)
International Classification System of Diseases, 10th Revision, Clinical Modification	ICD-10-CM	Diagnoses and disorders	National Center for Health Statistics

Source: Adapted from ASHA (n.d.-c): https://www.asha.org/practice/reimbursement/coding/code_intro/

- List of prognostic indicators that will be used to determine progress

- Barriers to progress

- Medications

Treatment encounter notes require the following:

- Documentation of every treatment day and of every treatment service

- Record of all skilled interventions and justification of need for billing purposes

- Identifying information, treatment provided, signature of professional providing the service

- Total treatment time

- Comprehensive information so that another clinician could conduct follow-up therapy with a reasonable expectation to progress in the therapeutic process

- Tip: Use SOAP note format (see Table 20–5).

- Tip: Include ICD-10 and CPT codes in notes to assist the reviewer.

Discharge notes require the following:

- A summary of all treatment provided

- A statement regarding progress or lack thereof and the reason for discharge

- A statement that the therapist agrees with discharge

The use of the following documentation tools are allowed to support claims:

- ASHA National Outcome Measurement System (NOMS)

- Functional Communication Measures (FCM) for reporting on the Physician Quality Reporting Initiative (PQRI)

- Continuity Assessment Record and Evaluation (CARE) as of October 2019

Plan of care and progress notes require the following:

- Inclusion in the clinical record

- Documentation of medical necessity and need for ongoing service

- Physician certification and approval of the care and treatment plan every 30 days

- Any changes to long-term and short-term goals, and the plan of care

- Completion after evaluation but before treatment begins; signed by treating physician

- Diagnosis, medical condition that relates to the speech/language diagnosis, long-term goals, frequency, and duration of treatment

- Tip: Be sure to include "PLAN OF CARE" on the note so the reviewer knows what it is.

(ASHA, n.d.-g; Hapner, 2008; Sutherland Cornett, 2006)

Coleman et al. (2008) report that denials of Medicaid claims are typically due to either failure to justify medical necessity (i.e., linking the medical diagnosis to the change in functioning abilities) or failure to justify the use of skilled services (i.e., making a skilled analysis and determining the need for treatment through a review of the objective data gathered from patient performance). For residents in skilled nursing facilities (SNFs), goal writing needs to be based on the requirements of the 1990 Omnibus Reconciliation Act, which calls for functional goals and outcomes for the resident. Specialized forms exist for these purposes. Use of SOAP notes, justification of medical necessity for treatment, and the previously stated requirements for progress notes are also suggested by these authors for use in the SNF. The advent of electronic medical records (EMRs) has created some improvements and efficiencies in documentation in health care settings (Swigert, 2018).

Although information provided here deals primarily with Medicare requirements, private health plans also cover speech-language and audiology services. As stated, many plans match or model Medicare requirements, but individual plans do vary in the amount, type, and conditions covered. Most services provided in hospitals are generally covered, but there are variations among plans (e.g., health maintenance organizations, preferred provider organizations, and individual, indemnity, or fee-for-service). The benefits authorized under any plan should always be researched prior to treatment (ASHA, n.d.-f). The writing guidelines are the same for both Medicaid and Medicare.

Documentation in Private Practice and University Clinics

Speech-language pathologists and audiologists working in private practice settings may have a variety of different types of clients and payers. Regardless of the type of client or who is funding the service, clinical notes are expected in accordance with the ASHA Code of Ethics (ASHA, 2016), although the type of client and payer may dictate the form of the notes.

Speech-language pathologists in private practice were not able to bill Medicare until July 1, 2009, following the passage of the Medicare Improvements for Patients and Providers Act of 2008 (MIPPA). An advisory on Medicare billing for speech-language pathologists in private practice is available at the CMS website (Centers for Medicare & Medicaid Services [CMS], n.d.-a).

Speech-language pathologists and audiologists in private practice who take private insurance may belong to networks within health maintenance organizations (HMOs) or preferred provider organizations (PPOs). Some private practitioners do not want to deal directly with insurance companies and the paperwork of billing. In these cases, private practitioners may require their patients or their families to pay directly for the service and then provide them with the appropriate forms with codes to bill for reimbursement.

Some speech-language pathologists may serve in other capacities, such as providing contract services to school districts; providing vendor services to early childhood agencies, courts, or other social service agencies; or establishing themselves as nonpublic agencies for specific contracting possibilities with public schools. Other speech-language pathologists may develop a relationship with a private school and take referrals from the private school or work with cases when students need services. In these situations, the private practitioner may be paid by the school or directly by the student's parent. In each of these situations, the type of documentation depends on who is paying for the service and that entity's documentation requirements. However, the professional requirements discussed in this chapter remain, regardless of who is paying for the service.

Private practice is the only setting in which direct fee-for-service may be received. In these cases, documentation for service is not established based on a third-party payer's requirements, but a client paying by fee-for-service, who still requires a billing statement. Therapy notes, including progress notes, should be maintained as part of keeping appropriate clinical records consistent with all of the reasons previously outlined in this chapter.

Services in university clinics may be provided by student clinicians or by university staff. Clients who receive services from students sign a contract indicating that they are aware that a student who is supervised will be providing the services. Universities use these clinics to teach students the art of documentation. If a faculty or staff member is providing services, the university may bill private insurance, Medicare, or Medicaid, or take private pay. Currently, university clinics billing Medicare

and Medicaid is a big issue. It is not within the scope of this chapter to discuss that issue, but students and faculty may find themselves involved in these discussions.

Documentation for Audiological Services

Audiologists who work in school settings follow all of the procedures discussed in the section on Documentation in Educational Settings. Audiologists in school settings typically provide testing such as hearing screening, pure-tone testing, otoacoustic emissions, and impedance audiometry. Additionally, educational audiologists provide consultative services and fitting and oversight of hearing aids, FM systems, and possibly mapping management of cochlear implants. Medically based audiological testing is not part of school-based services. Under Medicare, hearing and balance testing is covered under "other diagnostic tests," but Medicare has no provision to pay for routine hearing testing or audiological therapeutic services (CMS, n.d.-b). Audiology services must come from a physician's referral. Some private insurance providers require prior authorization, especially for certain procedures.

According to ASHA (n.d.-e), requirements include documenting the details of a physician's referral, services performed, and the follow-up provided to the physician. Requirements for documenting audiological testing are included in Chapter 15, section 80.3 of *The Medicare Benefit Manual* (CMS, n.d.-a), which includes the following:

Documenting for Audiological Tests. The reason for the test should be documented either on the order, and/or the audiological evaluation report, and/or in the patient's medical record. Examples of appropriate reasons include, but are not limited to:

- Evaluation of suspected change in hearing, tinnitus, or balance

- Evaluation of the cause of disorders of hearing, tinnitus, or balance

- Determination of the effect of medication, surgery or other treatments

Information on CPT codes and other requirements for audiology under Medicare can be found on the ASHA websites provided or from CMS. All of the information provided previously regarding Medicare documentation applies when appropriate to audiology services, but the specifics of documentation are too complex and lengthy for this chapter.

Audiologists who work in private practice or other clinical settings are often dispensing audiologists. Fitting and selling hearing aids involves documentation related to these activities. ASHA scope of practice documents, guidelines, and state licensure laws have information pertinent to any requirements and necessary documentation.

Summary

Learning to keep clear, concise, and complete documentation is one of the best habits a clinician can develop. The benefits of appropriate documentation extend first and foremost to providing appropriate clinical care to the student/client/patient, then to the employer and payer for compliance, and finally to the provider to ensure development of a legal record and to meet mandates for reimbursement. Lack of adequate documentation can lead to numerous types of problems, with time and energy then needed to contest, follow up, and challenge issues related to the lack of documentation.

This chapter attempted to define issues related to documentation in all settings in which speech-language pathologists and audiologists work. While each setting has its own requirements and standards, there is no doubt that conducting high-level professional services includes both the delivery of competent services as well as the documentation of these services because "if it's not documented, it didn't happen."

Critical Thinking

1. What skills do you think are important in writing good clinical evaluation reports versus other types of written documentation?

2. As a student, you are frequently required to write "lengthy" clinical evaluation reports, yet in the real clinical world, your reports will be more brief. What is the rationale for learning to write long, comprehensive reports?

3. How do technology and the internet affect documentation in our professions? What are the advantages and disadvantages of using technology for documentation?

4. Suppose you feel pressure from a parent to alter a report so that a child might access clinical services. What does our Code of Ethics say about fraudulent documentation? What would you do in this case?

5. What do you think when you read another clinician's reports that have obvious stylistic errors, numerous acronyms, and typographical errors? How should you ensure that you are using standard American English writing skills in your own documentation?

6. What federal laws guide our documentation in school and medical settings?

7. Ask to review a diagnostic report from your current clinic. What features do you like about the report? What could be improved? What would a professional from another discipline think about the report? Does it make a convincing case in a focused, clear, and succinct manner?

8. You work in the public schools, and a professor who teaches diagnostic methods has asked you to be on a panel and address her class about report writing in the educational setting. What would be five suggestions you would give students to help them write effective reports in the schools?

9. How do you think that electronic report writing has affected our report-writing skills in medical settings? What are the advantages and disadvantages of this style of report writing?

References

American Speech-Language-Hearing Association. (2015). *Speech-language pathology medical review guidelines*. Retrieved from http://www.asha.org/uploadedFiles/SLP-Medical-Review-Guidelines.pdf

American Speech-Language-Hearing Association. (2016). *Code of ethics* [Ethics]. Available from http://www.asha.org/policy/

American Speech-Language-Hearing Association. (n.d.-a). *Documentation in schools.* Retrieved from https://www.asha.org/PRPSpecificTopic.aspx?folder id=8589942597&section=Key_Issues

American Speech-Language-Hearing Association. (n.d.-b). *Individualized education programs.* Retrieved from https://www.asha.org/SLP/schools/IEPs/

American Speech-Language-Hearing Association. (n.d.-c). *Introduction to billing code systems.* Retrieved from https://www.asha.org/practice/reimbursement/coding/code_intro/

American Speech-Language-Hearing Association. (n.d.-d). *Medicare.* Retrieved from http://www.asha.org/public/coverage/medicare.htm

American Speech-Language-Hearing Association. (n.d.-e). *Medicare frequently asked questions:*

Audiology. Retrieved from http://www.asha.org/ Practice/reimbursement/medicare/audiology medicare-FAQs/

American Speech-Language-Hearing Association. (n.d.-f). *Private health plans: An overview.* Retrieved from http://www.asha.org/practice/ reimbursement/private-plans/overview/

American Speech-Language-Hearing Association. (n.d.-g). *Speech-language pathology and the Physician Quality Reporting System.* Retrieved from http:// www.asha.org/Members/research/NOMS/ PQRI/

American Speech-Language-Hearing Association. (n.d.-h). *Telepractice.* Retrieved from https:// www.asha.org/practice-portal/professional-issues/ telepractice/

Americans with Disabilities Act (ADA), 42 U.S.C. §§ 12101 *et seq.* (1990).

Association of California School Administrators. (2006). *Handbook of goals and objectives related to state of California content standards.* Sacramento, CA: Author.

Centers for Medicare & Medicaid Services. (n.d.-a). *Medicare billing for speech-language pathologists in private practice.* Retrieved from https://www.cms .gov/MLNProducts/downloads/ SpeechLangPath fctsht.pdf

Centers for Medicare & Medicaid Services. (n.d.-b). *Audiology services.* Retrieved from https://www.cms .gov/Medicare/Medicare-Fee-for-Service-Payment/ PhysicianFeeSched/Audiology.html

Code of Federal Regulations, Title 34, 504.3. Section 504 of the Rehabilitation Act of 1973.

Code of Federal Regulations, Title 34, 300.320. Individuals with Disabilities Education Improve-ment Act of 2004.

Coleman, J., Majerus, N. J., Meska, S., & Goulding, B. (2008). *Special challenges of documenting SLP services in the LTC setting.* Retrieved from http:// www.asha.org/Events/convention/ handouts/2008/ 2228_Goulding_Bill.htm

Elementary and Secondary Education Act (ESEA), 20 U.S.C. §§ 2701 *et seq.* (1965).

Every Student Succeeds Act (ESSA), 20 USC 6301 (2015).

Family Educational Rights and Privacy Act (FERPA), 20 U.S.C. §§ 1232g (1974).

Hapner, E. R. (2008, March). Documentation that works [Abstract]. *Perspectives on Voice and Voice*

Disorders, 33–42. Retrieved from http://div3per spectives.asha.org/cgi/content/ abstract/18/1/33

Health Insurance Portability and Accountability Act (HIPAA), 45 CFR Parts 160, 162, and 164 (2002).

Individuals with Disabilities Education Improvement Act of 2004 (IDEA), 20 U.S.C. §§ 614[d][A][i][I].

Medicare Improvements for Patients and Providers Act of 2008, Pub. L. No. 110-275. Retrieved from http://www.gpo.gov/fdsys/pkg/PLAW-110publ275/ pdf/PLAW-110publ275.pdf

Moore, B. J. (2010a). *Documentation for SLPs and audiologists in schools* [Audio program]. Rockville, MD: American Speech-Language-Hearing Association.

Moore, B. J. (2010b). If it's not documented, it didn't happen. *Perspectives on Administration and Supervi-sion*, *20*, 106–110.

Moore, B. (2018). Documentation and reimburse-ment in pediatrics: School settings. In N. Swiggert (Ed.), *Documentation and reimbursement for speech-language pathologists: Principles and practice.* Thorofare, NJ: SLACK, Inc.

Moore, B. J., & Montgomery, J. K. (2018). *Speech-language pathologists in public schools: Making a difference for America's children* (3rd ed.). Austin, TX: Pro-Ed.

National Governors Association Center for Best Practices, Council of Chief State School Officers. (2010). *Common core state standards.* Washington, DC: Author. Retrieved from http://www.corestan dards.org

No Child Left Behind Act of 2001, 20 U.S.C. SS 6311 *et seq.* (2002).

Omnibus Reconciliation Act of 1990, Pub.L. No. 101-508. Retrieved from http://www.law.cornell .edu/usc-cgi/get_external.cgi?type=pubL&target =101-508

Rehabilitation Act of 1973, 29 U.S.C. § 794, Section 504 (1973).

Rudebusch, J. (2008). *The source for RTI.* East Moline, IL: LinguiSystems.

Sutherland Cornett, B. (2006). Clinical documenta-tion in speech-language pathology: Essential information for successful practice. *ASHA Leader*, *11*(12), 8–25.

Swigert, N. (2003). Dollars and documentation. *Perspectives on swallowing and swallowing disorders (dysphagia)*, *12*(2), 32.

Swigert, N. (Ed.). (2018). Introduction. In *Documentation and reimbursement for speech-language pathologists: Principles and practice*. Thorofare, NJ: SLACK Inc.

U.S. Department of Education. (2011, February). *The Family Educational Rights and Privacy Act: Guidance for eligible students*. Retrieved from http://ed.gov/policy/gen/guid/fpco/ferpa/for-eligible-students.pdf

U.S. Department of Education. (n.d.). *Questions and answers about student records*. Retrieved from https://www2.ed.gov/about/overview/focus/daca-education-records.pdf

Wallach, G. P. (2008). *Language intervention for school-age students: Setting goals for academic success*. St. Louis, MO: Mosby Elsevier.

Resources

American Psychological Association. (2010). *Publication manual* (6th ed.). Washington, DC: Author.

American Speech-Language-Hearing Association. (2011). *Coding for reimbursement frequently asked questions: Speech-language pathology*. Retrieved from http://www.asha.org/practice/reimbursement/coding/coding_faqs_slp.htm

Association of California School Administrators. http://www.acsa.org/

Goldfarb, R., & Serpanos, Y. (2011). *Professional writing in speech-language pathology and audiology*. San Diego, CA: Plural Publishing.

Hacker, D. (2000). *Rules for writers*. Boston, MA: Bedford/St. Martin's.

Lamar University. (n.d.). *Professional writing*. Retrieved from http://dept.lamar.edu/cofac/deptspeech/files/professional_writing.pdf

NHIC Corp. (2010). *Physical, occupational & speech therapy billing guide*. Retrieved from http://www.medicarenhic.com/providers/pubs/Physical%20and%20Occupational%20therapy%20Guide.pdf

Purdue Online Writing Lab (OWL). http://owl.english.purdue.edu/

Shipley, K., & McAfee, J. (2008.) *Assessment in speech-language pathology* (4th ed.). Clifton Park, NY: Delmar Cengage Learning.

Stein-Rubin, C., & Fabus, R. (2012). *A guide to clinical assessment and professional report writing in speech-language pathology*. Clifton Park, NY: Delmar Cengage Learning.

21

Developing Leadership Skills

◇◇

Gail J. Richard, PhD

Introduction

We all function as leaders in our everyday lives, whether we realize it or not. As speech-language pathologists and audiologists, we assume responsibility for the well-being of our clients. They depend on us to evaluate and diagnose the communication disorder that is negatively impacting their lives. They trust us to determine an appropriate treatment plan to address the presenting deficits. The very nature of our professions requires that we responsibly communicate impressions and suggested interventions with confidence and authority to the clients we serve. In our clinical practice, research lab, or academic classroom, we function as a leader—influencing others to bring about change.

Wikipedia (2019) defines leadership as a practical skill regarding the ability to guide other individuals, teams or organizations. Yukl (1981) described leadership as the process of influencing or directing others to follow. Leadership is an interactive process to bring about change in working toward a common goal (Ebener, 2012).

The arena of leadership can be as small as our individual work setting or as large as a national platform. Leadership can be part of our work responsibilities, such as supervision of an assistant, student intern, or colleague. We might function as a department or division chair in a hospital or university. Other leadership experiences might be with volunteer service activities in the community or with a professional association at a regional, state, or national level. There are many steps and stages to developing expertise in leadership during our lifetime. There are different types of leadership opportunities, each requiring a certain skill set to be effective. We rely on individuals in leadership positions to make positive changes in our lives. We admire and respect their ability and commitment to make a difference. Most of us aspire to be effective when we are in a responsible leadership position. This chapter is intended to provide you with some inspiration and aspirational information to consider as you reflect on progressing down a pathway to leadership.

Roles of a Leader

"Leadership is a role or a function, not a person or a position" (Ebener, 2012). The goal of a leader is to facilitate a group effort to achieve certain objectives. Leadership style depends on the goal, the make-up of individuals in the group, and personality traits of the individual in charge. However, there are certain roles that a leader must assume when taking charge in a situation. How the role is fulfilled can vary, based on the individual, but effective leaders must be aware of the important role they play at various times. Five of those roles are discussed in the following section, specifically that of a motivator, organizer, influencer, mediator, and spokesperson. Aspects are also addressed in the discussion of leadership characteristics.

Motivator

Most individuals agree to serve in a leadership capacity because they have a vested interest or passion for the outcome. Even reluctant leaders accept the role of leadership because they believe an initiative is important and will make a positive difference. One of the challenges is to share that vision with clients, employees, colleagues, or members in an organization to inspire their cooperation in achieving the desired outcome. The leader must actively work to prevent discouragement or frustration when efforts stall or are not successful. Motivating others to become involved, coordinating efforts, and working cooperatively are important roles for the person in charge. Stay positive and maintain focus on the group's progress rather than on setbacks or problems.

Organizer

It is a leader's responsibility to ensure that people's valuable time is utilized effectively. Establish an agenda for meetings and maintain the timeframe. Gather relevant information and keep discussion focused by reiterating facts to minimize emotional statements. Don't allow tangents or personal topics to derail the meeting. Frame discussion by introducing background information, the issue at hand, and the desired outcome. Once discussion is over, clearly state the resulting action to bring closure to the topic. An example for framing discussion would be the following: "At the previous meeting there were some unresolved questions regarding possible placement options that could provide the necessary accommodations for this student to be successful. The case manager has done additional research and visited some programs. We'll let her share impressions and options. Please ask questions so we can reach a recommended decision before we adjourn today."

Influencer

Strategic thinking must always be aligned with the organization's priorities (Axelrod, 2016). An effective leader will anticipate potential problems and be prepared to address difficult issues. Information should be presented in an objective factual manner, and always consider all aspects of an issue to avoid bias. Individuals are more likely to resist suggestions if they feel that material is skewed or being presented from only one perspective. Constructive debate is important to explore divergent views, but the leader must guide the group back to a collective agreement on decisions. Listing advantages and disadvantages is one method to consider all perspectives while weighting the advantages toward the desired outcome. A skilled leader is able to subtly move opinions toward the objective without dictating the desired direction.

Mediator

Leadership is not without risk (Heifetz & Linsky, 2002). People will resist change and emotions can be intense when controversial decisions are introduced. Don't allow tensions to escalate or remain unresolved. The sooner a problem is addressed, the less likely it will grow out of proportion. Listen to where people are and help the group see the benefit of considering other options or compromising on a position. Manage a dominant personality by acknowledging his concern and then reiterate the follow-up options to bring closure to his turn at speaking. It is important to deal with conflict in a factual way and not take dissension personally. An effective leader will carefully avoid becoming defensive, will listen calmly and attentively, and try to resolve problematic issues in a reasonable and equitable manner.

Spokesperson

As a leader, you are often the spokesperson for the group you represent. Poise in front of a group is an important aspect of effective communication. A leader who uses lots of verbal fillers, such as "you know, um, like," can be annoying to listen to in a large group setting. Ineffective speaking can compromise the message. There is a great deal of research in communication studies and political science regarding the listener's focus on *how* the message is presented rather than the actual content. When speaking in front of a group, be articulate, clear, and focused. Prepare notes for reference to stay on topic and avoid rambling or going off on personal tangents. It is not about you; the communication is about the information you are sharing.

Effective Leadership Skills

There are a variety of characteristics that epitomize an effective leader. In fact, the list could be quite extensive. To organize and highlight some of the primary traits, the following list uses the acronym of *leadership* to discuss some of the important skills exemplified by effective leaders.

L	Listen
E	Efficient
A	Access
D	Dependable
E	Expectations
R	Responsive
S	Share
H	Hierarchy
I	Innovative
P	Prioritize

L: Engage in Active Listening

William Shakespeare said, "Give every man thine ear but few thy voice" (Sisson, 1960). Good advice for an effective leader! When facilitating a group, it is critically important to ask questions and listen carefully to the opinions being expressed. Committee members will not appreciate being told what to think or do. A leader who imposes his own agenda will usually fail to engage members in thoughtful discussion and participation in the project. An effective leader allows members to express their viewpoints and uses that information to subtly guide the group in the desired direction.

Active listening is a technique that focuses the group on the speaker (Kummer, 2011). As a leader, you set an example for courteous and respectful attention when others are expressing their thoughts. Principles of active listening suggest that you not interrupt and try to avoid imposing your own perspective on the speaker's comments. Acknowledge the speaker by showing interest nonverbally, such as nodding or maintaining an attentive body posture. Questions should be framed for clarification or additional information rather than challenging the speaker's viewpoint.

Careful listening allows the leader to gauge the position of a group and determine the necessary next steps to productively move an agenda item forward. Additional information might need to be generated or provided, or further clarification could be necessary if there is confusion. If the group seems comfortable and there is a general sense of consensus, then the leader should close discussion and move to resolution or the desired action.

E: Be Efficient

An effective leader needs to be efficient and organized. The leader's role is to facilitate the work of the group. Volunteers or employees who are dedicating their time to an initiative will not appreciate sitting in a meeting if they feel their time is being wasted. Good facilitation of a meeting requires extensive preparation and anticipation of all contingencies. An agenda and materials should be provided so members arrive confident and prepared for the work to be addressed. A leader who is disorganized and floundering in a meeting generates frustration and confusion, leading to other members trying to take control. As a result, little will be accomplished, and the group will lose confidence in the leader's ability to direct the actions of the group.

An aspect of efficiency in conducting a meeting is knowing when to continue discussion on an item and when to move on. It is not unusual for debate to become redundant, with multiple speakers reiterating the same point. It is also possible for one individual who disagrees with the group to continue emphasizing his point after other speakers express an opinion. The leader conducting the meeting can request that only new ideas be expressed and that individuals who have already spoken refrain from speaking again. This provides all participants with an opportunity to express their perspective without belaboring the same points.

A: Access Resources

An aspect of being organized is the ability to access appropriate resources to ensure that members have adequate information to make informed decisions. Good leadership doesn't function in a vacuum; it relies on data and knowledge from a variety of sources. Don't be afraid to say, "I don't know the answer to that, but I will find out and get back to you." It is not unusual for individuals to introduce statements to support their position that are not always grounded in fact. Rumor and innuendo can quickly derail a project and cause group members to question or lose confidence in an agreed upon plan. It is imperative that a leader gather information that is objective and factual so the group can make knowledge-based decisions.

An effective leader also consciously works on developing networks of support resources that can be accessed when questions arise. It is not necessary to reinvent the wheel if someone else has experience with a certain situation and can offer advice. The use of consultants or specialists can be extremely beneficial when a group is exploring new options and requires additional information. Engaging in multiple types of experiences over time will lead to building a network of colleagues that can be accessed for advice, questions, and guidance.

D: Be Dependable

Mark Twain said, "Always do what is right. This will gratify some people and astonish the rest." A leader must be dependable and responsible. It is difficult to follow the direction of a leader who isn't consistent and supportive of his co-workers. Simple actions, such as being on time or following through to complete expected tasks, can help to instill confidence in leadership.

Being dependable also implies that the actions of a leader are conducted with integrity. Colleagues need to be able to trust the individual in charge and rely on the fact that the leader will work cooperatively with them to accomplish joint initiatives. The leader should be a role model who instills trust and accepts responsibility for the actions taken by the group.

E: Establish Expectations

It is important for a leader to establish clear expectations. Colleagues working together need to know their responsibilities. Timelines should be established and reviewed on a regular basis to determine progress toward goals. Sequenced objectives or steps should be spelled out for general agreement and consensus. If an individual is not meeting his responsibilities, the leader should have a private conversation with him to clarify specific actions that need to be completed. One suggestion is to prepare a graph listing each action item, the date for completion, and name(s) of individuals responsible for addressing the item. The graph can be reviewed and modified as necessary, but it provides a concrete iteration to avoid any confusion regarding expectations for the group.

R: Respond in a Timely Manner

Procrastination and avoidance are banes to effective leadership. Persons in charge must be responsive to individuals with whom they are working. Questions and requests for information should be addressed as quickly as possible. If there are complications or issues that necessitate additional work, inform colleagues of the problem and reassure them that you will be back in touch as soon as possible. When colleagues complete assigned tasks, praise their efforts and acknowledge the work done. It is important that people feel rewarded and appreciated for their efforts.

S: Share Ideas

Consistent communication is essential in moving actions forward in an organization. Sharing ideas in a transparent way keeps everyone informed on progress and decisions. No one likes to feel like they aren't informed or included in information-sharing. Surprises regarding group initiatives are not necessarily a good thing in an organization.

Effective leaders communicate *with* other people, not to them. They bring a collaborative spirit to the group that encourages engagement of all members. There will be individual differences in the way that members participate, ranging from the very vocal to the quiet assimilators. But an effective leader is able to conduct discussion in a way that invites everyone to share her ideas and viewpoints. The exchange of ideas, both positive and negative, leads to healthy and robust debate that fosters better agreement when moving actions forward.

H: Develop a Hierarchy of Leadership Skills

Leadership is a skill that can be learned but requires patience and a variety of different experiences. As you have read through some of the characteristics discussed in this section, it should become apparent that not every leader will be well versed in all these skills, and certainly not during initial leadership activities. Individuals will have different strengths and weaknesses in their leadership attributes. An effective leader is aware of her strong points and knows how to compensate or work on improving areas in which she is not as proficient.

There are many types of opportunities to develop leadership skills. When I served as President of the American Speech-Language-Hearing Association in 2017, I overheard students commenting that they aspired to be ASHA president. That is a laudable goal, but not one that I ever anticipated for myself. Many volunteer opportunities preceded my achieving that prestigious position. I participated in numerous and varied volunteer service and employment positions before I felt ready to pursue that office. But in each activity, I had the opportunity to develop and improve the many leadership skills that are encompassed in effectively leading a national association. Some activities allowed me to focus on verbal presentation skills, some provided opportunities to learn how to deal with conflict and controversy, others taught me how to effectively organize and run meetings. There are numerous aspects to effective leadership. Small focused steps to develop leadership skills require a conscious effort to realistically evaluate our talents and specifically target areas to improve. Soliciting feedback from trusted colleagues who will provide constructive criticism is invaluable in promoting the continued evolution of leadership skills. The section on Pathways to Leadership further expands on this topic.

I: Be Innovative

"We can't solve problems by using the same kind of thinking we used when we created them." This quote attributed to Albert Einstein provides some insight regarding the importance of thinking creatively. One characteristic of an effective leader is the ability to be flexible in approaching issues. While there is merit to sharing a historical perspective on how things were addressed in the past, it is also important to explore different options. Problems can be approached as opportunities to try something new. Every obstacle has a solution if we have the patience and courage to take some risks with creative thinking.

As a leader, visionary thinking is a beneficial attribute. However, it is important to bring the group along for the journey. Sometimes the leader is far advanced from where other members are and needs to slow down and explain how she arrived at a new idea. A leader must also be open and flexible to alternative suggestions, giving them appropriate attention and discussion rather than just dismissing them. There can also be what are referred to as CAVE dwellers in the group—individuals who are *consistently against virtually everything*. An effective leader knows how to share innovative ideas in a positive non-threatening way so other members can embrace the possibilities and give them due consideration.

P: Prioritize

An effective leader is able to discriminate primary goals so that essential energy can be committed to achieving them. In any given day, there are many issues to be addressed. Leadership requires the ability to determine which items are most important, will have an impact, and will be a good investment of time and resources. Prioritizing within a leadership role is constant—agenda items, actions to be taken, discussion issues to introduce, delegation of assignments, etc. Efficiency is enhanced with effective prioritization in available time units.

Multiple ideas and initiatives can be part of any group's agenda. An effective leader knows how to prioritize and focus the members. The threat of not seeing the forest among the trees is a saying that resonates with leadership skills. Tangential discussion needs to be controlled and minimized. Off-target discussion tends to dilute energy and waste time, leading to frustration. The leader of a group maintains focus on the big picture, or main objective, so that members experience a sense of accomplishment for their efforts.

Reflection on Leadership Characteristics

The list of characteristics provided is intended to illustrate some of the primary skills that effective leaders demonstrate. It is certainly not exhaustive. It might be beneficial to take a moment and reflect on individuals who you believe demonstrate exceptional leadership.

What are the characteristics that you admire in their repertoire of abilities? Use that reflection to compile your own list of leadership traits that you aspire to develop and master. Individualize the list based on your personal strengths and areas that might need more attention.

Resources in the area of leadership are plentiful. Take time to access some of the many books and modules on leadership styles. Part of effective leadership is recognizing your own manner of interacting with people and utilizing a style that is comfortable and compatible with your personality. Don't try to become something that conflicts with your inherent nature. Adopting a certain leadership style because it sounds good doesn't mean it will work effectively for you. Strong leaders embrace their best attributes and acknowledge aspects that are challenging for them. For example, I am a "doer" and am very aware of the need to be patient and allow time for group members to assimilate information before pushing forward. Going a bit slower helps to prevent conflict, defensiveness, and having to go back and re-explain things. Making sure questions have been answered and everyone has the knowledge to move forward results in improved consensus and overall efficiency.

Pathways to Leadership

Developing leadership skills is a lifetime activity. Leadership develops over time as an individual participates in a variety of different types of experiences. There is a saying that most great leaders start out as great followers. The skills involved are developed and enhanced through modeling and mentoring.

I want to share an email I received from a student several years ago that helps to illustrate one of the most important first steps along the pathway to leadership —observing effective leaders. I've taken the liberty of modifying some wording to clarify, but the message is intact from this remarkable young woman. She was a student-athlete who served on one of my committees. She was then selected to be the student representative on a search committee that I served as Chair to hire a new Director of Athletics. She never spoke to me about her experience serving with me, but her email is one that I have kept and treasured for years.

Dr. Richard,

I wanted to tell you, whether you know it or not, about the impact you had on me while enrolled at the university. As a member of the Intercollegiate Athletic Board, I observed you leading meetings and organizing all of the work we accomplished. I also served on the Director of Athletics search committee. This is where I learned the most from you. I volunteered to be the student representative on the search committee to gain interview experience for my future. I asked my coach for advice and he told me to "watch Dr. Richard question the candidates and you will learn a lot." Not sure what to expect and a little intimidated, I went to the first on-campus interview looking forward to the experience. Watching you interview the candidates, observe their behavior and responses, and then listen to your evaluation of each candidate in post-interview discussion was invaluable and a priceless learning experience.

With this experience I was able to apply those skills to be selected for a paid internship at Boeing. Out of over 1,000 applicants, Boeing interviewed the top 20. Going into my first-ever interview, I felt surprising calm and prepared. Unbeknownst to you, "Coach Richard," I relate my success directly to you. I want you to know that you handed me an opportunity to learn and observe, and I am truly grateful for the experience.

My Pathway to Leadership

Strong leaders are not one-dimensional; they participate in a variety of different types of activities that broaden their perspective. Diverse interests provide opportunities to interact with people from all walks of life. Liberal arts colleges often focus their recruitment message on the importance of developing the mind, body, and spirit of students. An individual who only has one all-consuming interest can limit opportunities for that person to explore and appreciate a bigger picture, which is critical in effective leadership.

My pathway to leadership, summarized in Figure 21–1, was an exercise I completed for the ASHA Committee on Leadership Cultivation. My background included activities in theatre, athletics, and speech-language pathology. Theatre developed my skills in public speaking and poise in front of an audience. Athletics taught me the importance of collaboration and teamwork toward a common goal, as well as time management. Speech-language pathology required incredible organization and focus. Clinical skills required innovation, insight, communication, and strategic planning.

My first professional presentations were sharing results from my master's thesis. The topic was one that was familiar and comfortable for me to discuss with other professionals. My first employment position was in the public schools, where I volunteered to provide in-service presentations to teachers. After transitioning to a univer-

sity position, I became involved in committees on campus and volunteered to serve in my state speech-language pathology association. That led to chairing committees, serving on the Executive Board and eventually election to president of the state association. I wanted to learn more about our profession at a national level and was elected to represent my state on the ASHA Legislative Council, which led to leadership positions in that group. Committee membership and serving as committee chair led to the Board of Directors and, finally, President of ASHA.

While pursuing professional volunteer service opportunities, I was also involved in committees at the university, serving and then chairing committees such as Faculty Senate and the University Personnel Committee that makes tenure, retention, and promotion decisions. My involvement in athletics led to being appointed as the National Collegiate Athletics Association (NCAA) Faculty Athletics Representative for the university and serving on the NCAA Management Council for our athletic conference.

All of those experiences contributed toward building my hierarchy of leadership skills that kept me moving down a leadership pathway. I actively sought out some of those experiences due to my interest or passion for the topic. Other opportunities resulted from someone asking if I would serve in a leadership capacity. Not all were positive experiences, but I learned invaluable lessons in each and every activity. Be receptive and willing to participate in opportunities that cross your path.

Your Pathway to Leadership

Leadership allows you to have an impact. It provides an opportunity to choose where to commit your time, energy, and talent. Carefully choose the steps to take as you begin the journey on your leadership pathway. You want to experience success and engage in a positive, rewarding experience that fosters the desire to continue on the pathway.

Initial leadership experiences should focus on activities that you are comfortable and familiar with, or that you have a special passion or interest for. Volunteer service often grows out of frustration with an issue that needs to be addressed. An interest or passion for the topic provides the motivation to stay engaged with the responsibilities that will accompany the commitment. Rather than complain about the way something is being managed, jump in and make it better!

There are many opportunities for committee work as part of your undergraduate and graduate programs. The chance to work with colleagues might arise from fund-raising activities, National Student-Speech-Language-Hearing Association chapter events, or university sponsored events with the community. These are excellent

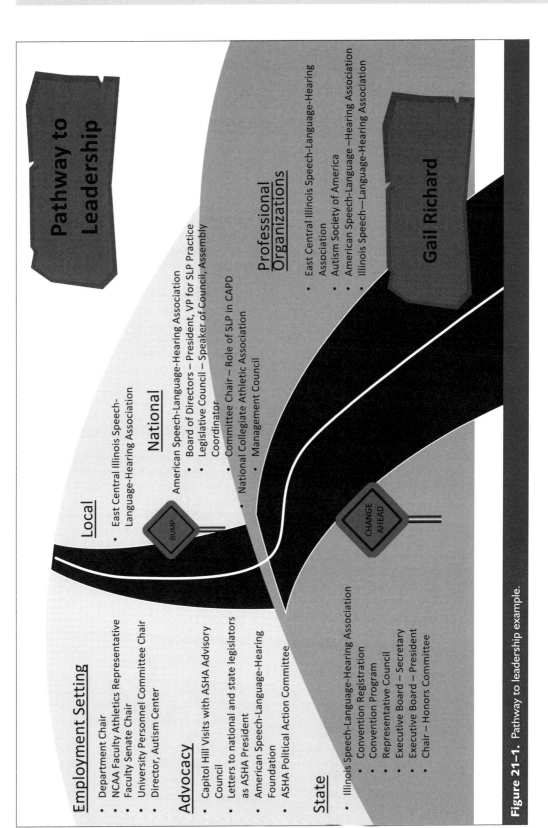

Pathway to Leadership

Employment Setting

- Department Chair
- NCAA Faculty Athletics Representative
- Faculty Senate Chair
- University Personnel Committee Chair
- Director, Autism Center

Advocacy

- Capitol Hill Visits with ASHA Advisory Council
- Letters to national and state legislators as ASHA President
- American Speech-Language-Hearing Foundation
- ASHA Political Action Committee

Local

- East Central Illinois Speech-Language-Hearing Association

National

- American Speech-Language-Hearing Association
  - Board of Directors – President, VP for SLP Practice
  - Legislative Council – Speaker of Council, Assembly Coordinator
  - Committee Chair – Role of SLP in CAPD
- National Collegiate Athletic Association
  - Management Council

State

- Illinois Speech-Language-Hearing Association
  - Convention Registration
  - Convention Program
  - Representative Council
  - Executive Board – Secretary
  - Executive Board – President
  - Chair – Honors Committee

Professional Organizations

- East Central Illinois Speech-Language-Hearing Association
- Autism Society of America
- American Speech-Language –Hearing Association
- Illinois Speech—Language-Hearing Association

Gail Richard

Figure 21–1. Pathway to leadership example.

ways to engage in observing campus leaders or serving as leaders with a support system in place and structure already provided.

Once you graduate, your employment setting will provide opportunities for committee engagement. It might be serving on a committee in the school, hospital, or agency where you work. Offering to provide an in-service for professional colleagues is another great chance to develop early presentation skills to build your repertoire of leadership skills. Share information you acquired by attending a conference in a department meeting. Submit a poster session to the state association convention, where you can interact with colleagues one-on-one. Explore opportunities in your local community or church to broaden the scope and type of volunteer service you participate in, such as Big Brothers, Big Sisters, helping with a fund-raising marathon, or United Way or Habitat projects. Community boards and councils are usually very grateful for volunteer participation.

As you become more skilled, transition to state level activities. Join the state professional association and volunteer to help with their annual meeting. Assist with advocacy and legislative efforts that impact professional services to clients. Committee or board membership often transitions to leadership positions over time. Active engagement in the state association activities gives you opportunities to observe seasoned leaders and begin demonstrating your own leadership.

Engagement with ASHA can be extremely stimulating and rewarding. Consider joining a Special Interest Group (SIG) on a professional topic of interest to you. Each SIG has a coordinating committee, community discussion site, and access to the *Perspectives* journal and sponsors continuing education sessions at the ASHA Convention. Go to the ASHA website and sign up to receive Headlines and Advocacy updates to stay apprised of current events and requests to provide input to legislators. Respond to calls for feedback on issues, attend Membership Forums at sponsored ASHA meetings, and complete the Volunteer Form to express interest in appointment to ASHA committees, boards, and councils. Explore similar activities with other related professional associations that are pertinent to your work setting or area of professional focus.

Take advantage of the many leadership development opportunities sponsored by ASHA. The 2018 Association Media & Publishing Excel Awards recognized ASHA with a bronze award for the Leadership Academy, citing the innovative commitment to providing leadership development activities for its members. The ASHA website for the Leadership Academy (https://community.asha.org/leadershipacademy/home) has training modules for beginning, intermediate, and advanced leadership skills. ASHA offers several leadership and mentoring programs that are designed for more individualized participation. The website includes assessment tools for an individual to examine leadership strengths and areas for improvement, as well as an evaluation of leadership styles and behaviors that are most natural for an individual and can then be incorporated into a personal plan for developing leadership skills. A community discussion site allows electronic interaction for questions, ideas, and insights to be shared. Additional resources and a tool kit are also provided. These resources are available to all members.

Use the example in Figure 21–1 to chart your own leadership pathway. The trail could be very winding with many twists and turns. Embrace the presented opportunities from a variety of sources. There is no right or wrong path and you won't get lost. Each activity will help you better understand and strengthen the traits in your leadership style. It is not unusual for some of our best learning experiences to result from failure or an incident that did not go as smoothly as expected. Observing poor leadership might help us recognize what we don't want to do when in a specific situation. Embrace every opportunity as an exercise to build additional leadership skills.

Fiduciary Responsibilities

As a member of a committee or board, you will be expected to meet fiduciary responsibilities. Fiduciary duty is defined as someone who holds something in trust for another. As a leader, other individuals are expecting the people with authority to act in the best interests of the organization. Decisions should be made on an informed basis, in good faith, and with the intention that the action is in the best interests of the individuals it affects (Gattuso, 2018). Fiduciary responsibilities are generally delineated in three areas:

- Duty of care
- Duty of loyalty
- Duty of fidelity to purpose

These three guiding principles are inherent in good leadership. They ensure that good judgment is exercised in all decisions, conflicts of interest are avoided, assets are used responsibly, and actions are taken using adequate oversight, reflection, and integrity. They are each discussed in more detail in the following section.

Duty of Care

Duty of care addresses the way in which persons should perform their responsibilities as leaders. The individual should be knowledgeable regarding discussion, actions, or decisions that will be made. This ensures that the leader is acting in an informed manner, by having read and reviewed provided data, materials, or other information. He has listened carefully to information presented to further inform the group that has the authority to make decisions.

In addition to being informed, duty of care implies that the individual acts in good faith. Directors must act in what they believe are the best interests of the group they are representing. Given similar circumstances, what decision would other individuals who have entrusted their well-being to this leader determine was the best option? Leaders are protected from personal liability under duty of care if they have acted with the best knowledge available at the time and in good faith that they were protecting the interests of their respective group (Gattuso, 2018).

Regular attendance at meetings is one obvious way to meet duty of care. But being present is not enough to fulfill this responsibility. As previously mentioned, preparation prior to attendance at the meeting is critical to ensure that you are an active engaged participant. Be prepared to ask clarification questions or clearly express an opinion with objective rationale to support your position. Don't be afraid to entertain opposing viewpoints that allow the group to feel that all aspects of an issue have been discussed and carefully considered. Utilize the expertise of others. Sometimes it is prudent to form a committee that is charged with developing an action plan or recommendation that can be brought back to a governing board or group.

Maintaining an official record of meetings is another aspect of duty of care. One mistake that can be made is to allow minutes to become a transcript of the meeting. Minutes should reflect the major agenda items that were addressed. Include specific decisions that were acted upon with appropriate justification or rationale, as well as subsequent steps for implementation. Detailed discussion attributed to specific individuals is not necessary. The minutes should reflect the consensus actions that occurred as a communication vehicle to inform members of the group represented by leaders at the meeting.

Duty of Loyalty

Duty of loyalty means that the individuals serving as leaders are obligated to be faithful to the organization's interest. The motivation to serve must be guided by the desire to function in the best interests of the constituency represented. An individual cannot advance personal interests above the interests of the organization. The focus of actions taken must be for the good of the whole, and not benefit any one particular constituency or individual at the expense of others.

An aspect of duty of loyalty often requires that individuals serving in a leadership capacity are asked to complete and sign a disclosure statement. The disclosure is to identify any potential conflicts of interest that could occur. The conflicts could be financial or personal. An example of a financial disclosure is when a speaker is presenting on a topic for which he has published materials that result in royalties or financial benefit. It is prudent to inform the audience of that financial relationship. An example of a personal conflict of interest would be if a leader advocates for doing business with a specific company that is owned by a family member. While that business arrangement might be in the best interests of the organization, it is imperative that the leader disclose the relationship and abstain from voting or influencing the decision in which he has a personal interest. Many employment settings, particularly state affiliated institutions and agencies, require employees to sign disclosure statements to raise awareness regarding the importance of avoiding any potential conflicts of interest.

Enhancing one's personal reputation or prestige by taking advantage of affiliation with an organization is also a violation of duty of loyalty. Individuals cannot advocate for themselves by using their leadership position in an organization to gain personal privileges or advantage. An example might be someone trying to secure personal favors by suggesting that she could influence a board's decision due to her position.

Confidentiality of non-public information is also inherent in duty of loyalty. Individual points of view discussed in a meeting should not be shared outside the setting unless they are part of the public record. While open, honest discussion is crucial to achieve effective results, the leader needs to emphasize the critical importance of maintaining confidential information. It is typical that the head of a group is designated as the public spokesperson; other members should defer to that individual in a public forum. The integrity of an organization can quickly be undermined if individual members are violating confidentiality.

Duty of Fidelity to Purpose

Fidelity to purpose requires that all group members act in accordance with the organization's governing documents, such as bylaws, mission and vision statements, as well as any applicable rules and legal regulations (Gattuso, 2018). All actions considered by the group should be guided by adherence to the designated purpose of the organization. This implies that members of the organization have access to and are familiar with the governing documents. Good governance standards recommend that bylaws be reviewed regularly and updated as necessary to ensure compliance with the direction of the association.

Fidelity to purpose also implies that assets or resources are used responsibly to accomplish the agreed upon mission, vision, and goals of the established organization. Each decision should be weighed carefully against the purpose of the organization. Will it benefit the greater good? Is it consistent with the best interests of members of the organization? While an action or direction might be laudable, leaders must always evaluate if an action is consistent with advancing the objectives of the organization.

Summary

Effective leadership requires excellent communication skills, strong interpersonal skills for interaction, active listening to hear all viewpoints, and the ability to set a vision and approach it in an organized way. It is also important to be practical and grounded in the reality of available resources in regard to finances and manpower.

Leadership is about investing your time and talent in an activity in order to make a difference. Mahatma Gandhi said, "The best way to find yourself is to lose yourself in the service of others." Leadership is not about power or being in control. It is about adding value and making a contribution. One of my favorite stories to share when I am encouraging people to become involved in volunteer service and leadership activities is the Story of the Starfish.

One day a man was walking along the beach when he noticed a boy picking something up and gently tossing it into the ocean. Approaching the boy, he asked, "What are you doing?" The youth replied, "Throwing starfish into the ocean. The surf is up and the tide is going out. If I don't throw them back, they'll die."

"Son," the man said, "Don't you realize there are miles and miles of beach and hundreds of starfish? You can't make a difference!" After listening politely, the boy bent down, picked up another starfish, and threw it back into the surf. Then, smiling at the man, he said, "I made a difference for that one."

—Adapted from Loren Eiseley, 1969

The desire to make a difference is a noble motivation. The decision to dedicate time and energy to a specific purpose is a significant investment for an individual. Leadership can be a conscious decision, but it can also be thrust upon you due to extenuating circumstances. There have been many reluctant leaders who found themselves faced with a situation that they could not, in good conscience, walk away from. They accepted the responsibility and executed the task to the best of their ability. Others embrace the challenge and seek opportunities to develop their leadership skills. Their mantra echoes the sentiment of Ralph Waldo Emerson: "Do not go where the path may lead. Go instead where there is no path and leave a trail."

Critical Thinking

1. As the leader of a committee, what are some of your primary responsibilities to facilitate success in meeting the committee's charge?

2. As leader of a Board with several vice-presidents, you want to plan and organize a mini-retreat to orient the Board. What types of agenda items should you plan to address?

3. You are interested in further developing your leadership skills. List some of the activities that you could pursue to engage in hands-on learning from experienced leaders.

4. One of your committee chairs is not meeting his expectations. Committee members are becoming frustrated and several have contacted you to voice complaints regarding disorganization and waste of time at meetings. The group as a whole is suffering because this committee's work is negatively affecting progress on several other committees. Outline your strategies and several options for addressing the issue with the committee chair.

5. You have a member of your Board who is very vocal and has an opinion on every issue. She tends to dominate discussion and keeps reiterating her point of view after each person speaks. Her opinion is sometimes biased by emotion and not always factual or accurate. How can you manage this member's behavior in a constructive way that won't disenfranchise her but maintain productive focus in discussion?

6. It has become apparent that a major initiative your group has been involved in will not be successful. How can you share this information with your members in a positive manner so they don't get discouraged from undertaking challenging tasks in the future?

7. What are some situations you might face as a leader that could present challenges in meeting fiduciary responsibilities and ethical behavior?

8. Your group has generated lots and lots of wonderful ideas to pursue. As the leader, you need to help the group prioritize goals because it is not feasible to pursue all of them. What parameters do you introduce to work toward focusing the group on activities that will have the most impact?

References

Axelrod, N. (2016). *Exceptional boards: Strengthening the governance team.* Meeting hosted by the American Society of Association Executives, Charleston, SC.

Ebener, D. (2012). *Blessings for leaders.* Collegeville, MN: Liturgical Press.

Gattuso, C. (2018). *Legal responsibilities of members of the Board of Directors.* Presentation to Board of Directors of the American Speech-Language-Hearing Association, Rockville, MD.

Heifetz, R., & Linsky, M. (2002). *Leadership on the line.* Boston, MA: Harvard Business Review Press.

Kummer, A. (2011). Successful leadership: Influencing others to follow your lead. In R. Lubinski & M. Huson (Eds.), *Professional issues in speech-language pathology and audiology* (4th ed., pp., 444–458). San Diego, CA: Plural Publishing.

Sisson, C. J. (1960). *William Shakespeare: The complete works.* New York, NY: Harper & Row.

Wikipedia. (n.d.). Retrieved March, 1, 2019 from https://en.wikipedia.org/wiki/leadership

Yukl, G. (1981). *Leadership in organizations.* Englewood Cliffs, NJ: Prentice Hall.

22

Safety in the Workplace

Cynthia McCormick Richburg, PhD and Donna Fisher Smiley, PhD

Introduction

Safety in the workplace is one of those topics that is often placed on the back-burner of employers' and employees' minds. However, safety is something we should all think about, especially in light of current times. Safety in the workplace involves multiple disciplines and can be described as the policies and procedures put in place to ensure the safety, health, and well-being of all employees and constituents associated with an employment setting. Workplace safety involves the identification of threats and hazards, as well as the implementation of controls and policies to counter those threats/hazards. A safe working environment reduces stress and health-related illnesses, improves productivity, and helps reduce absenteeism and job turnover. In essence, workplace safety is necessary for all employees to work in a safe and protected atmosphere.

Every workplace setting has safety concerns—some more than others. Because this book focuses on professional issues for audiologists and speech-language pathologists, this chapter's focus will concern the safety issues surrounding a professional practice setting. For audiologists and speech-language pathologists, that practice setting may be a hospital, a private practice, a school, a free-standing clinic, a nursing home, a manufacturing agency, or any other practice setting in which these professionals might be employed. Because it would become too cumbersome to address the specific safety concerns in each and every practice setting, the content in this chapter will focus on broad themes: (1) regulatory agencies, (2) policies, procedures, and trainings, (3) personal and environmental hazards, (4) infection control, and (5) confidentiality and Internet safety.

Workplace hazards have been categorized into six classifications: chemical, radiation, biological, physical, psychological, and ergonomic (Queensland Council of Social Services [QCOSS] Community Door, 2018). Hazards can also be classified as "acute" or "chronic" in nature (QCOSS Community Door, 2018; "What is the difference," n.d.). The controls are typically established by state or federal government standards, which necessitate the ongoing safety training and education of employees. It is the employer's responsibility to see that safety policies and procedures are implemented in the workplace, yet it is the employee's responsibility to abide by the policies and implement the procedures for the good of everyone in that environment.

Workplace safety should be important to audiologists and speech-language pathologists. These professionals should not think of workplace safety as something required for only employees in industrial or manufacturing jobs. As professionals, audiologists and speech-language pathologists should be concerned about safety and well-being for themselves, their fellow workers, as well as their clientele. These professionals should know what safety concerns are important to their specific setting, and to the people served within that setting. Simply knowing the policies and procedures within their own setting allows these professionals to carry out their responsibilities in a safe and effective manner.

Regulatory Agencies

Audiologists and speech-language pathologists should know which agencies regulate the safety concerns within their workplace environment. Knowing this information will assist in the development of that site's policies and procedures for safety and security measures, especially as they apply to the employees of that site. The following are international or national agencies that put specific regulations or mandates into effect to ensure the best possible safety outcomes for employers, employees, and constituents (e.g., clients, family members) associated with a particular work setting.

Occupational Safety and Health Administration

The Department of Labor has three agencies responsible for enforcing laws passed to protect the safety and health of workers/employees in the United States. These agencies include the Occupational Safety and Health Administration (OSHA), the Mine Safety and Health Administration (MSHA), and the Fair Labor Standards Act (FLSA). It is likely that OSHA would be the only one of these three agencies, therefore the only one further detailed in this chapter, to provide information and training guidelines relevant to the work environment of audiologists and speech-language pathologists. Although OSHA is typically thought of as an agency that regulates industries outside of health care, as of the early 1990s, OSHA has been responsible for overseeing and enforcing infection control programs and other safety hazards in the workplace (OSHA, 2016). Random inspections of health care facilities are accomplished to ensure that the employees, as well as the clients/patients seen in those facilities, are kept safe through compliance with current regulations. Most recently, OSHA has included information about "Emergency Preparedness and Response" to the information contained on its website (OSHA, n.d.-a).

Environmental Protection Agency

Although the Environmental Protection Agency (EPA) is not responsible for the safety and health of employees in a workplace environment to the extent that OSHA is responsible, the EPA, as part of their mission statement, works to ensure "that chemicals in the marketplace are reviewed for safety" (EPA, n.d.). The EPA is the agency responsible for ensuring that no significant risk is posed to the health and safety of those coming into contact with the chemicals used to clean, disinfect, and sterilize the equipment, probes, toys, and diagnostic/therapy items used by speech-language pathologists and audiologists.

Food and Drug Administration

The Food and Drug Administration (FDA) is a regulatory agency that has authority to regulate food, drugs, biologics (e.g., vaccines, gene therapies), medical devices (including surgical implants), electronic products that give off radiation, cosmetics, veterinary products, and tobacco products (FDA, n.d.). The role of the FDA is to protect and promote public health by ensuring the safety of products and food. The FDA ensures that the product labels and descriptions are accurate and specific enough for consumers to understand and use them properly. The FDA and EPA often work together to exchange information about the effects of chemicals, including the disinfectants and sterilization chemicals used by audiologists and speech-language pathologists.

Accrediting Agencies

Audiologists and speech-language pathologists should know which agencies license and/or accredit their workplace environment. Knowing this information will also assist in the development of that site's policies and procedures for safety and security measures, especially as they apply to the clients/patients of that site.

The Joint Commission

The Joint Commission has both national and international branches, with the branch located in the United States being responsible for accrediting U.S. health care organizations and programs (Joint Commission, n.d.-a). State governments recognize accreditation and certification by the Joint Commission as a reflection on an organization's commitment to maintaining certain performance standards. These standards often serve as a symbol of quality that consumers and third-party payers recognize for licensing and reimbursement purposes. The Joint Commission accredits hospitals, home health care, and nursing care centers, settings in which many audiologists and speech-language pathologists are employed. The Joint Commission regularly formulates National Patient Safety Goals, which include goals and updates meant to improve patient safety (Joint Commission, n.d.-b).

The Commission on Accreditation of Rehabilitation Facilities (CARF)

This international organization's mission is to provide accreditation standards for organizations working in the human-service professions, including services related to aging, behavioral health, child and youth services, employment and community services, medical rehabilitation, and opioid treatment programs (CARF, n.d.). The CARF is a system of rehabilitation facilities that monitors itself in order to maintain standards and state certifications/accreditations. Through accreditation, CARF assists service providers in improving the quality of their services and generating customized standards based on universal precautions for each department within a facility, such as rehabilitation (speech-language pathology, audiology, physical therapy, and occupational therapy), nursing, and nutrition services (CARF, n.d.).

Policies, Procedures, and Trainings

As described earlier, regulatory agencies help establish guidelines to be adopted and implemented by the employers/administrations within workplace settings in which audiologists and speech-language pathologists are employed. Each setting should have protocols and policies in place to describe the threats and hazards associated with that specific site. Those policies and procedures should include trainings provided at little or no cost to the employees in order to prevent or control the outcome of possible breaches in safety. The policies and trainings should allow an employee to implement the necessary controls to counter any safety threats with a minimum of negative impact.

Facility- and department-specific safety training protocols should be a part of any workplace environment's policies and procedures. Each workplace setting should have a set of operating procedures that describe in detail the plan for responding to emergencies. These plans should include trainings specific to the activities, threats, and population served within that facility. All facilities have the potential for threat from fire, power outage,

gas or water leaks, explosions, inclement weather, and environmental impacts. Some facilities will also have potential for threat from chemical spills, radiation leaks, or biohazard contamination. For example, if a speech-language pathologist is working in a hospital setting, he should know the emergency response plan for exposure to radiation or biohazardous materials. A plan should be accessible to all employees specifying how those hazards are to be communicated to the staff, how treatment for skin or eye contact should be handled, and how to dispose of the hazardous material appropriately (even if this means passing the responsibility off to another employee correctly). Likewise, if an audiologist is working in a school setting, she should know the emergency response plan for a bomb threat or gas leak. A plan should be accessible to all employees specifying how those hazards are to be communicated to the staff, how to account for and safely move away from the building with children under the audiologist's care, and when it is safe to re-enter the area/building and how that will be communicated.

All plans, policies, and trainings should be in written format and accessible as electronic documents. The information contained in the documents should be included in any new employee's orientation to the work setting. Knowledge of the information contained within the policies should be updated every 12 to 18 months, with trainings used to support and update past knowledge on the topics. In order to ensure that employees are informed properly, employers/administrations should have a method for documenting when and how employees obtained the information, and some sort of date/time-stamped information should be obtained and maintained in employee records.

Speech-language pathologists and audiologists should always inquire about the standard operating procedures and emergency plans in any work setting they enter, especially if they have an itinerant position that dictates they move from one setting to another. For example, if an audiologist starts the day in an ENT office setting in Kansas City, the audiologist is responsible for knowing what is contained within that setting's emergency plan, which may include a Hazardous Materials Management Plan, a Biohazards Management Plan, and the code for a Tornado Response Action. Then when that audiologist later drives to the local university's campus to teach a course on hearing aids, she becomes responsible for knowing the university's policies on campus safety (including policies on sexual violence, harassment, and active shooter threats).

There is a plethora of information from agencies and websites on the topic of workplace safety and trainings. Refer to Table 22–1 for a non-exhaustive collection of information on workplace safety websites.

Table 22–1. Examples of Available Online Workplace Safety Websites

Topic	Safety Trainings and Other Resources	Agency	Website
Active shooter	ALICE Training Program	ALICE Training Institute	https://www.alicetraining.com (Healthcare and Education options)
Active shooter/ campus intruder	Active Shooter and Campus Intruder Response Training (ASRP)	C.O.B.R.A. Defense System	https://www.cobradefensesystem.com
Active shooter. Mass attacks in crowded and public spaces	*Ready*	Department of Homeland Security	https://www.ready.gov/active-shooter https://www.ready.gov/public-spaces
Active shooter preparedness	Active Shooter Preparedness	Department of Homeland Security	https://www.dhs.gov/cisa/active-shooter-preparedness
Emergency preparedness	*Ready*	Department of Homeland Security	https://www.ready.gov/severe-weather https://www.ready.gov/tornadoes https://www.ready.gov/hazardous-materials-incidents
Workplace violence	Physical and Verbal Abuse Against Health Care Providers	Joint Commission	https://www.jointcommission.org/workplace_violence.aspx
Workplace safety & health	Workplace Safety Diseases and Conditions Emergency Preparedness & Response	Centers for Disease Control and Prevention	https://www.cdc.gov/features/workplacesafety.html https://www.cdc.gov/features/diseasesconditions.html https://www.cdc.gov/features/emergency.html

A topic not entirely related to policies, procedures, or trainings—yet one that needs to be addressed when discussing safety in the workplace—is the topic of background checks ("clearances") necessary for professional practice. The physical and emotional safety of clients should be paramount for audiologists and speech-language pathologists. One aspect for ensuring this safety is the utilization of background checks for potential new hires, students obtaining practical experiences, and current employees. The background checks should be appropriate for the job responsibilities and clientele, which may include children, youth, and/or vulnerable adults. Many state and local regulatory credentialing agencies, including licensure boards, may require an applicant to disclose relevant issues related to criminal history, employment history, and licensure history. It is likely that a new hire would be expected to disclose any prior misdemeanor or felony convictions. Similarly, employers would expect new hires to disclose if they had been disciplined or discharged from a professional position, as well as had a license suspended, denied, revoked, or annulled.

There are many types of background checks, each of which provide different information to the employer. Criminal background checks provide information on a person's criminal record. These types of checks can be completed using personal information, such as name, social security numbers, and/or fingerprints. These records can be obtained via the Federal Bureau of Investigations (FBI) database, state/local databases, and private vendor services. State and national sex offender and child abuse registries are also sources that may be checked for criminal activity.

In addition to criminal background checks, other types of background checks that may be of interest to employers include driving histories, education record/academic degree verification, and drug testing. The information from these types of background checks help to ensure that employees are providing services to clients safely and with competency.

Personal and Environmental Hazards

Physical Hazards

The workplace has many physical hazards, depending on the environment or setting. Physical hazards include such things as wet or slick floors, objects or obstructions in walkways, poor lighting, leaks of gas, fumes, dust, or vapors, as well as misused or unsafe machinery (e.g., sharp objects, exposed wires). Audiologists and speech-language pathologists working in all settings, but particularly pediatric settings, must be aware of the dangers associated with toys left out in waiting areas, other tripping hazards, exposed electrical outlets, small toy parts that pose a choking risk, dangling cords from window treatments, or cleaning agents that are not stored in child-locked cabinets. Likewise, these professionals must be aware of the dangers associated with sidewalk and parking lot hazards (e.g., door access, snow, ice, excessive heat, ramps) in clinical settings, especially in which the very young and/or elderly clients receive services.

Employees in all settings should be made aware of policies that prohibit the use of specific equipment in the building. For example, some settings prohibit the use of space heaters/fans, hotplates, coffee makers, or toaster ovens in individual offices due to the fire hazard risk they can create. Also, certain departmental safety procedure documents prohibit the use of extension cords or power strips that are "piggy-backed" on each other because of the risk of fire and/or tripping or using furniture (such as bookshelves) that are not mounted due to the risk of it tipping/falling over and injuring someone. Other regulations may be described more fully by the technology management team in a practice setting.

Ergonomic Hazards

For their own safety, clinicians should be instructed about ergonomic hazards, or physical conditions that may pose a risk for muscle, ligament, or tendon damage usually resulting from awkward/extreme postures or repetitive movements. "Ergonomics" is a term used to refer to the design of the work environment, with an intent for comfortably fitting workers' body size and capabilities, while supporting any limitations or restrictions (Claussen, 2011; OSHA, n.d.-b). The main objective of ergonomics in the workplace is to create a safe work environment that decreases fatigue, pain, and injury in workers (OSHA, n.d.-b).

Speech-language pathologists and audiologists are at risk for eye strain, lower back problems, and carpal tunnel syndrome because of the nature of their jobs (i.e., sitting at a computer or desk, typing or writing for long periods of time, etc.). Other aspects of these professionals' job responsibilities which could create physical distress might include carrying equipment (e.g., portable audiometers for screenings), lifting small children throughout the day, and transferring adults from wheels chairs or hospital beds. The employee's workplace is responsible for training staff on the proper use of body mechanics and the use of any special equipment for transferring. An example of a special piece of equipment would be a Hoyer Lift.

Behavioral Management and Restraints

Physical restraint may be necessary when a client's behavior poses a threat to himself, another person, or to the professional working with him. If an audiologist or speech-language pathologist finds herself providing services to a client who becomes combative, confused, or irrational, having been trained in behavioral management and restraint may make the difference between emerging from the situation with resultant injuries, or emerging from the situation injury free. Training instruction and videos (such as the one from Handle with Care, crisis intervention and behavior management training services found at http://handlewithcare.com/) may help to keep employees safe, as well as the clients and others within the practice setting. Each practice setting should have detailed instructions included in protocols and safety documents for addressing the use of restraints and behavioral management techniques. If an audiologist or speech-language pathologist is employed in a hospital or clinic setting, she must not only be knowledgeable of the codes for combative patients, but she must be able to use techniques for controlling the patient in a manner that allows both the clinician and the patient to maintain self-respect and emerge from the situation without harm (Gastmans & Milisen, 2006). This same scenario exists for speech-language pathologists and audiologists who work in school settings. Each school district should have operational plans and protocols established for behavioral management and/or physical restraint for students whose actions present a safety risk for those around them.

Regulations and policies exist at the local, state, and federal level to protect individuals from being unnecessarily or inappropriately restrained (CPI, 2009; U.S. DOE, 2013). For example, audiologists and speech-language pathologists who work in public school settings should be familiar with state and federal guidelines regarding when restraint of a student can and cannot be used. In other practice settings, such as a hospital, the rules and regulations will be different for when and how restraint may be used with patients. Regardless of the workplace, the use of restraints should be implemented only when necessary to protect the immediate physical safety of the student/patient, staff, and others.

De-escalation techniques are also important for audiologists and speech-language pathologists to become familiar with through trainings. De-escalation, also known as defusing, crisis or conflict resolution, or conflict management, can be described as a combination of strategies and techniques intended to reduce a patient's distress and aggression (Joint Commission, 2019). Audiologists and speech-language pathologists should obtain training that includes proper use of assessment, communication, and actions in order to reduce the risk of harm to patients and themselves. Examples of commonly used trainings can be obtained on the Crisis Prevention Intervention website (https://www.crisisprevention.com).

Workplace Violence

Information on workplace violence and prevention has become more common, and anyone can access information about this topic on the internet (see Table 22–1). For example, the ALICE Training Institute (an acronym to assist memory for *Alert, Lockdown, Inform, Counter, Evacuate*) has listed "10 Ways to Prevent Workplace Violence" (ALICE, 2015). The site stresses the need to make employees aware of what constitutes workplace violence, to establish training sessions to help employees act appropriately in cases of workplace violence, and to create policies that prevent threats, unacceptable behaviors, harassment, or retaliation. Speech-language pathologists and audiologists need to be encouraged to report any and all incidents to supervisors and employers.

Being informed about workplace violence is not the only step necessary for preventing these events. Making physical changes to a practice setting can also help discourage would-be attackers. For example, placing privacy screening (darkening or mirroring) on windows makes it impossible to see into rooms. Essentially, keeping an attacker unable to see through windows eliminates what is known as the "fishbowl effect" (Wyllie, 2010). Establishing a system of internal notifications (email, text, phones, and/or codes) provides a method for alerting workers about the presence of an attacker.

Making a plan and establishing protocols for all employees to follow is equally important. That plan should include what actions to take (by employees) for clients with disabilities, access limitations, or other functional needs. Any time an audiologist or speech-language pathologist enters a new work setting, she should identify the closest exits and visualize a path of escape should an active shooter or violent intruder enter the facility. Also, identifying a place to hide in any setting is prudent, should that be the only choice of action.

In addition to general information found on the ALICE website, information and videos can be found on the Joint Commission's website on the topic of Workplace Violence Prevention Resources for Health Care (Joint Commission, n.d.-b). For audiologists and speech-language pathologists who practice in a university clinic, there will be a plan for dealing with incidents of sexual violence, harassment, and theft. As with other places of employment, university employees typically must have proof of training completion on file with the Human Resources office. Every professional setting can tailor the recommendations and examples given on safety websites to accommodate the employee and client needs. Additional information laid out in a variety of educational and literacy levels and found in an assortment of written information, online training modules, and location-based training programs can be found in Table 22–1.

Signage and Catchy Acronyms

Every workplace setting should have highly visible emergency exits, along with signs, maps, and/or directions indicating the nearest exits. Emergency exits should lead directly out of the building. Other signage indicating additional dangerous conditions (e.g., what to do in the event of a chemical spill, an active shooter, or a dangerous weather event) should also be present and highly visible throughout hallways and areas in which employees and constituents are likely to congregate. Figure 22–1 provides an example of signage that must be located in all public areas.

Many employers or safety departments have established catchy or memorable acronyms for helping employees quickly remember specific protocol or processes for safety. For example, unless the hazard or threat is directly affecting an employee's work area, the use of the acronym S.N.O.W. may help hospital speech-language pathologists remember to "S—stay in place, N—notify the supervisor, O—operate normally, and W—wait for instructions." Likewise, a school-based audiologist may safely respond to a fire in a school by remember-

EMERGENCY INFORMATION:
- Do not use the elevators, use stairwells.
- Call **911** from any phone.

FIRE

- Evacuate building by nearest exit
- Move at least 300 feet away from building
- Get out of emergency responders' way

ACTIVE SHOOTER

RUN
- 1st Get out of shooter's path

HIDE
- 2nd Remain silent, still, and out of sight

FIGHT
- Only as a last resort, throw objects at them, distract them

TORNADO

- Go to the basement
- Do not leave if the tornado is coming toward your location

EARTHQUAKE

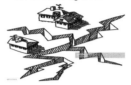

- Take cover under sturdy furniture
- Protect your head/neck with your arms
- Avoid windows, hanging objects, or tall furniture

Wait for "ALL CLEAR" before returning to activities

Figure 22–1. An example of emergency signage that must be located in all public areas.

ing the acronym R.A.C.E., which would remind him to "R—remove individuals from the immediate area, A—activate the alarm, C—contain the fire by closing all doors in the area, and E—extinguish the fire if it can be done safely or impedes evacuation/E—evacuate the area to your designated meeting location." Even active shooter trainings use a catchy, memorable phrase of "Run, Hide, Fight" to help workers remember what to do in times of stress and danger.

Infection Control in Clinical and Educational Settings

Minimizing and eliminating infectious disease contamination in the practice settings of speech-language pathologists and audiologists is another aspect of workplace safety. The pathogens commonly considered problematic in speech-language-hearing clinical settings include, but are not limited to, staphylococcus, influenza, common cold, tuberculosis, HIV, and the various forms of hepatitis. To learn more about these and other pathogens, it is recommended that the reader

go to the Centers for Disease Control and Prevention (CDC) webpage on Infection Control (CDC, n.d.). The CDC site, as well as book chapters written specifically on the topic of infection control in the speech-language-hearing clinical setting (e.g., Bankaitis & Kemp, 2008; Lubinski, 2013), will provide specific information for speech-language pathologists and audiologists to obtain knowledge and skills in the areas of (1) pathogen transmission, (2) infection prevention, (3) infection control plans for the specific settings, and (4) exposure protocols and reporting. Many workplaces will have specific documents outlining infection prevention and control for that setting. The ASHA website also has information about hand hygiene, isolation precautions, personal protective equipment, needle/sharps handling, as well as information specific to school-based professionals and practice guidelines (ASHA, 2019a, 2019b). The literature on the topic of infection control will enable professionals to become more knowledgeable about the various forms of pathogen transmission (e.g., contact, vehicle, airborne, and vector-borne transmission). Guidelines in the literature will help professionals learn to prevent and control contamination on the surfaces of equipment, toys, and diagnostic/therapy items. Knowing which chemicals are considered to be appropriate for cleaning on a topical level versus those chemicals that disinfect or sterilize will allow audiologists and speech-language pathologists to protect themselves and their clients. In addition, protocols addressing the handling and disposal of chemicals used for infection control should be part of the orientation and annual trainings provided for speech-language pathologists and audiologists.

Another element needed to be addressed in practice setting protocols (as they pertain to the protection of both professionals and constituents) includes pre-employment health screening documentation. As mentioned previously in the section containing information about background checks, new employees need to provide documentation of infectious disease immunizations/screenings (e.g., measles, mumps, rubella and tuberculosis tests) and/or clearance to work by a licensed physician. Additionally, many employers are now requiring annual flu vaccination, cardiopulmonary resuscitation (CPR) training, and defibrillator training as a condition for employment or continued employment.

Confidentiality of Client and Research Participant Information

Another aspect of workplace safety for audiologists and speech-language pathologists is the safeguarding and protection of client information. Additionally, when these professionals are involved in research projects using human participants, the professionals have both a legal and ethical obligation to protect the privacy of those participants.

Safeguarding Client Information

Prater (2014) outlines three entities that professionals must keep in mind when considering the safeguarding of information for clients: confidentiality, privacy, and security. Speech-language pathologists and audiologists need to consider each of these aspects as they reflect on safeguarding client information.

Confidentiality is the concept that the information a client reveals to a provider in a professional relationship is private and that there are limits on how and when the information may be disclosed to a third party (Confidentiality, n.d.). Information that a patient shares with a speech-language pathologist or audiologist in any format (i.e., written or verbal), as well as any documentation that results from the interaction between the patient and the professional, is confidential.

Privacy is the right of the patient to make decisions about when and how confidential information should be shared with a third party (USDHHS, 2003). Speech-language pathologists and audiologists will want to become familiar with rules/laws/regulations that affect their workplace and client population. These professionals must understand when and how they can release information on any given client. Many workplaces will have standardized forms for the client to sign that gives explicit permission as to who can receive confidential information and what information is to be released. Figure 22–2 is an example of a release of information form (ROI) that can be used to protect a patient's privacy.

Security (as it relates to patient information) refers to the method used to ensure that confidential information is protected, whether in paper or electronic format. For audiologists and speech-language pathologists who work in schools, hospitals, clinics, or large medical practices, decisions about security of client information may be made and enforced by administrators outside of their department. However, those professionals who are in private practice may possess the decision-making powers for determining how to ensure security of client information.

Regulations Regarding Patient Confidentiality, Privacy, and Security

Depending on their work settings and job responsibilities, audiologists and speech-language pathologists may be required to complete formal training regarding protection of client confidentiality, privacy, and security of data. Professionals working in hospital settings will most likely have annual trainings to ensure that they are aware of regulations and know how to report a data breach should it occur. For professionals involved in clinic, nursing homes, rehabilitation centers, and hospitals, the Health Insurance Portability and Accountability Act of 1996 (HIPAA) will very likely be among the regulations included in annual trainings. Regulations involving HIPAA required the Department of Human and Health Services (HHS) to adopt national privacy protection standards for electronic health care transactions because it was recognized that advances in electronic technology had the potential to create problems with maintaining privacy of health information (USDHHS, 2017). For professionals involved in educational settings, the Family Educational Rights and Privacy Act of 1974 (FERPA) will very likely be among the regulations included in annual trainings. Regulations involving FERPA apply to all schools that receive funds from the United States Department of Education, and these laws protect the privacy of educational records belonging to students (U.S. DOE, 2018).

AUTHORIZATION TO RELEASE HEALTH INFORMATION
All elements are required prior to information being released

Patient Name: _____ **Date of Birth:** _____

1. Who is authorized to disclose the information: _____

2. Who is authorized to receive the information:
   Name: _____
   Complete Address: _____
   City: _____ State: _____ Zip Code: _____

3. I understand that I will be charged for the costs of copying the information to be released.

4. The specific information to be requested or released is:
   List the dates of services: _____
   - □ Clinic Report   □ Operative Report   □ Radiology Films
   - □ Discharge Summary   □ Physical
   - □ ER Report   □ Shot Record
   - □ Lab   □ X-Ray Report
   - □ Medical Abstract   □ Other: _____

5. I understand that if the person or entity that receives the information is not a health care provider or health plan covered by federal privacy regulations, the information described above may be redisclosed and no longer protected by these regulations.

6. I understand that the [NAME OF SITE] will be paid for the cost of copying the information released.

7. I understand that I may refuse to sign this authorization and that my refusal to sign will not affect my ability to obtain treatment or payment or my eligibility for benefits. I may inspect or obtain a copy of any information used/disclosed under this authorization.

8. I understand that I may revoke this authorization in writing at any time by delivering a copy of my revocation to [NAME OF SITE] except to the extent that action has been taken in reliance on this authorization. This authorization expires: **1 year from date signed**

9. I understand that the information in my health record may include information relating to sexually transmitted diseases, acquired immunodeficiency syndrome (AIDS), or human immunodeficiency virus (HIV). It may also include information about behavioral or mental services and/or treatment for alcohol and drug abuse.

PLEASE INCLUDE A COPY OF A PHOTO ID

_____   _____
Signature of Patient or Representative   Date

_____   _____
Phone Number   Relationship to Patient

Witness: _____ Phone Number: _____ Date: _____

Figure 22–2. Sample of a release of information. *Source:* Adapted from Arkansas Children's (2019).

Speech-language pathologists and audiologists will find guidance concerning confidentiality, privacy, and security of patient information contained within their codes of ethics, state and federal regulations, and workplace-specific documents. According to the American Speech-Language-Hearing Association (ASHA, 2018), if there is inconsistency between these different documents, the professional should follow the most restrictive rule. One example of this inconsistency might be if the law seems to allow an action, but the ASHA Code of Ethics seems to prohibit that action. In this case, the professional should follow the ASHA Code of Ethics (refer to Chapter 5 for more information on ethical practice). Similarly, if there appears to be a conflict between documents/sources, the professional should abide by the law (e.g., when a workplace policy conflicts with legal requirements for the confidential handling of records, the law will take precedence [ASHA, 2018]).

Table 22–2 contains a list and short descriptions of several regulations and guidelines that speech-language pathologists and audiologists should be familiar with when considering how to safeguard client information.

Breaches of confidentiality and privacy may be due to carelessness, such as speaking about a patient in a public space or improperly safeguarding patient data around others. Breaches of this nature may also occur for malicious reasons, such as accessing the medical record of a patient who is well known when there is no relevant need to know that person's status to complete the work assignment. Regardless of the reason, breaches of confidentiality and privacy can result in disciplinary actions that range anywhere from disciplinary action by the

Table 22–2. Laws, Regulations, and Guidelines Regarding the Protection of Client Information

Law/Regulation/Guideline Name	Description
American Speech-Language-Hearing Association (ASHA) Code of Ethics	This document reflects the values of ASHA members regarding scientific and clinical practice based on principles of duty, accountability, fairness, and responsibility. This Code is modified, adapted, and updated as society and practices change. As of the writing of this chapter, the latest version of the ASHA Code of Ethics was published in 2016 (ASHA, 2016).
Health Insurance Portability and Accountability Act of 1996 (HIPAA)	This federal law was initially written to protect workers who changed jobs against the loss of health insurance or from encountering exclusions for pre-existing conditions in new health insurance coverage. Currently, standards and rules for how protected health information (PHI) may be used, disclosed, stored, maintained, and transmitted gets the most attention in the Administrative Simplification section of this act.
Family Educational Rights and Privacy Act (FERPA, 1974)	This federal law protects the privacy of student education records. In addition, the document requires schools that receive funding from the U.S. Department of Education to obtain written permission from the parent (or student once they turn 18 years of age) to release information from a student's education record. There are some exceptions and conditions that allow schools to share student education data without consent. See https://www2.ed.gov/policy/gen/guid/fpco/ferpa/index.html for those exceptions.
State and workplace-specific documents	These documents contain rules, regulations, and guidance on the protection of client information specific to each state and workplace. Speech-language pathologists and audiologists should make sure that they are familiar with these documents. Claiming "ignorance" will not protect a professional in a legal or ethical conflict when it comes to patient confidentiality, privacy, and security of data.

employer, to termination of employment, to criminal charges that may include monetary fines and/or imprisonment. In addition, audiologists and speech-language pathologists may have their Certificate of Clinical Competence (CCC) or American Board of Audiology (ABA) certification suspended or revoked, which in turn could lead to the suspension or revocation of their state license. At the least, these professionals could be reprimanded or censured by the Board of Ethics, which would also mean the state licensing board would be notified of the lapse in professional ethics (ASHA, 2019c). Therefore, these professionals are responsible for knowing and abiding by the laws and regulations that govern confidentiality, privacy, and security in their workplaces.

Computer and Internet Safety

In this digital age, most workplaces (if not all) will have computers, other electronic devices (e.g., tablets, smartphones), and internet access. Processes and procedures need to be put into place to safeguard both employees and clients as they relate to computer and internet safety.

In addition to the requirements of HIPAA and FERPA for protecting the security of client records, speech-language pathologists and audiologists need to be mindful of the use of computers and other electronic devices in public spaces. Guaranteeing that people are not able to access or view client data is critical. For example, if a speech-language pathologist writes client reports on a computer that is in a public work space, he will need to have a process for always logging out of that computer or locking the screen when he is away from that device. Logging out or using a screen lock will help to ensure that client information is safe from a breach of confidentiality.

Employees in any workplace need to use some basic online safety rules. Larger organizations may have specific rules in place to protect employees and electronic data. These rules should be outlined in employee orientation sessions and updated during annual trainings. All audiologists and speech-language pathologists, no matter how large or small their practice settings may be, should learn and practice skills for minimizing computer and internet safety breaches at work. One example of practicing online safety is avoiding the creation of generic passwords or easily guessable passwords. Avoid using a family name, birthdate, address, or even a pet's name as a password. The more random a password, the stronger it will be. Safety experts recommend that employees not use the same password for every situation that requires one. Additionally, employees should never have their passwords written down, especially in a location close to their computers or devices.

Lastly, email "phishing" scams often occur in the workplace. Suspicious-looking emails should not be opened. An email from an unknown source (especially one that promises quick money) should generate caution and cause a professional to think twice before looking at the contents. When the content of an email appears to be from someone known but contains suspicious or unusual requests, then workers should follow protocol to first report and then dispose of those emails appropriately. Speech-language pathologists and audiologists should be made aware that sophisticated hackers and spammers will use email addresses that appear to be legitimate but that are not. An email that appears to have been sent from a supervisor and asks the viewer to "click on a link and enter your username and password" should always be approached with skepticism. Again, workers should have specific protocol for reporting and handling emails that appear to be phishing for personal information; personal information of the worker as well as personal information of the client.

Modern-day technology, and access to information via the internet, can be necessary and beneficial. However, with the benefits of technology come the need to safeguard client confidentiality and privacy. Employees' use of email and other data sources require that precautionary measures be an element of today's workplace safety—now more than ever.

Summary

Workplace safety is a fairly new concept to modern society. Approximately 14,000 workers were killed on the job in 1970, the same year that the Williams-Steiger Occupational Safety and Health Act (1970) was signed into law by President Nixon. By 2009, the number of workers killed in the workplace dropped to under 4,400, yet the number of workers in the U.S. workforce had almost doubled (OSHA, 2010). We can thank OSHA, the National Institute of Occupational Safety and Health (NIOSH), and other agencies and policies dedicated to implementing safety practices for our modern workforce. Creating and fostering a culture of safety in the workplace leads to better performance within every organization and across all professions, including those of audiology and speech-language pathology. This culture of safety will result in better productivity from happier and healthier employees which will ultimately result in better patient outcomes.

Critical Thinking

1. How has the need for workplace safety changed the educational requirements and demands for employees and new hires?

2. Which of the six workplace hazard classifications (chemical, radiation, biological, physical, psychological, and ergonomic) would most likely be present in a speech, language, hearing clinic? in a manufacturer of assistive listening device lab area? in a school district employing speech-language pathologists and audiologists?

3. Consider your current employment or training setting. Which accrediting agency(ies) would provide the setting with the most comprehensive safety guidelines?

4. What infection precautions should you take if you provide services in a nursing home? If you provide services in a speech, language, hearing clinic?

5. Write up two policies that could be applied in your current employment or training setting on the topic of encountering an active shooter; on the topic of slipping and fall prevention.

6. What actions could be taken to de-escalate a confused and combative adult who enters your work setting's waiting room with a family member who is scheduled for services?

References

ALICE Training Institute (2015). *10 ways to prevent workplace violence.* Retrieved from https://www.alicetraining.com/resources-posts/blog/10-ways-to-prevent-workplace-violence/

American Speech-Language-Hearing Association. (2016). *Code of Ethics [Ethics].* Retrieved from http://www.asha.org/policy.

American Speech-Language-Hearing Association. (2018). *Issues in ethics: Confidentiality.* Retrieved from https://www.asha.org/Practice/ethics/Confidentiality/

American Speech-Language-Hearing Association. (2019a). *Infection control in speech-language pathology.* Retrieved from https://www.asha.org/slp/infectioncontrol/

American Speech-Language-Hearing Association. (2019b). *Infection control in audiology.* Retrieved from https://www.asha.org/aud/infection-control/

American Speech-Language-Hearing Association. (2019c). *How ASHA's Board of Ethics sanctions individuals found in violation of the Code of Ethics.* Retrieved from https://www.asha.org/practice/ethics/sanctions/

Bankaitis, A. U., & Kemp, R. J. (2008). Infection control. In H. Hosford-Dunn, R. Roeser, & M. Valente (Ed.), *Audiology practice management* (pp. 215–245). New York, NY: Thieme Medical.

Centers for Disease Control and Prevention. (n.d.). *Infection control.* Retrieved from https://www.cdc.gov/infectioncontrol/

Claussen, L. (2011, June). Recognizing hidden dangers: 25 steps to a safer office. *Safety + Health, 183*(6).

Commission on Accreditation of Rehabilitation Facilities. (n.d.). Retrieved from http://www.carf.org

Confidentiality. (n.d.). In *Miller-Keane encyclopedia and dictionary of medicine, nursing, and allied health* (7th ed.). Retrieved from https://medical-dictionary.thefreedictionary.com/confidentiality

Crisis Prevention Institute. (2009). *Joint Commission standards on restraint and seclusion/Nonviolent Crisis Intervention Training Program.* Retrieved from https://www.crisisprevention.com/CPI/media/Media/Resources/alignments/Joint-Commission-Restraint-Seclusion-Alignment-2011.pdf

Environmental Protection Agency. (n.d.). *Our mission and what we do.* Retrieved from https://www.epa.gov/aboutepa/our-mission-and-what-we-do

Family Educational Rights and Privacy Act (FERPA), 20 U.S.C. 1232g; 34 CFR Part 99. (1974).

Food and Drug Administration. (n.d.). Retrieved from https://www.fda.gov

Gastmans, C., & Milisen, K. (2006). Use of physical restraint in nursing homes: Clinical-ethical considerations. *Journal of Medical Ethics, 32*, 148–152. Retrieved from https://www.hhs.gov/hipaa/for-professionals/index.html

Health Insurance Portability and Accountability Act, Pub. L. No. 104-191, 45 CFR, Parts 160-164. (1996).

Joint Commission. (2019, Jan). De-escalation in health care. *Quick Safety, 47.* Retrieved from https://www.jointcommission.org/assets/1/23/QS_Deescalation_1_28_18_FINAL.pdf

Joint Commission. (n.d-a). Retrieved from https://www.jointcommission.org

Joint Commission. (n.d-b). *Workplace violence prevention resources for health care.* Retrieved from https://www.jointcommission.org/workplace_violence.aspx

Lubinski, R. (2013). Infection prevention. In R. Lubinski & M. Hudson (Ed.), *Professional issues in speech-language pathology and audiology* (pp. 460–476). Boston, MA: Cengage.

Occupational Safety and Health Act of 1970, 84 Stat. 1590, 29 U.S.C.A. § 651 et seq.

Occupational Safety and Health Administration. (2010). *OSHA celebrates 40 years of accomplishments in the workplace.* Retrieved from https://www.osha.gov/osha40/OSHATimeline.pdf

Occupational Safety and Health Administration. (2016). *Bloodborne pathogens.* CRF Title 29 Labor vol 6 part 1910.1030. Retrieved from https://www.osha.gov/laws-regs/regulations/standardnumber/1910/1910.1030

Occupational Health and Safety Administration. (n.d-a). *Emergency preparedness and response.* Retrieved from https://www.osha.gov/SLTC/emergencypreparedness/index.html

Occupational Health and Safety Administration. (n.d-b). *Ergonomics.* Retrieved from https://www.osha.gov/SLTC/ergonomics/

Prater, V. (2014). *Confidentiality, privacy and security of health information: Balancing interests.* Retrieved from https://healthinformatics.uic.edu/blog/confidentiality-privacy-and-security-of-health-information-balancing-interests/

Protection of Human Subjects, 45 C.F.R. pt. 46 (1991, rev. 2018, July 19). Retrieved from http://www.hhs.gov/ohrp/humansubjects/guidance/45cfr46.htm

QCOSS Community Door. (2018, December). *Types of hazards.* Retrieved from https://etraining.communitydoor.org.au/mod/page/view.php?id=216

United States Department of Education. (2013, October). *Seclusion and restraints: States and territories summary.* Retrieved from https://www2.ed.gov/policy/seclusion/seclusion-state-summary.html

United States Department of Education. (2018). *Family Education Rights and Privacy Act (FERPA).* Retrieved from https://www2.ed.gov/policy/gen/guid/fpco/ferpa/index.html

United States Department of Health and Human Services. (2003). *Office of Civil Rights summary of the HIPAA Privacy Rule.* Retrieved from https://www.hhs.gov/sites/default/files/privacysummary.pdf

United States Department of Health and Human Services. (2017). *Office of Civil Rights summary of HIPAA for professionals.* Retrieved from https://www.hhs.gov/hipaa/for-professionals/index.html

What is the difference between an acute hazard and a chronic hazard? (n.d.). Retrieved from https://www.safeopedia.com/7/4109/hazards/what-is-the-difference-between-an-acute-hazard-and-a-chronic-hazard

Wyllie, D. (2010, May). *Active shooters in schools: The enemy is denial.* Retrieved from https://www.policeone.com/school-violence/articles/2058168-Active-shooters-in-schools-The-enemy-is-denial/

23

Overview of Interprofessional Practice and Interprofessional Education

◇◇

Alex Johnson, PhD

Introduction

Interprofessional collaborative practice (IPCP) occurs "when health workers from different professional backgrounds work together with patients, families (caregivers), and communities to deliver the highest quality of care" (World Health Organization [WHO], 2010). Similarly, interprofessional education occurs when students from two or more disciplines learn from and with one another (WHO, 2010). On the surface, this simple statement suggests a level of cooperation and collaboration that is expected in every health transaction. Longitudinal evidence, however, suggests that these simple goals are frequently not achieved. Although our health care expenses and advances in technology both continue to grow, errors in judgment, practice, and collaboration lead to significant problems and growing cost of delivery of care. In the health care setting, the frequency of errors has led to the conclusion that failures in collaboration, communication, and teamwork provide an opportunity for resolution. A logical extension of this thinking is that improvement in these critical areas will improve the quality and cost of care.

Because speech-language pathology and audiology are delivered in school settings as well as health care, it is important to acknowledge that similar patterns of professional behavior can also result in challenges in the education setting. Failures in collaboration, communication, or teamwork result in delays or interruptions in needed services to children, conflicts with parents and educators, failures to achieve best outcomes, and costly litigation.

It seems reasonable to conclude that the contexts, primarily health care and education, where speech-language pathology services are delivered can be risk prone, complex, and at times challenging to the client/family complex and to those providing services. Because these concerns apply to individuals across settings, the generic term "client" will be used in this chapter. Hopefully, the reader can substitute their own setting-specific terminology (patient, client, student) accordingly.

Even though most clinicians strive to achieve the best quality outcomes, there are times when the needs of an institution or a provider can complicate the situation. Additionally, when the needs of the client are more complex, miscommunication or ineffective problem solving can lead to confusion and/or conflict. To be honest, the opportunities for error, dissatisfaction, and frustration in patient care are immense. In this brief chapter, we will focus on interprofessional collaborative practice (IPCP) as a mitigating approach to reducing risk, keeping the patient at the center, and enhancing communication with the patient and the health care team. Additionally, we will consider interprofessional education (IPE) as an approach to learning to work collaboratively. Readers should consider this discussion of an early primer on the topics of IPE and IPCP for two reasons. First, a broad set of available resources, some highlighted in this chapter, can provide important depth for those who are interested in learning more. Second, because this is a relatively new area of discussion in the field of *Communication Sciences and Disorders* (CSD), it is important to acknowledge that the evidence base is not yet extensive. Important and substantive scholarship is emerging to support this work but is just beginning to appear in the literature.

Interprofessional Practice

In order to further clarify this topic, the reader is invited to consider three clients from different settings. These cases highlight the types of issues that can arise when poor practices, miscommunication, or interpersonal conflict impact the care of the client.

Client I: Health Care

Mrs. Spinelli is an 88-year-old widow. She emigrated from Italy in her 30s, when she married her husband. Her primary language is Italian and while she understands common English terms and uses social language appropriately, her health literacy skills are weak. She was admitted to the hospital via the emergency department after suffering right-sided weakness, slurred speech, confusion, and difficulty speaking in either English or Italian. Her oldest daughter, Maria, has accompanied her mother and has been in the waiting room for several hours, hoping to see her mother soon. Maria has been gathering information via separate verbal reports from the emergency medicine physician, the neurologist, and the nurse practitioner. Her mother's condition stabilizes over the first 12 hours and she is more communicative, still has weakness, and some word finding difficulties, and appears to have difficulty swallowing. Mrs. Spinelli

is crying and says she just wants to go home. However, the team members think she should be admitted to the stroke unit at the hospital, as does her daughter. In the unit, Mrs. Spinelli is not allowed to eat or drink because of her apparent swallowing difficulty, and she is given intravenous fluids. She is complaining of being hungry and Maria (the daughter) doesn't understand why her mother can't eat. The nurse tells Maria that she can't have food until the speech-language pathologist evaluates her mother's swallowing. However, it's now 6 pm on Saturday. The speech-language pathologist (SLP) won't be available until sometime Monday morning to do the needed evaluation. Maria is very angry and frustrated with this situation and decides to get some soft foods and give it to her mother. After one or two swallows, Mrs. Spinelli starts to cough violently. The nurse walks into the room and begins to scold the daughter for feeding her mother. Both mother and daughter are upset and crying.

Consider this situation from the following perspectives. Answer these five questions:

1. What are the risks? What could go wrong?

2. Can you identify any issues that the health care team could have addressed in a more effective manner?

3. What are the complicating factors in this situation? How do they contribute to the manner in which the client could have received care?

4. Is there anything that could have been done to make this situation better from the client/family perspective?

5. What communication strategies could have been helpful?

Client 2: Public School Setting

Jamie is a 6-year-old boy who attends elementary school. At age three, Jamie was assessed by a speech-language pathologist and diagnosed with developmental stuttering. Her advice at that time was to wait and see if Jamie "grew out of it." Over time, Jamie's disfluencies became less frequent, but never totally disappeared. Now, in first grade, Jamie was placed on the caseload of the school-based SLP. His therapy has been focused on using fluency facilitating techniques. He is seen for one, 30-minute session per week. The SLP let the mother know that she doesn't have a lot of experience with children who stutter, but she will "give it a try." She also let the mother know that she has lots of children on her caseload with more complex speech and language problems, limiting the time available for Jamie.

Recently, Jamie has become less willing to participate in class or to play with other children. His mother has noticed that he is quieter than usual at home, especially when his siblings are involved in conversing. Jamie's teacher notes that he never volunteers to read aloud. She also notices that Jamie is starting to close his eyes when he speaks and seems to tense his shoulders and arms while speaking. The teacher suggests evaluation by the school psychologist. The SLP disagrees that this new referral is needed, saying these behaviors are exhibited by lots of children as they "begin to realize that they stutter." She thinks she can work with him on better coping skills and wants to enlist the teacher's support. The teacher is resistant and wants the referral. Jamie's mother wonders why he can't get more therapy at school, or if another SLP might seem more comfortable dealing with Jamie's problem.

Again, consider the same five questions used in the previous case:

1. What are the risks? What could go wrong?

2. Can you identify any issues that the team could have addressed in a more effective manner?

3. What are the complicating factors in this situation? How do they contribute to the manner in which Jamie could have been cared for?

4. Is there anything that could have been done to make this situation better from the client/family perspective?

5. What communication strategies could have been helpful?

Client 3: Child with Hearing Loss

Laura is a four-year old girl with severe speech-language and behavioral difficulties. Her mother brought her to the SLP for assessment and was referred by the pediatrician. At the evaluation, Laura engaged nicely in the speech and language assessment. When the SLP attempted to screen her hearing, Laura was uncooperative and exhibited loud crying, and seemed inconsolable. Because she was going to be enrolled in therapy, the SLP decided she would attempt to re-screen hearing in an upcoming session. The SLP forgot to document this in the plan and also forgot to follow up on the hearing assessment. Over the next six months of therapy, Laura became slightly more intelligible, but her progress was slow, and she exhibited problems with comprehension and with following directions. Laura's pediatrician suggested a more comprehensive neurodevelopmental assessment. Laura was then seen by a neurologist and a psychologist. The psychologist determined that Laura was developmentally behind in a number of cognitive and

language areas, but not in motor skills. He also noticed a number of behavioral difficulties. He indicated that a special education program might be needed, especially for these unexplained cognitive problems. The neurologist completed a thorough examination and indicated that she seemed neurologically intact but noted that a hearing assessment was not part of the record. He asked that she see an audiologist, who identified a significant hearing loss bilaterally. The team (neurologist, audiologist, psychologist) decided that the best approach would be to secure amplification for Laura and see if her other problems resolved and if this assisted her progress in speech and language therapy. Laura's mother called the speech-language pathologist and expressed her anger and frustration for the "waste of time" as a result of the missed hearing referral from the first examination. Also, Laura's mother's insurance required large co-payments on all of these medical appointments, which served as another trigger for her anger. She noted that she plans to pursue legal action. The SLP apologized and feels upset and embarrassed for her mistake. She is deeply concerned about the consequences.

Again, consider the same five questions used in the previous cases:

1. What are the risks? What could go wrong?

2. Can you identify any issues that the team could have addressed in a more effective manner?

3. What are the complicating factors in this situation? How do they contribute to the manner in which Jamie could have been cared for?

4. Is there anything that could have been done to make this situation better from the client/family perspective?

5. What communication strategies could have been helpful?

Hopefully, these cases highlight the need for improved care by those involved, improved communication with the client/family and within the team, the clarification of roles, and the best ways to manage disagreement or conflict. It is these areas (communication, role clarification, conflict/disagreement management) that are the core skills needed to effectively manage individuals in the context of health care or education. These skills do not replace the need or demand for clinical competency within a specific discipline. However, in the discussion of interprofessional collaboration, these skills are necessary; they complement good clinical skills and competency. And importantly, when an element within the system fails, there is opportunity for correction, and improvement of subsequent error.

There is an important caveat to this discussion. The cases above all present individuals with primary disorders of communication. Thus, the role of the audiologist or SLP in each discussion is quite clear and calls for a leadership perspective. It is not uncommon for SLPs and audiologists to be involved in clinical discussions and situations where the roles and concerns of the patient's communication disorder are not primary for another provider or family member or another provider. Consider the child in a school setting with a behavior disorder, complex health issues, social disadvantage, and a communication disorder. Or consider the patient in a skilled nursing facility (SNF) with hearing loss, dementia-related behavioral difficulties, language impairment, and an exhausted staff of caregivers. Understanding this larger context helps prioritize questions and resolve (or hopefully prevent) adverse outcomes.

Case scenarios such as those described above represent situations familiar to most speech-language pathologists and audiologists. Interprofessional collaborative practice represents an approach—a way of practicing—that addresses these potential failures and attempts to prevent them. At its center, interprofessional practice acknowledges the important role of information and best practices from each relevant discipline in ensuring that patient needs are met and at the same time coordinating and connecting to meet the patient's needs and doing so respectfully and with appreciation.

To the public, it might seem logical that the patient's health care or educational team would be coordinated, connected, orchestrated, and aligned. There is expectation that professionals talk to each other regularly, always put the client's issues first, and typically come to agreement about the desired approach to care or the expected outcome of treatment. The public audience might also assume that professionals educate each other, know (and appreciate) each other's roles, and are responsible in assuring a common set of health, education, or communication goals. Appreciation, respect, cooperation among providers would seem to be reasonable expectations. And as previously needed, these interprofessional competencies align with individual professional skills and knowledge.

While these goals are desirable and highly logical, they are often not fully achieved in today's health and education environments. Notably, speech-language pathologists and audiologists have an opportunity to impact the environment of care beyond their own practice. The client benefits in many positive ways when their SLP or audiologist is fully engaged with other team members. Table 23–1 provides examples of common technical and communication errors and potential interprofessional solutions. For purposes of this discussion, technical errors refer to errors carried out or observed by a professional that are tied to a mistake in judgment,

inferior competence, or poor supervision. Communication errors are errors that occur among members of the team of providers caring for the client or between providers and the client/family

Fortunately, the list of possible risks, errors, and complications as a result of poor care by specialists in communication disorders is limited and usually not life threatening. While a limited number of common procedures that are invasive (intraoperative monitoring, management of selected swallowing and voice issues) can produce serious complications when managed poorly, the consequences of errors in our discipline produce more long-term, insidious, and chronic challenges. Regardless of whether these errors are life threatening, their impact is significant in time, cost, quality of service (and communication). Many times, practice "mistakes" made by audiologists and SLPs are uncovered later in the trajectory of care, rather than at the initial point of services. Delays in discovery of clinical errors in audiology or SLP practices do not reduce importance or impact on quality of life.

On a more routine basis, colleagues in medicine, nursing, and pharmacy engage in procedures and decisions that contain greater risk and potentially more imminently dangerous outcomes. Appreciation for this risk and for insight into the varied approaches and types of decisions being made can be helpful in building relationships with these providers. At the same time, insightful feedback about their patients, especially any untoward consequences being observed, is usually greatly appreciated and can build trust and respect.

Understanding the collaborative context of nearly every client interaction in communication disorders shines light on interprofessionalism. Helping other professionals understand and appreciate the communication, hearing, and swallowing needs of a given patient provides an important foundation. Ensuring that practice is ethical, errors are avoided, and the needs of the patient always being at the center of the work contributes to quality care, but also to effectiveness and excellence of the team.

It is worth noting that there is no comprehensive, well documented taxonomy of errors related to service delivery in speech, language, and hearing settings. At such time as such a listing becomes available, the opportunity to understand and appreciate their impact will become useful in educating SLPs and audiologists. This has proven useful in other health fields and allowed for improved outcomes and quality (Clark, Derakhshan, & Desai, 2018; Cullen, Nath, & Marcus, 2010; Mu, Lohman, & Scheirton, 2006; Scheirton, Mu, Lohman, & Cochran, 2007). In the shorter term, reliance on practice guidelines, clinical experience, and risk mitigation approaches used by other professionals are necessary steps.

Table 23–1. Summary of Common Errors in Health Care and Education Settings: CSD Perspective

Example	Description/Effect	Potential Solutions Informed by Interprofessional Practice
Technical Errors		
Misdiagnosis	Mislabeling of a condition can lead to wrong treatment by another team member.	When in doubt, get supervision, advice, and always use best evidence. Confirm likelihood of diagnosis using information from your own background but also from other team members.
Medication error	Client receives wrong medication or wrong dose; can cause serious risks or failure to improve.	Ensure that patient and all providers understand; double check all medications; note any unexpected reactions or behaviors. When in doubt, speak up/ask. Circle back to team members when there is a question.
Child placed in wrong educational environment	Child fails to benefit from educational services being provided.	Observation of progress and frequent reassessment; input from all team members including parent and child. When in doubt, speak up.
Preventable injuries in an elderly person	Patient falls or is otherwise injured.	For high risk persons, ensure that all safety precautions are in place; involve appropriate professionals from other disciplines. Learn how to safely move patients. Know safety precautions made by others. When in doubt, ask.
Clinical competency errors	Errors in clinician judgment or skill cause unnecessary harm or inconvenience.	Ensure supervision at appropriate level for all providers, but especially those who are early in their careers; provide processes for review and feedback with difficult or challenging cases; always use available evidence; provide a practice environment that encourages questions and feedback, use best practice resources and guidelines and document their use. Acknowledge and learn from errors.
Communication Errors		
Misunderstanding among providers	Providers fail to implement necessary actions to affect benefit.	Avoid and challenge any assumptions by other providers that suggest misunderstanding; "speak up" with questions or clarifications as necessary; consider meaningful and efficient approaches to communicate about important issues.
Misunderstandings by client/family	Client/family fails to comply with recommendations.	Provide frequent opportunities (and time) for client/family to understand recommendations; contribute to reduced complexity of communication; use strategies for ensuring understanding and monitor compliance and follow-up.
Ignoring important information	Provider chooses to ignore information that may have been beneficial.	Use listening and reading skills to ensure that recommendations and clinical information from other members of the team are understood and appreciated. Ask questions to assist with understanding. Know the effects of medicines, treatments, therapies, or educational approaches that might have an effect on cognitive, communication, or swallowing behaviors.

continues

		Potential Solutions Informed by
Table 23–1. *continued*		
Example	**Description/Effect**	**Potential Solutions Informed by Interprofessional Practice**
Documentation failures	Provider fails to document an important finding or recommendation; can lead to unnecessary problems or expense.	Use best practices in documentation; develop mastery of the recording approach being used, particularly with electronic systems in common use; review before submitting final record. Check back to ensure that recommendations are considered or followed.
Failure to appreciate client's health literacy levels	Provider assumes client/family understanding of health or educational information.	Assess client's health literacy based on overall language abilities, use of standard and/or professional English or other language. Deliver information using tools to assist comprehension and compliance (interpreter, written and spoken, recorded materials, diagrams, visuals, etc.).
Contributing to conflict or confusion in any way	Provider allows conflict with another provider or the family to impact care.	Ensure that any disagreements, even healthy ones, are resolved prior to communicating with client/family. Avoid criticism or second guessing of another professional. When information seems confusing or conflicting, check in with other provider.

Interprofessional Education

IPE has been defined as occurring when "students from two or more professions learn about, from, and with each other to enable effective collaboration and improve health outcomes" (WHO, 2010).

The learner focus of IPE differentiates it from the professional practice focus of IPCP. A supposition has been made that if students began to learn together early in their professional formation that they may find it easier to practice interprofessionally as they enter their field. Interestingly, professional associations, academic institutions, and funders have gravitated to this approach in great numbers. Within the discipline of CSD, the American Speech-Language-Hearing Association (ASHA) has taken a leadership role. The ASHA website (www.asha.org/Practice/Interprofessional-Education-Practice) includes extensive resources providing basic information, ideas for infusion of IPE into the curriculum, videos and links to other relevant sites. An eBook developed by ASHA Special Interest Groups (Johnson, 2016) provides a comprehensive overview of IPE and IPP in CSD and highlights several examples for educators and practitioners to consider. A special issue of *Seminars in Speech-Language Pathology* (Johnson & Portney, 2017) included articles on a variety of topics related to interprofessionalism in CSD. The number of ASHA program sessions focusing on IPE/IPP totaled 106 in 2018 (source: http://www.asha.org/Practice/IPE-IPP-Activities-and-

Collaborations). Finally, the 2020 Council on Academic Accreditation (CAA) Standards encourages the use of interprofessional education within SLP and audiology graduate programs. The impact of the expanding interest in interprofessionalism has clearly found a home in CSD.

A wide variety of approaches exist for including interprofessional education as a component of communication disorders curricula. These models have been used in many health professions and the previously cited journals are filled with examples of a variety of novel approaches. Examples include shared practicum experiences with other professions, integration of core learning experiences within multi-professional schools and colleges, short term or intense learning experiences, simulation exercises, and team based or problem-based learning activities within the classroom. New approaches are emerging that address the obvious challenges of time and place, by instituting digital IPE opportunities. One of the obvious side benefits of these innovations in education has been the introduction of new active learning pedagogies in all of the health fields, including CSD. Table 23–2 provides a few examples of some of these new learning approaches that have been reported in the CSD literature.

However, in order to support these innovative learning approaches a wide variety of faculty development activities are being provided for instructors. Also, new approaches to assessment are being developed in order to determine the effectiveness of both teaching and

Table 23–2. Examples of Reported Interprofessional Education Activities That Have Included Students From SLP and Audiology

Topic	Brief Description	Author Reference
Shared media	Using popular media (film, book) to trigger a discussion with an interprofessional group about implications on care, roles, communication, etc.	(Doherty, Knab, & Cahn, 2018)
IPE simulations	Using pre-developed scenarios and/or standardized patient actors to elicit interprofessional discussions and decisions.	(Palaganas, Epps, & Raemer, 2014) (Decker et al., 2015) (Potter & Allen, 2013)
Community service learning	Using joint needs of a community to engage learners in a problem solving or hands on activity	(Bridges, Abel, Carlson, & Tomkowiak, 2010)
Shared practicum– IPE focus	Using a "real" patient/client care environment to practice interprofessional skills	(Palaganas, Epps, & Raemer, 2014) (Hoover, Caplan, Waters, & Carney, 2017) (Ker, Mole, & Bradley, 2003)
Immersive day-long experience	Using a complex simulated experience to integrate clinical skills and IP skills (e.g., natural disaster)	(Hall, Zoller, West, Lancaster, & Blue, 2011)
Hackathon	Using opportunities for students to come together in a time limited competitive experience to produce solutions to a health issue.	(Aungst, 2015)
Digital IPE	Using technology and a common platform to allow students to interact regarding a clinical problem	(Cain & Chretien, 2013) (Carbonaro et al., 2008)
Comprehensive approaches	Approaches that use a systematic approach to immersing IPE goals and activities across curricula and across professions	(Portney, Johnson, & Knab, 2017) (Cahn et al., 2018) (Knab, Inzana, Cahn, & Reidy, 2017)

learning. Finally, there is a growing archive of scholarly work, allowing for critical evaluation of interprofessional activities.

An enlightening membership survey by ASHA has been implemented recently and highlights the particular educational needs of current ASHA members. The most recent Interprofessional Practice Survey (ASHA, 2017) provided important information regarding the penetration of interprofessionalism into practice for audiologists and speech-language pathologists across settings. In this survey, 72% of audiologists and 94% of SLPs reported engaging in interprofessional practice. Despite this high level of participation, only 39% of audiologists and 60% of SLPs reported feeling prepared for IPP and even fewer (21%, 33%, respectively) felt prepared to lead interpro-

fessional teams. It will be important to track changes in these results as interprofessional education is expanded into graduate programs. These data suggest that education in interprofessionalism needs to extend beyond the entry level learner to include continuing education.

As the trend toward acknowledging the impact of interprofessionalism on quality care is relatively new in the broad health care discussion, it is important to acknowledge resources developed both within CSD and beyond. The opportunity to explore these resources presents a rich opportunity for those who wish to advance their understanding of interprofessionalism. Clinicians entering the field will benefit from the opportunity to develop familiarity with interprofessional collaborative practice. This will allow them to be prepared with the language and behaviors associated with interprofessional practice and in some cases to become the teacher of others.

It is important to acknowledge that the purpose of IPE is to prepare students to work in clinical settings with colleagues from other professions, to place the client's needs at the center of this work, and to improve outcomes (cost, efficiency, quality, satisfaction) in the health system. Again, these issues affect speech-language pathologists and audiologists in schools and health settings alike.

It is not possible to list all of the interactions for every clinical setting but consider the SLP or audiologist in the schools. Engaging administrators, special and regular educators, psychologists and social workers, families, and other colleagues are essential components of service delivery for most children on the caseload. Similarly, in a health care setting, interactions with both primary and specialty physicians, nurses, rehabilitation specialists are all important considerations. Working to appreciate the collective and unique goals with and for the client, determining obstacles to achieve outcomes, and addressing them are all parts of collaborative team practice.

National and International Organizations and Resources for IPE and IPCP

As noted above, a wide variety of resources are available to support interprofessional practice among health professions. For the reader interested in learning more and in accessing resources, some brief descriptions follow.

World Health Organization
(http://www.who.org)

WHO has been a leader in the discussion of interprofessionalism. While a particular focus on global health has been at the center of the WHO discussion (Gilbert, Yan, & Hoffman, 2010), the model and principles described can be useful to all health providers. WHO (2010) further explicates the details of their framework and is particularly useful in understanding the ways that best practices can come to scale nationally and internationally.

Interprofessional Education Collaborative
(http://www.ipecollaborative.org)

IPEC was formed in 2009 when six educational associations came together with the idea of collaborating across their varied education models. The focus was to improve and enhance team-based care of patients and improve health outcomes for populations. The organizations represented in the founding group included medicine, nursing, pharmacy, dentistry, and public health. In 2019, the IPEC membership was expanded to include 14 additional education members including ASHA. IPEC sponsors webinars and conferences to advance IPE.

American Interprofessional Health Collaborative (AIHC)
(http://www.aihc.org)

AIHC is an individual membership organization focused on broad and boundary spanning discussion of educational issues across professions. AIHC offers webinars and also partners the with Canadian Interprofessional Health Collaborative to jointly offer *Collaborating Across Borders* conferences biennially.

National Center for Interprofessional Practice and Education (NEXUS)
(http://www.nexusipe.org)

The most comprehensive resource for both educators and practitioners is the NEXUS. Resources include a large national conference (summit) held annually and a number of smaller conferences. The NEXUS also sponsors webinars and a number of publications to guide practice and education. There is a well-managed resource center that provides links to links and publications on a variety of related topics. The NEXUS platform includes an impressive learning system that provides extensive modules, webinars, and training materials. Faculty members and those interested in research in IPE/IPP may want to explore the extensive list of measurement tools provided.

Additionally, several journals exist that are specifically dedicated to reporting research and scholarly discussion around IPCP and IPE. Examples of some of these journals include *The Journal of Interprofessional Care, The Journal of Research in Interprofessional Practice in Practice and Education, The Journal of Interprofessional Education and Practice*, and *Health and Interprofessional Practice*. In addition, a number of health profession specific journals invite and publish articles on IPE and IPC. It is not uncommon to find audiologists and speech-language pathologists (and people with communication and swallowing disorders) represented in articles reported in these publications. Finally, two sources that focus on education in CSD include interprofessionally focused. *Perspectives of the ASHA Special Interest Groups* produces peer reviewed articles related to the various specialty interests with the discipline. The April 2019 issue produced three articles (Hall & Gilliland, 2019; Ludwig

& Kerins, 2019; Namazi Mahchid et al., 2019). A relatively new journal in our field, *Teaching and Learning in Communication Sciences and Disorders* also includes occasional papers on interprofessional activities involved in the education process. As both practice-focused and educational scholarship emerges in CSD it is likely that important new resources will be forthcoming.

Summary

The topics of interprofessional education and practice are emerging as important issues for all professionals in speech-language pathology and audiology. In this chapter, we have attempted to highlight some of the important features of IPE and IPCP. Additional resources and examples have been shared for the reader who wishes to pursue additional information on this topic.

Critical Thinking

1. How can interprofessional education and interprofessional practice be differentiated?

2. Using the three cases presented earlier in this chapter, lead a discussion with classmates that addresses the questions presented and then come to consensus with regard to a plan to prevent the key issues presented OR to develop a plan for resolving the problems resulting from the situation.

3. Discuss the role of speech-language pathologists and audiologists in teaching other professionals and consider the most effective ways to carry out this important task.

4. Identify a health profession about which you would like to learn more. Consider approaches to learning that would be most helpful to you.

5. Design a learning activity that could be useful in helping a team of providers reduce conflict, risk, or error in their practice.

References

American Speech-Language-Hearing Association (ASHA). (2017). *Interprofessional practice survey results*. Retrieved from https://www.asha.org/uploaded files/2017-Interprofessional-Practice-Survey-Results.pdf

Aungst, T. (2015). Using a Hackathon for interprofessional health education opportunities. *Journal of Medical Systems, 39*(5), 60. https://doi.org/10.1007/s10916-015-0247-x

Bridges, D., Abel, S., Carlson, J., & Tomkowiak, J. (2010). Service learning in interprofessional education: A case study. *Journal of Physical Therapy Education, 24*(1), 44.

Cahn, P., Tuck, I., Knab M., Doherty, R., Portney, L., & Johnson, A. (2018). Competent in any context: An integrated model of interprofessional education. *Journal of Interprofessional Care, 32*(6), 782–785. https://doi.org/10.1080/13561820.2018.1500454

Cain, J., & Chretien, K. (2013). Exploring social media's potential in interprofessional education. *Journal of Research in Interprofessional Practice and Education, 3*(2). https://doi.org/10.22230/jripe.2013v3n2a110

Carbonaro, M., King, S., Taylor, E., Satzinger, F., Snart, F., & Drummond, J. (2008). Integration of e-learning technologies in an interprofessional health science course. *Medical Teacher, 30*(1), 25–33. https://doi.org/10.1080/01421590701753450

Decker, S., Anderson, M., Boese, T., Epps, C., McCarthey, J., Motola, I., . . . Scolaro, K. (2015). Standards of best practice: Simulation Standard VIII: Simulation-Enhanced Interprofessional Education (Sim-IPE). *Clinical Simulation in Nursing, 11*(6), 293–297. https://doi.org/10.1016/j.ecns.2015.03.010

Doherty, R., Knab, M., & Cahn, P. (2018). Getting on the same page: An interprofessional common reading program as foundation for patient-centered care. *Journal of Interprofessional Care, 32*(4), 444–451. https://doi.org/10.1080/13561820.2018.1433135

Gilbert, J. H. V., Yan, J., & Hoffman, S. J. (2010). Interprofessional education and collaborative practice. *Journal of Allied Health, 39*(3, Pt. 2) (Special Issue).

Hall, K., & Gilliland, H. (2019). Changing the long-term care culture through interprofessional practice: A speech-language pathologist-led initiative. *Perspectives of the ASHA Special Interest Groups, 4*, 313–321. https://doi.org/10.1044/2019_PERS-SIG2-2018-0005

Hall, P., Zoller, J., West, V., Lancaster, C., & Blue, A. (2011). A novel approach to interprofessional education: interprofessional day, the four-year experience at the Medical University of South Carolina. *Journal of Research in Interprofessional Practice and Education 2*(1). https://doi.org/10.22230/jripe.2011v2n1a42

Hoover, E., Caplan, D., Waters, G., & Carney, A. (2017). Communication and quality of life outcomes from an Interprofessional Intensive, Comprehensive, Aphasia Program (ICAP). *Topics in Stroke Rehabilitation, 24*(2), 82–90. https://doi.org/10.1080/10749357.2016.1207147

Johnson, A. F., & Portney, L. (2017). Interprofessional education issue. *Seminars in Speech and Language, 38*(5), 333–334. https://doi.org/10.1055/s-0037-1607346

Ker, J., Mole, L., & Bradley, P. (2003). Early introduction to interprofessional learning: A simulated ward environment. *Medical Education, 37*(3), 248–255. https://doi.org/10.1046/j.1365-2923.2003.01439.x

Knab, M., Inzana, R., Cahn, P., & Reidy, P. (2017). Preparing future health professionals for interprofessional collaborative practice. Part 2: The student experience. *Seminars in Speech and Language, 38*(5), 342–349. https://doi.org/10.1055/s-0037-1607069

Ludwig, D. A., & Kerins, M. R. (2019). Interprofessional education: Application of interprofessional education collaborative core competencies to school settings. *Perspectives of the ASHA Special Interest Groups, 4*, 269–274. https://doi.org/10.1044/2018_PERS-SIG2-2018-0009

Mu, K., Lohman, H., & Scheirton, L. (2006). Occupational therapy practice errors in physical rehabilitation and geriatrics settings: A national survey study. *American Journal of Occupational Therapy, 60*(3), 288–297.

Namazi Mahchid, H., George P., McKenzie, S., Anuforo, P., Pax Jennifer, A., Knis-Matthews, L., & Marks, D. (2019). An exploratory survey study of grand rounds as an interprofessional education tool for graduate students in the health professions. *Perspectives of the ASHA Special Interest Groups, 4*(2), 299–306. https://doi.org/10.1044/2019_PERS-SIG2-2018-0007

Palaganas, J. C., Epps, C., & Raemer, D. B. (2014). A history of simulation-enhanced interprofessional education. *Journal of Interprofessional Care, 28*(2), 110–115. https://doi.org/10.3109/13561820.2013.869198

Portney, L., Johnson, A., & Knab, M. (2017). Preparing future health professionals for interprofessional collaborative practice. Part 1: The context for learning. *Seminars in Speech and Language, 38*(5), 335–341. https://doi.org/10.1055/s-0037-1607344

Scheirton, L. S., Mu, K., Lohman, H., & Cochran, T. M. (2007). Error and patient safety: Ethical analysis of cases in occupational and physical therapy practice. *Medicine, Health Care, and Philosophy, 10*(3), 301–311. (17310308).

World Health Organization. (2010). *Framework for action on interprofessional education and collaborative practice.* Geneva, Switzerland: Author.

24

Child Abuse and Elder Mistreatment

Carolyn Wiles Higdon, EdD

Introduction

During your employment as an audiologist or speech-language pathologist, you may suspect that a child or elder client is a victim of abuse or neglect. Child abuse and neglect are defined in federal and state laws. Federal legislation lays the groundwork in state laws by identifying a minimum set of acts of behaviors that define child abuse and neglect. The federal Child Abuse Prevention and Treatment Act (CAPTA), (42 U.S.C.A. $5106g), (P.L.100-294) as amended by the CAPTA Reauthorization Act of 2010 (P.L.111-320) defines child abuse and neglect as, at minimum: "Any recent act or failure to act on the part of a parent or caretaker which results in death, serious physical or emotional harm, sexual abuse or exploitation; or an act or failure to act which presents an imminent risk of serious harm" (https://www.childwelfare.gov). CAPTA was most recently amended by the Victims of Child Abuse Act Reauthorization Act of 2018 (P.L. 115-424, 1/7/2019). The law amends section 106(b)(2) (B)(vii) of CAPTA to provide immunity from civil and criminal liability (previously provided immunity from only prosecution) for people who make good-faith child abuse or neglect reports or who provide information or assistance, including medical evaluations or consultations, in connection with a report, investigation, or legal intervention pursuant to a good-faith report of child abuse or neglect.

As stated at the Childwelfare.Gov website (https://www.childwelfare.gov), child protection laws refer to cases of harm to a child caused by parents and other caregivers; generally do not include harm from other people; and some states include child witnessing of domestic violence as a form or neglect or abuse. Depending on the state in which you are employed, you will have either a professional and/or a mandated obligation to report incidences of suspected abuse. This chapter presents broad definitions and characteristics of various types of child abuse, possible causes for such mistreatment, the scope of the problem, and suggestions for what to do when indicators may be present. Similarly, various types of elder abuse and neglect are discussed. This chapter is intended to supplement and not replace individual state definitions, procedures, or requirements for coursework or certification on these topics. To find statute information for a particular state, go to https://www.childwelfare.gov/topics/systemwide/laws-policies/state/

The National Child Abuse and Neglect Data System (NCANDS) is a federal effort to organize annual data on child abuse and neglect. This national data collection and analysis effort was created as part of the CAPTA amendments with the data submitted voluntarily by the 50 states/District of

Columbia/Commonwealth of Puerto Rico to the Children's Bureau in the Administration on Children, Youth and Families, Administration for Children and Families, U.S. Department of Health and Human Services.

Child Abuse and Neglect

Clinicians must be able to identify the signs and symptoms of child abuse and neglect. In addition, you need to be aware of the potential causes and factors that put a child at risk for these forms of maltreatment. Finally, you need to know who may act as an abuser and how common child abuse and neglect are in our society.

Broadly defined, child abuse occurs when children under 18 years of age are physically or mentally harmed by a parent or other person legally responsible for their care. This may involve physical injury by other than accidental means, sexual offense against the child, or allowing the child to engage in such acts. Physical abuse involves the use of force, such as striking, beating, pushing, shoving, shaking, slapping, kicking, pinching, or burning, that results in injury, pain, or impairment. The abuse may or may not be executed with an object. The unjustifiable use of drugs and physical restraints may also be considered physical abuse. Child abuse may also include other forms of neglect such as malnutrition, dehydration, psychological mistreatment, and failure to treat mental or physical ills that may impair growth and development. Emotional abuse, also called mental cruelty, emotional neglect, or emotional maltreatment, occurs when there is some type of nonphysical actions toward a child that result in psychological stress and may lead to physical or psychological illness. Emotional abuse may entail threatening a child verbally or nonverbally, terrorizing, isolating or placing the child in a closed confinement, withholding nurturance and affection, and knowingly permitting the child's maladaptive behavior.

Victims in their first year of life tend to have the highest rate of abuse, and overall, boys of all ages tend to account for fewer than girls of all ages, and whites account for more reports and cases than individuals of Hispanic or African American heritage. However, these demographics are really unique to the exact time the data are collected and can vary over time in each category. There are more children who suffer from neglect than from physical and sexual abuse.

Parental substance abuse and/or abandonment in some states are also considered forms of child abuse. Approximately 38 states and American Samoa, Guam, the Northern Mariana Islands, Puerto Rico, and the Virgin Islands also include acts or circumstances that threaten the child with harm or create a substantial risk of harm to the child's health or welfare (Child Welfare Information Gateway, Children's Bureau/ACYF/ACF/HHS, 2016). The word "approximately" is used because state statues change. As of April 2016, the states are Alabama, Alaska, Arkansas, California, Colorado, Florida, Hawaii, Illinois, Indiana, Kansas, Kentucky, Louisiana, Maine, Maryland, Massachusetts, Michigan Minnesota, Montana, Nebraska, Nevada, New Jersey, New Mexico, New York, North Carolina, Ohio, Oklahoma, Oregon, Pennsylvania, Rhode Island, South Carolina, Tennessee, Texas, Utah, Vermont, Virginia, West Virginia, Wisconsin, and Wyoming. Seven states include human trafficking, labor trafficking, involuntary servitude, or trafficking of minors in the definition of child abuse. Those states are Hawaii, Illinois, Indiana, Louisiana, Mississippi, North Carolina, and Utah. Table 24–1 describes potential types and indicators of child abuse and neglect.

Maltreatment and Neglect

Maltreatment occurs when children under 18 years of age are neglected or have serious physical injury inflicted on them by other than accidental means. The parent or other person legally responsible for care fails to provide a minimum degree of care and the child's physical, mental, emotional, or educational well-being has been or is in danger of being impaired. Neglect is considered an act of omission.

According to the U.S. Department of Health and Human Services (2006), neglect can be categorized as physical, medical, inadequate supervision, environmental, emotional, and educational. Specific examples of neglect include when a responsible adult has not provided a child with adequate nutrition, clothing, shelter, protection from safety hazards, personal hygiene, nurturing or affection, or education, although financially able to do so or offered means to do so. Neglect also occurs when the responsible adult has not provided the child with proper supervision or guardianship. This may occur when this individual inflicts or allows harm to be inflicted, places the child at risk of harm, uses excessive corporal punishment, or uses substances that impair self-control.

A child who has been abandoned by his or her parents or other legally responsible person is also considered neglected. Emotional neglect occurs when there is a "state of substantially diminished psychological or intellectual functioning in relation to, but not limited to such factors as failure to thrive, control of aggression or self-destructive impulses, ability to think and reason, or acting out and misbehavior" (Center for Development of Human Services at Buffalo State College, n.d.,

Table 24–1. Types and Potential Indicators of Child Abuse and Neglect

Possible Signs of Physical Abuse

- Unexplained bruises or welts in different places, in clusters, in various stages of healing, and/or in shape of instrument used
- Unexplained burns
- Unexplained lacerations or abrasions
- Unexplained skeletal injuries, for example, bites, fracture, bald spots, detached retina
- Inappropriate clothing for weather to conceal injuries
- Extremes in behavior—aggressive to withdrawn
- Easily frightened or fearful—for example, of parents, adults, physical contact, going home, or when other children cry
- Self-destructive
- Hurts others
- Poor social relationships—craves attention
- Poor relationships with peers, manipulates adults
- Reports fear of parents, injuries, unbelievable reasons for injuries
- Poor academic performance
- Short attention span
- Language delays
- Runaway
- Truancy and or delinquency

Possible Signs of Sexual Abuse

- Difficulty walking
- Abnormalities in genital/anal areas—itching, pain, swelling, bruises, frequent infections, discharge, poor sphincter control
- Venereal disease
- Pregnancy
- Report of abuse

- Drop in academic performance
- Poor peer relationships
- Unwillingness to change, for example, gym clothing
- Unusually sophisticated sexual knowledge and behavior
- Depressed, apathetic
- Suicidal
- Sexually aggressive
- Regression to earlier developmental stages

Possible Signs of Emotional Maltreatment

- Failure to thrive in infancy
- Poor appearance
- Infantile or regressive behavior
- Developmental lags
- Extremes in behavior
- Poor self-concept
- Depressed, apathetic
- Suicidal

Possible Signs of Neglect

- Hunger and malnutrition, begs for or steals food
- Poor hygiene, lice, body odor
- Inappropriate clothing for weather and context
- Unattended physical problems or medical needs
- Lack of supervision especially in dangerous activities or contexts
- Constant fatigue
- Developmental lags
- Extremes in behavior
- Depressed, apathetic
- Seeks attention or affection
- Truancy or delinquency

p. 17). Such neglect may cause children to be permanently damaged or may be responsible for more deaths per year than abuse.

Per the Child Welfare Government website, approximately 25 states (Arkansas, Colorado, Connecticut, Delaware, Idaho, Indiana, Kentucky, Maine, Minnesota, Mississippi, Missouri, Montana, Nevada, New Hamp-

shire, New Jersey, New Mexico, Nevada, New York, North Dakota, Ohio, Pennsylvania, South Carolina, South Dakota, Utah, West Virginia, Wyoming), the District of Columbia, American Samoa, Puerto Rico, and the Virgin Islands include failure to educate the child as required by law in the definition of neglect (Child Welfare Information Gateway, Children's Bureau/ACYF/

ACF/HHS, 2016).Ten states (Arkansas, Florida, Mississippi, Iowa, North Dakota, Ohio, Oklahoma, Tennessee, Texas, West Virginia) and American Samoa define medical neglect as failing to provide any special medical treatment or mental health care needed by the child. Four states (Indiana, Kansas, Minnesota, Montana) define medical neglect as the withholding of medical treatment or nutrition from disabled infants with life-threatening conditions.

Continuum of Abuse and Neglect

Abuse and neglect range in severity from mild to moderate to severe (U.S. Department of Health and Human Services, 2006). Severity is determined by such factors as degree of harm or risk and the chronicity of the problem. Keep in mind that one occurrence of abuse or neglect may be serious and warrant identification and intervention. The professions of speech-language pathology and audiology over the years have not addressed and educated peers about abuse and neglect. In addition, many times we make excuses for situations we observe or are made aware of rather than identifying and intervening. The standards of reporting call for a report to be made when an individual knows or has "reasonable cause to believe or suspect that a child has been subjected to abuse or neglect." For example, in certain states, when a person suspects that a child is the victim of human trafficking, an abuse that is receiving much visibility in the legal and child protection arenas recently, a report is required.

Causes and Risks

There are numerous, interrelated possible causes of and risk factors for child abuse and neglect. Table 24–2 lists four major categories, including parent/caretaker characteristics, parent–child relationship characteristics, child characteristics, and environmental factors. It should be noted that these are potential risk factors, and the presence of any one is not an absolute predictor of child abuse or neglect. Further, it is likely that these factors are not mutually exclusive and do not all arise within the parent/caregiver. Finally, causes and risk factors must be considered within a framework of a cultural background of child-rearing practices and economic and political values. The origins of abuse and neglect should also be considered from a socio-ecological perspective. For example, poverty may contribute to a parent abusing a child, and thus, intervention would need to focus on both the parent and remediation of poverty (U.S. Department of Health and Human Services, 2006).

Several of these etiological factors bear more discussion. First, 40% of physical abuse of children is caused by people who themselves were abused as children (Check, 1989). These adults were inadequately parented during their own childhood and have carried over this negative child-rearing style to their own interactions with children.

Second, younger parents, particularly teenagers, appear more at risk for committing child abuse. Teenagers may be emotionally immature to take on the responsibilities of parenting and have limited parenting, coping, and homemaking skills. Teen mothers may be at greater risk for not completing their education, have limited work options, and face financial stress (U.S. Department of Health and Human Services, 2006).

Third, substance abuse contributes to drug-exposed newborns and inappropriate parenting styles. Substance abuse frequently co-occurs with other problems. For example, young parents may also be involved with substance abuse. Substance abuse is also a major contributor to criminal activity.

Fourth, parents under stress because of unmet internal needs, lack of support, unemployment, financial or familial crises, and their own health and emotional problems are more vulnerable to committing child abuse and neglecting their children.

Fifth, children who have challenging needs may be more susceptible to abuse and neglect. Children with a myriad complex of chronic needs may stress parents/caregivers beyond their limits, particularly when parents or caregivers have limited education, support, and respite and possibly face financial concerns. Parents may not know how to deal with challenging behavioral characteristics such as noncompliance and may resort to inappropriate measures to gain control. Children with communication disabilities pose double challenges. Parents may become frustrated by lack of meaningful intelligible communication. Further, children with communication problems may not be able to report their own abuse to parents or other caregivers/educators.

Statistics vary on the prevalence of child abuse among children with disabilities, but evidence does indicate that it may be at least 1.8 times greater than for children without disabilities (Hibbard & Desch, 2007; Sullivan & Knutson, 2000). As a comparison to the data reported in 2000, in 2012 more than 3.8 million children were the subjects of at least one report. This is a 3.5% increase from 2008, when an estimated 3.1 million children received a Child Protective Services (CPS) investigation. There is some indication that children with behavior disorders are at greater risk for physical abuse and those with speech/language disorders are at risk for neglect (Sullivan & Knutson, 2000).

Finally, as noted earlier in this chapter, very young children are at the highest risk for abuse and death from

---

Table 24–2. Possible Causes of Risks for Child Abuse and Neglect

Parent/Caretaker Characteristics

- Personal history of abuse
- History of family violence
- Single parenthood or absence of parent
- Social isolation and lack of emotional support
- Parental/caregiver immaturity or lack of parenting knowledge
- Marital problems of parents
- Physical or mental health problems
- Life crises such as financial problems, unemployment or underemployment, death of spouse
- Substance abuse
- Adolescent parents
- Lack of knowledge in areas of housekeeping, nutrition, and medical care
- Expectation that child act like an adult (e.g., leaves young child alone or to care for other younger children)
- Has low frustration tolerance and poor judgement; cannot delay gratification
- Lack of motivation to learn productive child-raising practices
- Does not believe there is a problem, is unconcerned, or refuses to cooperate

Child Characteristics

- Infant/child with special needs (e.g., intellectual disability, health problems, sensory impairments, learning difficulties, communication difficulties)

- Twins or multiple births
- Premature baby
- Baby born during time of family trauma
- Baby or young child who cries excessively (colicky), has feeding difficulties, resists being held
- Stepchild
- Child of unplanned or unwanted pregnancy
- Adolescence, teenager's striving for independence, teenager's dependency on teenage culture

Parent–Child Relationship Characteristics

- Parent's unrealistic expectations for development, achievement, or responsibility
- Lack of nurturing child-rearing skills
- Use of violence as an accepted means of personal interaction
- Inadequate bonding between parent and child
- Delay or failure to seek needed health care
- Perception that child is evil or different

Environmental Factors

- Lack of social support
- Homelessness
- Poor or inadequate housing
- Large family in crowded housing
- Poverty
- Withdrawal of governmental social, housing, and economic support

---

abuse. According to the National Center on Child Abuse and Neglect, children less than 1 year old are more likely to be neglected than at any other time of their lives (U.S. Department of Health and Human Services, 2018). The demands of infant care may tax parents or caregivers, particularly those with limited parenting skills, support, or patience.

Child fatalities are the most tragic outcome of neglect and abuse. The Department of Health and Human Services (2018) reports the following data: "The national rate of child fatalities was 2.20 deaths per 100,000 children. Nearly three-quarters (70.3%) of all child fatalities were younger than 3 years of age. Boys had a higher child fatality rate than girls at 2.54 boys per 100,000

boys in the population. Girls died of abuse and neglect at a rate of 1.94 per 100,000 girls in the population. Nearly 90% (85.5%) of child fatalities were comprised of [sic] White (38.3%), African-Americans (31.9%) and Hispanic (15.3%) victims. Four-fifths (80.0%) of child fatalities were caused by one or both parents."

Munchausen by Proxy

Munchausen syndrome is a disorder in which an individual deliberately creates fictitious physical and/or mental health symptoms to gain attention and sympathy, particularly from medical personnel. When this pattern of exaggeration, fabrication, and inducement is applied to the symptoms of others (usually children), it is called Munchausen by proxy (MBP). This is considered a recognized type of maltreatment that may involve physical, sexual, or emotional abuse, neglect, or a combination (Lasher, 2004). MBP perpetrators are usually mothers who appear to be good caretakers, may have extensive health care knowledge and experience, and are convincing in their concern. Some may change health care providers frequently to avoid suspicion and subject their child to unneeded medical tests and procedures. Some may inflict injury to magnify the symptomatology. Most will deny the maltreatment even when confronted with evidence.

Possible indicators of MBP include some combination of the following: frequent emergency room admissions, recurrent episodes of the same complaint, treatment that does not produce expected results, a pattern of the problem arising in the perpetrator's presence and disappearing in his or her absence, and recurrences when the child goes home after treatment. The parent exhibits characteristics commensurate with the pattern described (Lasher, 2004). Confirmation of this diagnosis is difficult but necessary because of the potential for serious harm to a child. SLPs and audiologists who work in medical settings should be alert to this category of child abuse.

Who Is an Abuser?

Child abuse spans all ethnic, social, economic, and racial lines. Abusers may be parents, guardians, relatives, or friends. Eighty percent of abusers are parents, and women (53.8%) are the majority of abusers (U.S. Department of Health and Human Services Bureau, 2009). In 2009, a typical profile of an abuser is a young adult in his or her mid-20s, with limited education, living at or below the poverty level, and depressed. In 2012, the data remained fairly consistent, although our measures continued to be more refined if reporting is reliable. Fifty states reported unique perpetrators, meaning data were tallied only once, regardless of the number of times the perpetrator was identified. Four fifths of the perpetrators were between the ages of 18 and 44 years. More than half were women (53.5%), 45.3% were men, 1.1 % were unknown sex. Four-fifths of the perpetrators were parents (80.3%) and of those, 88.5% were the biological parents (U.S. Department of Health and Human Services, 2018). Nearly all child abusers were inadequately parented in their own childhood, and most were abused as children (Andrews University, 1999). It should be noted that child–child abuse also occurs, such as adolescent–child sexual abuse, sibling incest, and cousin–cousin incest.

Extent of the Problem

Each year, the U.S. Department of Health and Human Services Children's Bureau (2018) publishes data on child maltreatment that are collected and analyzed by the National Child Abuse and Neglect Data System (NCANDS). Note that these data are aggregate as a child may be reported as a victim of one or more types of abuse or neglect. In 2012 there were about 3.3 million referrals to Child Protective Services (CPS) in the United States involving the alleged maltreatment of 6.0 million children. About one-quarter of these were found to be victims with substantiated cases. Children from birth to 1 year had the highest rate of victimization. Boys presented as 48.2% of the victims and girls 51.1%. Whites accounted for 44% of the cases; African Americans, 22.3%; and Hispanics, 20.7%. Neglect accounted for the highest percent of maltreatment (78.3%), followed by physical abuse (17.8%), sexual abuse (9.5%), and psychological maltreatment (7.6%). Eighty-one percent of abuse cases were committed by parents, and women constituted 53.8% of perpetrators as compared with 44.4% male. Four-fifths of perpetrators were between the ages of 20 and 49 years. The national data estimate that 1770 children died from abuse or neglect. Most of these child fatalities involved children younger than 4 years and boys, and were attributable to neglect or multiple maltreatments. Table 24–3 lists some signs and signals of the presence of child abuse or neglect. The table is not all the signs of abuse or neglect so it is necessary to be vigilant about any behaviors that appear to be unusual or concerning. More details specific to signs of physical abuse, neglect, sexual abuse, and emotional maltreatment are discussed at the following website: https://www.childwelfare.gov/pubs/factsheets/whatiscan.cfm

Effects of Child Abuse and Neglect

Child abuse and neglect have numerous negative effects that may be obvious immediately or may be more covert and manifest themselves later in life. There may be some combination of social, emotional, behavioral, academic, and physical consequences. Each of these negative effects may in some way influence communicative and cognitive development. For example, child neglect has been associated with the failure of the brain to develop and impoverished cognitive and social skills (U.S. Department of Health and Human Services, Children's Bureau, 2018). The Children's Bureau states:

> Children who are neglected early in life may remain in a state of "hyperarousal" in which they are con-

Table 24–3. Signs and Signals of the Presence of Child Abuse or Neglect

In the Child

- Child demonstrates sudden changes in behavior or school performance
- Parents, although notified (sometimes repeatedly), have not obtained help for physical or medical problems
- Child demonstrates potential learning or attention problems without specific physical or psychological causes
- Child demonstrates anxiety about something bad happening, leading to continual hypervigilance
- There is a lack of adult supervision when it would be normal for supervision at the particular chronological age
- Child is noted to be overly compliant, or passive, or withdrawn
- Child does not want to go home, is reticent to leave a safe environment
- Child shows reluctance to be around a particular parent, rarely touching or looking at parent
- Child reports problems or maltreatment at home, or reports parent does not like the child. Sometimes the comments are subtle and infrequent because the child is embarrassed about the differences between himself/herself and peers

In the Parent

- Parent blames the child for problems at school or home
- Parent expects teachers or caregivers to administer harsh physical punishment if child misbehaves
- Parent does not see the child's value or indicates the child is a burden
- Parent demands levels of academic or sports performance the child cannot achieve
- Parents' emotional needs are primarily dependent on the success of the child
- Parent has no real concern for the child, sees the relationship as negative, states dislike for the child
- Parent rarely touches the child

stantly anticipating threats, or they may experience dissociation with a decreased ability to benefit from social, emotional, and cognitive experiences. To be able to learn, a child's brain needs to be in a state of "attentive calm," which is rare for maltreated children. (p. 22)

The brain of abused or neglected children may be as much as 20% smaller than that of non-abused children. Abuse particularly affects the development of language skills. Effects in the education realm include lower IQ; poorer scores on reading, language, and math skills; and overall lower academic performance. Children who are abused or neglected may be diagnosed with oppositional defiant disorder, conduct disorder, post-traumatic stress disorder, depression, anxiety, and sexual abuse of others. They also may be at a higher risk for health problems as an adult.

It is important to note that child abuse and neglect do have long-term implications for victims, even after the physical wounds heal, but that a child's or youth's ability to cope and to even thrive after trauma relates to the child's resilience. With identification and help, these children can overcome the negative experiences.

The estimated annual financial costs are extremely high, totaling more than $103.8 billion (Wang & Holton, 2007). Direct costs are estimated to be at least $33 billion and include costs for hospitalization, chronic health problems, mental health services, child welfare, and law enforcement and judiciary. The remaining indirect costs are related to special education, mental health, juvenile delinquency, lost productivity to society, and adult criminality.

Societal consequences go beyond the financial. Indirect effects include increased child and adult criminal activity, mental illness, substance abuse, and domestic violence. The fact that one-third of neglected children are likely to maltreat their own children creates a vicious cycle that affects generations (U.S. Department of Health and Human Services, Children's Bureau, 2018).

What to Do If You Suspect Abuse

In 2018, the most recent compilation of data this writer could locate, professionals (a person who had contact with the child as part of his or her job) made three-fifths (58.7%) of the reports of alleged child abuse and neglect. Professionals include teachers, police officers, lawyers, social service workers, therapists, education administrators, and clergy. Nonprofessionals (friends, neighbors, relatives) submitted one-fifth of the reports (18.0%) per the data prepared by the Children's Bureau (Administration on Children, Youth, and Families, Administration for Children and Families) of the U.S. Department of Health and Human Services (2018). The report is available on the Children's Bureau website at http://www.acf.hhs.gov/programs/cb/research-data-technology/statistics-research/child-maltreatment

You cannot ignore signs of abuse. First, you must know if you are a mandated reporter of abuse in your state. You must also know what constitutes abuse in your state, what reasonable cause is, and what to do when you suspect abuse. Your confidentiality will be protected if you have made the report in good faith. If you work in a larger organization, policies and procedures will be in place to guide you in the steps to take when reporting abuse. You are advised to inform your supervisor of your suspicions.

Who Is a Mandated Reporter of Abuse?

Each state has specific people who are required by law to report suspected child abuse or neglect. In approximately 48 states, the District of Columbia, American Samoa, Guam, the Northern Mariana Islands, Puerto Rico, and the Virgin Islands, specific professionals are mandated to report child abuse and child neglect. This list includes social workers, teachers, principals, and other school personnel, physicians, nurses, and other health care workers, counselors, therapists and other mental health professionals, child care providers, medical examiners or coroners, and law enforcement officers. In some states other specific professionals are mandated to report. Examples include commercial film or photographic processors, substance abuse counselors, pro-

bation or parole officers, directors and/or employees of camps, youth centers, and recreation centers, domestic violence workers, animal control or humane officers, court appointed special advocates and clergy. And recently, some states have designated faculty, administrators, athletic staff, and other employees at private and public colleges, universities, and vocational and technical schools as mandatory reporters. Some states have started to require anyone suspecting child abuse or child neglect, without specifying professions, to report.

For example, according to New York State Law Chapter 544, Identification and Reporting of Child Abuse and Maltreatment (Explaining Reporting Requirements, Study Requirements for Licensing) (1989), speech-language pathologists and audiologists are not specifically named in this category. They may, however, be considered under some other mandated personnel category such as a school official; a day care center worker; or a member of hospital personnel engaged in the admission, examination, care, or treatment of patients. It is best to review your school, hospital, or agency's policy and procedure manual for precise guidelines in your facility, locality, and state. Note that if you are a mandated reporter, you can face criminal and civil liability for not reporting suspected abuse (U.S. Department of Health and Human Services, 2018). It is your responsibility to know the reporting laws in the state in which you practice (Child Welfare Information Gateway Children's Bureau, 2019; https//www.childwelfare.gov/topics/systemwidelaws-policies/state/); however, even if you are not a mandated reporter, you have an ethical responsibility to document in writing possible signs of abuse or neglect and report these to your supervisor or immediate superior.

What Is Reasonable Cause?

Circumstances for making a report may vary from state to state. The key words for the need to report in any official capacity, are "suspects" or "has reason to believe" that a child has been abused or neglected. Another benchmark is if the reporter has "knowledge of" or "observes a child being subjected to, conditions that would reasonably result in harm to the child." The facts and circumstances are reported, without the burden of providing proof that the neglect or abuse has occurred. This is true for anyone reporting, either professional or nonprofessional.

When and to Whom to Report

Suspected child abuse or neglect should be reported immediately by telephone, at any time of day, seven days a week. Each state, on its state human services or Department of Children and Family Services websites, will have a phone number to report child abuse or child neglect. If additional information is needed, the Child Help 800 number is a resource (800-422-4453). Depending on the state, a written report may be required within a specified time limit, typically 24 to 48 hours after the initial phone report. In addition, national phone numbers are listed in the Resources section at the end of this chapter. Your agency, hospital, or school will have specific guidelines for policies and procedures regarding reporting of possible child abuse.

Immunity and Confidentiality

When reporting, you will need to provide the name, address, and age of the child, the name(s) and address(es) of the parents or guardians, and the nature of the abuse. If possible, the name of the perpetrator and that person's relationship to the child are helpful but not mandatory. If you are a mandatory reporter by your state laws, you will need to provide your name; however, this information typically is confidential and protected by law. You have immunity from any civil or criminal liability if you or your agency has reported a suspected case of child abuse or neglect in good faith.

Most mandatory reporting laws specify how and when communication is privileged. "Privileged communications" is the right, by law, to maintain confidential communication between professionals and clients and patients. At the time of this writing, all but three states and Puerto Rico address the issue of privileged communication, affirming the privilege or denying it (i.e., not allowing privilege to be grounds for failing to report) per Child Welfare Information Gateway (2019). Connecticut, Mississippi, and New Jersey do not currently address privileged communication within their reporting laws but this information may be in rules of evidence dealing with other statutes in these states. It is wise to know the definitions and laws pertaining to privileged communication in your state, but not knowing this information does not protect you from reporting child abuse or child neglect.

Consequences for Failing to Report

As noted earlier in the chapter, if you are a mandated reporter and willfully fail to report a case of suspected child abuse or maltreatment, you may be guilty of a misdemeanor and have a civil liability for damages caused by such failure. More importantly, failure to report your suspicion may result in continued and/or traumatic harm to a child.

Elder Abuse, Neglect, and Exploitation

Elders are among the most vulnerable members of our society. There are 75 million baby boomers who will retire, and for the next 20 years an average of 10,000 people per day will reach 65 years of age, moving into their retirement phase of their lives. Aging is one of the most important demographic trends in the United States (U.S. Administration on Aging, 2006). In 1965, the Older Americans Act (OAA) was signed into law to meet the diverse needs of an aging population. This law had specific objectives for maintaining the dignity and welfare of older individuals. In 2016, the Older Americans Reauthorization Act "OAA as amended" was approved by Congress. As we go to press, the OAA expires on September 30, 2019. A bipartisan reauthorization is the top priority of the National Association of Area Agencies on Aging. The OAA reauthorizes services and strengthens the law by providing better protection for vulnerable elders, promoting evidence-based support, improving nutritional services, and aligning senior employment services with the workforce development system.

Aging can be complicated by the onset of chronic illnesses and disabling conditions, which can increase the likelihood of functional loss and disability. Elderly persons' ability to protect themselves may be hampered by physical, cognitive, and communication problems. As with child abuse, you need to be aware of the signs and symptoms of elder abuse and what to do if you suspect such maltreatment. Remember that elder abuse or neglect can take place in the home or in formal care settings.

Elder Abuse

Elder abuse is a general term that describes intentional and neglectful actions by a person(s) in trust or a caregiver who causes harm to an elder (National Center on Elder Abuse, 2010). A second definition of elder abuse is "the willful infliction of injury, unreasonable confinement, intimidation, or cruel punishment with resulting physical harm, pain, or mental anguish; or deprivation by a person including a caregiver, of goods or services that are necessary to avoid physical harm, mental anguish, or mental illness" (Older Americans Act Section 102 [13][A][B]). For an action to be classified as elder abuse, a person either does something or fails to do something that harms an elder. Elder abuse may occur in the home or in institutional settings, or it may be self-imposed (Administration on Aging, 1998). In 2002, Weinrich stated that a research agenda as well as community awareness are needed because elder abuse is now considered a serious health concern for the older population.

The most common forms of elder abuse include physical abuse, sexual abuse, emotional or psychological abuse, neglect, abandonment, financial or material exploitation, and self-neglect. Many types of elder abuse are similar to those of child abuse, including physical abuse involving injury, pain, or impairment and sexual abuse, whereby individuals receive inappropriate and unwanted sexual activities imposed on them. Several other types of abuse are particular to elders or have different characteristics and are described in the following sections. The following list provides a summary of the major types of elder abuse and potential signs of treatment of each type.

Physical Abuse. This type of abuse involves the non-accidental use of force that results in pain, injury, or impairment (Helpguide, 2010). Physical abuse may also include the inappropriate use of drugs, restraints, or confinement.

Emotional or Psychological Abuse. Elders who experience undue emotional pain or distress are said to be emotionally abused. A common type of emotional abuse is administered verbally through verbal attacks, insults, threats, intimidation, humiliation, or harassment or by giving the elder the "silent treatment." Nonverbal abuse involves ignoring or terrorizing the older person. Other forms of emotional abuse include infantilizing of the elder and isolation from people and activities of choice.

Neglect. Elder neglect is defined as "an act of omission, of not doing something, of withholding goods or services" (Quinn & Tomita, 1986, p. 34). Neglect involves deliberately ignoring the needs of an elder and may take the form of financial neglect, by failing to attend to financial obligations, and physical neglect, when the elder receives inadequate food, water, clothing, shelter, personal hygiene, medicine, comfort, or personal safety (Administration on Aging, 1998). Neglect can be intentional (active), characterized by a conscious effort to inflict harm, or unintentional (passive), which is associated with laziness or lack of knowledge (Cicirelli, 1986).

Self-Neglect. Self-neglect occurs when elders harm themselves. For example, elders may improperly or inadequately care for their own health, safety, clothing, nutrition, hygiene, or shelter. Potential factors that lead to self-neglect include long-term chronic self-neglect through adulthood, dementia, illness, malnutrition, overmedication, depression, substance abuse, poverty, and isolation (Woolf, 1998).

Abandonment. Abandonment is the deliberate desertion of an elder by a person who has responsibility for that elder. Abandoned elders are left alone frequently and for extended time periods in their home or other setting by caregivers. This is particularly dangerous for those elders who cannot provide for their own daily needs such as food, personal care, and medications. In addition, the loss of socialization opportunities may have a deleterious effect on the elder and contribute to cognitive and emotional decline.

Financial or Material Exploitation. This type of abuse occurs when an elder's funds, property, or material assets are illegally or improperly used, usually without authorization or permission. Examples of financial or material exploitation include fraudulent check cashing or use of a credit card; forgery of a signature; misuse or theft of money, property, or other possessions; coercion into signing a document (e.g., a will); identity theft; or the improper use of conservatorship, guardianship, or power of attorney (Administration on Aging, 1998; Helpguide, 2010).

Decision-Making Ability and Risk of Elder Mistreatment

Changes in the brain and cognition and social functioning affect the decision-making ability of older people, resulting in decisions that affect an older person's ability to pay bills, drive, follow recipes, adhere to medication schedules, or refuse medical treatment (IOM, 2015). Individuals can show lack of decision-making ability in one area while retaining ability in other areas. Impaired ability may lead to an increased risk for abuse in older people (Spreng et al., 2016). The natural process of aging, including cognitive aging, and the social aspects of decision making may be the first consideration. Psychosocial factors such as depression, reduced feelings of well-being, less social support, and increased risk of financial vulnerability also lead to increased risk of elder abuse.

Cognitive aging (memory, decision making, processing speed, wisdom and learning) includes structural and functional brain changes that may impact daily tasks. Cognitive aging may not be able to be avoided, but there is evidence that effects can be reduced with physical exercise, reducing and managing cardiovascular disease risk factors, and medication management (IOM, 2015). Cognitive aging may be associated with the potential for financial fraud and abuse and poor consumer decision making (IOM, 2015). Decisions that require a person to understand his/her decision and be able to take responsibility for the consequences of the decision (Falk et al., 2014, p. 853) may be affected by situations that involve new learning or stressful situations.

Moye and Marson (2007) identified medical decision-making capacity and financial decision-making capacity as two major clinical domains of capacity fundamental to personal autonomy and independent functioning that have received the most research attention. A person's ability to make decisions regarding her/his medical treatment is a fundamental aspect of autonomy. Moye and Marson (2007) identify the four core abilities associated with consent capacity as understanding, appreciation, expressing a choice, and reasoning. Understanding is the ability to comprehend diagnostic and treatment-related information that may include risks and benefits of proposed treatments. Appreciation is the ability to relate medical information and related consequences to one's own personal situation. Expressing a choice is the ability to convey relatively consistent treatment choices. Reasoning is ability to rationally evaluate and compare treatment alternatives. Although these four core abilities are not just used in medical decision-making capacity, speech-language pathologists may be the first to see changes occurring in these areas and should be vigilant when working with the elderly.

If changes are noticed in an older person's decision-making ability, it is important to seek further evaluations to assess an individual's physical and psychological status to identify any conditions that may require therapy or medical treatment. A speech-language pathologist is trained in assessment processes to analyze information and make recommendations that will allow an older person to maintain independence and decision-making abilities protecting the individual against abuse and exploitation. A trusted support team is critical in supporting the individual at this stage.

Who Is Abused?

According to the National Center on Elder Abuse (2010), the majority of elder abuse victims are female (67.3%) with about 1 in 10 elders becoming the victims of elder abuse. National data indicate that there may be between 1 million and 2 million older Americans who have been abused or neglected. The median age of elders abused by others is 77.9 years and 77.4 years for elders who neglected themselves. Two-thirds of the victims of domestic abuse are white, 18.7% are African American, and 10% are Hispanic.

The World Health Organization (WHO) (2019) estimates that 15.7% of the individuals 60 years or older (around one in six people) may have experienced elder abuse. The number may be higher for people in "at risk" categories, including older people with physical or mental incapacity and people living in institutional settings. Abuse within institutions is more likely to occur where standards for health care are low, staff are poorly trained/overworked, the physical environment is deficient, and policies prioritize institution needs over resident needs.

WHO states that rates of elder abuse are high in nursing homes and long-term care facilities with two in three staff reporting they have committed abuse in the past year (WHO, 2019). As the global population of people age 60 and older will more than double to about 2 billion in 2050, elder abuse is predicted to increase in many countries, leading to serious physical injuries and long-term psychological consequences. These data are considered gross underestimations of the true number of cases but are much higher in institutions than in community settings. It is predicted that for every reported incident of elder abuse, five go unreported. Reliable statistics on elder abuse and neglect are difficult to find but as more agencies collect data, we will have an improved accounting of elder abuse cases.

Who Is at Risk?

Any elder is at risk for abuse, although those who have mental or physical disabilities are at the greatest risk, but overall elder abuse is becoming an important public health problem that is underreported and underestimated. Recent data (2017) indicate that about 67% of elders with substantiated reports of abuse were female, 43% were over age 80, and 77% were Caucasian; 89% of incidents occurred in the home (National Center on Elder Abuse, 2010). Elders are at risk when their caregivers over- or underestimate their abilities and thus have unreasonable expectations for performance. Elders are also at risk if there is a history of domestic abuse in their family or in that of a professional caregiver. The likelihood of abuse increases when caregivers have difficulty with temper control; physical, mental, or substance abuse problems; and immature personalities. Elders themselves may increase their risk for abuse if they verbally insult or psychologically taunt their caregivers, especially with threats of withholding inheritances (Quinn & Tomita, 1986). Other factors that place elders at risk include dependency and isolation, family conflict, and financial stress. Those elders with dementia and mental disorders are at significant risk for abuse, as care for these individuals is particularly stressful and time-consuming (National Center on Elder Abuse, 2011).

Risk factors have been identified by the World Health Organization (2019) as individual risks, relationship risks, community risks, and sociocultural risks. Table 24–4 lists possible risk factors in each of these categories. Table 24–5 gives readers a list of types and potential indicators of elder abuse, neglect, and exploitation.

Who Is an Abuser?

Those who abuse elders come from all racial, economic, educational, and socioeconomic strata (Quinn &

Table 24–4. Individual, Relationship, Community, Socio-Cultural Risk Factors

Individual Risk Factors

- Poor physical health of the individual
- Mental health problems of the individual
- Mental health disorders of the abuser
- Substance abuse of the abuser
- Gender of the victim
- Shared living situation of individual and abuser
- Inferior social status of women in some cultures
- Marriage status of women in some cultures

Relationship Risk Factors

- A shared living situation between two parties
- An abuser who is financially dependent on the older person
- A history of challenging family relationships
- Female or male family members' expectation but inability to care for older family members

Community Risk Factors (specifically toward social isolation)

- Caregivers and older persons' social isolation
- A person's loss of physical or mental capacity
- The loss of close family and friends

Sociocultural Risk Factors

- Older adults depicted as frail, weak, or dependent, promoting ageist stereotypes
- A breakdown in the bonds in and between generations in the family
- Situations affecting distribution of power and goods in families, specifically affecting plans for inheritance or land rights
- In societies where older persons were traditionally cared for by their children, adult childrens' attitudes and migration plans leave older parents alone
- Older adults are realizing a lack of personal funds, changes in funding of medical care, and changes in funding for long-term care affecting individuals' ability to pay for the needed care and services

Tomita, 1986). In 2004, the National Center on Elder Abuse (2010) reported that 52.7% of alleged perpetrators of abuse were female and three-quarters were under the age of 60. It also found that adult children are the most frequent abusers of the elderly (34.6%), followed by other family members (21.5%). Formal caregivers who have poor working conditions, low salary, and limited education are at higher risk for becoming abusers.

Most Common Types of Abuse

The most common types of elder maltreatment are, in decreasing order of frequency, neglect (49%), emotional/psychological abuse (35%), financial/ material exploitation (30%), physical abuse (27%), abandonment (4%), sexual abuse (3%), and other (1.4%). These frequency data are not mutually exclusive, as more than one type of abuse may be reported for an incident.

Table 24–5. Types and Potential Indicators of Elder Abuse, Neglect, and Exploitation

Possible Signs of Physical Abuse

- Cuts, wounds, punctures, choke marks
- Unexplained fractures, broken bones, skull fractures
- Bruises, welts, discolorations on face or body
- Bedsores or significant skin problems
- Detached retina, hematomas
- Injuries left untreated or improperly cared for
- Poor skin hygiene or condition
- Dehydration without illness-based cause
- Malnourishment without illness-based cause
- Loss of weight
- Cigarette or rope burns
- Soiled clothing or bed
- Broken eyeglasses, hearing aids, other assistive devices
- Signs of being restrained
- Sudden change in elder behavior
- Elder report of physical abuse
- Death or murder

Possible Signs of Sexual Abuse

- Bruises around breasts or genital area
- Unexplained sexually transmitted diseases
- Unexplained vaginal or anal bleeding
- Torn, stained, or bloody underclothing
- Inappropriate display of affection by caregiver
- Elder report of sexual abuse

Possible Signs of Psychological/ Emotional Abuse

- Hesitancy to express feelings in public
- Ambivalence, deference to others, passivity, cowering
- Lack of eye contact
- Clinging, trembling
- Depression
- Confusion or disorientation
- Fear
- Withdrawal

- Denial
- Helplessness, hopelessness
- Severe anxiety or agitation
- Anger
- Confabulations
- Elder report of verbal or emotional mistreatment
- Extreme withdrawal
- Elder becomes non-communicative, especially in presence of caregiver
- Attempted suicide

Possible Signs of Financial or Material Exploitation

- Improper signatures on financial documents
- or unusual activity in bank accounts
- Identity theft
- Financial statements do not come to elder's home without explanation
- Power of attorney given or changed without explanation
- Change(s) in will or other documents without explanation
- Financial mismanagement of funds, including unpaid bills
- Elder states that he or she has been signing papers without understanding their content
- Missing personal items
- Heightened concern by elder regarding financial management
- Lack of amenities, including appropriate clothing, entertainment, and so on that elder could afford
- Promises of care by caregiver or family
- Provision of unnecessary services or purchase of items
- Unauthorized withdrawal of funds using an ATM or credit card
- Elder receives eviction notice from house he or she owned
- Elder report of financial or property mismanagement
- Caregiver concerned that too much money is spent on the elder

continues

Table 24–5. *continued*	
Possible Signs of Abandonment	**Possible Signs of Self-Neglect**
■ Desertion of an elder at a hospital, nursing home, or other institution	■ Inability to handle activities of daily living,
■ Desertion of an elder at a public location	■ including personal care and meal preparation
■ Report by elder of being abandoned	■ Suicide attempts
	■ Inadequate financial management
Possible Signs of Neglect	■ Dirty, unsafe living environment
■ Dirty environment	■ Homelessness
■ Fecal or urine smell	■ Refusing medical or personal care
■ Environmental safety hazards	■ Willful isolation
■ Rashes, sores, lice, or other infestation	■ Alcohol or other drug abuse
■ Untreated medical condition	■ Slovenly appearance
■ Malnourishment or dehydration	■ Malnourishment or dehydration
■ Inappropriate or inadequate clothing and grooming	■ Not keeping medical or other important personal appointments

Why Does Elder Abuse Occur?

Elder abuse and neglect are generally attributed to the following factors:

- Physical and mental impairment of the elder
- Psychological abuse
- Financial abuse
- Neglect
- Sexual abuse
- Caregiver stress
- Violence as a problem-solving strategy
- Individual problems of the abuser
- Society's negative portrayal of the elderly
- Greed (Quinn & Tomita, 1986)

It is likely these hypothesized causes work in tandem rather than individually. Meeting the needs of frail, physically and/or mentally challenged elders is a time- and effort-consuming, especially for caregivers with limited personal resources and reduced or immature psychological stamina. In some cases, a "triggering crisis" may instigate an incident of abuse. In other cases, long-term, unrelieved stress and physical fatigue may result in an explosion of violence. Some families may routinely use abuse as a problem-solving strategy.

Some elders may purposely antagonize their caregivers, whereas others with reduced cognitive abilities may not understand or appreciate the care received. Finally, society stigmatizes the disabled and their caregivers. Limited financial or social incentives are available for caregivers, who may sacrifice career and social lives for their elder family member. Some caregivers may deliberately hasten the progression of decline because it will result in a greater or earlier financial inheritance. Reinharz (1986) commented that elder abuse is not a modern problem and represents "twin cultural themes of honor and contempt" toward the elderly.

Certain caregiving contexts appear to trigger abuse, and many of these are related to the stress involved. For example, feeding, incontinence, interrupted sleep, and incessant vocalizations are all extremely stressful for caregivers, especially when they occur repeatedly and without respite. These situations become even more problematic if the caregiver is an alcohol or drug abuser or has a history of being abused or abusive.

Elders may be afraid to report abuse because of their fear of what will happen to them if their caregiver is removed. Many elders greatly fear they will be forced to leave their home and relocate to an institutional setting where there will be less independence, loss of control, and loss of familiar surroundings and property. Thus, many elders refrain from mentioning incidents of abuse because they perceive the alternative of institutionalization to be worse than the abuse they receive in their home.

Elder Abuse in Long-Term Care Facilities

Working with elders in long-term care facilities can be a challenging job, particularly when residents have demanding physical and psychological needs, salary, and societal regard are low, and training is minimal. The list of examples of abuse is long and growing longer to include physically restraining patients; depriving them of their dignity (not meeting bathroom needs, leaving them in dirty clothes); not allowing them to make decisions within their ability levels about daily activities or decisions about personal affairs; not providing sufficient care, which then results in medical issues such as pressure sores, infections, torn skin, broken bones, dehydration, loss of weight; over- or under-medicating or withholding medications, and emotional neglect and abuse, leading, at times, to psychological consequences including depression, anxiety, or premature death.

Pillemer and Moore (1990) state that possible risk factors for staff abuse of elders in long-term care settings include patient aggression and provocation, staff burnout, staff age, and conflict regarding daily routines. In their confidential interviews of 577 nurses and aides, Pillemer and Moore found that more than 75% of staff had observed psychological abuse, 41% admitted to committing such abuse, about 33% had observed physical abuse, and 10% had committed physical abuse. Physical abuse is the most commonly reported abuse against elders in nursing homes, followed by sexual abuse, neglect, and monetary abuse. Male nursing aides committed two-thirds of the reported cases of abuse. Prevention undoubtedly lies in higher qualifications for staff, more staff training, and enforcement of mandatory abuse reporting (Quinn & Tomita, 1997).

What to Do?

The World Health Organization (2019) has identified strategies to prevent or react quickly to take action against elder abuse but attention and support come primarily from high(er) income countries. Prevention steps include caregiver training on dementia, school-based intergenerational programs, awareness programs for the public and professional communities, screening of potential victims and abusers, support interventions for caregivers including respite and stress management, and improving residential care policies to define and improve standards of practice and care.

To prevent or respond in a timely manner to reports of abuse, procedures for reporting abuse to authorities and helplines to provide information and referrals need to be clearly defined and accessible to all. Self-help groups, safe houses, emergency shelters should be highly visible and available to all individuals. Caregiver support interventions and psychological programs for abusers should be available to all who need these resources. In addition, the courts, legal system, and medical community need to be better educated and quicker to react to potential problems to avoid serious outcomes as well as to establish legal, financial, and housing support. The World Health Organization (2019) also shows evidence that adult protective services and home visitation by police and social workers for victims of elder abuse may in fact increase elder abuse.

There is a five-step approach to dealing with elder abuse. The guidelines for action are listed below. Although these steps appear to be linear, they can occur simultaneously.

1. Identify whether abuse is taking place. Ask questions to find out further information such as "is someone hurting you?" or "are you frightened by anyone?" If this appears to be an emergency, jump to Step 3. Responding to an emergency such as serious assault or ongoing criminal act should be first priority to protect the older person.

2. Provide emotional support. Listen, acknowledge, and validate. Listen to what the person is saying. Acknowledge what they are saying. Validate their feelings.

3. Assess risk and plan safety. Determine the level of response needed. Is it an emergency? Call 911. Follow procedures by notifying managers and administrators, take safeguards to protect the older person and others.

4. Refer. Contact the appropriate service or agency with reference to the level of risk to the older person and others. If it is not an emergency, obtain the person's consent and make appropriate referrals. If the person does not want assistance, attempt to provide them with contact information for services.

5. Document. Record concerns, communication with the person, and whatever actions have been taken.

Table 24–6 is a list of intervention steps to consider based on the Alliance for Prevention of Elder Abuse Western Australia publication (Elder Abuse Protocol, 2017). Several factors increase the risk that an older person will be abused. These include dependency, family dynamics and living arrangements, social isolation, health and cognitive impairments, addictions, caregiver stress, language and cultural barriers, and ageism. Each state determines whether audiologists and speech-lan-

Table 24–6. Intervention Principles

- Do no harm.
- Accept what the elder person is saying.
- Do not escalate action unnecessarily.
- Assess safety and risks and implement safety management plans.
- Uphold older persons' rights in all actions and interactions and respect their right to autonomy and self-determination.
- If you have doubts about the older person's decision-making ability, make appropriate referrals.
- Recognize the importance of preserving family relationships where possible.
- Responses should take into account the needs of the older person in relation to disability, culture, language, religion, gender, sexuality, and historical abuse and reporting experiences.
- Know your organization's policies and procedures, including duty of care responsibilities.
- Be aware of the potential for conflict of interest, especially in small communities or within service settings.
- Be clear about your role in supporting the older person and do not be co-opted into other people's agendas.
- Be informed about elder abuse and engage in training where available.

guage pathologists are mandated to report child or elder abuse. If you suspect elder abuse, it is best to document in writing the indicators and discuss the policy and procedure of your setting for reporting these potential signs of elder abuse.

In most states, the Adult Protective Services (APS) agency is the major site responsible for both investigation of reported cases of elder abuse and for providing help to victims and their families. This agency is often contained within the county department of social services. Other organizations that have primary roles in investigation and follow-up of elder abuse referrals include the Area Agency on Aging, county departments of social services, the local law enforcement agency, the medical examiner/coroner's office, hospitals, the state long-term care ombudsman's office, mental health agencies, and facility licensing or certification organizations. Investigations may lead to provision of community supportive services, financial or legal assistance, counseling referrals, or guardianship. Alleged perpetrators may face criminal investigations and prosecution.

What to Report

When reporting suspected abuse, the reporter should have as much information as possible. The purpose of an investigation is to determine if abuse actually occurred and how/if the case will be prosecuted for abuse. The following information is needed when reporting abuse: the

supposed abused person's name, address, date of birth and gender as well as the same information of the alleged abuser; a description of the incident; name, address, phone number of next of kin, guardian or representative payee; names and information of any parties with whom the older person resides, and any information that adds further clarity to the cause or how the abuse has been occurring. It is important to remember that you should first report the suspected abuse to your supervisor but any individual is able to report directly to the state APS department. It is not wise for a reporter to attempt to intervene in cases of suspected abuse, and you need to keep in mind that the older person may be traumatized or may not want the abuse reported. Neither, however, alleviate you of your legal responsibility to report the suspected abuse (World Health Organization, 2019). Individuals who have lived with abuse over time may believe that it is better to put up with the abuse than to leave their environment and possessions at this age of life. This can create a very sad and negative lifestyle for this person, as well as the danger of something more serious occurring.

If the person who is allegedly doing the abusing is made aware of the identification of abuse or the reporting of abuse, the abuse may escalate. Confidentiality and anonymity are important considerations but it is never alright not to report suspected abuse. The practice of speech-language pathology and audiology has increased in settings and with individuals in the aging and elder population, thus increasing the likelihood of identification of individuals who are being abused. With life expectancies increasing, with our evidence-based research showing more need for speech, language, swallowing, hearing assessments, treatment with the aging population, and with the establishment of longer-term relationships with these individuals, SLPs and audiologists have more opportunities to be watchdogs for elder abuse.

The World Health Organization adopted, in 2019, a global strategy and action plan on ageing and health that provides guidance for coordinated action to prevent elder abuse through the following initiatives that help to identify, quantify, and respond to the problem (WHO, 2019). These include building evidence on the scope and types of elder abuse in different settings (to understand the magnitude and nature of the problem at the global level), with an emphasis on low and middle income countries where there are little data, developing evidence and providing prevention guidance to member states, supporting national efforts to prevent elder abuse, and collaborating with international agencies and organizations to deter the problem globally.

There are three case studies in Appendices 24–A, 24–B, and 24–C to represent child neglect and elder abuse issues that occur. Although these are real cases, the names and events have been altered to protect the anonymity of the individuals.

Summary

When providing intervention services in home, community, or institutional settings, audiologists and speech-language pathologists need to be vigilant for signs of abuse. Young children and elders with communication problems and other disorders are particularly vulnerable to abuse because of their high-intensity needs. Abuse can take a variety of forms, including physical, psychological, sexual, financial, or neglect. Abuse or neglect can occur in any age, ethnic, or economic group; in urban, suburban, or rural settings; and in any type of setting by paid caregivers, family members, or others. Globally too little is known about child and elder abuse, how to prevent it, and consequences, and evidence of what works to prevent both is very limited. Speech-language pathologists and audiologists need to know their individual state regulations regarding mandated reporting of child or elder abuse and should know their agency's particular guidelines for reporting suspected cases of child abuse. Identification of abuse against those with whom we work may help prevent further abuse and provide abusers with the help they need to refrain from this type of dangerous and humiliating behavior.

Critical Thinking

1. What steps would you take if you suspected child or elder abuse?

2. How would you consider cultural differences in child-raising practices in deciding if a child had possibly been abused?

3. What might be the effects if you do not report a suspected case of child or elder abuse?

4. Should speech-language pathologists and audiologists be legally described as "mandated" reporters of child abuse in every state? Why or why not?

5. When visiting a home for an early intervention evaluation, you notice that the children in the home are dirty, dressed inappropriately for the heating conditions in the home, and frequently scratch themselves. The physical environment of the home is also filthy. The mother, however, is an excellent informant and greatly interested in the speech and language development of her children. The mother and children appear to have a warm relationship. What would you do?

6. You are hired by a private practice on an hourly wage to provide clinical services in a long-term care facility. You notice some signs of resident neglect in the facility but are reluctant to say anything because it may jeopardize your position in the facility. What would you do? What would the Code of Ethics of the American Speech-Language-Hearing Association or American Board of Audiology say about this issue?

7. Review the cases in Appendices 24–A, 24–B, and 24–C. Consider what you should do in each situation.

References

Administration on Aging. (1998). *The national elder abuse incidence study: Final report September 1998.* Retrieved from http://www.aoa.gov/AoARoot/ AoA_Programs/Elder_Rights/Elder_Abuse/docs/ ABuseReport_Full.pdf

Andrews University. (1999). *Child abuse.* Available from http://www.andrews.edu/

Center for Development of Human Services at Buffalo State College. (n.d.). *Identification and report of child abuse and maltreatment: A course for mandated reporters.* Buffalo, NY: Author.

Check, W. (1989). *Child abuse.* New York, NY: Chelsea House.

Child Welfare Information Gateway: Children's Bureau/ACYF/ACF/HHS. (2016). Retrieved from https://www.childwelfare.gov

Child Welfare Information Gateway. (2019). *Mandatory reporters of child abuse and neglect.* Retrieved from https://www.childwelfare.gov

Child Welfare Information Gateway. (2019). Retrieved from https://www.childwelfare.gov/pubs/factsheets/whatiscan.cfm

Child Welfare Information Gateway. (2019). Retrieved from https://www.acf.hhs.gov/programs/cb/research-data-technology/statistics-research/child-maltreatment.

Child Welfare Information Gateway. (2019). Retrieved from https://www.childwelfare.gov/topics/systemwide/laws-policies/state/

Child Welfare Information Gateway. (2019). *About CAPTA: A legislative history.* Washington, DC: U.S. Department of Health and Human Services, Children's Bureau.

Cicirelli, V. (1986). The helping relationship and family neglect in later life. In K. Pillemer & R. Wolf (Eds.), *Elder abuse conflict in the family* (pp. 49–66). Dover, MA: Auburn House.

Elder Abuse Protocol. (2017). APEA: *Western Australia Alliance for Prevention of Elder Abuse: Western Australia publication.* https://www.advocare.org.au/aged-care-sector/apeawa/

Falk, N., Norris, K., & Quinn, M. (2014). The factors predicting stress, anxiety, and depression in parents of children with autism. *Journal of Autism Developmental Disorder, 44*(12), 3185–3203. https://doi.org/10.10007/S10803-014-2189-4

Helpguide. (2010). *Elder abuse and neglect.* Retrieved from http://www.helpguide.org/mental/elder_abuse_physical_emotional_sexual_neglect.htm

Hibbard, R., & Desch, L. (2007). Maltreatment of children with disabilities. *Pediatrics, 119,* 1018–1025.

IOM/(renamed) National Academies of Medicines. (2015). *Improving diagnosis in health care.* Washington, DC: National Academies Press. Retrieved from https://www.ncbi.nim.nih.gov/books/NBK 3385961

Lasher, L. (2004). *MBP overview and definitions.* Available from http://www.mbpexpert.com/

Moye, J., & Marson, C. (2007). Assessment of decision-making capacity in older adults: On emerging area of practice and research. *Journal of Gerontology Series B Psychological Sciences and Social Sciences, 62*(1), P3–P11.

Multiple Approaches to Understanding and Preventing Elder Abuse: Proceedings of the Cross-Disciplinary National Institute of Health Workshop. (2016). *Journal of Elder Abuse & Neglect, 28*(4–5). Retrieved from https://www.tandfonline.com/toc/wean20/28/4-5?nav=tocList

National Center on Elder Abuse. (2010). *Why should I care about elder abuse?* National Center on Elder Abuse, 1201 15th Street, N.W., Suite 350, Washington, DC 20005–2842.

National Center on Elder Abuse. (2011). *Risk factors for elder abuse.* Retrieved from http://www.ncea.aoa.gov/NCEAroot/Main_Site/FAQ/Basics/Risk_Factors.aspx

New York State Law Chapter 544 (1989). Identification and Reporting of Child Abuse and Maltreatment— Explaining Reporting Requirements—Study Requirements for Licensing.

Pillemer, K., & Moore, D. (1990). Highlights from a study of abuse of patients in nursing homes. *Journal of Elder Abuse & Neglect, 2,* 5–29.

Quinn, M. J., & Tomita, S. (1986). *Elder abuse and neglect.* New York, NY: Springer.

Quinn, M. J., & Tomita, S. (1997). *Elder abuse and neglect* (2nd ed.). New York, NY: Springer.

Reinharz, S. (1986). Loving and hating one's elders: Twin themes in legend and literature. In K. Pillemer & R. Wolf (Eds.), *Elder abuse conflict in the family* (pp. 25–48). Dover, MA: Auburn House.

Spreng, R., Karlawish, J., & Marson, D. (2016). Cognitive, social, and neural determinants of diminished decision making and financial exploitation risk in ageing and dementia: A review and new model. *Journal of Elder Abuse & Neglect, 28*(4–5), 320–344.

Sullivan, P., & Knutson, J. (2000). Maltreatment and disabilities: A population-based epidemiological study. *Child Abuse and Neglect, 24,* 1257–1273.

U.S. Administration on Aging. (2017). *U.S. Department of Health and Human Services. Strategic action plan (2007–2012).* Retrieved from https://acl.gov/about-acl/authorizing-statutes/older-americans-act

U.S. Department of Health and Human Services, Administration for Children and Families. (2006). *Child neglect: A guide for prevention, assessment, and intervention*. Washington, DC: U.S. Government Printing Office.

U.S. Department of Health and Human Services, Children's Bureau. (2009). *Child maltreatment 2009*. Retrieved from http://www.acf.hhs.gov/ programs/cb/stats_research/index.htm#can

U.S. Department of Health and Human Services, Children's Bureau. (2010). *Child maltreatment 2008*. Retrieved from http://www.acf.hhs.gov/ programs/cb/pubs/cm08/index.htm

U.S. Department of Health and Human Services/ Children's Bureau (2018). Retrieved from https:// www.act.hhs.gov/cb/research-data-technology/ statistics-research

U.S. Department of Health and Human Services, National Center on Child Abuse and Neglect. (1994). *Child maltreatment 1992: Reports from the states to the National Center on Child Abuse and Neglect*. Washington, DC: U.S. Government Printing Office.

Wang, C., & Holton, J. (2007). *Total estimated cost of child abuse and neglect in the United States*. Chicago, IL: Prevent Child Abuse America. Retrieved from http://www.preventchildabuse.org/about_us/ media_ releases/pcaa_pew_economic_impact_ study_final.pdf

Weinrich, D. (2002). Elder abuse: A hidden tragedy. *Perspectives on Gerontology, 7*(1), 5–10. Retrieved from https://pubs.asha.org/doi/10.1044/gero7.1.5

Woolf, L. (1998). *Elder abuse and neglect*. Retrieved from http://www.webster.edu/~woolflm/abuse.html

World Health Organization. (2019). *Elder abuse*. Retrieved from https://www.who.int/news-room/ fact-sheets/detail/elder-abuse.html

Resources

NOTE: The web addresses and phone numbers of these resources are fluid and should be checked for accuracy at time of use.

Administration on Aging
   U.S. Department of Health and Human Services
   330 Independence Avenue, SW
   Washington, DC 20201
   Telephone: 202-401-4634
   Website: https://acl.gov/about-acl/adminstration-aging

Adult Protective Service (APS)
   Call directory assistance and request the number for the department of social services or aging services in your county.

American Academy of Pediatrics
   Check this website for information on what to know about child abuse developed by the American Academy of Pediatrics.
   Website: http://www.aap.org/en-us/search/pages/ results.aspx?k=child%20abuse

Area Agency on Aging
   Look in the government section of your telephone directory under the terms aging or elderly services. This agency can provide the phone number for the local ombudsman for long-term care in your area.

Child Help USA Hotline
   Telephone: 800-422-4453 (24 hours)
   Website: http://www.childhelp.org

Elder Abuse Resources
   Website: https://www.cdc.gove/violenceprevention/ elderabuse/resources.html

Eldercare Locator
   For those who want to identify aging services in specific communities, call this Administration on Aging agency.
   Telephone: 800-677-1116

Medicaid Fraud Control Units (MFCU)
   Every State Attorney General's Office has an MFCU to prosecute Medicaid provider fraud and patient abuse in long-term care or home health care settings.

Mental Help Net
   Provides information and referral numbers for numerous national hotlines.
   Website: http://mentalhelp.net/

National Center for Missing and Exploited Children
   Helps families and professionals.
   Telephone: 800-843-5678

National Center on Child Abuse and Neglect. (1993). Washington, DC: U.S. Department of Health and Human Services.
   A report on the maltreatment of children with disabilities.

National Center on Elder Abuse
   State directory of help lines, hotlines, and elder abuse prevention resources.
   Website: http://www.ncea.aoa .gov/NCEAroot/ Main_Site/Find_Help/Resources/ Elders_Families .aspx

National Committee to Prevent Child Abuse
Website: http://preventchildabuse.org/

National Domestic Violence Hotline
Helps children, parents, friends, and offenders of family violence.
Telephone: 800-799-7233

National Parent Hotline
Call for support from trained persons. Part of Parents Anonymous.
Telephone: 855-4APARENT
Website: http://www.nationalparenthelpline.org

National Respite Locator Service
Helps parents, caregivers, and professionals caring for children with disabilities, terminal illnesses, or those at risk of abuse.
Telephone: 800-677-1116

Youth Crisis Hotline
Helps individuals reporting child abuse of children ages 12 to 18.
Telephone: 800-448-4663

Websites

AARP: Coping with Grief and Loss
http://www.aarp.org/griefandloss

Administration on Aging—Department of Health and Human Services
https://acl.gov/about-acl/adminstration-aging

Agency for Health Care Research and Quality
http://ahcpr.gov

Aging Life Care Association
http://www.aginglifecare.org

AGS Foundation for Health in Aging
http://www.healthinagingfoundation.org/

Alzheimer's Association
http://www.alz.org

Alzheimer's Disease Education and Referral Center at the National Institute of Aging
https://www.nia.nih.gov/alzheimers

American Association of Homes and Services for the Aging
http://www.aahsa.org

American Association of Retired Persons (AARP)
http://www.aarp.org

American Geriatrics Society
http://www.americangeriatrics.org

American Society on Aging
http://www.asaging.org

Association for Gerontology in Higher Education
http://www.aghe.org

Benefits Checkup
http://www.benefitscheckup.org

Brookdale Center for Health and Longevity
http://www.brookdale.org

Caregiver Survival Resources
http://www.caregiver.com

Caregiving Online
http://www.caregiving.com

Careguide@Home—Elder Care
http://www.eldercare.com

Clinical Trials
http://www.clinicaltrials.com

The Eldercare Directory
http://www.eldercaredirectory.org

ElderCare Online
http://www.ec-online.net

Eldercare Workforce Alliance
https://eldercareworkforce.org/

Elder Support Network Association of Jewish Family and Children Agencies
http://www.ajfca.org

Elderweb—Center for Eldercare
www.seniorliving.org

Family Caregiver Alliance—National Center on Caregiving
http://www.caregiver.org

Fisher Center for Alzheimer's Research Foundation
http://www.alzinfo.org

Gerontology Society of America
http://www.geron.org

GriefNet
http://www.griefnet.org

Health and Age
http://www.healthandage.com

Health Care Financing Administration
https://www.federalregister.gov/agencies/health-care-finance-administration

Healthfinder
http://www.healthfinder.gov

Health Policy and Management
http://www.hpm.umn.edu

Hospice Foundation of America
http://www.hospicefoundation.org

Institute for Aging Research
https://www.instituteforagingresearch.org/
resources/news

Medicine Program
http://www.themedicineprogram.com

National Academy of Elder Law Attorneys
http://www.naela.org

National Asian Pacific Center on Aging
http://www.napca.com

National Association for Hispanic Elderly
http://www.anppm.org

National Association of Area Agencies on Aging
http://www.N4A.org

National Association of State Units on Aging
http://www.nasua.org

National Caregivers Library
http://www.caregiverslibrary.org

National Center on Addiction and Substance Abuse
http://www.centeronaddiction.org/

National Council on the Aging
http://www.ncoa.org

National Institutes of Health
https://www.nih.gov/

National Institute on Aging
https://www.nia.nih.gov/

National Policy Resource Center on Nutrition
Physical Activity and Aging
http://nutritionandaging.org

National Rehabilitation Information Center
https://www.justiceinaging.org

Senior Link: Innovation in Care Collaboration
http://www.seniorlink.com

SeniorNet
http://www.seniornet.org

Social Security Administration Online
http://www.ssa.gov

Web of Care
http://www.webocare.com

Appendix 24–A

◇◇

Case I: Joshua

Joshua lived with his father. The father's then-wife informed the county police that the father was physically abusing Joshua, who was around 3 years old at the time. The county department of social services investigated the claim, but the father denied the allegations, and the inquires stopped. A year later, Joshua presented to the hospital with multiple bruises and abrasions covering his body leading the treating physician to suspect child abuse and he reported the injuries to the department of social services. The hospital was then granted temporary custody of Joshua, and a multidisciplinary team examined the case. The team concluded that there was not enough evidence to keep Joshua away from his father's custody but implemented the following protective measures: the father was required to enroll Joshua in a preschool program and participate in counseling services. Joshua was returned to his father. The department of social services started making monthly visits to the home, and noted suspicious injuries on Joshua's head and observed he was not enrolled in school as was previously agreed upon. Despite all of this, the department of social services took no further action. When Joshua was 4 years old, his father beat him so badly that he suffered a massive brain hemorrhage and fell into a coma. The child underwent emergency neurosurgery, which revealed older brain hemorrhages, consistent with shaken baby syndrome. Given his permanent brain damage, Joshua was expected to live the rest of his life institutionalized. The father pled no contest to felony abuse charges and was sentenced to four years in prison.

The mother, on behalf of Joshua, filed a lawsuit against the county and the department of social services, claiming a lack of intervention to protect Joshua. The legal decision was in favor of the individual state laws, allowing each state to determine liability in cases where the state has failed to act.

However, the Supreme Court saw this case otherwise. The state was not the agent who physically beat Joshua into a coma, but the state did play an indirect role in the child's fate. A state is to be held accountable because under the current structure mandated reporters' responsibility is to report the suspected child abuse. A state assumes a special relationship with child abuse victims since it is the epicenter for dealing with mandated reporters, alleged child abuse victims, and suspected abusers. Mandated reporters are compelled to report suspected child abuse cases to state entities, and would be held accountable for failing to report; therefore states should be held accountable for what happens after the report is made.

The author's reason for including this case is to show that all parties need to take reporting suspected abuse very seriously, and that even then, there are a series of steps in the justice system, creating complex outcomes. The first and very necessary piece is to watch for and report suspected abuse, initiating the system responses.

Appendix 24–B

◇◇◇

Case 2: Sam

Sam Smith has an intellectual disability and mental health problems. He lived with his grandmother, who managed his life for him until her death a year ago. Sam's only time away from his grandmother was the couple of years he spent in a vocational training program. After Sam's grandmother died, he moved into a licensed Board and Care home. The owner of the facility made Sam clean the house and do all the yard work without receiving adequate food and nutrition. When the neighbors reported this to the proper agency, they discovered the inadequate care the residents were receiving and the facility's license was revoked.

The agency tried to help Sam move to a safer, better environment, but he was fearful and declined to move at that time. The agency continued to contract and work with Sam for the next year before Sam was willing to relocate to another facility.

The agency assisted by:

- Locating an assisted living facility that could provide a healthy and safe living environment for Sam

- Assisting Sam in moving to his new home

- Helping Sam apply for medical benefits and attendant care benefits, and assisting him in completing applications for caregiving services

- Arranging primary medical care for Sam, as he hadn't seen an MD in a decade

- Transporting Sam to all follow-up medical appointments

- Arranging for Sam to participate in an Arts Program to enhance his social activities

After three months, Sam had adjusted nicely to his new home. He had made friends with many of the other residents and was participating in new activities through the Arts Program. He had started to attend his local church, participate in outings offered by the assisted living program, and was engaging with the other residents.

Appendix 24–C

<><><><><><><><><><><><><><><><><><><><><><><><><><><><><><><><><><><><><><><>

Case 3: Miriam

The local elder care agency received a report on Saturday afternoon from a hospital regarding Mrs. Miriam Wiles, a frail 95-year-old female. On Thursday, the hospital determined that Mrs. Wiles was ready to be discharged following a fall in her home. She had remained in inpatient and skilled rehabilitation care in the facility for five months. At the point of discharge from therapy and the facility, she was weak, had difficulty lifting her weight from sitting to standing, and difficulty maintaining her balance. The hospital was recommending that Miriam move to a rehabilitation center to regain her strength. Miriam refused, so the hospital discharged her to her home. She lived in an accessible one level home with a son and daughter living within a five-mile radius of the home. She accepted home health services with providers coming for an hour at breakfast, lunch, and dinner to assist with meals and dressing.

On Saturday following the week of her discharge from the hospital, the hospital telephoned Miriam to monitor her medications but could not get an answer to their call. They called the local elder care agency to investigate. The agency worker was unable to reach Miriam by telephone, so he went directly to her home. There was no answer despite repeated knocking on her door and ringing the doorbell.

The agency worker called a family member who was unable to come, so the agency worker called emergency services and the police were dispatched. When the police arrived, the agency worker entered with the police and located Miriam sitting in her recliner chair, where she had been stationary for six hours because she was too weak to stand up by herself. Mrs. Wiles was overjoyed that someone had discovered her, because she did not have her emergency alert button in a location what she could access and call for help, and was otherwise too isolated for anyone to hear or come to assist her.

The agency assisted by:

- Calling the paramedics to transport Miriam to the hospital for further evaluation

- Following Miriam to the hospital and making sure she was readmitted there

- Working with the hospital to ensure that adequate home care services were in place before Miriam was discharged home

- Advocating to make sure that Miriam accepted the in-home care services and that they addressed her needs

Miriam was very thankful for the agency's help and was happy to be safe in her home.

25

Working with Culturally and Linguistically Diverse Populations

Shirley Huang, MS and Pui Fong Kan, PhD

Introduction

Speech-language pathologists' (SLPs) and audiologists' (AuDs) clinical work with culturally-linguistically diverse (CLD) populations must be discussed within the context of a larger ecosystem, which includes the social environment, political and economic factors, and community values—all of which are subject to change over time. Therefore, clinicians must be prepared to work within this dynamic system. According to the American Speech-Language-Hearing Association (ASHA, 2017), "culture and cultural diversity can incorporate a variety of factors, including but not limited to age, disability, ethnicity, gender identity (encompasses gender expression), national origin (encompasses related aspects such as ancestry, culture, language, dialect, citizenship, and immigration status), race, religion, sex, sexual orientation, and veteran status. Linguistic diversity can accompany cultural diversity." While the majority of this chapter will focus on ethnic and racial diversity accompanied by linguistic diversity, we will also address other characteristics of diversity (e.g., Deaf/hard-of-hearing, transgender) throughout this chapter. CLD populations may include immigrants, or children of immigrants, who are bilingual and speak more than one language. With recent demographic changes to the immigrant population in the United States, SLPs and AuDs are more likely to work with people whose cultural-linguistic background is different from their own. Clinicians who are not bilingual will need to be prepared to work with culturally diverse and bilingual populations.

Additionally, clinicians must be aware of how our clinical work is influenced by larger institutions or systems-level work. This includes health care and special education policies, government programs like early intervention, funding for rehabilitation and social service programs, or health insurance coverage for clinical services. Changes at the systems level will have cascading effects on the clinical services we provide to CLD populations—populations that have historically been considered vulnerable. Common barriers include difficulty accessing and navigating the health care system and limited standardized bilingual tools for accurate and appropriate diagnosis. As health care providers, whose scope of practice spans across different disorders, age populations, and clinical settings, we hold a responsibility to be informed consumers of current events and understand how these systems-level changes impact our clinical work with individuals from diverse backgrounds. In this chapter, we will cover the following topics:

1. CLD populations in the United States,

2. Some characteristics of language differences in language-diverse learners,

3. Assessment and intervention issues for clients/patients/students from CLD backgrounds,

4. Systems-level constraints affecting CLD populations, and

5. Ways to prepare now for working with and supporting CLD populations.

Demographic Profiles

Over the past twenty-first century, the cultural and linguistic landscape of the United States has been changing steadily, resulting in a rich makeup of traditions, beliefs, and values. As cultural and linguistic diversity in our nation continues to increase, SLPs and AuDs must be prepared to work sensitively and competently with clients/patients/students/families, as well as with their colleagues, who may come from a variety of CLD backgrounds and characteristics.

Overview of Cultural-Linguistic Populations

Population Estimates. Every 10 years, the U.S. Census Bureau collects demographic information on population and language use, and their projections, to know how to best provide and allocate appropriate services and resources to people from different cultural and linguistic backgrounds (Ryan, 2013). Minority groups are projected to grow significantly by 2060, with CLD groups constituting a majority of the U.S. population (Colby & Ortman, 2015). According to the U.S. Census Bureau population estimates (2018), the two largest minority groups are the Hispanic/Latino and black/African American populations, who comprise about 18% and 13.4% of the U.S. population, respectively (Table 25–1 provides demographic breakdown). The Asian population comprises about 5.8% of the U.S. population, but this group is growing quickly and is projected to nearly double its population count by 2060 (Colby & Ortman, 2015). While the U.S. Census Bureau provides a large breakdown of the U.S. population, it is still limited in that it does not further divide different cultural-linguistic subgroups within the larger racial/ethnic group. For example, in the latest U.S. Census Bureau 2010, the data broadly aggregated all people of Asian ethnicity into one ethnic group, as opposed to disaggregating the data into other types of Asians such as Vietnamese, Japanese, Korean, Cambodian. It is especially important that SLPs and AuDs working with CLD groups recognize and are knowledgeable of the client/patient/student/family's ethnic, racial and language backgrounds. Since each racial and ethnic subgroup could speak different languages or language dialects, or have cultural values that differ from one another, clinicians must be cautious not to make broad assumptions about someone's cultural experiences simply because they belong to a larger racial or ethnic group. Overgeneralizing or adhering to stereotypes may have negative consequences in interpreting assessment

Table 25–1. U.S. Population Estimates in 2018

Population Estimate	327,167,434
Race	**Percentage**
White	76.6%
Hispanic or Latino	18.1%
Black or African American	13.4%
Asian	5.8%
American Indian and Alaska Native	1.3%
Native Hawaiian and Other Pacific Islander	0.2%

Source: U.S. Census Bureau (2018). *Quick Facts, Population Estimates 2018.* Retrieved from https://www.census.gov/quickfacts/fact/table/US/PST045218

results, making diagnoses, providing therapy, or building therapist–client rapport.

Cultures, Subcultures, and Inclusivity. Differences in cultural views and worldviews between the clinician and the client/patient/student/family may have far-reaching implications on our provision of services and on their perception of health care and interpretation of medical conditions (ASHA, 2013; Dyches, Wilder, Sudweeks, Obiakor, & Algozzine, 2004; Napier et al., 2014; Sue, 2006). Culture has been defined as "the set of distinctive spiritual, material, intellectual and emotional features of society or a social group . . . [which] encompasses . . . lifestyles, ways of living together, value systems, traditions and beliefs" (UNESCO, 2001). Culture is not solely linked to groups of people who share the same racial and ethnic background. Indeed, there are various cultural groups that originated based on their neurodiverse backgrounds such as Deafness and hard-of-hearing, autism spectrum disorder, gay, lesbian, bisexual, and transgender (Clark, Landers, Linde, & Sperber, 2001; Correll, 2005; Davidson, 2008; Holcomb, 2013; Whitmarsh & Jones, 2010). Another important aspect of cultural diversity is that culture is dynamic and is influenced by the changing environment. For example, immigrants from diverse cultures gradually adopt certain aspects of the mainstream culture (Schwartz, Unger, Zamboanga, & Szapocznik, 2010). Thus, clinicians should be aware that individuals from the same backgrounds might have different levels of experiences within the mainstream culture, and be cautious not to overgeneralize or make stereotypes.

The term "linguistically diverse" is often assumed to refer to spoken languages; however, individuals in the Deaf community who have a shared communication system using American Sign Language are also linguistically diverse. The term big 'D' Deaf recognizes that the Deaf community is a distinct culture with values, traditions, history and social norms like other ethnic and racial cultures (Grosjean, 1992; Holcomb, 2013). American Sign Language is an autonomous language, distinct from English, and possesses its own rules of phonology, morphology, syntax and social-pragmatics (turn-taking, topic initiation and maintenance) (Holcomb, 2013). According to ASHA (2019), there are only 702 registered ASHA-certified bilingual service providers who communicate using American Sign Language. SLPs and AuDs working with the D/deaf or hard-of-hearing populations who do not use American Sign Language should work with interpreters or make referrals to clinicians who do have specialized knowledge and skills in American Sign Language and Deaf culture.

The cultural and service needs of transgender minority groups are relevant to SLPs and AuDs. According to the most recent population-based survey (Herman, Flores, Brown, Wilson, & Conron, 2017), there are an estimated 0.6% of adults, about 1.4 million, who identify as transgender in the U.S. Less is known about the demographics of children who identify as transgender in the U.S. Transgender people may want voice therapy and communication services from SLPs to safely modify the way they talk and sound (Coleman, Bockting, & Botzer 2012). Our scope of practice includes supporting and counseling transgender people and developing goals with them to address their wants and needs (ASHA, 2016). It is important that clinicians stay informed of political discussions that affect transgender people because changes in federal and state laws and regulations will impact health care policies, our service provision, and research. Clinicians working with this population should have specific training and respectful attitudes in order to provide culturally sensitive and competent care.

Linguistic Diversity, Accents, Dialects and Status. As the number of immigrants entering the U.S. continues to grow, so does the diversity of languages. There are at least 350 languages spoken in the U.S. (U.S. Census Bureau, 2015). While the exact number of immigrant children and adults in the U.S. is not available, it was estimated that 13.4% of the U.S. population was foreign born between 2013 and 2017 (U.S. Census Bureau, 2018). About 21% of people in the U.S. who are 5 years and older speak a language other than English at home (U.S. Census Bureau, 2015). Of that group, about 62% of the population speak Spanish and 16% speak an Asian language (e.g., Chinese, Japanese, Korean). SLPs and AuDs are more likely to work with individuals who may be immigrants or from immigrant families, and who speak a home language other than English. It is critical then that clinicians be culturally and linguistically knowledgeable in order to provide appropriate and respectful services and resources to these populations.

Linguistic diversity includes language accents and dialects. A language accent refers to the unique way that groups of people who speak the same language pronounce or stress certain sounds in words (ASHA, n.d.-a). An accent is not a language disorder. Everyone speaks with an accent because it is a natural part of spoken language. Regional accents are influenced by geographical regions. For example, individuals from Boston may pronounce the 'r' phoneme differently (e.g., Harvard Yard → *Hahvahd Yahd*) compared with individuals from California. Foreign accents are common in English language learners because they are borrowing the sounds in their home language when trying to pronounce sounds in English words. A dialect is a variety of language that is defined by historical, social, geographical factors, in addition to linguistic factors such as vocabulary words and grammar rules. For example, African American English, also known as "Black English," "Ebonics," or "African American Vernacular English," is a dialect of English. African American English is recognized as a legitimate rule-governed language system (ASHA, 2003). Clinicians evaluating individuals who speak an English dialect other than mainstream Standard American English should know how to distinguish the difference between a language disorder and a language difference.

Speech-Language Pathologists and Audiologists from Diverse Backgrounds

ASHA has a total of 191,904 certified speech-language pathologists, audiologists, scientists, and clinical support personnel, and 6% of them indicated they are bilingual service providers (i.e., native or near native proficiency in a language other than English) (ASHA, 2019). The language use information reported includes 81 spoken languages other than English, 702 individuals who use American Sign Language, and 64% of bilingual service providers who are Spanish-language service providers. ASHA-certified SLPs who are bilingual service providers are not evenly distributed across the U.S., but rather they are concentrated in Texas, New York, California,

and Florida. Therefore, this poses a major challenge for CLD families in getting access to bilingual service providers if they don't live in these states. Figure 25–1 presents a U.S. map of ASHA's bilingual service providers by state. The majority of ASHA bilingual service providers were white (80%), and only about 20% belong to a racial group other than white (or multiple racial groups). Hispanic or Latino ethnicity comprised about 42% of bilingual service providers.

Given that about 20% of the U.S. population speaks a home language other than English, there is a growing need for more clinicians who are bilingual. It is important to point out that recruitment of bilingual SLPs and AuDs should not be the only solution when improving how we serve CLD populations. Professionals who are not bilingual or do not come from ethnically or racially diverse backgrounds can provide culturally and linguistically appropriate services when working with these populations.

Bridging the Gap: Clinical Cultural Competency in Practitioners

Cultural-linguistic competency involves the general ability to understand the diversity of cultural variables that contribute to the interactions between the clinician and

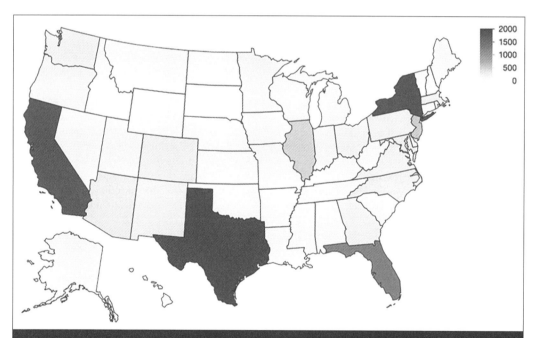

Figure 25–1. U.S. map of ASHA's bilingual service providers by state. *Source:* Based on data from American Speech-Language-Hearing Association. (2019). Demographic profile of ASHA members providing bilingual services, year-end 2018. Available from http://www.asha.org.

the client/patient/student/family (ASHA, 2013). In line with evidence-based practice, providing clinical services to CLD populations must take into consideration their values, needs, cultural practice, and choices (ASHA, 2005). Cultural-linguistic competence recognizes that differences do not mean disorders or deficiencies. The ability to work effectively with individuals whose experiences are different from our personal and professional experiences becomes critical in order to provide high quality services (ASHA, 2013; Kritikos, 2003). It is important to understand that cultural-linguistic competency is not a final product. Rather, it is an active ongoing effort to increase our cultural awareness, cultural knowledge, and skills (ASHA, 2013). By understanding our client/patient/student/family's needs, we could better understand communication disorders and hearing loss within their sociocultural contexts.

According to the standards and implementation procedures for the Certificate of Clinical Competence in speech-language pathology and in audiology (ASHA, 2018b, 2018c), SLPs and AuDs are required to have the basic knowledge of how linguistic and cultural factors affect human communication and swallowing processes as well as the cultural-linguistic knowledge and clinical skills in the areas of speech, language, hearing, and swallowing. While some graduate programs offer specific courses on working with CLD populations, many programs incorporate the issues regarding working with CLD in various courses and practicum experiences. Many clinicians continue to develop their cultural competence through continuing education, in their community, and from their clinical caseloads (ASHA, 2018a; Stockman, Boult, & Robinson, 2008).

Language Difference: Language Characteristics in Typical Bilinguals

In this section, we focus on the general language characteristics of typical bilinguals who have different language experiences. Bilingual individuals may be simultaneous bilinguals who learn two languages since birth, or sequential bilinguals who are exposed to their home language at birth and then learn a second language (e.g., English) later in school. Because of bilinguals' unique language learning experience in each language, bilinguals' language knowledge fluctuates over time (Kohnert, 2010). As a result, bilinguals' language skills in each language might look different from their monolingual peers (Bialystok & Luk, 2012; Bialystok, Luk, Peets, & Yang, 2010; Hoff & Core, 2015; Nicoladis, Song, & Marentette, 2012). Certain characteristics in typically developing children who are in the process of learning

two languages or bilingual adults who are from diverse language backgrounds might potentially be confused with symptoms of language disorders (Bedore & Peña, 2008; Kohnert, 2010; Muñoz & Marquardt, 2003). In what follows, we describe five general characteristics of typically developing bilingual children: (1) silent period, (2) code-switching, (3) distributed language knowledge across two languages, (4) language attrition, and (5) cross-language interference and transfer. It is important for clinicians to understand these characteristics when making clinical decisions, and not confuse them with a language impairment.

(1) Silent Period

The silent period (also called silent stage or silent phase) is a period of time when second language learners (L2) refuse to talk at the early stage of L2 learning (Bligh, 2014; Roberts, 2014). The silent period, which could last for months, is considered as an important stage of L2 acquisition (Bligh & Drury, 2015; Clarke, 2009). The silent period is not a sign of a disorder. Rather, it is an important learning experience for these children. For early sequential bilinguals from minority families, early school experience involves the transition from first language (L1) interactions in homes to L2 instructions in school settings (Duursma et al., 2007; Pearson, 2007). Receiving instructions in L2 in school settings, children may appear to be unwilling to interact or to speak (Siraj-Blatchford & Clarke, 2000). Although they might appear to be quiet, they might be focusing on comprehending the new language and figuring out the new language and learning environment (Bligh & Drury, 2015; Roberts, 2014).

Not all young bilingual learners encounter a silent period; and there is great variability in the language patterns of children who are in a silent period. Some typically developing bilingual children who are in a silent period might be thought to have a "language delay" or "selective mutism" (Clarke, 2009). Language impairment is typically present in both languages (Bedore & Peña, 2008). In order to determine whether a CLD child is going through a silent period or has a language disorder, clinicians should ask the family about whether and how much the child uses L1 at home and gather information about the child's L1 and L2 use over time and across home and school settings (Kohnert, 2010).

(2) Code-Switching

Code-switching refers to the alternation of two languages (or dialects) during various communicative activities such as conversations or telling stories (Grosjean, 1995; Paradis, Genesee, & Crago, 2011). Code-switching is a type of natural communication among bilinguals (Grosjean,

1995; Miccio, Hammer, & Rodríguez, 2009). The amount of code-switching depends on many contextual factors (e.g., communicative contexts and partners), language input, and language proficiency in each language (Beatty-Martínez & Dussias, 2017; Gutiérrez-Clellen, Simon-Cereijido, & Erickson, 2009). Code-switching serves many communicative functions, such as facilitating comprehension, avoiding miscommunication, expressing specific language concepts, and establishing membership in a social group (Hughes, Shaunessy, Brice, Ratliff, & McHatton, 2006; Pavlenko, 2009). In school settings, code-switching is used by developing bilingual children to promote communication, to enhance peer interaction, and to facilitate learning (Hughes et al., 2006; Moore, 2002; Reyes, 2004). Research shows that bilingual children with developmental language disorders did not use more atypical code-switching patterns compared with their typically developing bilingual peers (Gutiérrez-Clellen et al., 2009). Thus, code-switching should not be considered as a symptom of language deficits (Kohnert, Yim, Nett, Kan, & Duran, 2005; Miccio et al., 2009).

(3) Distributed Language Knowledge Across Two Languages

Bilinguals use their two languages with different partners (parents vs. teachers; spouse vs. co-workers) in different contexts (home vs. school; home vs. workplace). Because of their unique language experience in each language, they are likely to have uneven and distributed language knowledge across two languages (Kohnert, 2010; Oller, Pearson, & Cobo-lewis, 2007; Pearson, Fernandez, & Oller, 1993). Some concepts are lexicalized in one language, some in the other, while some in both languages. Clinically, language input and the distributed nature of bilingual knowledge may explain the low language scores in bilinguals (Muñoz & Marquardt, 2003; Pearson et al., 1993). Thus, when assessing language skills in bilinguals, clinicians should assess bilinguals' linguistic knowledge in both languages as well as their opportunities to use two languages.

(4) Language Attrition

Language attrition (or language loss) is the nonpathological loss of language ability (Ecke, 2004; Köpke & Schmid, 2004). Language loss could occur in either language (L1 or L2). For example, L1 attrition is documented in immigrant children who do not have frequent opportunities to use L1 (Karayayla & Schmid, 2019) and in internationally adopted children who are adopted by a family who do not speak their L1 at home (Anderson, 2001). Language attrition could be at the phonological,

morphological, lexical, syntactic, and/or semantic levels (Ecke, 2004). Language loss is not a disorder. Many factors are associated with language attrition, including the age of L1 and L2 acquisition, infrequent use of one language (e.g., the L1 of immigrant children), and incomplete acquisition of L1 or L2 (Fillmore, 1991; Karayayla & Schmid, 2019; Nicoladis, & Grabois, 2010; Proctor, August, & Carlo, 2010). Thus, when assessing children or adults from diverse language backgrounds, clinicians should examine their language knowledge holistically by considering various factors, such as language input and social-linguistic variables.

(5) Cross-Language Interference and Transfer

Interference is the negative effect of cross-language interaction, and transfer involves a facilitative effect of one language on performance in another (Grosjean, 2012; MacWhinney, 2005). Cross-linguistic interference and transfer have been observed in bilinguals in the areas of phonology, lexical–semantics, and morphosyntax (Goldstein & Bunta, 2012; Kaushanskaya & Marian, 2007; Nicoladis, 2006). For example, Goldstein and Bunta (2012) reported that a typical bilingual preschooler transferred Spanish phonemes such as /u/ to English (e.g., [bʊk] → [buk]). Adult L2 learners (e.g., adult immigrants) may exhibit L1 interference when speaking English (Flege et al., 2006), such as accents. The patterns that are the result of interference or transfer are not indicators of language impairment. Clinicians should work with the interpreter to determine if certain error patterns in L2 are influenced by the individual's L1 or vice versa.

Service Delivery for Children and Adults

SLPs and AuDs have a primary responsibility for providing clinical services to children and adults with communication disorders. The two primary goals of clinical service delivery for bilinguals include (1) making accurate differential diagnosis between normal language variations and communication disorders and (2) designing intervention programs that would enhance habilitation or rehabilitation. To serve CLD populations, clinicians should understand that the cultural-linguistic differences between the client/patient/student/family and the clinician could critically affect the assessment and treatment outcomes (Kritikos, 2003). Clinicians should also understand that other related factors such as education levels, poverty, and level of acculturation could influence bilinguals' performance (Hoff, 2013; Kohnert, 2013;

Zhang, Dennis, & Houseman, 2018). Knowledge about the differences would help clinicians to ask the right questions, such as whether the client/patient/student/family is familiar with the assessment processes (e.g., the idea of a diagnosis), whether the testing materials and procedures (e.g., telling story, naming pictures) are culturally appropriate, and whether intervention strategies are in line with the family's values (e.g., level of family involvement). For example, a clinical diagnosis, which is common in the Western culture, might be considered a stigma in another culture (Padilla, Palmer, & Rodríguez, 2018; Zuckerman et al., 2018). Some strategies (e.g., following the child's lead) that are recommended to facilitate young children's communicative interactions in intervention programs may not be consistent with the cultural values for some families from other cultural backgrounds (Simmons & Johnston, 2007; Soto & Yu, 2014; van Kleeck, 1994). For example, swallowing and feeding therapy is critical for young children with swallowing and feeding disorders. However, there are significant cross-cultural differences in feeding practices and beliefs about child nutrition (Davis-McFarland, 2008). Clinicians should be aware of and knowledgeable about their own culture and the cultural biases they bring when delivering services. By working with cultural brokers, interpreters, or the minority community leaders, clinicians can identify the cultural gap between the client and the clinician, and adopt a training program to fit the family's needs (Wing et al., 2007).

Assessment and Diagnosis

One of the main goals of assessment is differentiating typical from atypical communication skills. Early identification of communication disorders and hearing loss is critical for providing effective intervention and reducing negative long-term consequences (Durán, Hartzheim, Lund, Simonsmeier, & Kohlmeier, 2016). When assessing the language skills of bilinguals, both languages should be taken into consideration. However, there are many challenges in assessing the two languages of bilinguals. One critical issue is the lack of valid and reliable bilingual standardized tests (Bedore & Peña, 2008). To date, only a handful of tests report normative data of Spanish-English bilingual children (e.g., Spanish versions of the Preschool Language Scales–5; Zimmerman, Steiner, & Pond, 2012; the Clinical Evaluation of Language Fundamentals–4; Wiig, Semel, & Secord, 2006). Although there are published tests in various languages (e.g., Spanish, Chinese), many of these tests are merely translations of measures from English, with questionable construct or content validity. Another challenge is that children's language skills may fluctuate in relation to the use of and exposure to two languages.

Bilinguals' language learning experience cannot be easily quantified in the assessment process. For example, some children may start to lose their skills in their home language (L1), while some maintain their L1 while learning L2 (Kohnert, 2010). Because of these limitations, bilingual children are oftentimes either over-identified or under-identified as having language impairment (Bedore & Peña, 2008). Overidentification occurs when an individual's language variation is mistakenly identified as a speech-language impairment. For example, the U.S. Department of Education (2017) reported that school-age Native American and African American children were 1.5 and 1.4 times, respectively, more likely to be enrolled in special education. In contrast, under-identification occurs when an individual's language impairment has not been captured in the assessment process. Failure to differentiate language difference and language disorders delays intervention for bilingual children and could lead to a long-term negative impact on their development.

The American Speech-Language-Hearing Association adopted the International Classification of Functioning, Disability and Health (World Health Organization, 2001) as the framework for assessment and intervention in our Scope of Practice (ASHA, 2016), which contains components of health conditions (body functions and structures; activity and participation) and contextual factors. In the context of identifying developmental language impairment in CLD populations, clinicians need to have clear understanding of typical and atypical language performance under diverse circumstances. Three aspects of skills should be examined in the assessment process: (1) general knowledge and functional skills in both languages, (2) diverse language learning environments, and (3) learnability.

(1) Measuring General Knowledge and Functional Skills in Both Languages. Several tools can be used to measure general knowledge and functional skills in both languages. Speech and language samples in both languages (conversation or narrative) are useful for assessing bilinguals. It allows clinicians to analyze bilinguals' morphological, syntactic, phonological, and lexical systems in both languages. Criterion-referenced assessment tools that are designed by clinicians can be used to examine a client's strengths and weaknesses in both languages. In addition, although there are many limitations in many standardized tests, standardized measures may be administered and interpreted in a non-standardized format (Kohnert, 2010). For example, clinicians could modify the test items with the assistance of interpreters or translators, modify the task instructions, provide additional training items and feedback, and use alternate scoring rubrics (Laing & Kamhi, 2003). Even though

the normative data are not informative for bilinguals, raw scores and additional item analyses may be useful for documenting progress over time. It is important to note that assessment tools are not culture free. Formal and informal testing procedures could be biased and affect the performance of individuals who have not had exposure to the mainstream educational contexts. Thus, clinicians should document the clients' verbal and non-verbal responses and consult with cultural brokers about the responses.

(2) Gather Information about Bilinguals' Diverse Language Learning Environments. The contextual factors can be examined using questionnaires and ethnographic interviews. Questionnaires (e.g., parent questionnaires), with open-ended questions, are useful tools to obtain information about the individual's communication characteristics and specific knowledge of the views of clients and their families (Bedore, Peña, Joyner, & Macken, 2011; Gutiérrez-Clellen & Kreiter, 2003). Ethnographic observations and interviewing are effective ways to learn about the culture of the family (e.g., their worldview, values, and beliefs, and about the strengths and needs of the client and his/her family [Soto & Yu, 2014; Westby, 1990]).

(3) Probing Learnability. "Learnability" measures focus on the difference between the learner's current independent functioning level and the level of functioning when a communicative partner supports his/her performance (zone of proximal development) (Vygotsky, 1978). Different from traditional tests, dynamic assessment emphasizes the learning process of the learner. Dynamic assessment involves three components: pretest, teach, and post-test (Gutiérrez-Clellen & Peña, 2001; Kapant-zoglou, Restrepo, & Thompson, 2012). The mediated learning experiences involves the examiner's effort to teach, observe the child's responses, and adjust teaching strategies. Focusing on the learning process rather than knowledge, dynamic assessment has been considered a tool that reduces assessment bias that is more likely to occur in the traditional standardized test environment.

Intervention

After a diagnosis of a communication disorder or a hearing loss is confirmed, an intervention plan is developed in conjunction with other members of the intervention team. The plan includes intervention outcomes, approaches, methods, and settings. According to the International Classification of Functioning, Disability and Health (WHO, 2001), the intervention should involve both health conditions and contextual factors (ASHA, 2016). For CLD clients/patients, planning

intervention requires the consideration of their history with both languages, his/her current and future needs for using each language across settings, as well as the family's values, cultures, and needs (Dyches et al., 2004; Soto & Yu, 2014; Westby & Washington, 2017).

(1) Goal Setting. It is important to keep in mind throughout intervention that the family of a patient/client already has patterns of communication at home, in school, or at work. Understanding the existing interaction across settings and the cultural practice is critical when designing an intervention program (Parette, Huer, & Brotherson, 2001). For example, dysphagia can negatively affect the pleasure of eating and, thus, can have an impact on quality of life. The effects can be further influenced by patients' cultural views about disease and disorder (Sharp & Genesen, 1996). In setting an effective treatment plan, clinicians need to include the family's input about their communication needs, their views on the patient's communicative functions, and their culture about family involvement (ASHA, 2013; Soto & Yu, 2014).

(2) One Language or Two? There is a growing body of evidence supporting intervention in bilingual children's home language (Durán, Hartzheim, Lund, Simons-meier, & Kohlmeier, 2016; Lim, O'Reilly, Sigafoos, Ledbetter-Cho, & Lancioni, 2019). Supporting home language is important not only for improving communication outcomes but also for helping children and adults maintain communication with their families, who may primarily speak the minority language (Durán et al., 2016; Yu, 2013). In a systematic review, Lim and colleagues examined 18 studies on treatment outcomes for individuals with neurodevelopmental disorders. Interventions delivered in the home language led to slightly better outcomes than the interventions delivered solely in the majority language (Lim et al., 2019). Two approaches have been proposed to provide intervention to bilinguals: bilingual approach and cross-linguistic approach (Kohnert, 2010; Kohnert, Yim, Nett, Kan, & Duran, 2005). The bilingual approach focuses on cognitive processing skills that are common to both languages. The intervention emphasizes the aspects that are shared by the two languages (e.g., cross-linguistic cognates) and the metalinguistic processing skills. The cross-linguistic approach targets specific linguistic features or communicative functions in L1 and L2. For the SLP who does not speak both of the child's languages, Kohnert (2010) suggested working with the interpreter or recruiting parents or siblings to mediate interactions with the clients in their home language.

Relatively fewer studies have examined treatment outcomes for bilinguals with acquired language disorders. The overall goal of SLP service for bilinguals is to improve their social participation and quality of life (see ASHA, 2016). The major issue related to social participation for bilinguals is whether the client/patient is able to communicate with his/her family whose native language is not English. Thus, one major question is whether to treat bilinguals in one language or two. Intervention language for bilinguals depends on their proficiency with both languages, their current and future needs for both languages across home and work settings, and recovery phases. Families' values, cultures, and needs are also critical for designing the goals of the intervention (Lorenzen & Murray, 2008). In contrast with intervention research on developmental disorders, intervention for bilinguals with acquired language disorders tends to focus on one language. Although more research needs to be done on bilingual treatment approaches, research shows that patients with aphasia showed improvement in both L1 and L2 after treatment in only one language (Kiran, Sandberg, Gray, Ascenso, & Kester, 2013).

(3) Cultural Consideration of Intervention. Clinicians serving CLD populations may or may not share the language or culture of their clients/patients/families. Due to the shortage of bilingual-bicultural clinicians, the mismatch between clients and professionals will likely be expected. One challenge is to facilitate the knowledge and skills of a language that the clinician does not speak. Another challenge is to ask the family members to complete tasks that are not consistent with their cultural practice. To overcome these limitations, clinicians can recruit family members, peers, and paraprofessionals to implement certain facilitation strategies in the client's home language (Kohnert, 2013). This process should take the patient's cultural background into consideration. For example, in some cultures, play-based child–parent interaction is not a common practice (Dyches et al., 2004; van Kleeck, 1994). Thus, it is important to gather information about the level of involvement with which the family members feel comfortable and consider the daily activities that family members are familiar with.

Systems-Level Constraints Affecting Culturally-Linguistically Diverse Populations

In addition to clinical barriers when providing services, CLD populations often face larger systems-level issues that impede their ability to access appropriate health care or special education services in a timely manner. The first is gaining access to the health care system. The second is accessing and obtaining accurate language trans-

lation and interpreter services. The third issue, which impacts school-age children, is getting effective bilingual education to support academic success. The remainder of this chapter will address these issues and suggest how SLPs and AuDs can support children, adults, and their families in overcoming these systems-level barriers.

(1) Accessing the Health Care System

Culturally-linguistically diverse populations, especially racial and ethnic minority groups, experience major disparities when accessing and navigating the health care system (Betancourt, Green, Carrillo, & Ananeh-Firempong, 2003). One of the Healthy People 2020 goals is to eliminate health care inequality in order to improve access to comprehensive, quality health care services (Healthy People, 2020). Having health insurance coverage is essential in gaining access to timely health care services (National Quality Forum, 2017). Health insurance can provide financial access to a broad range of covered clinical services, including diagnostic and intervention services. In the U.S., racial and ethnic minorities continue to have lower rates of health insurance coverage compared with non-Hispanic whites (Berchick, Hood, & Barnett, 2018). Moreover, the health insurance coverage they do have may not be comprehensive enough, and so speech, language, hearing, or swallowing intervention services may be discontinued due to lack of coverage. SLPs and AuDs are in a position to advocate to insurance companies for continued coverage of more services for their clients/patients. Clinicians can make a case by providing data that show progress and improved quality of life as a result of therapy.

(2) Language Access and Rights

Another major systems-level barrier to getting health care or special education services is the lack of translated written materials or interpreters (Barr & Wanat, 2005). The term *translator* refers to someone who translates from one language to another in writing, while an interpreter does so with spoken language. Three federal laws—Title VI of the Civil Rights Act of 1964, the Americans with Disabilities Act, and the Affordable Care Act—require that health care providers who receive federal funds (e.g., Medicare, Medicaid) provide spoken or signed interpreters and translated written materials to limited English proficiency and Deaf/hard-of-hearing clients/patients/families (Chen, Youdelman, & Brooks, 2007). At the state level, the National Health Law Program has secured language access laws in all 50 states. Communication is a human right. Access to appropriate methods of communication—both in written and spoken language—is a right of every individual.

There are three important reasons why SLPs and AuDs should know the laws in the state where they work. First, clinicians will be legally compliant in providing their clients/patients/families with language access. Second, clinicians can advocate for their clients/patients/families and demand for translators and interpreters. Third, clinicians can educate their clients/patients/families about their language rights and empower them to obtain language access.

Even after obtaining access to translators and interpreters, CLD populations may face another systems-level barrier of getting culturally-linguistically appropriate and accurate translations (Flores, 2006). The process of translating from one language to another may appear to be straightforward, but that is not the case. Rather, it is a complex and sensitive process that must take into consideration cultural and linguistic nuances between languages. Written documents, such as special education documents (e.g., Individualized Education Plans [IEPs]) or clinical documents (e.g., evaluation reports, therapy notes), are often translated using computer translation programs, which may not be sensitive to cultural differences in word choice, or linguistic differences in syntax and morphology. Consequently, the documents are unreadable and not useful to clients/patients/families, or worse, critical health care and special education documents are misinterpreted. As for interpreters, it is not always possible for them to directly translate an English word into another language because that target word may not exist in the other language. For example, the diagnostic label "autism" in Chinese could be translated into "loneliness disease" or "closed-self disease"—both of which convey different meanings (Hussey 2013). Inaccurate translation of a word or phrase during a diagnostic feedback may be confusing at best, and stigmatizing at worst. SLPs and AuDs working with translators should have a two-way relationship: clinicians educate translators on the definition of medical terms commonly used in our field (e.g., autism, IEPs, language disorder), while translators educate us on the linguistically equivalent terms or phrases. Additionally, SLPs and AuDs can collaborate with cultural brokers in the communities they serve. Cultural brokers are knowledgeable about the sociocultural norms and expectations in a cultural group within the community, and can be an invaluable resource for translation and interpretation services.

(3) Bilingual Education in a School System

The term 'bilingual education' is frequently used when clinicians make recommendations about school programming, yet its meaning is ambiguous and not obvious.

Bilingual education is an overly simplistic label for a rather complex academic program (Baker & Wright, 2017). This section aids SLPs and AuDs in understanding the range of bilingual education programs, and deconstructing how they support bilingual students in schools.

Under the umbrella term 'bilingual education,' we must first distinguish between formal instruction that uses and promotes two languages versus a relatively monolingual education in the second language (English). The major typologies of bilingual programs each have different societal and educational aims, and language outcomes (Baker & Wright, 2017). Table 25–2 provides examples of bilingual education programs across a spectrum. In submersion programs, or the more notorious label "sink or swim," language minority students are submersed in English-only classrooms, and expected to learn English as quickly as possible (Baker & Wright, 2017). The societal and educational aim of submersion programs is to assimilate language minority students to the mainstream classroom, with the language outcome being monolingualism. On the opposite end of the bilingual education spectrum is maintenance/heritage language programs, which is considered a strong form of bilingual education. The language of instruction in the classroom includes both minority and majority languages, with a greater emphasis on the home language. The goal of the program is to maintain the home language, while learning and using the majority language in order to achieve bilingualism and biliteracy. Bilingual education is not just about education. There are sociocultural, political, and economic issues imbued in the debate over the provision of bilingual education (Garcìa & Kleifgen, 2010). SLPs and AuDs working with school-age bilingual children or work in the school system should be knowledgeable of how these bilingual education programs range and how educational policies and programs change in response to current events.

Behind these bilingual education programs is the highly influential belief that the language learning process of dual language learners is broadly divided into two categories: Basic Interpersonal Communication Skills (BICS) and Cognitive Academic Language Proficiency (CALP) (Baker & Wright, 2017; Cummins, 1979). BICS is contextualized language often used in social settings and conversations and is supported by social cues. CALP is a different set of language abilities needed in academic settings to engage in classroom discourse and understand written texts (Cummins, 1979). While this distinction has helped educational professionals recognize that dual language learners need different kinds of language support, the BICS/CALP dichotomy oversimplifies the complex and dynamic nature of learning a second language. Social and academic language are not

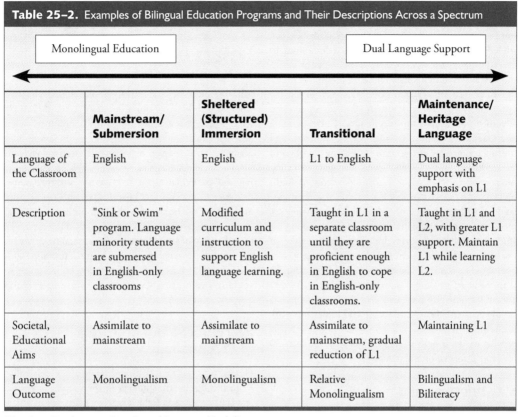

Table 25–2. Examples of Bilingual Education Programs and Their Descriptions Across a Spectrum

Monolingual Education   Dual Language Support

	Mainstream/ Submersion	**Sheltered (Structured) Immersion**	**Transitional**	**Maintenance/ Heritage Language**
Language of the Classroom	English	English	L1 to English	Dual language support with emphasis on L1
Description	"Sink or Swim" program. Language minority students are submersed in English-only classrooms	Modified curriculum and instruction to support English language learning.	Taught in L1 in a separate classroom until they are proficient enough in English to cope in English-only classrooms.	Taught in L1 and L2, with greater L1 support. Maintain L1 while learning L2.
Societal, Educational Aims	Assimilate to mainstream	Assimilate to mainstream	Assimilate to mainstream, gradual reduction of L1	Maintaining L1
Language Outcome	Monolingualism	Monolingualism	Relative Monolingualism	Bilingualism and Biliteracy

Note. L1 = First language, L2 = Second Language (English).

Source: Adapted from Baker, C., and Wright, W. E. (2017). *Foundations of Bilingual Education and Bilingualism* (6th ed.). Bristol, UK: Multilingual Matters.

mutually exclusive, but rather they interact synergistically both in and outside the classroom (Aukerman, 2007; deJong, 2011). Clinicians working with dual language learners in the school setting must be aware of the relationship between social and academic language skills in order to support students' language and communication skills.

Moving the Field Forward

Looking ahead to the future, students in speech, language, and hearing sciences should be aware that our responsibilities as speech-language pathologists and audiologists encompass more than providing clinical intervention and evaluation services. As the demographic landscape in the U.S. continues to change, SLPs and AuDs must be prepared to hold multiple roles and responsibilities when working with and supporting our clients/patients/students/families from culturally-

linguistically diverse backgrounds. We are advocates and leaders in our clinical settings and communities, informed consumers and educators, and community collaborators and partners. The final section of this chapter will discuss what students in the field can do now to prepare for working with CLD populations and to fulfill these roles and responsibilities. Lastly, we will discuss recruiting and retaining SLP and AuD students from diverse backgrounds in an effort to promote greater cultural and linguistic diversity in our field.

Advocacy and Leadership Roles

Speech-language pathologists' and audiologists' clinical roles provide us with a platform to advocate for the children, adults, and families we serve, especially those from culturally-linguistically diverse backgrounds. There are a multitude of activities you can do at various levels to develop your advocacy and leadership skills. At the grassroots level, SLP and AuD graduate students can promote greater awareness of multicultural issues and health care disparities in and outside the classroom. This can be done informally through conversations between students and professors within and across disciplines, or more formally through departmental events or workshops open to all. Graduate students in clinical placements, clinical fellows, and externs have an invaluable opportunity to learn from their clinical supervisors' advocacy and leadership experiences. Undergraduate and graduate students studying speech, language, and hearing sciences are encouraged to become members of either the National Student Speech Language Hearing Association (NSSLHA) or Student Academy of Audiology (SAA). These national organizations will provide students with access to more educational opportunities, including workshops, conferences, and networking, or student leadership skill development. Additionally, at the state and national levels, ASHA suggests voicing support about legislative issues that ASHA is advocating for with members of Congress, or participating in ASHA's annual Capitol Hill Day visit. SLP and AuD students should be aware that our advocacy and leadership work is not in addition to our clinical work, but rather a part of what we do as health care providers. See Chapter 30 for more information on advocacy.

Stay Informed and Disseminate Knowledge

The field of speech, language, and hearing sciences functions within a larger dynamic social, political, and economic system. SLPs and AuDs must stay informed of current events and policies, especially as it relates to their work setting (e.g., hospitals, schools, private practice) and the populations they serve. In turn, clinicians have a responsibility to disseminate their knowledge back to underserved communities to empower and educate them. SLP and AuD students now can stay informed about our profession's current health care initiatives by visiting ASHA's Take Action web page, following ASHA Advocacy social media pages, or subscribing to email news updates on ASHA advocacy issues. Additionally, ASHA Special Interest Group 14, Cultural and Linguistic Diversity (ASHA, n.d.-b), provides excellent opportunities for SLPs and AuDs to continue to advance their knowledge about cultural and linguistic diversity. In addition to ASHA sources, SLP and AuD students can listen to or watch local and national news channels to stay up-to-date on how changes in the community and in national and federal policies affect our field's provision of work and the CLD populations we serve. In addition to staying informed, students are encouraged to go into the community and share their knowledge. Students can reach out to the local community where they attend

school or in their hometown and volunteer their time and efforts.

Engaging and Collaborating with Communities

Additionally, SLP and AuDs should engage and collaborate with local communities to understand precisely what multicultural issues are most important to them. Students can attend parent support groups, community organization meetings, or town hall meetings to learn from communities. Students can begin by volunteering and participating in local community programs, and over time develop a relationship with community members. Collaborating with communities in clinical work and research projects can occur at different levels, including initial formulation of ideas, ongoing consultation, or full partnership. Establishing relationships with community members and organization leaders is key to working together to address systems-level issues in health care and education.

Recruitment and Retention of CLD Students

Finally, we need to recruit and retain more culturally-linguistically diverse students in the speech, language, and hearing sciences field. There are many scholarships, fellowships, and mentorship opportunities available to minority students through ASHA, NSSLHA, SAA, universities, and state- and national-level organizations. The ASHA Minority Student Leadership Program (MSLP), which is available to both undergraduate and graduate students, focuses on building and enhancing leadership skills in students from historically underrepresented racial and ethnic backgrounds. The American Speech-Language-Hearing Foundation has the Minority Student Scholarship to support master's or doctoral-level graduate students' academic careers. Students who come from CLD backgrounds are encouraged to attend their university's graduate student fairs to actively recruit other minority students. Additionally, student organizations such as NSSLHA and SAA should consider collaborating with other interdisciplinary fields such as occupational therapists, physical therapists, teachers, or psychologists to develop events and workshops together. By interacting with other disciplines, CLD students may form more connections with CLD students in other fields, and begin building a support system to empower one another. Lastly, SLPs and AuDs who have neurodiverse backgrounds such as autism, language and learning disorders, ADHD, or anxiety disorder are encouraged to pursue a career in the speech, language, and hearing sciences field as clinicians and/or researchers. Those who have these diverse characteristics may understand the disorders on a deeper and more personal level, and are more likely to provide services that align best with the needs of their clients/patients/students/families.

Summary

In this chapter, we provided an overview of challenges that individuals from CLD backgrounds experience, and how we as speech-language pathologists and audiologists can provide appropriate services and become advocates to help our clients/patients/students/families overcome these challenges. First, we presented the demographic profiles of and linguistic diversity among CLD populations. Second, we described language differences and development in bilinguals. Third, we discussed clinical issues related to assessing and treating clients/patients/students from culturally-linguistically diverse backgrounds. Fourth, we highlighted larger systems-level issues that impact CLD populations from accessing and navigating health care or special education services. Each of these issues has an impact on the quality of services we provide and on how our patients/clients/families perceive health care services. Lastly, in an effort to shape the future of the speech, language, and hearing sciences field, we suggested steps that students can do now to prepare for working with and supporting CLD populations.

Critical Thinking

1. There are different types of bilinguals (e.g., sequential vs. simultaneous) and different bilingual processes (e.g., silent period, code-switching) that come with bilingual language learning and development. How do you think knowing this will inform our clinical services?

2. In addition to clinical barriers in assessment and intervention, what are some systems-level barriers that impact how clients/patients/families access and navigate services and resources?

3. Cultural-linguistic competence is a lifelong process. What do you think health care professionals can do to continue developing their cultural-linguistic competency skills? Think about what they can do at different levels of their career, including student level, clinical fellow level, or clinical educator level.

4. How do you think we can recruit and retain students and clinicians from culturally-linguistically diverse backgrounds in the speech, language,

and hearing sciences field? What do you think are barriers preventing students from entering or staying in the field?

References

American Speech-Language-Hearing Association. (2003). *American English dialects* [Technical report]. Available from http://www.asha.org/policy

American Speech-Language-Hearing Association. (2005). *Evidence-based practice in communication disorder*s. https://doi.org/10.1044/policy.PS 2005-00221

American Speech-Language-Hearing Association. (2013). *Issues in ethics: Cultural and linguistic competence.* https://doi.org/10.0144/policy.ET 2013-00340

American Speech-Language-Hearing Association. (2016). *Scope of practice in speech-language pathology.* https://doi.org/10.1044/policy.SP 2016-00343

American Speech-Language-Hearing Association. (2017). *Issues in ethics: Cultural and linguistic competence.* Retrieved from http://www.asha.org/ Practice/ethics/Cultural-and-Linguistic-Competence/

American Speech-Language-Hearing Association. (2018a). http://2018-Schools-Survey-Summary-Report.pdf

American Speech-Language-Hearing Association. (2018b). *2020 audiology certification standards.* Retrieved from https://www-asha-org.colorado .idm.oclc.org/certification/2020-audiology-certification-standards/

American Speech-Language-Hearing Association. (2018c). 2020 *Certification standards in speech-language pathology.* Retrieved from https://www.asha.org/ Certification/2020-SLP-Certification-Standards/

American Speech-Language-Hearing Association. (2019). *Demographic profile of ASHA members providing bilingual services, year-end 2018.* Available from http://www.asha.org

American Speech-Language-Hearing Association. (n.d.-a). *Accent modification* [Practice portal]. Retrieved from http://www.asha.org/Practice-Portal/Professional-Issues/Accent-Modification/

American Speech-Language-Hearing Association. (n.d.-b). *Special Interest Group 14, cultural and*

linguistic diversity. Retrieved from http://www.asha
.org/SIG/14/

Anderson, R. T. (2001). Lexical morphology and
verb use in child first language loss: A preliminary
case study investigation. *International Journal of
Bilingualism, 5*(4), 377–401. https://doi.org/10.11
77/13670069010050040101

Aukerman, M. (2007). A culpable CALP: Rethinking
the conversational/academic language proficiency
distinction in early literacy instruction. *The Reading
Teacher, 60*(7), 626–635. Retrieved from http://
www.jstor.org/stable/20204516

Baker, C., & Wright, W. E. (2017). *Foundations of
bilingual education and bilingualism* (6th ed.).
Bristol, UK: Multilingual Matters.

Beatty-Martínez, A., & Dussias, P. E. (2017). Bilingual
experience shapes language processing: Evidence
from codeswitching. *Journal of Memory and
Language, 25*, 173–189. https://doi.org/10.1016/j
.jml.2017.04.002

Bedore, L. M., & Peña, E. D. (2008). Assessment of
bilingual children for identification of language
impairment: Current findings and implications
for practice. *International Journal of Bilingual
Education and Bilingualism, 11*(1), 1–30. https://
doi.org/10.2167/beb392.0

Bedore, L. M., Peña, E. D., Joyner, D., & Macken,
C. (2011). Parent and teacher rating of bilingual
language proficiency and language development
concerns. *International Journal of Bilingual Education and Bilingualism, 14*(5), 489–511. https://doi
.org/10.1080/13670050.2010.529102

Berchick, E. R., Hood, E., & Barnett, J. C. (2018).
*Health insurance coverage in the United States: 2017.
Current population reports* (pp. 60–264). Wash-
ington, DC: U.S. Government Printing Office.

Betancourt, J. R., Green, A. R., Carrillo, J., &
Ananeh-Firempong, O. (2003). Defining cultural
competence: A practical framework for addressing
racial/ethnic disparities in health and health care.
Public Health Reports, 118(1), 293–302.

Bialystok, E., & Luk, G. (2012). Receptive vocabulary
differences in monolingual and bilingual adults.
Bilingualism: Language and Cognition, 15(2), 397–
401. https://doi.org/10.1017/S136672891100040X

Bialystok, E., Luk, G., Peets, K. F., & Yang, S. (2010).
Receptive vocabulary differences in monolingual
and bilingual children. *Bilingualism: Language and*

Cognition, 13(4), 525–531. https://doi.org/10.1017/
S1366728909990423

Bligh, C. (2014). *The silent experiences of young
bilingual learners: A sociocultural study into the silent
period.* Rotterdam, Netherlands: Springer.

Bligh, C., & Drury, R. (2015). Perspectives on the
"silent period" for emergent bilinguals in England.
Journal of Research in Childhood Education, 29(2),
259–274. https://doi.org/10.1080/02568543.201
5.1009589

Chen, A., Youdelman, M. K., & Brooks, J. (2007).
The legal framework for language access in health
care settings: Title VI and beyond. *Journal of
General Internal Medicine, 22*(2), 362–367.

Clark, M. E., Landers, S., Linde, R., & Sperber, J.
(2001). The GLBT Health Access Project: A state-
funded effort to improve access to care. *American
Journal of Public Health, 91*(6), 895–896. Retrieved
from https://www.ncbi.nlm.nih.gov/pmc/articles/
PMC1446464/

Clarke, P. M. (2009). *Supporting children learning
English as a second language in the early years (birth
to six years).* Retrieved from http://www.vcaa.vic
.edu.au/earlyyears/supporting_children_learning_
esl.pdf

Colby, S. L., & Ortman, J.M. (2014). *Projections of the
size and composition of the U.S. population: 2014
to 2060,* Current Population Reports, P25-1143.
Washington, DC: U.S. Census Bureau.

Coleman, E., Bockting, W., Botzer, M., Cohen-Ket-
tenis, P., DeCuypere, G., Feldman, J., . . . Zucker,
K. (2012). Standards of care for the health of transsexual, transgender, and gender-nonconforming
people, version 7. *International Journal of Transgen-
derism, 13*(4), 165–232.

Correll, J. (2005). Review of inside deaf culture.
Deafness and Education International, 7(4),
223–224. http://dx.doi.org.colorado.idm.oclc
.org/10.1002/dei.17

Cummins, J. (1979). Cognitive/academic language
proficiency, linguistic interdependence, the
optimum age question and some other matters.
Working Papers on Bilingualism, 19, 121–129.

Davidson, J. (2008). Autistic culture online:
Virtual communication and cultural expression on the spectrum. *Social and Cultural
Geography, 9*(7), 791–806. https://doi.org/
10.1080/14649360802382586

Davis-McFarland, E. (2008). Family and cultural issues in a school swallowing and feeding program. *Language, Speech, and Hearing Services in Schools, 39*(2), 199–213. https://doi .org/10.1044/0161-1461(2008/020)

deJong, E. J. (2011). *Foundations for multilingualism in education.* Philadelphia, PA: Caslon.

Durán, L. K., Hartzheim, D., Lund, E. M., Simons-meier, V., & Kohlmeier, T. L. (2016). Bilingual and home language interventions with young dual language learners: A research synthesis. *Language, Speech, and Hearing Services in Schools, 47*(4), 347–371. https://doi.org/10.1044/2016_LSHSS-15-0030

Duursma, E., Romero-Contreras, S., Szuber, A., Proctor, P., Snow, C., August, D., & Calderón, M. (2007). The role of home literacy and language environment on bilinguals' English and Spanish vocabulary development. *Applied Psycholinguistics, 28*, 171–190. https://doi.org/10.1017/S014271 6406070093

Dyches, T. T., Wilder, L. K., Sudweeks, R. R., Obiakor, F. E., & Algozzine, B. (2004). Multi-cultural issues in autism. *Journal of Autism and Developmental Disorders, 34*(2), 211–222. https:// doi.org/10.1023/B:JADD.0000022611.80478.73

Ecke, P. (2004). Language attrition and theories of forgetting: A cross-disciplinary review. *International Journal of Bilingualism, 8*(3), 321–354. https://doi .org/10.1177/13670069040080030901

Fillmore, L. W. (1991). When learning a second language means losing the first. *Early Childhood Research Quarterly, 6*(3), 323–346. https://doi .org/10.1016/S0885-2006(05)80059-6

Flege, J. E., Birdsong, D., Bialystok, E., Mack, M., Sung, H., & Tsukada, K. (2006). Degree of foreign accent in English sentences produced by Korean children and adults. *Journal of Phonetics, 34*(2), 153–175. https://doi.org/10.1016/j.wocn .2005.05.001

Flores, G. (2006). Language barriers to health care in the United States. *New England Journal of Medicine, 355*(3), 229–231. https://doi.org/10.1056/NEJM p058316

García, O., & Kleifgen, J. A. (2010). *Educating emergent bilinguals: Policies, programs, and practices for English language learners.* New York, NY: Teachers College Press.

Goldstein, B. A., & Bunta, F. (2012). Positive and negative transfer in the phonological systems of bilingual speakers. *International Journal of Bilingualism, 16*(4), 388–401. https://doi.org/ 10.1177/1367006911425817

Grosjean, F. (1992) The bilingual and bicultural person in the hearing and in the deaf world. *Sign Language Studies, 77*(1), 307–320.

Grosjean, F. (1995). A psycholinguistic approach to code-switching: The recognition of guest words by bilinguals. In *One speaker, two languages: Cross-disciplinary perspectives on code-switching.* https:// doi.org/10.1017/CBO9780511620867.012

Grosjean, F. (2012). An attempt to isolate, and then differentiate, transfer and interference. *International Journal of Bilingualism, 16*(1), 11–21. https://doi .org/10.1177/1367006911403210

Gutiérrez-Clellen, V. F., & Kreiter, J. (2003). Under-standing child bilingual acquisition using parent and teacher reports. *Applied Psycholinguistics, 24*(2). https://doi.org/10.1017/S0142716403000158

Gutiérrez-Clellen, V. F., & Peña, E. D. (2001). Dynamic assessment of diverse children: A tutorial. *Language, Speech, and Hearing Services in Schools, 32*(4), 212–224. https://doi.org/10.1044/0161-1461(2001/019)

Gutiérrez-Clellen, V. F., Simon-Cereijido, G., & Erickson L. (2009). Code-switching in bilingual children with specific language impairment. *International Journal of Bilingualism, 13*(1), 91–109. https://doi.org/10.1177/1367006909103530

Healthy People. (2020). Washington, DC: U.S. Department of Health and Human Services, Office of Disease Prevention and Health Promo-tion. Retrieved from https://www.healthypeople .gov/2020/about/foundation-health-measures/ Disparities.

Herman, J. L., Flores, A. R., Brown, T., Wilson, B., & Conron, K. J. (2017). *Age of individuals who identify as transgender in the United States.* Los Angeles, CA: The Williams Institute.

Hoff, E. (2013). Interpreting the early language trajectories of children from low-SES and language minority homes: Implications for closing achieve-ment gaps. *Developmental Psychology, 49*(1), 4–14. https://doi.org/10.1037/a0027238

Hoff, E., & Core, C. (2015). What clinicians need to know about bilingual development. *Seminars* in Speech and Language, 36(2), 89–99. https://doi .org/10.1055/s-0035-1549104

Holcomb, T. K. (2012). Introduction to American Deaf culture. Oxford, UK: Oxford University Press.

Hughes, C. E., Shaunessy, E. S., Brice, A. R., Ratliff, M. A., & McHatton, P. A. (2006). Code switching among bilingual and limited English proficient students: Possible indicators of giftedness. Journal for the Education of the Gifted, 30(1), 7–28. Retrieved from https://eric.ed.gov/?id=EJ750758

Hussey, M. (2013, May 28). Autism in transla- tion. The world of Chinese. Retrieved from http://www.theworldofchinese.com/2013/05/ autism-in-translation/

Kapantzoglou, M., Restrepo, M. A., & Thompson, M. S. (2012). Dynamic assessment of word learning skills: Identifying language impairment in bilingual children. Language, Speech, and Hearing Services in Schools, 43, 81–96. https://doi.org/10.1044/0161- 1461(2011/10-0095)a

Karayayla, T., & Schmid, M. S. (2019). First language attrition as a function of age at onset of bilingualism: First language attainment of Turkish–English bilinguals in the United Kingdom. Language Learning, 69(1), 106–142. https://doi .org/10.1111/lang.12316

Kaushanskaya, M., & Marian, V. (2007). Bilingual language processing and interference in bilinguals: Evidence from eye tracking and picture naming. Language Learning, 57(1), 119–163. https://doi .org/10.1111/j.1467-9922.2007.00401.x

Kiran, S., Sandberg, C., Gray, T., Ascenso, E., & Kester, E. (2013). Rehabilitation in bilingual aphasia: Evidence for within- and between- language generalization. American Journal of Speech-Language Pathology, 22(2), S298–S309. https://doi.org/10.1044/1058-0360(2013/12- 0085)

Kohnert, K. (2010). Bilingual children with primary language impairment: Issues, evidence and implications for clinical actions. Journal of Communication Disorders, 43(6), 456–473. https:// doi.org/10.1016/j.jcomdis.2010.02.002

Kohnert, K. (2013). Language disorders in bilingual children and adults. San Diego, CA: Plural Publishing.

Kohnert, K., Yim, D., Nett, K., Kan, P. F., & Duran, L. (2005). Intervention with linguistically diverse preschool children: A focus on developing home

language(s). Language, Speech, and Hearing Services in Schools, 36(3), 251–263.

Köpke, B., & Schmid, M. S. (2004). Language attrition: The next phase. In M. S. Schmid, B. Köpke, M. Keijzer, & L. Weilemar (Eds.), Studies in bilingualism (Vol. 28, p. 1). https://doi .org/10.1075/sibil.28.02kop

Kritikos, E. (2003). Speech-language pathologists' beliefs about language assessment of bilingual/ bicultural individuals. American Journal of Speech- Language Pathology, 12(1), 73–91. https://doi.org/ 10.1044/1058-0360(2003/054)

Laing, S. P., & Kamhi, A. (2003). Alternative assess- ment of language and literacy in culturally and linguistically diverse populations. Language, Speech, and Hearing Services in Schools, 34(1), 44–55. https://doi.org/10.1044/0161-1461(2003/005)

Lim, N., O'Reilly, M. F., Sigafoos, J., Ledbetter-Cho, K., & Lancioni, G. E. (2019). Should heritage languages be incorporated into interventions for bilingual individuals with neurodevelopmental disorders? A systematic review. Journal of Autism and Developmental Disorders, 49(3), 887–912. https://doi.org/10.1007/s10803-018-3790-8

Lorenzen, B., & Murray, L. L. (2008). Bilingual aphasia: A theoretical and clinical review. American Journal of Speech-Language Pathology, 17(3), 299–317. https://doi.org/10.1044/1058- 0360(2008/026)

Lugo-Neris, M. J., Bedore, L. M., & Peña, E. D. (2015). Dual language intervention for bilinguals at risk for language impairment. Seminars in Speech and Language, 36(2), 133–142. https://doi .org/10.1055/s-0035-1549108

MacWhinney, B. (2005). A unified model of language acquisition. Retrieved from http://scholar.google. com/scholar?hl=en&btnG=Search&q=intitle:A+Un ified+Model+of+Language+Acquisition#0

Miccio, A. W., Hammer, C. S., & Rodríguez, B. (2009). Code-switching and language disorders in bilingual children. In The Cambridge handbook of linguistic code-switching. https://doi.org/10.1017/ CBO9780511576331.015

Moore, D. (2002). Code-switching and learning in the classroom. International Journal of Bilingual Education and Bilingualism, 5(5), 279–293. https:// doi.org/10.1080/13670050208667762

Muñoz, M., & Marquardt, T. (2003). Picture naming and identification in bilingual speakers of Spanish and English with and without aphasia. *Aphasiology, 17*(12), 1115–1132. https://doi.org/10.1080/02687030344000427

Napier, A. D., Ancarno, C., Butler, B., Calabrese, J., Chater, A., & Chatterjee, H. (2014). Culture and health. *The Lancet, 384*(9954), 1607–1639. https://doi.org/10.1016/S0140-6736(14)61603-2

National Quality Forum. (2017). *A roadmap for promoting health equity and eliminating disparities: The four I's for health equity.* Retrieved from https://www.qualityforum.org/Publications/2017/09/A_Roadmap_for_Promoting_Health_Equity_and_Eliminating_Disparities__The_Four_I_s_for_Health_Equity.aspx

Nicoladis, E. (2006). Cross-linguistic transfer in adjective–noun strings by preschool bilingual children. *Bilingualism, 9*(01), 15. https://doi.org/10.1017/S136672890500235X

Nicoladis, E., & Grabois, H. (2010). Bilingualism learning English and losing Chinese: A case study of a child adopted from China. *International Journal of Bilingualism, 6*, 441–454. https://doi.org/10.1177/13670069020060040401

Nicoladis, E., Song, J., & Marentette, P. (2012). Do young bilinguals acquire past tense morphology like monolinguals, only later? Evidence from French-English and Chinese-English bilinguals. *Applied Psycholinguistics, 33*, 457–479.

Oller, D. K., Pearson, B. Z., & Cobo-lewis, A. B. (2007). Profile effects in early bilingual language and literacy. *Applied Psycholingustics, 28*, 191–230.

Padilla, A. H., Palmer, P. M., & Rodríguez, B. L. (2018). The relationship between culture, quality of life, and stigma in Hispanic New Mexicans with dysphagia: A preliminary investigation using quantitative and qualitative analysis. *American Journal of Speech-Language Pathology.* https://doi.org/10.1044/2018_AJSLP-18-0061

Paradis, J., Genesee, F., & Crago, M. B. (2011). *Dual language development and disorders: A handbook on bilingualism and second language learning* (2nd ed.). Baltimore, MD: Brookes.

Parette, H. P., Huer, M. B., & Brotherson, M. J. (2001). Related service personnel perceptions of team AAC decision-making across cultures. *Education and Training in Mental Retardation and Developmental Disabilities, 36*(1), 69–82.

Pavlenko, A. (2009). Conceptual representation in the bilingual lexicon and second language vocabulary learning. In A. Pavlenko (Ed.), *The bilingual mental lexicon interdisciplinary approaches.* https://doi.org/10.21832/9781847691262-008

Pearson, B. Z. (2007). Social factors in childhood bilingualism in the United States. *Applied Psycholinguistics, 28*(3). https://doi.org/10.1017/S014271640707021X

Pearson, B. Z, Fernandez, S., & Oller, D. K. (1993). Lexical development in bilingual infants and toddlers: Comparison to monolingual norms. *Language Learning.* https://doi.org/10.1111/j.1467-1770.1993.tb00174.x

Proctor, C., August, D., & Carlo, M. (2010). Language maintenance versus language of instruction: Spanish reading development among Latino and Latina bilingual learners. *Journal of Social Issues, 79*–94. https://doi.org/10.1111/j.1540-4560.2009.01634.x

Reyes, I. (2004). Functions of code switching in schoolchildren's conversations. *Bilingual Research Journal, 28*(1), 77–98. https://doi.org/10.1080/15235882.2004.10162613

Roberts, T. A. (2014). Not so silent after all: Examination and analysis of the silent stage in childhood second language acquisition. *Early Childhood Research Quarterly, 29*(1), 22–40. https://doi.org/10.1016/j.ecresq.2013.09.001

Ryan, C. (2013). *Language use in the United States: 2011.* American Community Survey Reports, ACS-22. Washington, DC: U.S. Census Bureau.

Schwartz, S. J., Unger, J. B., Zamboanga, B. L., & Szapocznik, J. (2010). Rethinking the concept of acculturation. *The American Psychologist, 65*(4), 237–251. https://doi.org/10.1037/a0019330

Sharp, H. M., & Genesen, L. B. (1996). Ethical decision-making in dysphagia management. *American Journal of Speech-Language Pathology.* Retrieved from http://pubs.asha.org/doi/abs/10.1044/1058-0360.0501.15

Simmons, N., & Johnston, J. (2007). Cross-cultural differences in beliefs and practices that affect the language spoken to children: Mothers with Indiana and Western heritage. *International Journal of Language and Communication Disorders, 42*(4), 445–465. https://doi.org/10.1080/13682820600988926

Siraj-Blatchford, I., & Clarke, P. (2000). *Supporting identity, diversity and language in the early years.* Buckingham, UK: Open University Press.

Soto, G., & Yu, B. (2014). Considerations for the provision of services to bilingual children who use augmentative and alternative communication. *Augmentative and Alternative Communication, 30*(1), 83–92. https://doi.org/10.3109/07434618.2013.878751

Stockman, I., Boult, J., & Robinson, G. C. (2008). Multicultural/multilingual instruction in educational programs: A survey of perceived faculty practices and outcomes. *American Journal of Speech-Language Pathology, 17*(3), 241–264. https://doi.org/10.1044/1058-0360(2008/023)

Sue, S. (2006). Cultural competency: From philosophy to research and practice. *Journal of Community Psychology, 34*(2), 237–245. https://doi.org/10.1002/jcop

UNESCO. (2001). *Universal declaration on cultural diversity.* Retrieved from http://portal.unesco.org/en/ev.php-URL_ID=13179&URL_DO=DO_TOPIC&URL_SECTION=201.html

U.S. Census Bureau. (2015). *Detailed languages spoken at home and ability to speak English.* Retrieved from https://www.census.gov/data/tables/2013/demo/2009-2013-lang-tables.html

U.S. Census Bureau. (2018). *Quick facts, Population estimates 2018.* Retrieved from https://www.census.gov/quickfacts/fact/table/US/PST045218

U.S. Department of Education. (2017). *39th Annual Report to Congress on the implementation of the Individuals with Disabilities Education Act, 2017.* Washington, DC.

van Kleeck, A. (1994). Potential cultural bias in training parents as conversational partners with their children who have delays in language development. *American Speech-Language-Hearing Association, 20*(3), 67–78.

Vygotsky, L. S. (1979). *Mind in society: The development of higher psychological processes.* Boston, MA: Harvard University Press.

Westby, C. E. (1990). Ethnographic interviewing: Asking the right questions to the right People in the right ways. *Journal of Childhood Communication Disorders, 13*(1), 101–111. https://doi.org/10.1177/152574019001300111

Westby, C., & Washington, K. N. (2017). Using the International Classification of Functioning, Disability and Health in assessment and intervention of school-aged children with language impairments. *Language, Speech, and Hearing Services in Schools, 48*(3), 137–152. https://doi.org/10.1044/2017_LSHSS-16-0037

Whitmarsh, I., & Jones, D. S. (Eds.). (2010). What's the use of culture? Health disparities and the development of culturally competent health care. In *What's the Use of Race?* https://doi.org/10.7551/mitpress/8360.003.0014

Wiig, E. H., Semel, E., & Secord, W. A. (2006). *Clinical evaluation of language fundamentals®— Fourth edition, Spanish.* Retrieved from https://www.pearsonclinical.com/language/products/100000436/clinical-evaluation-of-language-fundamentals-fourth-edition-spanish-celf-4-spanish.html

Wing, C., Kohnert, K., Pham, G., Cordero, K. N., Ebert, K. D., Fong, P., & Blaiser, K. (2007). Culturally consistent treatment for late talkers. *Communication Disorders Quarterly, 29*(1), 20–27. https://doi.org/10.1177/1525740108314862

World Health Organization. (2001). *International Classification of Functioning, Disability and Health (ICF) framework to facilitate interprofessional education and collaborative practice.* Retrieved from http://www.who.int/hrh/news/2014/hrh_icf_framework/en/

Yu, B. (2013). Issues in bilingualism and heritage language maintenance: Perspectives of minority-language mothers of children with autism spectrum disorders. *American Journal of Speech-Language Pathology, 22*(1), 10–24. https://doi.org/10.1044/1058-0360(2012/10-0078)

Zhang, J., Dennis, J. M., & Houseman, C. (2018). The role of family and community bicultural socialization in the bilingual proficiency of immigrant young adults. *International Journal of Intercultural Relations, 67*, 44–57. https://doi.org/10.1016/j.ijintrel.2018.09.003

Zimmerman, I. L., Steiner, V. G., & Pond, R. E. (2012). *Preschool Language Scales, Fifth Edition Spanish.* Retrieved from https://www.pearsonclinical.com/language/products/100000401/preschool-language-scales-fifth-edition-spanish-pls-5-spanish.html

Zuckerman, K. E., Lindly, O. J., Reyes, N. M., Chavez, A. E., Cobian, M., Macias, K., . . . Smith, K. A. (2018). Parent perceptions of community autism spectrum disorder stigma: Measure validation and associations in a multi-site sample. *Journal of Autism and Developmental Disorders, 48*(9), 3199–3209. https://doi.org/10.1007/s10803-018-3586-x

Resources

Bialystok, E. (2009). Bilingualism: The good, the bad, and the indifferent. *Bilingualism-Language and Cognition, 12*(1), 3–11. https://doi.org/10.1017/s1366728908003477

Fenner, D. S. (2013). *Advocating for English learners.* Thousand Oaks, CA: Corwin Press.

Genesee, F., & Nicoladis, E. (2006). Bilingual acquisition. In E. Hoff & M. Shatz (Eds.), *Handbook of language development.* Oxford, UK: Blackwell.

Goldstein, B., & Oller, D. K. (Eds.). (2011). *Bilingual language development and disorders in Spanish-English speakers* (2nd ed.). Baltimore, MD: Brookes.

Gonzalez-Mena, J. (2014). *50 strategies for communicating and working with diverse families* (3rd ed.) Boston, MA: Pearson.

Grosjean, F. (1989). Neurolinguists, beware! The bilingual is not two monolinguals in one person. *Brain and Language, 36*(1), 3–15.

Grosjean, F. (2008). A wholistic view of bilingualism. In F. Grosjean (Ed.), *Studying bilinguals.* Oxford, UK: Oxford University Press.

Kohnert, K. (2013). *Language disorders in bilingual children and adults.* San Diego, CA: Plural Publishing.

Kroll, J. F., Dussias, P. E., Bice, K., & Perrotti, L. (2015). Bilingualism, mind, and brain. *Annual Review of Linguistics, 1,* 377–394.

Rubin, R., Abrego, M. H., & Sutterby, J. A. (2012). *Engaging the families of ELLs: Ideas, resources, and activities.* Larchmont, NY: Eye on Education.

Internet Resources

American Speech-Language-Hearing Association. (ASHA). Minority Student Leadership Program https://www-asha-org.colorado.idm.oclc.org/Students/MSLP-Award/

American Speech-Language-Hearing Foundation Minority Student Scholarship https://www.ashfoundation.org/apply/#Grants

ASHA Advocacy https://www-asha-org.colorado.idm.oclc.org/advocacy/

ASHA Multicultural Affairs and Resources https://www.asha.org/practice/multicultural/

ASHA Special Interest Group 14, Cultural and Linguistic Diversity https://www-asha-org.colorado.idm.oclc.org/SIG/14/

ASHA Special Interest Group 17, Global Issues in Communication Sciences and Related Disorders https://www-asha-org.colorado.idm.oclc.org/SIG/17/

ASHA Take Action https://takeaction.asha.org/asha/?3

Awesome Library: Multilingual Lesson Plans https://www.awesomelibrary.org/Classroom/English/Languages/Languages.html

Collaborating with Interpreters https://www-asha-org.colorado.idm.oclc.org/PRPSpecificTopic.aspx?folderid=8589935334&section=Key_Issues

Colorín Colorado: A bilingual site for educators and families of English language learners http://www.colorincolorado.org/

Foundation for Child Development https://www.fcd-us.org/

International Children's Digital Library: hosting a collection of books from around the world. http://en.childrenslibrary.org/

National Student Speech Language Hearing Association, Student Leadership https://www.nsslha.org/student-leadership/

Student Academy of Audiology https://saa.audiology.org/

We Need Diverse Books™ https://diversebooks.org/

26

Supervision and Mentoring

Melanie W. Hudson, MA and Mary Sue Fino-Szumski, PhD, MBA

Introduction

This chapter is written by supervisors for both supervisees and supervisors in audiology and speech-language pathology. The information in this chapter is based on both the literature and personal experiences in supervising and in training supervisors in a variety of professional contexts. Good sources for more in-depth discussion of supervision in general and in speech-language pathology and audiology in particular include Anderson (1988) and McCrea and Brasseur (2003). The chapter begins with an overview of the foundations of the supervisory process including a description of the Dreyfus Model of Skill Acquisition (1980) and Anderson's Continuum Model (1988). It includes a model of supervision that can be applied across all levels of experience and settings, and moves to practical issues discussions. Specific discussion is directed to current issues such as the Clinical Fellowship Experience and the audiology externship, ethics, cultural, linguistic and generational differences, technology, training, accountability, and research needs.

A Brief History of Supervision and Mentoring

An appreciation of the history of supervision and mentoring is as important to the pre-professional as it is to the seasoned clinician. Supervision and mentoring have been integral parts of both professions from their early beginnings. It is safe to state that each member of the professions of speech-language pathology and audiology has participated in the supervisory process during the course of his or her clinical training, certainly as a supervisee and perhaps also as a supervisor. In her book *Science of Successful Supervision and Mentorship*, Carozza (2010) explains the importance of knowledge of the history of supervisory education and research and how such knowledge relates to providing effective supervision. As interest in supervision and mentoring increases, and as they continue to play such a significant role in professional growth and development, it is helpful to understand the evolutionary progress of this distinct area of practice.

It was not until the last quarter of the twentieth century that a true understanding of supervision as a process in clinical education was established. Anderson (1988), Farmer and Farmer (1989), and Ulrich (1985) provide informative summaries of the early development of the supervisory process when the professions of speech pathology and audiology were in their infancy. During the 1960s and 1970s, conferences and publications devoted exclusively to issues pertaining to supervision began to appear on the professional horizon (Anderson, 1970; Halfond, 1964; Kleffner, 1964). In 1970 the Council of College and University Supervisors was established, expanding in 1974 into the Council of University Supervisors in Speech-Language Pathology and Audiology (CCSPA). In 1975 the American Speech and Hearing Association (ASHA) Committee on Supervision was established and some Communication Science Disorders (CSD) programs began course offerings in supervision. In 1985 The American Speech-Language-Hearing Association (ASHA) adopted a position statement describing competencies associated with appropriate supervision, with an emphasis on supervision of students (ASHA, 1985). As interest continued to grow, there were several national conferences devoted to the topic resulting in more publications, along with major books that continue to define the knowledge base (Anderson, 1988; Casey, Smith, & Ulrich, 1988; Crago & Pickering, 1987; Farmer & Farmer, 1989). During the 1990s, there was a move toward combining theory and practice in supervision, and the ASHA Certification and Membership Handbook was revised to document the requirements for the Clinical Fellowship Year (CFY) (ASHA, 1997).

At the beginning of the new millennium, there was more emphasis placed on quality clinical education for audiologists and speech-language pathologists. ASHA developed new standards for students' courses of study that required documentation of knowledge and skills, including both formative and summative assessment in addition to new standards for academic program accreditation and certification of personnel (ASHA, 2000). Further research on the topic of merging theory and practice in supervision led to the publication of two major books (Dowling, 2001; McCrea & Brasseur, 2003). With the publication of these books, supervisors had a better understanding of how to implement effective supervisory practices supported by evidence and research.

Several factors during the preceding decade stimulated interest in supervision, including expanded scope of practice, personnel shortages, and sustained influx of new professionals (O'Connor, 2008). For example, supervisors may find themselves in situations where they do not feel qualified to provide supervision because an individual case is out of their scope of practice. This feeling of lack of qualification to supervise may also apply to situations where the scope of practice has expanded beyond the specific skill set of a supervisor. Or, due to a shortage of qualified clinicians in a facility, a supervisor does not have the appropriate amount of time to provide the required supervision and mentoring, thus jeopardiz-

ing the supervisee's ability to meet certification and/or licensure requirements. These and other types of similar situations may also present ethical dilemmas for both the supervisor the supervisee.

In keeping with some of these variables, ASHA revised its certification guidelines for the Clinical Fellowship (CF) experience (Council for Clinical Certification, 2005). You will note that this revision includes discontinuing the "Y" designation for "year" to denote the adjustment in the length of time to complete requirements. These revised guidelines also include replacing the term "supervisor" with "mentor" to reflect the higher degree of autonomy now placed on the clinical fellow or audiology extern. Policy documents regarding CF mentoring (ASHA, 2007) and ethical issues pertaining to supervision of student clinicians (ASHA, 2010), a technical report (2008a) and a document addressing knowledge and skills for clinical supervision (ASHA, 2008b) were also published.

During this same time-period, ASHA audiology certification standards were updated in response to the transition to the doctoral degree as the entry level degree to the profession. The 2007 audiology certification standards specified that the clinical experience required for certification was included in the educational program. There was no longer a post-graduation clinical fellowship required for audiology certification and the minimum number of supervised clinical practicum hours was increase to the equivalent of one-year of full-time experience (1,820 hours). The 2007 audiology standards also removed the minimum percentage of supervision requirement and gave discretion to supervisors on this based on a student's training, education, experience, and competence (Allen, Cosby, Figueroa, & Allen, 2008).

In more recent years, many professionals involved in the supervisory process use the terms **clinical educator** and **clinical instructor** to more accurately reflect their work (CAPCSD, 2013). The term **clinical educator** is typically used in conjunction with the clinical training, education, *and* supervision of audiology and speech-language pathology graduate students. The term **preceptor** most commonly refers to audiologists who supervise audiology students in their final externship. The role of the clinical educator is to integrate theoretical, evidence-based knowledge with clinical practice to prepare student clinicians to provide quality services (ASHA, 2013a).

In 2013, ASHA's Ad Hoc Committee on Supervision (ASHA, 2013c) acknowledged that supervision is a distinct area of practice and discounted the faulty assumption that competency in clinical service delivery translates into effective clinical supervision. Experts in clinical education have long recognized that effective supervision requires a unique set of knowledge and skills and as such, individuals must receive training to gain competence before engaging in the activity. The committee identified five constituent groups for supervision including clinical educators of graduate students, preceptors of audiology externs, mentors of clinical fellows, supervisors of support personnel, and supervisors of those in transition, with each of these groups requiring specific knowledge and skills in supervision. In 2016, ASHA's Ad Hoc Committee on Supervision Training identified topics for supervision training for each of these constituent groups.

The 2020 ASHA certification standards for audiology (Council for Clinical Certification in Audiology and Speech-Language Pathology of the American Speech-Language-Hearing Association, 2018a) and speech-language pathology (Council for Clinical Certification in Audiology and Speech-Language Pathology of the American Speech-Language-Hearing Association, 2018b) recognize the need for training and experience for supervisors/clinical educators working with students, CFs, and audiology externs. The 2020 ASHA certification standards require the equivalent of a minimum of nine months of clinical experience after securing ASHA certification as a prerequisite for being involved in clinical education/supervision. In addition, two hours of professional development in topics related to supervision/clinical education must be completed.

Many states now have specific supervision requirements in place to ensure appropriate levels of supervision and/or mentoring for the beginning clinician working toward being fully credentialed. In some states, licensing boards have enacted regulations regarding supervision of audiology externs. Further guidance related to the role and responsibilities of an audiology preceptor is provided in the position statement on clinical education guidelines for audiology externships that resulted from the American Academy (AAA) Taskforce on Supervision (AAA, 2006). The Council on Academic Accreditation in Audiology and Speech-Language Pathology (CAA) sets out specific standards for clinical education for training programs (CAA, 2017) and the Council for Clinical Certification in Audiology and Speech-Language Pathology (CFCC) has established standards that incorporate supervision requirements for individuals seeking certification (CFCC, 2018a, 2018b). Individuals who enter into a supervisory or mentoring relationship need to become familiar with regulations and guidelines applicable to their specific circumstances. Whether you are a supervisor, mentor, preceptor, clinical fellow, or audiology extern or hold a provisional certificate or license, the success of the experience depends on assuming this responsibility. Regulations, standards, and guidelines will be covered in more detail later in this chapter.

Supervision and mentoring have played significant roles in the development of speech-language pathology and audiology since the early history of both professions. Over the years, research and evidence have demonstrated how effective supervision and mentoring support service delivery and positive outcomes. As a result, university programs, professional organizations, and government agencies have learned to recognize the value of effective supervision and mentoring of the new clinician. Their attempts to address this need by establishing regulations, guidelines, and training for clinical supervisors and mentors are evidence of this belief.

The Supervisory Process

Supervision as a process is more easily understood when presented in the context of learning or acquiring clinical skills and knowledge in audiology and speech-language pathology. The insightful student of supervision will be able to draw a parallel between supervisee performance and supervisor expectations when such a process is taken into consideration.

The Dreyfus Model of Skill Acquisition

The Dreyfus Model of Skill Acquisition (1980) describes a learning process consisting of five stages: *novice, advanced beginner, competent, proficient,* and *expert.* It is used as a means of assessing and supporting progress in the development of skills. It also provides a definition of acceptable level for the assessment of competence. Similar in its design to a developmental continuum, the learner, or supervisee progresses from one stage to the next as the level of clinical knowledge and skills increases.

At the *novice* stage, the learner has minimal knowledge connected to practice. Because supervisees at this stage have no experience in the application of rules, behavior is predictably inflexible. The novice needs to be closely supervised and cannot be expected to use discretionary judgment. The supervisor would naturally need to incorporate a more direct style of supervision, such as modeling behaviors for supervisees.

At the *advanced beginner* stage, supervisees are able to demonstrate marginally acceptable performance, but with limited situational perception. They are beginning to treat knowledge in context, but still treat attributes and aspects separately and with equal importance. For example, they may not perceive the relationship between a hypernasal vocal quality and restricted movement of the mandible, thus viewing them as distinct areas for treatment.

At the *competent* stage, supervisees are able to plan with more independence, deliberately using analytical assessment to treat problems in context. Competent supervisees can view actions in terms of long-term goals and are able to incorporate conscious, deliberate planning to achieve those goals. These supervisees are also able to use standardized and routine procedures while recognizing their relevance to a given situation. For example, after conducting pure-tone audiometric testing, supervisees would be able to assess the necessity of impedance testing or the use of a bone oscillator to help determine type of hearing loss.

At the *proficient* stage, supervisees are able to see the situation as a whole in terms of long-term goals. This holistic understanding improves decision making, as maxims are used for guidance and they are now able to modify plans in terms of what should be expected. Proficient supervisees perceive deviations from what is typical and, as a result, are able to make clinical judgments more easily. These supervisees are also able to see what is most important in a situation and to take responsibility for their own decisions. If working with a non-verbal child with autism, for instance, these supervisees would recognize the value of joint attention training before attempting to initiate a system of picture exchange for communication.

At the *expert* stage, clinicians are able to make decisions not only based on a set of rules, but using their experience to manipulate these rules to achieve the end goal. Expert clinicians have an intuitive grasp of situations and only rely on an analytical approach to problem solving when unfamiliar situations occur. Expert clinicians are able to see the end-goal and know just how to achieve it. They see the big picture and are able to consider various alternatives, possibly going beyond existing standards in order to achieve the end result.

The goal of a supervisor is to ensure that the supervisee progresses from one stage to the next while employing effective strategies that promote increasing levels of independence. Implementation of models of the supervisory process that utilize such strategies will help achieve this goal.

Anderson's Continuum of Supervision

Jean Anderson's book *The Supervisory Process in Speech-Language Pathology and Audiology* (1988) had a major impact in the area of supervision. The profound influence of her work is reflected in the fact that her approach to the supervisory process is reflected in the current accreditation standards for academic programs in Communication Sciences Disorders (CSD) (ASHA, 2017). Anderson (1988) defines supervision as "a process that consists of a variety of patterns of behavior, the appropriateness of which depends on the needs, competencies, expectations and philosophies of the supervisor and supervisee and the specifics of the situation (tasks, cli-

ent, setting, and other variables)" (p. 12). This definition supports flexibility, self-evaluation, and critical thinking. It also promotes collaboration, a key component of the process. Prior to the publication of this book, supervisory style was characterized by stricter control and higher levels of direction on the part of the supervisor. There was very little, if any, collaboration between the supervisor and the supervisee.

Anderson's *Continuum of Supervision* (1988) is the most widely recognized supervision model in speech-language pathology and audiology (Dowling, 2001). This continuum model was influenced by the theoretical framework of Cogan (1973), whose ongoing cycle of supervision was designed to improve the performance of teachers. Anderson employs different strategies and styles that may be incorporated at different stages of the supervisory process, depending on the situation. The continuum model allows for the eventual competent independence of the supervisee while the degree of involvement of both the supervisor and supervisee shifts as they move along the continuum.

The continuum consists of three stages, *evaluation-feedback, transitional,* and *self-supervision* (Figure 26–1). It is important to understand that the stages are not time-bound, but allow for the supervisee to be at any given stage, or point along the continuum, depending on circumstances, including knowledge and skills. An important feature of this model is that it also promotes the professional growth of the supervisor. As the supervisee progresses along the continuum, the supervisor learns to adjust her supervisory style according to the needs of the supervisee. The supervisor may choose to become more or less directive as appropriate, according to the knowledge and skills of the supervisee.

Students and entry level clinicians with minimal knowledge and skill work closely with their supervisors at the *evaluation-feedback stage* of the continuum. The supervisee who is a marginal student or who is working in a new setting would be most likely seen in this stage where the supervisor has a dominant role and employs a more direct style of supervision. The goal at this initial stage is for the supervisee to move as quickly as possible from a level of dependence on the supervisor to one that is more consultative in nature (McCrea & Brasseur, 2003). As the student or new clinician begins to demonstrate the ability to employ critical thinking skills and principles of reflective practice (self-evaluation), then movement to the *transitional stage* is appropriate.

At the *transitional stage*, supervision is a shared process and the supervisee is moving toward more independence. Supervisors now use a less direct style of supervision and employ methods that include the supervisee as an active participant in the supervisory process. Supervisors encourage the development of problem-

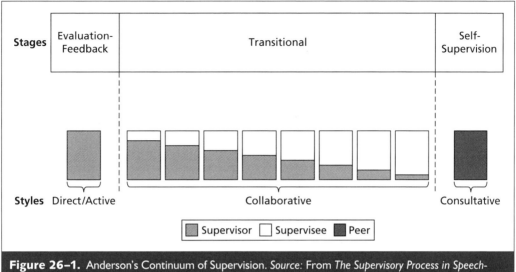

Figure 26–1. Anderson's Continuum of Supervision. *Source:* From *The Supervisory Process in Speech-Language Pathology and Audiology* (p. 27), by E. S. McCrea and J. A. Brasseur, 2003, Boston, MA: Allyn & Bacon. Reprinted with permission.

solving skills, critical thinking, and reflective practice to guide the supervisee to higher levels of independence and competence. Individual circumstances and situations will necessitate a fluidity of movement within this stage as dictated by experience, comfort level, and skill of the supervisee (McCrea & Brasseur, 2003).

The *self-supervision stage* is attained when supervisees no longer rely upon the feedback of their supervisors to analyze their work but are able to self-analyze their clinical behavior. The relationship between supervisor and supervisee becomes more of a peer interaction. At this stage, supervisees are truly competent, independent clinicians, having assumed complete responsibility for their own professional development, although they still desire peer interaction (McCrea & Brasseur, 2003).

Key Elements of the Supervisory Process

We learn from Anderson's continuum (1988) that an effective supervisory model should have a framework for systematic development of the process of supervision. The key components of such a framework should include collaborative planning, observation and data collection, analysis of data, and evaluation and feedback. Each of these elements should support principles of reflective practice that lead to self-supervision. Although professional demands and responsibilities may vary from setting to setting, these key elements are universal and not specific to any particular setting or profession.

Planning. Supervisors need to consider more than just the relationship with the supervisee as part of the planning process. McCrea and Brasseur (2003) describe the concept of "fourfold planning" (p. 106) for all participants, including the client, the clinician, the supervisee, and the supervisor, as the foundation of the ongoing supervisory process. When setting goals, the needs of each of these participants should be considered and addressed appropriately. Thus, supervisors must balance helping supervisees plan for their clients and for their own clinical and professional growth. In all cases, goals should be measurable, serve as a guide for action, and serve as a source of motivation. The supervisee will more likely achieve specified goals if the supervisor offers continued support and recognizes effort and success.

Observation and Data Collection. The purpose of the observation is to collect data on some aspect(s) of the clinical work being done. Anderson (1988) described observation as the point at which supervision changes from being solely an art to more of a science and stressed that it must be an active process if it is to be of value. She also stated that "observation without data is a waste of time" (p. 123). Objectivity in the supervisory process is achieved through clinical observation and data collection.

A supervisor may want to gather information about the supervisee's communication skills, or monitor a specific clinical activity to assess quality of service delivery. Data may also be collected by the supervisees themselves, depending on the objectives set as part of the planning process. These data would typically be centered on client or patient behavior and organized in such a way that they can be related to actions of the supervisee. In any case, data collection should correspond to the goals established in relation to expected clinical activities and professional growth.

There are a variety of tools used to observe and collect data in audiology and speech-language pathology. Casey, Smith, and Ulrich (1988) identified seven types of data collection including verbatim recording, selective verbatim, rating scales, tally, interaction analysis, nonverbal analysis, and those that are individually designed. To facilitate self-supervision, or reflective practice, the Kansas Inventory of Self-Supervision (Mawdsley, 1987) is an excellent example of an individually designed system for collecting specific data. New clinicians should become familiar with several data collection tools to diversify their clinical skills. Whichever methods are employed, the resulting data are analyzed so that they become logical and meaningful, and have a specific purpose.

Analysis. Analysis of collected data allows supervisees to observe the relationship of their behavior to that of the client. It also affords an opportunity for supervisors to observe how their actions may influence the behavior and performance of their supervisees. As cited in McCrea and Brasseur (2003, p. 193), Cogan (1973) listed the purposes of analyzing data:

- Determining if objectives from the planning stage were met

- Identifying salient patterns in the teacher's (supervisee's) behavior

- Identifying unanticipated learning by the student (client/patient)

- Identifying critical incidents in the interaction (behavior that significantly affects the learning or relationship between teacher and student)

- Organizing the data to determine what was learned

- Determining if what was planned was carried out

- Developing a database for the rest of the supervision program

The results of analyzed data may yield information that provides an opportunity for supervisors to improve their interactions and become more effective at their job. The results may also yield information that informs the clinician whether or not certain clinical procedures are effective. Objective data must be collected so that events can be reconstructed for accurate analysis (Goldhammer, Anderson, & Krajewski, 1980). The reconstruction of the collected data also promotes accountability and thus maintains compliance with codes of ethics for both professions. Before an objective evaluation of performance or effectiveness can occur, data must be carefully examined and interpreted. The process of analysis also provides supervisors with an opportunity to examine and interpret their own behavior to see how it influences the supervisory relationship. For instance, if the supervisor has been employing a more direct style of supervision, the supervisee may not have demonstrated sufficient confidence in determining if a certain clinical procedure would be appropriate in treatment for the client. In this situation, the supervisor would need to move from a direct style of supervision to a more flexible one that affords the supervisee more input in the decision-making process.

Evaluation. The importance of collection of objective data is underscored when an evaluation component is being considered. Current literature on supervisor accountability discounts the acceptability of a totally subjective evaluation on the part of the supervisor (Anderson, 1988). When the supervisory relationship is based on a collaborative and consultative model, the effective supervisor relies on the results of analysis of objective data as part of the evaluation process. Objective data support the observations that the supervisor shares with the supervisee. Dowling (2001) states that "if supervisees are truly self-evaluating, they are aware of their levels of performance and assessment becomes a joint sharing of known information" (p. 227). The process of evaluation is ongoing in nature, and the supervisee always has an understanding of his strengths and weaknesses. The effective supervisor assists the supervisee in describing and measuring his or her own progress and achievement as part of this ongoing process (ASHA, 2008b). In other words, there would be no surprises at a prescribed evaluation conference with the supervisor using a collaborative model that employs tools for self-assessment.

Principles of active learning support engaging students in written self-analysis of their discrete and nonverbal clinical behaviors (Gillam, Roussos, & Anderson, 1990). Many university CSD programs have developed their own tools for self-assessment of clinical knowledge and skills to support these principles. Weltsch and Crowe (2006) studied the effectiveness of a supervisory approach designed to facilitate self-analysis by graduate clinicians. They concluded that having student clinicians complete written self-analyses of recorded target intervention behaviors may lead to greater clinical competency. The Supervisee Performance Assessment Instrument (SPAI) (Fall & Sutton, 2004) is an example of an instrument used for self-assessment by the supervisee. Its design supports collaboration by allowing the supervisor and supervisee to target specific areas for evaluation that can be tailored to certain individuals or groups. The format uses a nonhierarchical type of scaling and a large number of evaluation criteria.

Professionals in both educational and healthcare settings have developed a variety of self-assessment tools, including rating scales and performance checklists. Many of these may be adapted for use by audiologists and speech-language pathologists. Dowling (2001) discusses the importance of evaluation but states that overemphasis on this component of the process may be destructive to the supervisory relationship. The use of self-assessment tools may serve to place the evaluation component of the supervisory process in the proper context to support a collaborative supervisory relationship.

CORE Model of Supervision and Mentoring

Hudson (2010) describes the CORE Model of Supervision and Mentoring incorporating these key elements of the supervisory process. Based on the combined works of individuals who have made significant contributions to the knowledge base of the supervisory process, including Anderson (1988), McCrea and Brasseur (2003), Cogan (1973), and Dowling (2001), the model is a cycle comprising four major components: *Collaboration, Observation, Reflection,* and *Evaluation.*

The goal of the first component of this model, *Collaboration,* is to establish an effective and trusting working relationship between supervisor and supervisee, emphasizing the joint nature of the supervisory relationship. ASHA (2008a) describes supervision as a collaborative process, with shared responsibility for many of the activities throughout the supervisory experience. This is where the supervisor sets the stage for growth in relation to the supervisory process by explaining policies and procedures, performance expectations and assessment procedures, including data collection. In addition, the supervisor guides the supervisee in establishing performance goals and objectives to promote clinical knowledge, personal improvement, productivity, and self-directed learning.

The *Observation* component allows the supervisor to record data that will be used during the processes of analysis and evaluation. McCrea and Brasseur (2003) states that observation is the place where real objectivity begins in the supervisory process. The observation and data collection are based on the goals and objectives that were established during the collaboration component of the model. The supervisor should specify the purpose

for each observation, and on what supervisee behavior data will be collected. For instance, the supervisor may be collecting data on the number of times the supervisee uses the phrase "good job" when the goal was to use appropriate positive reinforcement consistent with client performance of targeted skills.

The *Reflection* component is where evidence-supported strategies to promote reflective practice are specifically identified to promote self-supervision and independence. These strategies may include the use of journals, portfolios, and self-evaluation checklists (Hudson, 2010). As in Anderson's model, the ultimate goal of this component is for the supervisee to engage in critical thinking for solving professional problems as an independent, competent clinician (McCrea & Brasseur, 2003). The supervisor plays an important role in supporting guided reflection as the supervisee implements pre-determined goals, tackles new situations, embraces challenges, and meets expectations.

The purpose of the *Evaluation* component is to provide the supervisee with feedback that is objective, data-based, verifiable, and systematic. It is designed to confirm or reinforce behavior, correct behavior, and should be designed to motivate and enhance performance (Nottingham & Henning, 2014). Dowling (2001) states that managing feedback is a fundamental issue in building constructive supervisory relationships. Self-assessment tools that support principles of reflective practice are an important ingredient of this component. As specific skills in need of improvement are identified, or as new situations occur as part of this process, they are addressed by rotating to the *Collaboration* component and then proceeding through the remaining components of the cycle.

Supervisory Style and Communication Skills

What do you think of when you hear the word "style"? In the context of supervision, definitions that have been offered include "A distinctive manner of responding to supervisees" (Ladany, Walker, & Melincoff, 2001, p. 263) and "The way in which the personality and convictions of the supervisor are demonstrated in the supervisory relationship" (Leighton, 1991; Long, Lawless, & Dotson, 1996, p. 589). Anderson (1988) discusses the influence of personal characteristics and interpersonal style on the type of supervisory style chosen by the supervisor. She also refers to supervisory style as it applies to stages of her continuum model: direct-active style at the evaluation-feedback stage, collaborative style at the transitional stage, and consultative style at the self-supervision stage. In a study of supervisory styles in nursing, two styles were revealed by clinical nurse supervisors: emotional style and cognitive style (Severinsson, 1996; Severinsson & Hallberg, 1996). Research tells us that supervisors tend to use one style even when they think they do not (McCrea & Brasseur, 2003). Experience tells us that certain styles are more effective in some situations than in others. Supervisors should be aware of the supervisory style that they choose and develop an appreciation of how various styles affect the supervisory relationship.

Most of us recognize the role that communication style can play in our interpersonal relationships. The influence of interpersonal communication skills on the supervisory process has been widely studied, and research demonstrates that the communication skills of the supervisor play a key role in the clinical performance of the supervisee and the overall success of the supervisory relationship (McCrea & Brasseur, 2003). Essential components of effective communication may include active listening, asking purposeful questions, and responding appropriately to questions when asked. Each of these has both verbal and nonverbal aspect. Verbal behaviors that support active listening include saying "fine," "I see," "good," "mmm," or "uh-huh" (Shipley, 1997). Nonverbal behaviors that support active listening include facing the listener, maintaining eye contact, and using appropriate facial expressions and head movements. Purposeful questions are well thought out, and are formulated to encourage the supervisee to think creatively and develop problem-solving skills. In a study on questioning behaviors of supervisors, Smith (1979) found that when supervisors dominated the questioning process by asking for factual information, they deprived supervisees of the opportunity to problem-solve, self-analyze, and self-direct their own behavior. This type of communication style on the part of the supervisor would certainly present a challenge for the new clinician who is striving for independence.

The effective supervisor promotes self-supervision as the supervisee grows toward competence and independence. Strategies that encourage critical thinking on the part of the supervisee are an important part of this growth. The clinical educator must not only teach critical thinking skills but also nurture the *disposition* toward clinical thinking (Gavett & Peapers, 2007), and knowing how to *ask* questions is an essential communication skill for the supervisor when facilitating these skills. Cunningham (1971) developed a category system for questioning by dividing questions into broad and narrow categories. The narrow category includes cognitive memory questions, (recall, identify/observe, yes/no, define, name, designate) and convergent questions (explain, state relationships, compare, and contrast). The broad category includes divergent questions (predict, hypothesize, infer, reconstruct) and evaluative questions (judge, value, defend, justify, choice). Supervisors need to consider the types of questions they employ when facilitating critical thinking as part of the supervisory process.

The manner in which the supervisor *responds* to questions also plays an important role in interpersonal communication style and has an effect on the supervisory relationship. Carin and Sund (1971) stress the importance of a diplomatic reply to questions that are answered incorrectly by redirecting, helping the respondent move closer to a better answer, and not blocking communication by responding negatively. In a study of classroom teacher behavior, they reported that when wait-time was extended for students to reply to questions, it resulted in longer responses, less "I don't know" answers, more whole sentences, and increased speculative thinking. Supervisors should learn to adjust their wait-time when asking questions to afford the supervisee the opportunity to reflect and formulate considered responses.

Providing feedback is a key element of supervision and mentoring, typically linked to the evaluation component of the supervisory process. Supervisors and supervisees alike may even consider "supervising" and "providing feedback" as synonymous. But, no matter how much of a role feedback may play, it is a fundamental expectation of both parties in the supervisory relationship. In a traditional supervisory model, feedback is usually provided in written form, or it may be spontaneous or unscheduled verbal interaction (Anderson, 1988). Feedback may also be provided as a scheduled conference, either in person or by telephone or other real time electronic method. These sessions typically consist of the supervisor giving suggestions, reviewing expectations, and discussing overall performance while the supervisee listens and perhaps provides clarification and asks questions.

In a collaborative/consultative model, supervisors should encourage supervisees to seek feedback as part of an ongoing process, thereby reducing the number of formal feedback sessions. Feedback-seeking behavior is an important educational strategy and can facilitate an individual's adaptation, learning, and performance (Bose & Gijselaers, 2013; Crommelinck & Anseel, 2013). Ashford and Cummings describe such behavior as a conscious effort to determine the correctness and adequacy of one's own behavior for the purpose of attaining a goal (1983).

The supervisee is more likely to be receptive to feedback if it is constructive. Pfeiffer and Jones (1987, p. 121) list ten characteristics of constructive feedback:

1. It is descriptive rather than evaluative.

2. It is specific rather than general.

3. It is focused on the behavior rather than the person.

4. It takes into account the needs of both the receiver and the giver of the feedback.

5. It is directed toward performance rather than personal characteristics.

6. It is well timed.

7. It involves sharing of information rather than giving advice.

8. It involves the amount of information the receiver can use, rather than the amount of information we would like to give.

9. It is checked to insure clear communication.

10. It is checked to determine the degree of agreement of the receiver.

In order to be effective, feedback should be part of an ongoing process, supported by careful analysis of data and related to the goals developed as part of the initial collaborative planning phase of the supervisory process. Feedback should always serve to promote critical reflection on the parts of both the supervisor and the supervisee. It should enable both parties to explore why some strategies worked and others did not. To respect the supervisee's privacy and promote dialogue, it should be delivered in a confidential, non-confrontational way. This will naturally lead to the collaboration involved in outlining specific, measurable, action-oriented, realistic, and time-bound goals for improvement.

Both supervisors and supervisees need to recognize how their individual communication styles affect the supervisory relationship. There is a great deal of literature pertaining to communication style among the realms of counseling, education, self-improvement, career development and management, to name a few. There are also course offerings available at professional conferences on this topic, sometimes with an emphasis on the influence of cultural, linguistic, and generational issues on communication skills in the professional setting. Taking advantage of professional development opportunities in this area will enhance not only the supervisory relationship, but any other professional relationships that occur in the work setting.

Transition: Supervisor to Mentor/Preceptor

As students, you have come to expect a certain degree of dependency on your clinical supervisor for most, if not all aspects of your clinical activities. Your supervisor reads your reports, reviews your audiograms, observes you counseling family members, watches how you fit a hearing aid, sees you perform an oral-peripheral examination, helps you introduce a new therapy activity to a client, and so on. There is very little you have done as a student clinician that was not observed and/or evaluated by a supervisor. It is no wonder that as your knowledge and skills develop, and your supervisor naturally becomes less directly involved in your clinical activities, that you may, on occasion, develop a sense of uncertainty and/or panic. As you approach graduation, and your first professional employment, you are told that you will have a mentor or preceptor instead of a supervisor. Now, the sense of panic may really begin to set in. You were accustomed to working with a supervisor as a student and were familiar with your role as a supervisee. So, just what is the difference between a supervisor and a mentor/preceptor?

Consider this fact: as a paid professional, your employer has rightfully assumed that your clinical knowledge and skills are worth whatever you are being paid. If that is the assumption, why would the employer feel the need to assign someone to work closely beside you, watching you perform daily tasks that your resume indicates you know how to do independently? On the other hand, you just graduated and are new to the job, so it is understandable that some sort of coaching or even some direction on occasion would be in order. Hence, the mentor or preceptor is put in place, and you are now entering into a special relationship that will assist you in your quest for further professional growth through learning. This relationship is a valuable resource in your commitment to lifelong learning.

Shea (1997) describes the mentor as someone whose role is to gently guide the new clinician by offering knowledge, insight, perspective, or wisdom. ASHA (2008) describes mentoring as a collaborative process of shared responsibility. This concept of shared responsibility sets the stage for a relationship that offers more give and take, more exchange of ideas, and more working as a team than was the case in the student–supervisor relationship. If your previous supervisory relationships were truly collaborative, and you were guided in the art of reflective practice, the transition from supervisor to mentor/preceptor will feel quite natural. Mentors/preceptors are expected to lead by example and their example should facilitate your professional growth and learning. As role models, they will demonstrate ethical conduct, responsibility, perspective-taking, and have knowledge of strategies that foster self-evaluation. They will appreciate learning styles, personality types, and consider how race, culture, gender and age may influence personal interactions. Your mentor/preceptor will guide you to proficiency, where you will obtain a greater understanding and appreciation of the big picture, the holistic view of a situation. You and your mentor/preceptor will discuss why some strategies worked and some did not as you continue to develop confidence in your current knowledge and skills and to take the initiative to try new strategies on your own. In this strategic partnership, you will feel empowered to explore new territory and stretch your skills with the knowledge that you have a foundation of support, your mentor/preceptor.

Regulations, Standards, and Guidelines

At the pre-professional level, the Council on Academic Accreditation (CAA) standards state that academic programs are required to demonstrate that "the type and structure of the clinical education is commensurate with the development of knowledge and skills of each student" (Standard 3.7A & 3.7B; CAA, 2017). Before providing direct services in any setting, supervisors, mentors, preceptors, student clinicians, clinical fellows, and audiology externs need to be aware of professional association standards for certification, state licensure laws, and federal/state reimbursement programs such as Medicaid and Medicare. State licensure boards and state boards of education have their own regulations and requirements, and supervision requirements may not match those of certification bodies. Thus it is important to refer to all applicable sources. Each state has information that is readily available on requirements for certification and licensure and is easily obtainable on their internet websites. ASHA has information on its website on the certification process for speech-language pathologists and audiologists. ABA also has information available on its website regarding board certification. For audiologists, ASHA certification and certification through ABA do not require membership in a professional organization.

Supervisors and mentors/preceptors are fully responsible for the behavior, clinical services, and documentation of their supervisees. This means that supervisors and mentors/preceptors must be aware of the professional competence of the supervisee in specific area/scope of practice, not only to protect themselves but to protect the welfare of the clients and to foster the growth of the supervisee (ASHA, 2008b). If you find yourself in a situation where you do not feel qualified, competent, physically or emotionally safe, or if you are in a situation that involves an ethical dilemma, it is absolutely imperative that you inform your supervisor or mentor/preceptor of the situation. If it is the supervisor or mentor/preceptor who has placed you in this situation, you should contact your university program, professional association, or employer for direction and guidance.

Clinical Fellowship Experience and Audiology Externship

Upon completion of the required academic coursework and clinical practicum experiences and after the graduate degree has been conferred, speech-language pathologists advance to the next stage of their professional career development by beginning a Clinical Fellowship (CF) experience in accordance with the ASHA standards for certification for speech-language pathology. Since the change in entry level degree to a doctorate, audiology students complete an extended externship, usually 10 to 12 months, after completion of coursework and prior to graduation, instead of a CF experience postgraduation. This long practicum placement is often called the fourth-year externship, because it takes place in the final year of the graduate program. The ASHA certification standards for both professional areas of practice are defined by members of the Council for Clinical Certification in Audiology and Speech-Language Pathology (CFCC), a semi-autonomous body of ASHA The American Board of Audiology (ABA) also offers a certification avenue for audiologists. Because the clinical experiences of speech-language pathologists and audiology students diverge at this point, they will be addressed separately in this chapter.

Speech-Language Pathology Clinical Fellowship (SLPCF)

ASHA (2018) describes the Clinical Fellowship (CF) experience as a transition between being a student and being an independent provider of clinical services that involves a mentored professional experience. The purposes of the CF experience are:

- to promote excellence in the practice of the professions of audiology and speech-language pathology through the development and implementation of standards;

- to identify individuals who meet standards established as necessary to provide clinical services; and

- to protect and inform the public by recognizing individuals who meet the certification standards.

It is the responsibility of the Clinical Fellow (CF) to identify a mentor who holds a current Certificate of Clinical Competence (CCC) that meets mentor requirements (experience, continuing education in supervision) and if applicable, state licensure. Some states do not require the completion of a CF experience but have their own provisional licensure requirements that include supervision by a licensed speech-language pathologist who may or may not be required to hold a CCC. In those instances, the CF will need to determine if the supervisor can also serve as a CF mentor. If not, the ASHA website has information on how to find a CF mentor. The CF should find out what the requirements are for the state in which he or she is going to be working and verify this information before the start of the CF experience. This may be done by contacting the ASHA National office and by checking with state licensure boards, as appropriate.

It is important that both the CF and the CF mentor are familiar with the ASHA Code of Ethics, Scope of Practice, and the ASHA Certification and Membership Handbook, all of which are available on the ASHA website, and any and all applicable state licensure/certification requirements in order not to jeopardize the certification or licensure status of the CF. The CF and the CF mentor need to discuss at the very beginning of the CF experience how the monitoring activities will be completed, including frequency and method of documentation, and how his or her performance will be evaluated. Both parties should maintain copies of all written feedback and other documentation, including the required forms submitted to ASHA and the state. The specific requirements for completion of the CF experience are provided in Chapter 12.

Finally, the CF and the mentor need to be aware of possible ethical misconduct on the part of the CF mentor. Although these events are not typical, they may include arbitrary termination of the mentoring relationship, failure to complete and sign the required paperwork in a timely manner, failure to provide the required amount and type of mentoring, or recruitment of the CF as independent practitioners. Should any of these or other unfortunate situations occur, the CF should consult with a certification manager at the ASHA National office immediately.

Audiology Externship

The profession of audiology has gone through changes in recent years that impact credentialing requirements. There are two professional certifications available to audiologists: ASHA (CCC-A) and ABA (ABA Certified or ABAC). Both are voluntary and do not require membership in a professional organization. Certification reflects a higher standard of professional practice and may be required as a minimum job qualification for certain employers or in certain settings. In addition, individual states continue to have their own requirements for licensure which may or may not mirror either of the professional certification programs available to audiologists. Audiology students should carefully consider the requirements for certification early in their graduate career to ensure that they are on a path to meet all requirements prior to graduation or within the timeframe specified by the credentialing body. More information about requirements for ASHA certification and ABA Board Certification is provided in Chapter 3.

The audiology externship has been adopted by many academic training programs to provide students with an extended clinical experience where they can further develop their knowledge and skills and prepare for independent practice. Accredited academic training institutions are not specifically required to include an externship as part of their curriculum, but many have elected to do so. Externships are offered in many work settings and locations. A preceptor plays a key role in the externship experience. The academic institution and the student extern should ensure that clinical supervision provided by the preceptor meets all credentialing requirements at an externship site. This includes certification and licensure requirements. Securing an externship is usually the result of a competitive process where students complete applications and submit transcripts, cover letters, and resumés. Interviews are commonly part of this process, also. Students should check externship postings and ask questions during the application process to verify their assigned preceptor will meet credentialing requirements. Licensure and certification in almost all cases can be verified online through the website of the credentialing body. These sites will also indicate if the preceptor is in good standing and meets any requirements necessary for providing supervision.

Externship preceptors/supervisors and externs are responsible for completing all licensure requirements in a timely manner. This may include registration with the appropriate licensing board(s) or securing temporary or provisional licensure. If a state has hearing aid dispenser and audiologist requirements that are handled separately by different regulatory bodies, all requirements must be investigated and met. Requirements vary from state to state, so this requires investigation.

Finally, the audiology extern and the preceptor need to be aware of possible ethical misconduct on the part of the externship preceptor. Although these events are not typical, they may include failure to complete evaluations and verify clock hours, failure to complete required licensure paperwork related to the extern in a timely manner, failure to provide the required amount and type of supervision, treating the extern as an independent practitioner, or failure to maintain their professional credentials. Should any of these or other unfortunate situations occur, the extern should consult with their academic training institution immediately.

Supervision Post-Certification

Now that you have earned your Certificate of Clinical Competence, or Board Certification, what can you expect in the way of supervision? The answer to that question will depend on your individual circumstances, including your work setting and the nature of your assigned duties. You should expect to have someone to whom you report directly, perhaps a rehabilitation director, clinic or private practice owner, service coordinator, school principal, or regional supervisor. This individual may or may not share your professional credentials. This supervisor's main goal is to ensure the well-being of the patients, clients, or students whom you serve, and to ensure the quality of the services you provide in that setting. As such, you can expect to have some type of supervision and receive an evaluation of your performance by someone in a supervisory capacity. A more detailed discussion of the employee evaluation process is provided in Chapter 12, but the employee evaluation process bears some mention in this chapter as you will most likely continue to be in a supervisory or mentoring/preceptor-type of relationship. The fundamental principles of supervision and mentoring still apply, so you may want to review those principles at this next stage of your career. You may also be asked to provide supervision to a graduate student or an assistant (support personnel). Now you become the supervisor.

Supervision of Students and Support Personnel

Graduate programs require students to accrue clinical practicum hours in a variety of settings in order to prepare them for the professional work environment. You may be asked very early in your post-certification career to supervise a student in your work setting. If that is the case, remember above all other considerations that you are a role model to this individual. You need to keep in mind that your opinions and impressions may carry a great deal of weight, and that this student will look to you for guidance and direction in many areas, including clinical skills, ethical behavior, interpersonal skills, and work habits. Typically, the student's university Program Director or Clinic Director will have made the necessary arrangements between the university and your work site for the student placement. You should determine who your contact at the university will be and what type of documentation is expected of you as the student's supervisor. You should also discuss your professional liability with your work-site supervisor and verify that your current licensure and certification will meet the needs of the university.

It is both a responsibility and a privilege to play a part in the early professional growth of a student clinician. The rewards of creating the professional climate in which a student can thrive are well worth the challenges that this unique supervisory relationship will present to you. The opportunity that this relationship will provide will also make a significant contribution to your own professional growth and development.

Supervision of support personnel, including speech-language-pathology assistants (SLPAs) and support personnel in audiology presents a unique challenge, particularly for the new clinician who may just be learning how to do his or her first job. One of the most important issues has to do with the amount of supervision that is required and the documentation associated with that supervision. Typically, the more complex cases will necessitate increased levels of supervision. As in any supervisory relationship, the basic principles apply to the supervisor of the SLPA or support personnel in audiology, particularly in the areas of ethical behavior, communication, and documentation.

ASHA (2013a) developed a Scope of Practice for Speech-Language Pathology Assistants to provide guidance for SLPAs and their supervisors regarding ethical considerations related to the SLPA practice parameters. The document addresses how SLPAs should be utilized and what specific responsibilities are within and outside their roles of clinical practice. In addition, ASHA offers an affiliation category for individuals who work in speech-language pathology and audiology and anticipates launching the Assistants Certification Program and examination to establish standards on a national level by the end of 2020. Assistants are required to have the necessary skills to work in a support position, and their duties are performed under direct supervision of an ASHA-certified speech-language pathologist or audiologist. The topic of support personnel in speech-language pathology and audiology is covered extensively in Chapter 13.

Ethical Issues

Professional codes of ethics are established to provide the standards of conduct that guide the behavior of members of the professions of speech-language pathology and audiology. Both ASHA and ABA have codes of ethics that serve this purpose, and supervisors have the responsibility to ensure that they and their supervisees adhere to ethical principals in every aspect of their clinical activities.

The ASHA Code of Ethics (2016) specifies compliance with certification and licensure for members and certificate holders as required by their employers, their states, governmental agencies, and by ASHA in the area of their clinical or supervisory work, regardless of the work setting. The primary responsibility of ASHA-certified individuals who are engaged in supervision is to hold paramount the welfare of persons they serve professionally and to ensure that services are provided competently by individuals under their supervision. Whether the title used is **supervisor**, **clinical educator**, **mentor**, or **preceptor**, each of these individuals exercises professional authority or power over the supervisee and ensures the trust that is an integral part of any supervisory relationship. There are several sections in the Code of Ethics that pertain to supervision:

- *Principle I:* Individuals shall honor their responsibility to hold paramount the welfare of persons they serve professionally or who are participants in research and scholarly activities, and they shall treat animals involved in research in a humane manner.

- *Principle I, Rule A:* Individuals shall provide all clinical services and scientific activities competently.

- *Principle I, Rule D:* Individuals shall not misrepresent the credentials of aides, assistants, technicians, support personnel, students, research interns, Clinical Fellows, or any others under their supervision, and they shall inform those they serve professionally of the name, role, and professional credentials of persons providing services.

- *Principle I, Rule G:* Individuals who hold the Certificate of Clinical Competence may delegate to students tasks related to the provision of clinical services that require the unique skills, knowledge, and judgment that are within the scope of practice of their profession only if those students are adequately prepared and are appropriately supervised. The responsibility for the welfare of those being served remains with the certified individual.

- *Principle II, Rule A:* Individuals who hold the Certificate of Clinical Competence shall engage in only those aspects of the professions that are within the scope of their professional practice and competence, considering their certification status, education, training, and experience.

- *Principle IV, Rule H:* Individuals shall not engage in sexual activities with individuals (other than a spouse or other individual with whom a prior consensual relationship exists) over whom they exercise professional authority or power, including persons receiving services, assistants, students, or research participants.

- *Principle IV, Rule I:* Individuals shall not knowingly allow anyone under their supervision to engage in any practice that violates the Code of Ethics.

- *Principle IV, Rule L:* Individuals shall not discriminate in their relationships with colleagues, assistants, students, support personnel, and members of other professions and disciplines on the basis of race, ethnicity, sex, gender identity/gender expression, sexual orientation, age, religion, national origin, disability, culture, language, dialect, or socioeconomic status.

Supervisors also need to be aware of the issue of *vicarious liability* that describes the supervisor's responsibility concerning the behavior of the supervisee (Newman, 2001). The legal and ethical responsibility for persons served remains with the certified individual, so responsibility for clinical decision making and management should not be delegated to the supervisee. However, as part of the educational process, supervisees should be encouraged to make clinical recommendations and decisions that are commensurate with their knowledge, experience, and competence and fall within the scope of practice for their specific profession.

Supervisors also need to be aware of the dual relationship that can develop between the supervisor and the supervisee (Newman, Victor, & Zylla-Jones, 2009). When the relationship between the supervisor and the supervisee becomes more personal than professional, it can compromise the integrity of the supervisory process. For example, if a supervisor and a supervisee develop a personal friendship, will the supervisor be able to maintain objectivity when evaluating the supervisee's ability to assume responsibility? This new relationship now presents its own set of problems that can adversely affect the supervisory relationship. Supervisors assume the responsibility of maintaining the proper balance in the relationship and of setting and maintaining appropriate boundaries as needed.

Situations involving ethical misconduct, including abuse of power, may also occur on the part of the supervisor. For example, a supervisor may fail to provide a sufficient amount of supervision based on the performance of the supervisee, fail to educate and monitor the supervisee's protection of patient confidentiality, fail to verify appropriate competencies before delegating tasks to supervisees, fail to demonstrate benefit to the patient based on outcomes, and fail to provide self-assessment tools and opportunities to supervisees (King, 2003). The astute supervisee will learn to recognize possible ethical misconduct on the part of the supervisor and should seek appropriate consultation. Good sources of reference are ASHA's Issues in Ethics statements of *Supervision of Student Clinicians (2017) and Issues in Ethics: Responsibilities of Individuals Who Mentor Clinical Fellows in Speech-Language Pathology* (ASHA, 2017).

Adherence to principles of ethical conduct transcends all aspects of clinical practice and professional behavior. The supervisory relationship provides the supervisor with the opportunity to model behaviors necessary for life-long ethical practice. See Chapter 5 for a more in-depth discussion of ethical issues.

Cultural, Linguistic, and Generational Issues

As we become more diverse as a nation, supervisors will have more and more opportunities to work with individuals from backgrounds different from their own. Because values, behaviors, and beliefs may vary according to age, disability, ethnicity, gender identity, national origin, race, religion, sex, and sexual orientation, supervisors will need to learn to appreciate the effect that these factors have on communication, behavior, and learning styles. Linguistic diversity can accompany cultural diversity (ASHA, 2017), and supervisors and mentors should encourage an understanding of linguistic differences. They are also obligated to prevent discrimination against persons who speak with an accent and/or dialect in educational programs, employment, or service delivery (ASHA, 1998).

Coleman (2000) noted that differences in cultural values have an impact on the nature and effectiveness of all aspects of clinical interventions, including supervisee relationships. He added that in order for interactions with supervisees to be successful, supervisors must consider learning styles and culturally based behaviors of their supervisees. Researchers who have studied clinical intervention strategies related to cultural issues (Anderson, 1992; Battle, 1993; Langdon & Cheng, 1992) promote the use of self-inventory of cultural competence awareness and sensitivity. Munoz, Watson, and Yarbrough (2011) state that the roles and responsibilities of the supervisor can still be met even when observing sessions in a language one doesn't speak, while ASHA (2008b) recommends that supervisors provide culturally appropriate feedback to supervisees. It is also important to know when it may be appropriate to use a cultural mediator or advisor concerning effective strategies for interactions with individuals (clients and supervisees) from specific backgrounds. Development of self-

awareness on the part of the supervisor sets the stage for increased sensitivity and understanding of situations that may occur during the supervisory process that are solely related to cultural differences. Carozza (2011) offers a cogent discussion of cross-cultural issues in supervision.

McCready (2007) reviewed the research on generational differences in the workforce and noted that the disparities between generations are more complex today than in the past. The experiences of each generation shape the values, beliefs, attitudes, and behaviors that may have a significant effect on the supervisory relationship. For example, a 22-year-old AuD student is in a meeting with his 56-year-old clinical supervisor to discuss a patient with unilateral Meniere's disease. The student checks his cell phone several times and begins replying to a text message while the supervisor is describing the testing and how the pattern of results relates to the patient's condition. The supervisor is rather offended, believing that the student is not listening, and decides to stop speaking until the student has finished looking at his phone. The student looks up suddenly, and asks the supervisor to continue the discussion, quite surprised that she appeared to be offended. The supervisor believes that the student should give her his undivided attention, assuming he can only focus on one thing at a time, while the student believes that multi-tasking is typical behavior and that his texting while listening should be no reason for the supervisor to take offense.

In order to bridge this type of generation gap, McCready suggests the formation of smaller study groups within the work setting to investigate the research in this area that can then be presented to the larger group as a whole. She also suggests that the supervisor engage in discussions about generational differences pertaining to a particular work setting or situation and how those differences may or may not apply to that specific setting. In the scenario provided, the supervisor could use the situation to explain the philosophical differences between her generation and that of the AuD student regarding perceptions of multi-tasking. Where cultural, linguistic, and generational issues are considered, supervisors have a responsibility for their own professional development in order to increase their knowledge and sensitivity. Demonstration of this desire to learn may also motivate the supervisee to develop a plan for his or her own growth in this area.

Supervision of Challenging Supervisees

In graduate CSD programs, there are those students who may present special challenges during the supervisory process (Shapiro et al., 2002) and are often referred to as "marginal" students. Dowling (1985, as cited in

Dowling, 2001) described marginal students as individuals who "cannot work independently, are unable to formulate goals and procedures, have basic gaps in conceptual understanding, and cannot follow through with suggestions" (p. 162). Understanding how to work effectively with marginal students deserves serious and systematic consideration (Shapiro et al., 2002). By the time these "marginal" students have graduated, they have completed the necessary requirements in their academic courses and clinical work to begin employment. However, new clinicians who experienced some of these challenges as students may need to be carefully monitored by their supervisors once they are in the work setting. In particular, these new clinicians may have difficulty evaluating their skill level accurately (Kruger & Dunning, 1999, as cited in McCrea & Brasseur, 2003). The initial collaborative planning phase of the supervisory process should address this and any other potential areas of concern and goals should be developed to target those areas specifically. Schober-Peterson and O'Rourke (2008) describe using a formative assessment when working with the "at-risk" student, and describe how this type of ongoing assessment encouraged students to take responsibility for their learning and to be active participants in the assessment of their knowledge and skills. This type of ongoing assessment, including providing specific feedback based on objective data collection, can support these new clinicians as they achieve the ultimate goal of self-supervision.

Technology and Supervision

The use of technology in supervision, referred to as telesupervision is not necessarily a new concept although the variety of forms to support the supervisory process has expanded significantly in recent years. The internet has made it possible for supervisors to use email, instant messaging, social networks, and videoconferencing to communicate with supervisees in real time. Webinars, blogs and podcasts can store information for access at a later time and may be shared with a large number of individuals. The use of audio and video recordings will likely reveal behaviors that supervisors and supervisees may use for the development of goals for improvement (McCrea & Brasseur, 2003). For example, the supervisor and supervisee may view a video-recorded treatment session to verify data, review and discuss subtle behaviors that were not easily observable in real time, or evaluate the success of a treatment technique. The ability to self-analyze behaviors after they have occurred is an extremely effective tool in promoting reflective practice.

Although many universities use videoconferencing routinely for course delivery, it is also an effective technology to support required supervisory visits that may be challenged by time factors and/or geographical distance. It should not, however, be used solely for the convenience of the supervisee or the supervisor. Distance supervision, or telesupervision, was described by Dudding (2002) as the use of two-way interactive videoconferencing technology for supervision of graduate students. Dudding (2006) reports that in a later study she found that there was no significant difference in graduate student perceptions of the effectiveness of the traditional versus distance supervision models. She reports that the graduate students "indicated that they felt more in charge of the session and less distracted than when the supervisor was physically in the therapy room" (p. 17).

Tellis, Cimino, and Alberti (2010) described a novel video-capture technology, the Landro Play Analyzer, to supervise clinical sessions and to train students to improve their clinical skills. They were able to observe four clinical sessions simultaneously from a central observation center. In addition, speech samples were analyzed in real time, saved on a CD, DVD, or flash/jump drive, viewed in slow motion, paused, and analyzed with Microsoft Excel. The use of this technology for clinical supervision allowed the authors to monitor multiple sessions as well as provide their student clinicians with specific feedback. Students indicated that they improved their clinical skills because they had the opportunity to review their sessions. Clinicians also reported using this technology successfully with their clients.

Advances in technology have played an important role in the area of supervision and are likely to continue to do so. The opportunities, as well as the challenges, that technology presents and the role that it will continue to play are important issues for supervisors and supervisees alike. ASHA (2008a) stresses the importance of following regulatory guidelines involving confidentiality when using technology in supervision (e.g., videoconferencing). The integral concerns related to ethics, etiquette, access to technical support, licensure board rules, state and federal laws and regulations, university and/or clinical setting policies, and capital resources should also be considered in any discussion of technology and its application to the supervisory process. See Chapter 27 for a more in-depth discussion of technology.

Training in Supervision

Achieving clinical competence does not necessarily mean one has the ability to be an effective supervisor. All too often, clinicians are placed in a supervisory role with limited or no supervisory experience. They may be clinically experienced and available, but they do not necessarily have an interest or the knowledge and skills to be effective supervisors. Both ASHA (2013c) and the Council of Academic Programs in Communication Sciences and Disorders (CAPCSD) have recognized that clinical supervision is a distinct area of expertise and practice, and, as in other distinct areas, individuals must receive training to gain competence before engaging in the activity (ASHA, 2013c; CAPCSD, 2013).

The ASHA Ad Hoc Committee on Supervision (2013c) identified the knowledge and skills required of supervisors.

Overarching Knowledge and Skills

- Knowledge of clinical education and the supervisory process, including teaching techniques, adult learning styles, and collaborative models of supervision

- Skill in relationship development, including the creation of an environment that fosters learning

- Ability to communicate, including the ability to define expectations and engage in difficult conversations

- Ability to collaboratively establish and implement goals, give objective feedback, and adjust clinical education style when necessary

- Ability to analyze and evaluate the student clinician's performance, including gathering data, identifying areas for improvement, assisting with self-reflections, and determining if goals are being achieved

- Skill in modeling and nurturing clinical decision making, including (a) using information to support clinical decisions and solve problems and (b) responding appropriately to ethical dilemmas

- Skill in fostering professional growth and development

- Skill in making performance decisions, including the ability to create and implement plans for improvement and to assess the student's response to these plans

- Ability to adhere to the principles of evidence-based practice and conveying research information to student clinicians

Knowledge and Skills Specific to Student Training in the University Clinic or Off-Site Setting

- Ability to connect academic knowledge and clinical application

- Ability to sequence the student's knowledge and skill development

Knowledge and Skills Specific to the Clinical Educator Working With Students in the Culminating Externship in Audiology

- Ability to provide a multifaceted experience across the scope of the profession

- Ability to serve as a liaison between the facility, student, and university

- Skill in guiding the student in reflective practice

- Skill in facilitating the development of workplace navigation skill (e.g., being part of a team and adhering to policies and procedures)

The Ad Hoc Committee also noted the importance of early education in the supervisory process, including an introduction to the subject as part of the graduate curriculum and more advanced training for practicing and aspiring supervisors (2013b).

ASHA certification standards for audiology and speech-language pathology are established by the Council for Clinical Certification in Audiology and Speech-Language Pathology (CFCC), a semi-autonomous credentialing body of ASHA. Both ASHA (2013c) and CAPCSD (2013b) suggested the need for systematic approaches to the training and preparation of clinical educators. As a result of these recommendations, the 2020 Standards and Implementation Procedures for the Certificate of Clinical Competence require clinical supervisors to have a minimum of 2 hours of professional development (training) in the area of supervision and 9 months of clinical experience post-certification before serving as a clinical supervisor or CF mentor.

ABA requires that preceptors for externs hold a state license and may be a certified ABA audiologist. However, some states (e.g., California) or settings may require specific coursework or credentials before being granted supervisory status. Although the availability for training in the form of coursework and continuing education (CE) in supervision may not always meet the demand, there are opportunities for continuing education in supervision. ASHA and CAPCSD provide CE sessions at their annual convention as well as webinars and teleconferences on supervision. Many state associations and related professional organizations also provide CE sessions on supervision. Special Interest Group 10–Higher Education, and 11–Administration and Supervision publish "Perspectives" throughout the year and afford opportunities to earn CE credit. There are also several noteworthy books available to those who have an interest in learning more about supervision (Carozza, 2010; Dowling, 2001; McCrea & Brasseur, 2003).

Supervisor Accountability

The evaluation of a supervisor should be based on the demonstration of skills and competencies associated with the supervisory process. Supervisees are often asked to participate in the evaluation process of their supervisors. Do most supervisees have the knowledge required to know what to expect from a supervisor if asked to provide feedback? Even if they did, would they provide feedback that is honest and objective? The answers to these questions support self-evaluation by the supervisor relative to the supervisory process (ASHA, 2008). However, there are no validated guidelines for the outcomes achieved by supervisors, thus making it necessary for supervisors to use informal measures to evaluate their own supervisory skills and competencies (McCrea & Brasseur, 2003).

Supervisors may consider using items from a self-assessment guide developed by Casey, Smith, and Ulrich (1988) to assist their effectiveness in acquiring the 13 tasks and 81 associated competencies contained in the ASHA position statement (ASHA, 1985). Supervisors may also consider using the more recent ASHA (2016) "Self-Assessment of Competencies in Supervision" developed by the 2016 ASHA Ad Hoc Committee on Supervision Training (AHCST) to assess supervisory knowledge and skills identified by the Ad Hoc Committee on Supervision (ASHA, 2013c). This tool is used to rate competencies and to develop goals for training for clinical educators, preceptors, mentors, and supervisors. A performance appraisal that employs multiple sources of input is referred to as a *360 Degree Assessment* (U.S. Department of Personnel Management, 1997). This appraisal includes self-assessment, and some aspects of a supervisor's performance may also be evaluated by a professional peer, support staff, and an administrator to whom the individual reports. This type of performance appraisal focuses on subjective impressions of global aspects of supervisor behavior and will not necessarily provide insight into the efficiency and effectiveness of an individual supervisor's practice (McCrea & Brasseur, 2003).

The results of a successful evaluation of one's own behavior present an opportunity for quality assurance to ensure accountability. Making a decision to improve as a supervisor promotes job satisfaction, self-fulfillment, and ethical behavior and prevents burnout (Dowling, 2001). Self-assessment is a key ingredient of reflective practice, and the supervisor who engages in this activity is also providing the supervisee an effective role model.

Future Needs in Supervision and Mentoring

Supervision and mentoring are required components of clinical training and credentialing for professional organizations in speech-language pathology and audiology. Because of its pervasive nature in the professions, supervision is universally recognized as a distinct area of practice. What research is needed to ensure evidence-based practices in the distinct area of supervision? Data collection and analysis as part of the supervisory process provide the foundation for research and evidence to support effective supervisory practice. Anderson (1988) stated: "When the clinical supervision process proceeds as inquiry, personal discoveries have the potential for becoming collective discoveries" (p. 298). These discoveries are made after careful examination of the effects of certain supervisory practices, forming the basis of research.

In recent years, audiologists and speech-language pathologists have been involved in interdisciplinary research, training, and practice examining how workers from a variety of professional backgrounds work together with clients, students, patients, families, caregivers, and communities to provide the highest quality and most comprehensive services possible. However, the final report of ASHA's (2013b) Ad Hoc Committee on Interprofessional Education noted that the focus on interprofessional education to increase value in health care delivery has primarily involved the disciplines of medicine, nursing, pharmacy, and public health. Interprofessional education (IPE) is an essential first step in preparing professionals to work collaboratively in response to client/student/patient needs, and clinical educators play a key role in reinforcing best practices in this area. Supervisors of audiologists and speech-language pathologists should examine their own competencies in this area, and learn how to facilitate learning on the part of the supervisee as part of a collaborative service delivery model that centers on the individual and the family/caregivers. There are several resources available for clinical educators and CF mentors in this area including *Core Competencies for Interprofessional Collaborative Practice*, a report published by an expert panel of the Interprofessional Education Collaborative (IPEC, 2011), as well as ASHA's *Interprofessional Education (IPE): Final Report, Ad Hoc Committee on Interprofessional Education* (ASHA, 2013b).

Both supervisors and supervisees alike have the responsibility to learn about issues in clinical supervision. The most effective supervisors will approach the supervisory relationship with the understanding that each supervisee brings not only certain skills, knowledge and clinical experience to a situation, but also his or her own individual talents, perceptions, and life experiences. They will also appreciate how each of these factors can influence both the supervisory relationship and the overall clinical experience itself. For supervisees to develop critical knowledge and skills leading to competency, they must also learn to analyze their own behaviors to see how their actions influence the supervisory relationship and their clinical experiences. This shared responsibility for supporting the principles of reflective practice will lead to self-supervision of the independent clinician who is committed to lifelong learning and professional growth.

Summary

Supervision plays a major role in the professions of speech-language pathology and audiology because of its pervasive nature. This chapter presented a model of skill acquisition that forms the basis of successful models of supervision including a continuum model and a model comprised of four key components of the supervisory process. It also provided an overview of regulations and guidelines leading to professional certification in both speech-language pathology and audiology. Current issues in supervision that are relevant across settings, including professional ethics, cultural competence, technology, training, and accountability, were also discussed. Finally, it set the stage for further exploration of research and training, particularly in interprofessional education and practice, in this essential area within the scope of practice in the professions.

Critical Thinking

1. What are some of the dynamic differences you should anticipate as you move from working with a clinical supervisor in a university setting to a mentor/preceptor in your professional workplace? What role do interpersonal communication skills play in this relationship?

2. You are a clinical fellow in an elementary school and have just been asked to supervise an SLPA. What responsibilities do you plan to assign her? How will you evaluate her performance?

3. Suppose your supervisor during an externship gave you more clinical responsibility than you thought you were prepared to implement. How would you approach your supervisor about this issue?

4. You had limited hands-on experience doing vestibular testing prior to your audiology externship. Shortly after beginning your externship, your supervisor advises that he will be at another clinic location one day a week and that you will need to independently complete vestibular evaluations on your own on while he is at the other site. How would you handle this situation?

5. How would videotaping a treatment session assist the supervisor in promoting self-assessment? What

other forms of technology do you think facilitate supervision? Why?

6. One of the difficult issues university programs face is when a student has excellent academic ability but clinical skills are poor or very slow in developing. What evidence should a supervisor present to document clinical skill achievement in such a situation?

7. You work for a large community speech and hearing center and are about to hire a clinical supervisor who can mentor both those in his clinical fellowship and also manage the hearing impaired pre-school program. What qualities would you look for in this professional? What are some questions you might pose to the professional during an interview for this position?

8. Suppose you have completed half of your audiology externship and you discover that one of your supervisors that approved about one-third of your hours is not ASHA certified. What would you do?

9. Suppose your supervisor abruptly ended the supervisory relationship before you had met the requirements for certification and/or licensure. What would you do?

10. In what specific area(s) of training do you think supervisors should be required to have training before they can become supervisors?

References

Allen, R., Cosby, J., Figueroa, C. M., & Allen, R. L. (2008). Differences between the 1993 and 2007 standards for the Certificate of Clinical Competence in Audiology. *Perspectives on Administration and Supervision, 18*(2), 44–49.

American Academy of Audiology. (2006). American Academy of Audiology Clinical Education Guidelines for Audiology Externships. *Audiology Today, 18*(2), 29–31.

American Board of Audiology. (2011). *Board certification in Audiology.* Retrieved from http://www.americanboardofaudiology.org/.../faqs_board_certification.html

American Speech-Language-Hearing Association. (1985). Committee on Supervision in Speech-Language Pathology and Audiology: Clinical supervision in speech-language pathology and audiology. A position statement. *ASHA, 27,* 57–60.

American Speech-Language-Hearing Association. (1996). Guidelines for the training, credentialing, use, and supervision of speech-language pathology assistants. *Asha, 38*(Suppl. 16), 21–34.

American Speech-Language Hearing Association. (1997). *ASHA membership and certification handbook.* Rockville, MD: Author.

American Speech-Language-Hearing Association. (1998). *Students and professionals who speak English with accents and nonstandard dialects: Issues and recommendations* [Position statement]. Available from http://www.asha.org/policy

American Speech-Language-Hearing Association. (2000). *Background information and standards for implementation for the certificate of clinical competence in speech-language pathology.* Rockville, MD: ASHA, Council on Professional Standards in Speech-Language Pathology and Audiology.

American Speech-Language-Hearing Association. (2007). *Responsibilities of individuals who mentor clinical fellows* [Issues in ethics]. Available from http:// www.asha.org/policy

American Speech-Language-Hearing Association. (2008). *Clinical supervision in speech-language pathology* [Position statement]. Available from http://www.asha.org/policy

American Speech-Language-Hearing Association. (2008a). *Clinical supervision in speech-language pathology* [Technical report]. Available from http:// www.asha.org/policy

American Speech-Language-Hearing Association. (2008b). *Knowledge and skills needed by speech-language pathologists providing clinical supervision* [Knowledge and skills]. Available from http://www.asha.org/policy

American Speech-Language-Hearing Association. (2010a). *Supervision of student clinicians* [Issues in ethics]. Available from http://www.asha.org/policy

American Speech-Language-Hearing Association. (2010b). *Certification.* Retrieved from http://www.asha.org/about/membership-certification/

American Speech-Language-Hearing Association. (2013a). *Speech-language pathology assistant scope of practice* [Scope of practice]. Available from http://www.asha.org/policy

American Speech-Language-Hearing Association. (2013b). *Ad Hoc Committee on Interprofessional Education Final Report.* Available from https://www.asha.org/uploadedFiles/Report-Ad-Hoc-Committee-on Interprofessional-Education.pdf

American Speech-Language-Hearing Association. (2013c). *Knowledge, skills and training considerations for individuals serving as supervisors* [Final report, Ad Hoc Committee on Supervision]. Retrieved from http://www.asha.org/uploadedFiles/Supervisors-Knowledge-Skills-Report.pdf

American Speech-Language-Hearing Association. (2016). *Code of ethics* [Ethics]. Retrieved from https://www.asha.org/Code-of-Ethics/

American Speech-Language-Hearing Association. (2017). *Issues in ethics: Ethical issues related to clinical services provided by audiology and speech-language pathology students.* Retrieved from https://www.asha.org/Practice/ethics/Ethical-Issues-Related-to-Clinical-Services-Provided-by-Audiology-and-Speech-Language-Pathology-Students/

American Speech-Language-Hearing Association. (2017). *Issues in ethics: Responsibilities of individuals who mentor clinical fellows in speech-language pathology.* Retrieved from https://www.asha.org/Practice/ethics/Responsibilities-of-Individuals-Who-Mentor-Clinical-Fellows-in-Speech-Language-Pathology/

American Speech-Language-Hearing Association. (2017). *Issues in ethics: Cultural and linguistic competence.* Available from https://www.asha.org/Practice/ethics/Cultural-and-Linguistic-Competence/

American Speech-Language-Hearing Association. (2018). *2018 Speech-language pathology certification handbook of the American Speech-Language-Hearing Association.* Retrieved from https://www.asha.org/uploadedFiles/SLP-Certification-Handbook.pdf

Anderson, J. (Ed.). (1970). *Proceedings of conference on supervision of speech and hearing programs in the schools.* Bloomington: Indiana University.

Anderson, J. L. (1988). *The supervisory process in speech-language pathology and audiology.* Austin, TX: Pro-Ed.

Anderson, N. B. (1992). Understanding cultural diversity. *American Journal of Speech-Language Pathology, 1,* 11–12.

Ashford, S. J., & Cummings, L. L. (1983). Feedback as an individual resource: Personal strategies of creating information. *Organizational Behavior and Human Performance, 32,* 370–398.

Battle, D. (1993). *Communication disorders in multicultural populations.* Boston, MA: Butterworth-Heinemann.

Bose, M. M., & Gijselaers, W. H. (2013). Why supervisors should promote feedback-seeking behaviour in medical residency. *Medical Teacher, 35*(11), e1573–e1583.

Carin, A., & Sund, R. (1971). *Developing questioning techniques.* Columbus, OH: Charles E. Merrill.

Carozza, L. (2011). *Science of successful supervision and mentorship.* San Diego, CA: Plural Publishing.

Casey, P. (1985). *Supervisory skills self-assessment.* Whitewater, WI: University of Wisconsin.

Casey, P., Smith, K., & Ulrich, S. (1988). *Self-supervision: A career tool for audiologists and speech-language pathologists* (Clinical Series No. 10). Rockville, MD: National Student Speech-Language-Hearing Association.

Cogan, M. (1973). *Clinical supervision.* Boston, MA: Houghton Mifflin.

Coleman, T. J. (2000). *Clinical management of communication disorders in culturally diverse children.* Needham Heights, MA: Allyn & Bacon.

Council on Academic Accreditation in Audiology and Speech-Language Pathology. (2004). *Standards for accreditation of graduate education programs in audiology and speech-language pathology programs.* Available from http://www.asha.org/policy

Council on Academic Accreditation in Audiology and Speech-Language Pathology. (2017). *Standards for accreditation of graduate education programs in audiology and speech-language pathology (2017).* Retrieved from http://caa.asha.org/wpcontent/uploads/Accreditation-Standards-for-Graduate-Programs.pdf

Council for Clinical Certification in Audiology and Speech-Language Pathology. (2005). *Membership and certification handbook of the American Speech-Language-Hearing Association.* Retrieved from www.asha.org/about/membership-certification/handbooks/slp/slp_standards.htm

Council for Clinical Certification in Audiology and Speech-Language Pathology of the American Speech-Language-Hearing Association. (2018a). *2020 Standards for the Certificate of Clinical Competence in Audiology.* Retrieved from http://www.asha.org/certification/2020-Audiology-Certification-Standards/

Council for Clinical Certification in Audiology and Speech-Language Pathology of the American Speech-Language-Hearing Association. (2018b). *2020 Standards for the Certificate of Clinical Competence in Speech-Language Pathology.* Retrieved from https://www.asha.org/certification/2020-SLP-Certification-Standards.

Crago, M., & Pickering, M. (Eds.). (1987). *Supervision in human communication disorders: Perspectives on a process.* San Diego, CA: Little Brown-College Hill Press.

Crommelinck, M., & Anseel, F. (2013). Understanding and encouraging feedback-seeking behaviour: A literature review. *Medical Education, 47,* 232–241.

Cunningham, R. (1971). Developing question-asking skills. In J. Weigand (Ed.), *Developing teacher competencies.* Englewood Cliffs, NJ: Prentice Hall.

Dowling, S. (2001). *Supervision: Strategies for successful outcomes and productivity.* Boston, MA: Allyn & Bacon.

Dreyfus, H. I., & Dreyfus S. E. (1986). Five steps from novice to expert. In *Mind over machine.* New York, NY: Free Press.

Dudding, C. (2002). The use of videoconferencing in supervision of graduate clinicians. *Perspectives on Administration and Supervision, 12*(1), 8–12.

Dudding, C. C. (2006). Distance supervision: An update. *Perspectives on Administration and Supervision, 16*(1), 16–18.

Fall, M., & Sutton, J. M. (2004). *Clinical supervision: A handbook for practitioners.* Auckland, NZ: Pearson Education New Zealand.

Farmer S., & Farmer, J. (1989). Supervision *in communication disorders.* Columbus, OH: Merrill.

Gavett, E., & Peapers, R. (2007). Critical thinking: The role of questions. *Perspectives on Issues in Higher Education, 10,* 3–5.

Gillam, R. B., Roussos, C. S., & Anderson, J. L. (1990). Facilitating changes in supervisees' clinical behaviors: An experimental investigation of supervisory effectiveness. *Journal of Speech and Hearing Disorders, 55*(4), 729–739.

Goldhammer, R., Anderson, R., & Krajewski, R. (1980). *Clinical supervision* (2nd ed.). New York, NY: Holt, Rinehart, and Winston.

Halfond, M. (1964). Clinical supervision-stepchild in training. *ASHA, 6,* 441–444.

Hudson, M. W. (2010). *Supporting professional performance in the clinical workplace.* Proceedings of a short course held at Philadelphia, PA: American Speech-Language-Hearing Association.

Hudson, M. W. (2010). Supervision to mentoring: Practical considerations. *Perspectives on Administration and Supervision, 20*, 71–75.

King, D. (2003, May 27). Supervision of student clinicians: Modeling ethical practice for future professionals. *The ASHA Leader, 8*, 26.

Kleffner, F. (Ed.). (1964). *Seminar on guidelines for the internship year*. Washington, DC: American Speech and Hearing Association.

Ladany, N., Walker, J. A., & Melincoff, D. S. (2001). Supervisory style; Its relation to the supervisory working alliance and supervisory self-disclosure. *Counselor Education and Supervision, 40*, 263–275.

Langdon, H. W., & Cheng, L. (1992). *Hispanic children and adults with communication disorders*. Gaithersburg, MD: Aspen.

Leigton, J. (1991). Gender stereotyping in supervisory styles. *Psychoanalytic Review, 78*, 347–363.

Long, J., Lawless, J., & Dotson, D. (1996). Supervisory styles index: Examining supervisees' perceptions of supervisory style. *Contemporary Family Therapy, 18*(4), 589–606.

Mawdsley, B. (1987). Kansas inventory of self-supervision. In S. Farmer (Ed.), *Clinical supervision: A coming of age*. Proceedings of a national conference on supervision held at Jekyll Island, GA: Las Cruces, New Mexico State University.

McCrea, E., & Brasseur, J. (2003). *The supervisory process in speech-language pathology and audiology*. Boston, MA: Allyn & Bacon.

McCready, V. (2007). Generational differences: Do they make a difference in supervisory and administrative relationships? *Perspectives in Administration and Supervision, 17*(3), 6–9.

Munoz, M. L., Watson, J. B., & Flahive, L. K. (2011). Monolingual supervision of bilingual student clinicians: Challenges and opportunities. *ASHA Leader, 16*, 5.

Newman, W. (2001, June/July). The ethical and legal aspects of clinical supervision. *CSHA [California Speech-Language-Hearing Association] Magazine, 30*(1), 10–11, 27.

Newman, W., Victor, S., & Zylla-Jones, E. (2009). *Tools for the first-time supervisor*. Proceedings of a session held at New Orleans, LA: American Speech-Language-Hearing Association.

Nottingham, S., & Henning, J. (2014). Feedback in clinical education, Part I: Characteristics of feedback provided by approved clinical instructors. *Journal of Athletic Training, 49*(1), 49–57.

O'Connor, L. (2008). A new focus on supervision: Looking to the future. *Perspectives on Administration and Supervision, 18*, 17–23.

Pfeiffer, J. W., & Jones, J. E. (1987). *A handbook of structured experiences for human relations training*. San Diego, CA: University Associates.

Schober-Peterson, D., & O'Rourke, C., (2008). Identifying and assisting at-risk graduate students: Process and outcome factors. *Perspectives on Administration and Supervision, 18*, 94–98.

Severinsson, E. (1996). Nurse supervisors' views of their supervisory styles in clinical supervision: A hermeneutical approach. *Journal of Nursing Management, 4*, 191–199.

Severinsson, E., & Hallberg, I. (1996). Clinical supervisors' views of their leadership role in the clinical supervision process with nursing care. *Journal of Advanced Nursing, 24*, 151–161.

Shapiro, D. A., Ogletree, B. T., & Brotherton, W. D. (2002). Graduate students with marginal abilities in communication sciences and disorders: Prevalence, profiles, and solutions. *Journal of Communication Disorders, 35*, 421–451.

Shea, G. F. (1997). *Mentoring: A practical guide* (2nd ed.). Lanham, MD: Crisp Publications.

Shipley, K. (1997). *Interviewing and counseling in communicative disorders—principles and procedures* (2nd ed.). Boston, MA: Allyn & Bacon.

Smith, K. (1979). *Supervisory conferences questions: Who asks them and who answers them*. Paper presented at the annual convention of the American Speech and Hearing Association, Atlanta, GA.

Tellis, G., Cimino, L., & Alberti, J. (2010). Advanced digital technology for supervising graduate clinicians. *Perspectives on Administration and Supervision, 20*, 9–13.

Ulrich, S. (1985). Continuing education model of training. In K. Smith (Moderator), *Preparation and training models for the supervisory process*. Short course presented at the annual convention of the American Speech-Language-Hearing Association, Washington, DC.

U.S. Department of Personnel Management. (1997). *360 degree assessment: An overview*. Retrieved from http://www.opm.gov/perform/wppdf/360asess.pdf

Victor, S. (2010). Coordinator's column. *Perspectives on Administration and Supervision, 20*(3), 83–84.

Weltsch, B. R., & Crowe, L. K. (2006). Effectiveness of mediated analysis in improving student clinical competency. *Perspectives on Administration and Supervision, 16,* 21–22.

Williams, A. L. (1995). Modified teaching clinic: Peer group supervision in clinical training and professional development. *American Journal of Speech-Language Pathology, 4,* 29–38.

Resources

Bartlett's Action Plan

Bartlett, S. (2003). In E. McCrea & J. Brasseur (Eds.), *The supervisory process in speech-language pathology and audiology* (pp. 154–156). Boston, MA: Allyn & Bacon.

Council of Academic Programs in Communication Sciences and Disorders eLearning Courses: https://www.capcsd.org/clinical-education-courses/

Hurst, B., Wilson, C. & Cramer, G. (1998). Professional teaching portfolios. *Phi Delta Kappan, 79*(8), 578–582. EJ 563 868

Knowles, M. (1975). *Self-directed learning: A guide for learners and teachers.* New York, NY: Association Press.

McCarthy, M. P. (2009). *Promoting independence through self-evaluation and formative assessment in clinical education.* Presentation at Chicago, IL: American Speech-Language and Hearing Association.

Pultorak, E. G. (1993). Facilitating reflective thought in novice teachers. *Journal of Teacher Education, 44*(4), 288–295.

Rahim, M. A. (1989). Relationships of leader power to compliance and satisfaction with supervision: Evidence from a national sample of managers. *Journal of Management, 15,* 495–516.

Schon, D. A. (1996). *Educating the reflective practitioner: Toward a new design for teaching and learning in the professions.* San Francisco, CA: Jossey-Bass.

27

Technology for Student Training, Professional Practice, and Service Delivery

◇◇

Carol C. Dudding, PhD and Susan B. Ingram, PhD

Any sufficiently advanced technology is indistinguishable from magic.
—Arthur C. Clarke, Profiles of the Future: An Inquiry into the Limits of the Possible, 1962

Introduction

This chapter provides you with an introduction to the uses of technologies as they are used by both students and professionals in communication sciences and disorders (CSD). It offers insights into the technologies themselves as well as ways in which they change how we train students, conduct business, diagnose, treat, and interact with the clients we serve. This chapter will explore web-based tools, simulations, virtual and augmented reality, and teleconferencing technologies as they apply to each of these areas.

The Digital Revolution

We are living in a time referred to as the digital revolution. Smartphones, texts, and viral videos are likely to have always been part of your experience. As a *digital native* you are thought to be fluent in your use of technologies, impatient with linear thinking, and possess the ability to multitask (Jones, Ramanau, Cross, & Healing, 2010; Prensky, 2001). You have expectations for how you receive and share information, acquire knowledge, and interact with other people. You view learning as best achieved through action and exploration within a given context (Brown, n.d.). This contrasts with many of your instructors, clinical educators, and employers who are known as digital immigrants, those individuals exposed to digital technologies later in life. As you, the digital natives, are the future of our professions, it is important that we all have a shared understanding of the promises and pitfalls of the use of technologies as we move forward in research, education, and service delivery.

Instruction and Training

Classroom Technologies

Terms like learning management system (LMS), cloud sharing, web-conferencing, and electronic response systems have transformed the way we teach and learn at the university level. Students have come to expect that every course come with an LMS. Canvas (Canvas, 2011) and Blackboard (Blackboard®, 1997) are two of the more common examples of an LMS. LMSs are used to post lectures, assignments, and quizzes. They also allow for peer to peer (P2P) collaboration. An example of P2P is when students meet and share information virtually. This can be done with web-conferencing applications (apps) embedded within the LMS. More and more students are using free web-based apps for collaboration outside of the classroom system. Slack (2013) is a good example of an application that allows students to control how, what and when they share and collaborate. The rapid emergence of collaborative technologies and apps has university Help Desks struggling to keep pace. BYOD (Bring Your Own Device) is a term referring to the technologies students bring into the classroom including the hardware (e.g., smartphones, tablets, laptops) and the countless apps and software programs.

Online Learning

Recent federal reports have indicated that online learning is the fastest growing segment of higher education. Currently 31.6% of all students now take at least one distance education course (a total of 6,359,121 students) and on-campus enrollments have dropped by over 1 million between 2012 and 2016. This growth has been consistent over the last 14 years and shows no signs of slowing (Seaman, Allen, & Seaman, 2018).

The disciplines of speech-language pathology and audiology are experiencing similar growth rates in the use of distance education technologies in the academic and clinical training of future professionals. A search using the American Speech-Language-Hearing Association's (ASHA) EdFind (ASHA, 2019a) revealed that 17 institutions offer fully online degree programs, while 63 programs offer prerequisite coursework online. These numbers do not include graduate courses that are offered as hybrid or blended, that is, courses that employ both face-to-face and online delivery methods.

Previous versions of this chapter included detailed descriptions of the kinds of technologies used in online learning (e.g., chatrooms, discussion boards, web conferencing, electronic gradebook) and key terms (e.g., synchronous, asynchronous, hybrid). These technologies and vocabulary are now ubiquitous not only in higher

education but are heard in pre-school and elementary school classrooms. Online learning has been fueled by the ability to provide access to millions who could not attend traditional courses on a brick and mortar campus. Massive open online courses (MOOCS) spiked in numbers and popularity in 2012 as a way of offering access to high quality education free of cost. This initiative was wildly successful in enrolling 81 million students in 9,400 courses (Shah, 2018). There is little doubt that online learning will have an evolving role in higher education. Assuredly the next generation of online learning will look very different from what we have available today, perhaps occurring within immersive, virtual classrooms.

In addition to the education and training of future professionals, online and distance technologies have impacted professional development and training in both audiology and speech-language pathology. Beginning in 2003 for audiology and 2005 for speech-language pathology, professionals certified by ASHA are required to obtain 30 hours of continuing education activities each three-year certification period. A number of companies have emerged to meet this need by offering online professional development. Additionally, the Council of Academic Programs in Communication Sciences and Disorders (CAPCSD) offers free online continuing education for those who provide supervision to students, clinical fellows and other professionals.

E-Supervision and E-Mentoring

Graduate programs in speech-language pathology and audiology recognize the significance of supervision as a means of producing quality clinicians. Bernard and Goodyear (1992) state the importance of supervision as a "means of transmitting the skills, knowledge, and attitudes of a particular profession. It also is an essential means of ensuring that the clients receive a certain minimum of quality of care while trainees work with them to gain their skills" (p. 2).

Many professional organizations (e.g., American Board of Audiology [ABA], ASHA) and state licensing boards require student clinicians to complete practicum requirements under the supervision of accredited and/or licensed professionals. Graduate programs in audiology and speech-language pathology are facing dwindling availability of clinical placements for their students. This is a result, in part, of workplace demands and restrictions handed down from insurance companies that greatly limit the ability of a working professional to supervise a student, even if motivated to do so (Dudding, McCready, Nunez, & Procaccini, 2017).

The rise in the number of nontraditional graduate students, including those enrolled in online programs, requires substantial resources to provide supervision to students at a distance from the campus (Dudding & Justice, 2004). E-supervision, the use of digital video-conferencing for supervision, provides a means for students at geographically distant sites to be supervised by clinical educators located at a college campus or selected base sites. E-supervision offers many benefits, including cost-effectiveness and productivity of clinical instruction (Dudding & Justice, 2004). As web conferencing technologies and high-speed internet access have developed, more institutions are considering the benefits of e-supervision. E-supervision is distinct from online learning and professional webinars in that it often necessitates observing clients/patients as well as the supervisee. This brings into play considerations of the Health Insurance Portability and Accountability Act (HIPAA). The HIPAA Privacy Rule is a national standard to protect individuals' medical records and other personal health information (United States, 2004). Therefore, application of e-supervision must consider these very important patient protections. Refer to Chapter 14 for a full explanation of HIPAA.

Our professional learning does not end after the first years of practice. The mentoring process is recognized as an integral part of professional growth and development. Audiologists seeking certification from the ABA must receive a minimum of 2,000 hours of mentored professional practice as audiologists following completion of the clinical doctorate in audiology. Professionals seeking ASHA certification in speech-language pathology must complete a clinical fellowship post-graduation from an accredited graduate program. The Clinical Fellow (CF) must receive ongoing mentoring and formal evaluations from a CF mentor for a minimum of 1260 hours. The mentor must be able to provide direct observation in real time and must be available to consult with the CF. In some instances when traditional onsite mentoring is not possible, e-mentoring may be used with prior approval (CFCC, 2018).

See Chapter 26 in this text for an in-depth discussion of clinical education and mentoring.

Virtual Simulations for Instruction and Learning

In 2014, ASHA's Council for Clinical Certification (CFCC, 2013) changed the implementation language for Speech-Language Pathology Standard V-B to allow up to 20% of the required 375 direct clinical hours to be obtained through simulation. This change has resulted in an eruption of interest in simulations in audiology and speech-language pathology. Simulations, more specifically health care simulations, are a way to provide students with a realistic learning environment, allow-

ing them to practice and learn without risk to patients/clients. Simulations allow students to perform a clinical skill, develop critical thinking, and practice communication in a simulated professional health care setting. Programs in CSD are using simulations (e.g., Simucase™) for instruction in the classroom and clinic, for student remediation, and as a method of authentic assessment (Dudding, Brown, Estis, Szymanski, & Zraick, 2018).

A key principle to keep in mind is that simulations are more than a type of technology. They are a learning tool for students and professionals. Simulations can take several forms and utilize a range of technologies. They range in the level of fidelity (i.e., realism) and cost. Standardized patients, the use of a trained person or persons to portray a patient or family member, have a long history of use in CSD and other health care arenas. The use of manikins (whole body) and task trainers are often found in simulation labs on medical campuses and hospitals. High-tech manikins can simulate a patient experiencing a number of medical conditions including stroke, cardiorespiratory arrest, and even childbirth. Some advanced human patient simulators can be programmed to cry, breathe, sweat, and bleed. Many of us were trained in cardiopulmonary resuscitation (CPR) using Rescuci-Anne® (Laerdal Medical, n.d.). This is an example of a task trainer. Task trainers are dedicated to training a very specific skill such as cerumen removal. Emerging technologies in virtual and augmented reality are being explored to offer immersive and realistic simulation experiences for learning. The possibilities have yet to be imagined.

Simulations provide another opportunity for students enrolled in speech-language pathology programs to obtain the required minimum 25 guided clinical observation hours. Accrual of these hours generally precedes direct contact with clients/patients and should reflect varied disorders across work settings. Simulations provide an alternative method for students to gain observation hours for individuals presenting with a variety of disorders across the lifespan. Reflective debriefing/discussion of clients/patients led by ASHA-certified clinical educators following each simulation experience completes this introductory clinical requirement (CFCC, 2018).

Impact on Professional Practice Settings

Speech-language pathologists and audiologists are employed in a variety of work settings including early intervention, health care, schools, and/or private practice. Each of these settings is greatly influenced by technology trends. In addition to the need for electronic billing and reporting functions, including speech-recognition software, practice settings rely on technology to offer collaboration tools and to provide services to patients at a distance.

The health care arena is seeing a surge in health information technologies, such as electronic health records (EHR) or electronic medical records (EMR), electronic billing, and clinical point of care technologies. Eighty-one percent of health care payer executives indicate their company is "investing in technology to improve member experience (PwC, 2018)" (CDW Healthcare, 2018, p. 5). Perhaps you have heard the term "personalized health care." This refers to a movement to provide health care specific to the needs and history of a patient. This is possible, in part, due to a health information technology known as clinical decision support system (CDSS; American Physical Therapy Association, 2010). This technology allows physicians and other health care workers to access information and health care records to aid in clinical decision making. Another way that medical care is becoming more personalized is with the inclusion of tablets, smart TVs, and interactive digital whiteboards in patients' rooms aiming to improve patient satisfaction/participation, quality of care, and lower readmission rates (CDW Healthcare, 2018).

Hospitals and health care clinics are not the only work settings to be impacted by technology. Public and private schools have certainly been impacted by educational technologies used in teaching (e.g., SMART Board®, n.d.); data management systems that assist tracking student progress; online and web-based therapy portals; computerized assessments and analysis programs; various assistive technologies including augmentative-alternative communication (AAC) systems; hearing aids and cochlear implants; and service delivery through telepractice.

Through several commercially available programs, speech-language pathologists and audiologists based in public schools can access scheduling calendars and student records. They can share information with family members given signed consent, and other professionals and track and report progress toward goals. Many public school systems use dedicated, password protected online programs such as IEP Online (PCG Education, n.d.) to create, track, and share students' Individualized Education Programs (IEPs), thereby streamlining the cumbersome documentation process and securing educational records. When sharing educational records and/or medical information it is paramount to follow the employment setting's policies and procedures related to information security. In addition to the HIPAA Privacy Rule governing health care information, clinicians should be familiar with the regulations protecting educational records as outlined by the Family Educational

Rights and Privacy Act (FERPA) of 1974. Failure to comply with these safeguards may result in civil penalties and fines and criminal charges (ASHA, 2019b). Breaches of information security may also result in loss of employment. Safeguarding of information will be addressed later in this chapter and more fully detailed in Chapter 5, "Professional Ethics."

It is no longer prudent or best-practice to provide services in isolation from other professionals. Indeed, interprofessional practice and collaboration are becoming mandates of many professions, including audiology and speech-language pathology. Consider the use of web-conferencing software programs such as Skype™ (2003) and WebEx™ (1995) for collaborating on a research project or discussing a challenging case. These applications, and others like them, allow for real-time communication through use of text, voice, and/or video communication. Desktop sharing allows all participants to view and modify shared documents and applications in real time. With the use of the aforementioned technologies, practitioners are able to consult with an expert located across the country or indeed across the world. They can virtually meet in real time to discuss a client, view videos of a client's performance, and/or share test results. Now imagine that the same expert is researching a rare or complex condition but has access to a limited number of clients. Once again, through the use of web-conferencing technologies, the professionals can now collaborate and share information to advance research in this area.

Another way that professionals and students can collaborate and share information is through P2P file-sharing programs and document-sharing websites and cloud applications. Cloud computing allows users to store electronic files on a password protected site on the internet. Cloud computing provides users access to files and applications through browsers, without housing software or files on a computer. There are a number of web- and cloud-based applications to support professional collaboration. Current examples of cloud applications are Google Drive (2012), Google Calendar (2009), and Dropbox (2008). Some applications have meeting schedulers, shared calendars, and web-conferencing capabilities for members to discuss the project. This type of technology is particularly useful for students and professionals working as a team to create a research paper, procedure manual, or other text-based project. These technologies, used individually or together, support and enhance collaboration and research for practicing professionals, students, and researchers in speech-language pathology, audiology, and the speech-hearing sciences. No doubt you can imagine any number of scenarios in which the sharing of information among professionals would be beneficial not only to the clients but to the advancement of the professions.

Service Delivery

Technology is incorporated into the assessment and intervention for communication disorders in myriad ways across work settings. Audiologists and speech-language pathologists have access to a number of non-imaging instrumentation and imaging technologies for use in diagnostics. In the area of intervention, web-based applications and software programs allow for the creation of individualized therapy materials. Game-based activities and virtual simulations can be incorporated into treatment sessions. Assistive technology devices benefit those with speech, language, and hearing disorders. Web-conferencing technologies allow for the provision of services through telepractice. It is beyond the scope of this chapter to discuss all of the technologies in detail, but an effort is made to provide an overview of the current applications with an eye toward future development and trends.

Prevention/Assessment

Consider some of the tools used by health care professionals that are important to audiologists, speech-language pathologists, and speech, language, and hearing scientists. For example, imaging technologies such as magnetic resonance imaging (MRI), functional magnetic resonance imaging (fMRI), diffusion tensor imaging (DTI), near-infrared spectroscopy (NIRS), and noninvasive brain stimulation procedures such as transcranial magnetic stimulation (TMS) and transcranial direct current stimulation (tDCS) have greatly advanced the understanding of brain functioning and aid in the diagnosis and treatment of communication disorders.

Technological advancements have aided in the accurate diagnosis of communication disorders. For audiologists, assessment is driven by instrumentation technologies. In addition to using audiometers to conduct pure-tone hearing screenings, audiologists use otoacoustic emissions (OAEs) and auditory brainstem responses (ABRs) to screen the hearing of newborns/infants. Diagnostic assessment measures include audiometry (pure-tone air/bone conduction and speech recognition), otoscopy, immittance testing, OAEs, ABRs, and electrocochleography. Technology also supports the audiologist's vestibular diagnostic battery, including testing procedures such as videonystagmography (VNG), vestibular evoked myogenic potential (VEMP), and rotational chair assessment.

For speech-language pathologists, digital-recording devices are commonplace in assessment procedures. Basic audio-recorders and iPads assist the SLP in recording and transcribing speech-language samples for speech sound production and subsequent language analyses, using a computer-assisted language sample analysis software package such as Systematic Analysis of Language Transcripts (SALT; Miller & Nockerts, n.d.). More sophisticated recording hardware like the Computerized Speech Lab™ (CSL™, n.d.) and freeware programs such as PRAAT (Boersma & Weenink, 2019) often aid the SLP in the analysis of acoustic speech signals for clients with voice disorders, for example.

Furthermore, technology allows for digital administration, scoring, and reporting for numerous common pediatric speech and language assessment measures (Pearson Education, Inc., n.d.). The *Clinical Evaluation of Language Fundamentals–Fifth Edition* (CELF-5; Wiig, Semel, & Secord, 2013) and the *Goldman-Fristoe Test of Articulation–Third Edition* (GFTA-3; Goldman & Fristoe, 2015) are among the numerous digital assessment tools offered by Pearson. For assessment of adult clients with swallowing concerns, imaging technologies including modified barium swallow tests (MBS), flexible endoscopic evaluation of swallowing (FEES), and laryngoscopy add significant diagnostic information.

Intervention

Assistive Technology. Assistive technology (AT) refers to assistive, adaptive, and rehabilitative devices to improve or enhance the functioning of an individual with a disability. AT is a specialized area shared with many other professionals such as occupational therapists, physical therapists, and rehabilitation engineers. Intervention for individuals with speech, language, or hearing disorders utilizes AT devices such as programmable digital hearing aids, hearing assistive technology systems (HATS), cochlear implants/osseointegrated devices, and AAC devices.

The audiology profession has experienced rapid growth in hearing aid technologies since 1987, when the first digital hearing aids were manufactured. Present-day digital aids offer advantages in terms of wireless technology, feedback cancellation, directional microphones, and improved environmental noise control. According to the ASHA 2018 Audiology Survey (ASHA, 2019c), over 80% of audiologists fit and dispense hearing aids on a daily/weekly basis.

HATS are devices that provide additional help in specific listening situations such as talking on the phone, communicating in noise, or socializing in small or large groups and can be used with or without hearing aids or cochlear implants. These technologies include FM (frequency modulation) systems, in which the speaker wears a microphone and the listener wears a receiver; infrared systems, whereby light waves send sounds across a room; induction loop systems, which are beneficial for large group areas; and one-to-one communicators, in which the speaker wears a microphone and the listener wears a hearing aid or headset (ASHA, 2019d). Devices that increase the intensity of phones and answering machines, loud doorbells, computers, and wake-up alarms also fall within this category of assistive technology. Based on responses to the ASHA 2018 Audiology Survey (ASHA, 2019c), approximately 68% of audiologists demonstrate, fit, or dispense hearing assistive technology on a daily/weekly basis.

The terms TTY (TeleTYpe), TDD (Telecommunications Device for the Deaf), and TT (Text Telephone) are used interchangeably to refer to any type of text-based telecommunications device. This technology, utilized by individuals with significant hearing and/or speech-language impairment when using the telephone, can communicate directly with one another through speech and/or text, or they may communicate via a live relay operator who conveys the messages between the users.

Perhaps no technology has impacted the profoundly deaf and hearing-impaired community more than the development of the cochlear implant. A cochlear implant is a device that is surgically implanted in the individual with profound sensorineural hearing loss and provides direct electrical stimulation to the auditory nerve. A cochlear implant is not a cure for deafness, but it does provide people who cannot benefit from hearing aids the perception of the sensation of sound. Similarly, osseointegrated devices are treatment options for individuals with conductive or mixed hearing loss. These implants are surgically embedded to the outside of a person's skull, behind the ear, and transmit sounds to the inner ear through skull vibrations. Recent technological advancement in this area of intervention includes FDA approval for a new nonsurgical option for the traditional bone conduction implant surgery. ADHEAR (MED-EL, 2016; ASHA, 2018a) utilizes a disposable adhesive adapter (placed on the skin behind the ear) in place of surgical implantation.

Another major area of assistive technologies is the use of AAC systems. These unaided (no-tech) and aided devices (low- and high-tech) are considered "augmentative" when used to supplement existing speech and "alternative" when used in place of speech that is absent or not functional. ASHA (2019e) defines AAC as "a variety of techniques and tools, including picture communication boards, line drawings, speech-generating devices (SGDs), tangible objects, manual signs, gestures, and finger spelling, to help the individual express thoughts, wants and needs, feelings, and ideas." Examples of no-tech AAC include gestures and manual signs. Low-tech communication systems include pictures (e.g., Picture Exchange Communication System [Bondy & Frost, 1994]), writing, and communication boards/books that may be made commercially or by a clinician or family member. These systems also include devices operated by electromechanical switches. High-tech communication systems use specialized software with some form of technology hardware (e.g., computer, tablet, smartphone) and have the capacity to provide printed and/or voice output. A device that has voice output is referred to as an SGD and the output may be digitized (recorded human voice) or synthesized (produced from stored digital data). Artificial phonation devices (e.g., electrolarynx devices and speech valves for individuals with tracheostomies or ventilators) are also considered high-tech devices to augment speech.

AAC devices have evolved from expensive and cumbersome devices that required special mounting on wheelchairs, to small, compact, and powerful communication aids. Apple's iPad technology is increasingly popular as an AAC device due to its affordability, cultural acceptance, and the emerging number of apps that are being developed for this specific purpose.

Assistive technology devices will undoubtedly play a larger role as the U.S. population ages. Elderly people with cognitive and language disabilities may benefit from signaling devices to alert others of their needs; identification aids to convey biographical information; voice amplifiers to increase speech loudness; alphabet and pacing boards to clarify speech communication; and alerts, environmental organizers, and memory books to serve as external memory aids.

Apps. Many digital immigrants recall days when "Xeroxing" or photocopying materials were the mainstays of speech-language intervention programs. In this earlier time, worksheets and clinician-created activities required considerable time and planning. Today, a number of web-based commercially available applications exist, such as Boardmaker® (2014), TheraSimplicity® (1998), and LessonPix (2011), that allow clinicians to create customized materials in little time. Furthermore, through the development of apps on mobile devices, non-dedicated touch-screen technologies such as the iPhone and iPad have made their way into intervention services in CSD. ASHA (2019f) has identified numerous advantages of integrating apps in intervention including increasing motivation, monitoring progress, serving as support tools, and addressing specific communication targets such as written language and literacy. A common communication app for any communicator is Proloquo2Go (AssistiveWare B.V., 2008). Children with speech sound disorders may benefit from use of the app, Articulation Station (Little Bee Speech, 2018) and Epic! (StoryMagic, Inc., 2017), a digital library for children. The LAMP Words for Life language system (Prentke Romich Company, 2019) is useful for clients with language based disorders such as those diagnosed on the autism spectrum, while Spaced Retrieval Therapy (Tactus Therapy Solutions Ltd., 2012) can be a helpful app for clients with dementia.

Digital Games. An extensive number of computer and video games are available for use in intervention. Some programs have been designed for individuals with a speech-language impairment, while others can be adapted for this purpose. The better examples of these commercially available programs allow for interactivity, provide specific feedback, and are motivating to the user. Digital games for intervention offer advantages by incorporating the concepts of conflict, cooperation, rules, and constraints while targeting specific communication skill development. Several popular blogs and websites offer a listing of available games, along with suggestions on how to incorporate them into intervention programs.

Children are not the only population that can benefit from the use of computer and video games. An internet search reveals several applications intended for adults with cognitive deficits, including those who have aphasia, dementia, or head injury. Some of these digital applications focus on rehabilitation of skills and encompass the areas of cognitive retraining, word retrieval, and memory drill and practice. Other applications, such as planners, organizers, and altering systems, serve as external memory aids. Research is being conducted on the use of virtual gaming systems for remediation of vestibular and balance problems.

Consideration should be given to the design, quality, and appropriate application of any technology employed. While digital games offer benefits to both clinicians and clients, you are cautioned to carefully evaluate the claims of any program employed in treatment. It is important to consider the population that the program was designed to address (i.e., age, diagnosis, prerequisite skills, motor, and intellectual ability). Just as one treatment approach does not apply to all types of clients, a single digital game or program cannot address the needs of all clients. The professional should be guided by evidence-based practice in assessing the efficacy of a program employed in intervention. Highly interactive, visually appealing video games do not replace the skills of a highly trained communication disorders professional.

Virtual Simulations. Another application of technology is the use of virtual simulations for intervention. Virtual simulations involve practice within an environment developed to imitate or estimate how events might occur in real world situations. Advantages of simulations include opportunities for meaningful contextual learning and exposure to real-life challenges. Simulations encourage repeated practice within a safe environment that is challenging and motivating and promotes gener-

alization of skills (Williams, 2008). Proposed ways that virtual simulation environments could be used in the area of language and literacy intervention include the following:

- Immersion of students in a variety of learning environments to explore and practice curricular content such as space, lost civilizations, and historic moments

- Reading skill development with virtual characters and settings

- Animation of stories written by students

- Demonstration of appropriate types of speaking in virtual environments (e.g., negotiation, persuasion, public speaking) (Williams, 2008)

Specialized Software

Provision of feedback to our clients is an important component of intervention. Available technology includes low-cost software programs that conduct voice and sound analyses and are invaluable to the clinician in both diagnosis and treatment of a variety of speech disorders. Programs such as Waveforms Annotations Spectrograms and Pitch (WASP; Huckvale, 2012), WaveSurfer (WaveSurfer, 2012), and PRAAT (Boersma & Weenink, 2019) provide basic spectral analysis of the client's speech and in some cases may be used to provide feedback to our clients with speech and voice disorders. A more sophisticated technology used for providing feedback to clients relative to speech and voice production is the Computerized Speech Lab™ (CSL, n.d.). Clinicians, too, may find the IOPI System (IOPI®, 2011) useful for providing feedback to clients working on improved tongue and lip strength. These and other specialized software have allowed practitioners to provide in-depth analysis and feedback that was formerly only possible in research laboratories.

Carryover/Generalization of Skills

The transfer of communication skills gained within the therapy setting to other contexts is an important part of the intervention process. This transfer of knowledge is otherwise known as carryover or generalization of skills. Vayo, Ingram, Doyle, and Ingram (2018) found the use of an app, HP Reveal (Aurasma, 2018), helpful in facilitating the transfer of speech-language goals for children from the clinic setting to the home environment. The app allows clinicians to create videos that are subsequently launched by trigger images on mobile devices. They serve to remind parents and clients of the therapy goals, provide verbal and visual prompts to encourage accuracy, and provide activities to facilitate sound production and language use at home. Similar apps for skill transfer include Seesaw (Seesaw Learning, Inc., 2019), which serves as a digital portfolio of the client's progression in intervention, and Bitsboard (Happy Moose Apps, Inc., 2019), which aids clinicians in developing games to target communication goals for clients of all ages.

Telepractice for Service Delivery

New professionals can expect to be involved either professionally or personally in telehealth. *Telehealth* is a term used to describe the delivery of health care services through telecommunication technologies. In 2001, ASHA adopted the term *telepractice* to describe delivery of "a range of services provided through telecommunications technology that are not exclusively health related, including clinical services for communication enhancement, and education and supervision" (ASHA, 2005, p. 1). Telepractice as a delivery method is meeting several critical needs within the professions. Telepractice provides improved access to services that may not otherwise be available due to geographic limitations, mobility of the client, and/or accessibility to a qualified professional (ASHA, 2005). Populations served through telepractice include: children within the public schools, survivors of combat-related brain injury (Mashima, 2010); persons requiring audiological services, early hearing detection and intervention (Houston & Muñoz, 2010; Krumm, 2005; Krumm, Ribera, & Froelich, 2002); and those with swallowing disorders (Georges, Belz, & Potter, 2006; Houn & Trottier, 2006).

When considering the use of telepractice, it is essential to ensure that the services provided are cost-effective, in compliance with state and national standards, meet regulatory requirements for reimbursement and licensure, and do not violate interstate licensure laws. It is important that delivery of services through telepractice is acceptable to the clients and families and yields outcomes at least equal to those of face-to-face delivery methods.

There are various models of telepractice and types of equipment employed in delivery of services through telepractice. One model is known as "store and forward" in which information, such as test results and images, obtained at one site is electronically forwarded to a practitioner at a distant site for consultation. This model is currently not eligible for reimbursement by many insurance carriers. "Face to face" provision of services refers to the use of digital videoconferencing technologies (using web-based or digital videoconferencing units) to provide services in real time, with interaction between the client and the practitioner. This model is gaining acceptance with a number of insurance carriers and regulatory agen-

cies for reimbursement of services. Telepractice may also involve remote monitoring devices and the use of distance learning technologies. Considerations for selection of technology for telepractice are similar to those discussed in the section on e-supervision and e-mentoring.

Government and regulatory agencies have created a series of documents to ensure that the provision of services through telehealth and/or telepractice meets the same standards as those provided in face-to-face service delivery. The American Telemedicine Association (ATA) is a great resource for policy and national trends on telehealth practices. In response to these national trends, ASHA's Practice Portal (2019g) provides numerous resources for those involved in telepractice. These documents delineate responsibilities of professionals in terms of confidentiality, ethics, and reimbursement. Those interested in networking with other telepractitioners are encouraged to join a special interest group as part of several associations dedicated to telemedicine/telepractice (ATA and ASHA).

Ethical Considerations

As we continue to integrate existing and emerging technologies into audiology and speech-language pathology, whether it is through collaboration, training, and/or provision of services, it is critical to our professions and to the clients we serve that we maintain the integrity and quality of the services provided. As new technologies continue to emerge, speech-language-hearing practitioners are charged with gaining requisite knowledge for proper and ethical application of these technologies.

ASHA's Code of Ethics, Principle II, Rule G and Rule H directly address the use of technology by stating, "Individuals shall make use of technology and instrumentation consistent with accepted professional guidelines in their areas of practice. When such technology is not available, an appropriate referral may be made" and "Individuals shall ensure that all technology and instrumentation used to provide services or to conduct research and scholarly activities are in proper working order and are properly calibrated" (ASHA, 2016, p. 7). These rules directly address the use of instrumentation and other clinical equipment. Ethical responsibilities are an inherent part of clinical practice and research regardless of the use of technology. While not specifically aimed at technology, other rules of the ASHA Code of Ethics can be applied when it comes to the use of technology: Principle 1, Rule A, states, "Individuals shall provide all clinical services and scientific activities competently," and Principle 1, Rule B states: "Individuals shall use every resource, including referral and/or interprofessional collaboration when appropriate, to ensure that quality service is provided" (ASHA, 2016, p. 4). When employing alternative service delivery models, clients and caregivers should be given a clear and concise explanation of the technologies employed, along with the mention of benefits, limitations, and risks. They should be given an opportunity to ask questions and opt out of services. In the event that the speech-language-hearing professional is dispensing a technology, such as a hearing aid or AT device, the client should be provided with information regarding the full cost, along with a description of the return policy.

Although the benefits of technology use for the disciplines of audiology and speech-language pathology are astounding, ASHA's Healthy Communication & Popular Technology Initiative (ASHA, 2018b) serves to remind professionals and consumers of the critical need for inclusion of ample face-to-face interaction for young children's communication development. We know that speech, language, and social skills are fostered by conversation and interaction with varied communication partners versus exposure to screen time alone. Encouraging safe listening practices with technology use and promoting hearing protection are also objectives supported by this initiative.

In addition to ASHA's Code of Ethics, practitioners are bound by the directives of other agencies such as state licensing boards, federal agencies, insurance carriers, and employers. As previously mentioned, the federal regulation known as HIPAA necessitates that practitioners meet stringent privacy and confidentiality requirements that apply to use of many of the technologies discussed in this chapter, including document-sharing technologies and email. Additionally, FERPA regulations must be addressed when accessing and sharing educational records for students in K–12 and higher education. Reimbursement agencies may also have guidelines for use of technologies. For example, the Centers for Medicare & Medicaid Services provide guidelines for reimbursement for the use of technology in service delivery. Read Chapter 5 for a more in-depth discussion of professional ethics.

Summary

This chapter offers an introduction to the application of technologies in communication sciences and disorders within the digital age. It includes a description of various technologies, including web-conferencing, assistive technology, apps, digital games, and virtual simulations. In addition, it offers information about current application in the areas of online learning, collaboration, e-supervision/e-mentoring, and telepractice. The chapter includes information on service delivery models with

consideration of the technologies, security, and ethical considerations.

More important, this chapter encourages students and professionals in audiology and speech-language pathology to embrace emerging technologies as opportunities to enhance education, collaboration, assessment, and intervention. We want to explore the potential of new and emerging technologies to help better the lives of those that we serve, but to do so with an understanding and appreciation of their strengths and limitations so as not to become enslaved by them.

Critical Thinking

1. How might digital technologies assist audiologists and speech-language pathologists in areas related to prevention?

2. How could learning based on virtual simulations, apps, and digital games be incorporated into the training of audiologists and their clinical practice?

3. What kinds of opportunities does telepractice open to audiology?

4. How might the development of communication technologies (e.g., text, email, video chat) and social networks (e.g., Facebook, Twitter, Instagram) either assist or hinder people with language and literacy disorders?

5. How does the experienced practitioner best keep informed about the latest technological developments in the field? What role might professional organizations play? What conflicts might arise?

6. What measures would you put in place to ensure security and confidentiality of client information when utilizing the various technologies discussed in this chapter?

7. What is meant by health literacy and what is our role as audiologists, speech-language pathologists, and speech, language, and hearing scientists?

8. How might the high prevalence of digital technologies in our society assist those with communication disorders in reducing perceived disabilities and impairments?

9. Consider the learning, social, and cultural characteristics of today's digital native. What are the implications for the future speech-language pathology and audiology clinical workforce?

10. In what ways do online technologies present a challenge for copyright and fair-use laws?

References

American Physical Therapy Association. (2010, February). Health care technology today. *PT in Motion, 2*(1), 41–43.

American Speech-Language-Hearing Association. (2005). *Speech-language pathologists providing clinical services via telepractice* [Technical report]. Available from http://www.asha.org/policy

American Speech-Language-Hearing Association. (2016). *Code of ethics* [Ethics]. Available from http://www.asha.org/policy/

American Speech-Language-Hearing Association. (2018a). FDA approves new nonsurgical bone conduction hearing technology. *ASHA Leader, 23*(7), 8. https://doi.org/10.1044/leader.NIB1.23072018.8

American Speech-Language-Hearing Association. (2018b). *Healthy communication & popular technology initiative.* Retrieved from https://communicationandtech.org/

American Speech-Language-Hearing Association. (2019a). *Frequently requested EdFind lists.* Retrieved from https://www.asha.org/students/edfind/browse/

American Speech-Language Hearing Association. (2019b). *Health information privacy: Frequently asked questions.* Retrieved from https://www.asha.org/practice/reimbursement/hipaa/privacy/

American Speech-Language-Hearing Association. (2019c). *2018 Audiology survey. Survey summary report: Number and type of responses.* Available from http://www.asha.org

American Speech-Language-Hearing Association. (2019d). *Hearing assistive technology.* Retrieved from https://www.asha.org/public/hearing/Hearing-Assistive-Technology/

American Speech-Language-Hearing Association. (2019e). *Augmentative and alternative communication.* Retrieved from https://www.asha.org/Practice-Portal/Professional-Issues/Augmentative-and-Alternative- Communication/

American Speech-Language-Hearing Association (2019f). *Applications (Apps) for speech-language pathology practice.* Retrieved from https://www.asha.org/SLP/schools/Applications-for-Speech-Language-Pathology-Practice/

American Speech-Language-Hearing Association. (2019g). *The practice portal.* Retrieved from https://www.asha.org/practice-portal/

AssistiveWare B.V. (2008). Proloquo2Go (6.1) [Mobile application software]. Retrieved from https://itunes.apple.com/us/app/proloquo2go/id308368164?mt=8

Aurasma. (2018). HP Reveal (6.0.1) [Mobile application software]. Retrieved from https://itunes.apple.com/us/app/hp-reveal/id432526396?mt=8

Bernard, J. M., & Goodyear, R. K. (1992). *Fundamentals of clinical supervision.* Boston, MA: Allyn & Bacon.

Blackboard. (1997). [Computer software]. Retrieved from https://www.blackboard.com/index.html

Boardmaker. (2014). [Computer software]. Retrieved from https://goboardmaker.com/pages/boardmaker-online/

Boersma, P., & Weenink, D. (2019). Praat: Doing phonetics by computer [Computer program]. Version 6.0.49. Retrieved from http://www.praat.org/

Bondy, A. S., & Frost, L. A. (1994). The picture exchange communication system. *Focus on Autistic Behavior, 9*(3), 1–19. https://doi.org/10.1177/108835769400900301

Brown, J. S. (n.d.). *Learning in the digital age.* Retrieved from http://net.educause.edu/ir/library/pdf/ffpiu015.pdf

Canvas. (2011). [Computer software]. Retrieved from https://www.canvaslms.com/

CDW Healthcare. (2018). *Next-generation engagement technology enhances patient outcomes* [White paper]. Retrieved from https://www.cdwg.com/content/cdwg/en/industries/healthcare-technology.html?cm_mmc=Vanity-_-Healthcare-_-NA-_-012019

Clarke, A. C. (1962). *Profiles of the future: An inquiry into the limits of the possible.* London, UK: Indigo.

Council for Clinical Certification in Audiology and Speech-Language Pathology of the American Speech-Language-Hearing Association. (2013). *2014 Standards for the Certificate of Clinical Competence in Speech-Language Pathology.* Retrieved from http://www.asha.org/Certification/2014-Speech-Language-Pathology-Certification-Standards/

Council for Clinical Certification in Audiology and Speech-Language Pathology of the American Speech-Language-Hearing Association. (2018). *2020 Standards for the Certificate of Clinical Competence in Speech-Language Pathology.* Retrieved from https://www.asha.org/certification/2020-SLP-Certification-Standards

CSL. (n.d.). [Computer software]. Retrieved from https://www.pentaxmedical.com/pentax/en/99/1/Computerized-Speech-Lab-CSL

Dropbox. (2008). [Computer software]. Retrieved from https://www.dropbox.com/

Dudding, C. C., & Justice, L. (2004). A model for e-supervision: Videoconferencing as a clinical training tool. *Communication Disorders Quarterly*, *25*(3), 145–151.

Dudding, C. C., McCready, V., Nunez, L. M., & Procaccini, S. J. (2017). Clinical supervision in speech-language pathology and audiology in the United States: Development of a clinical specialty. *The Clinical Supervisor*, *36*(2), 161–181. https://doi.org/10.1080/07325223.2017.1377663

Dudding, C. C., Brown, D. K., Estis, J. M., Szymanski, C., & Zraick, R. (2018). *Best practices in healthcare simulations in communication sciences and disorders* [E-reader Version]. Retrieved from http://www.capcsd.org/wp-content/uploads/2018/05/Simulation-Guide-Published-May-18-2018.pdf

Family Educational Rights and Privacy Act of 1974, 20 U.S.C. § 1232g (1974).

Georges, J., Belz, N., & Potter, K. (2006). Telepractice program for dysphagia: Urban and rural perspectives from Kansas. *ASHA Leader*, 11(15), 12–13. Retrieved from http://www.asha.org/Publications/leader/2006/061107/061107d.htm

Goldman, R., & Fristoe, M. (2015). *Goldman-Fristoe Test of Articulation–Third Edition* (GFTA-3). Circle Pines, MN: American Guidance Service.

Google Calendar. (2009). [Computer software]. Retrieved from https://www.google.com/calendar

Google Drive. (2012). [Computer software]. Retrieved from https://www.google.com/drive/

Happy Moose Apps, Inc. (2019). Bitsboard Flashcards & Games (36.8.1) [Mobile application software]. Retrieved from https://itunes.apple.com/us/app/bitsboard-flashcards-games/id516842210?mt=8

Houn, B., & Trottier, K. (2006). Telepractice brings treatment to rural North Dakota. *ASHA Leader*, *11*(16), 16–17. Retrieved from http://www.asha.org/Publications/leader/2006/061128/061128f/

Houston, K. T., & Muñoz, K. (2010). Workshop features telepractice programs for EHDI. *ASHA Leader*, 15(6), 5–6. Retrieved from http://www.asha.org/Publications/leader/2010/100518/Telepractice-Programs-EHDI.htm

Huckvale, M. (2012). Waveforms Annotations Spectrograms and Pitch (WASP) [Computer program]. Version 1.54. Retrieved from https://www.phon.ucl.ac.uk/resource/sfs/wasp.php

IOPI. (2011). [Medical device]. Retrieved from https://iopimedical.com/

Jones, C., Ramanau, R., Cross, S., & Healing, G. (2010). Net generation or digital natives: Is there a distinct new generation entering university? *Computers & Education*, *54*(3), 722–732.

Krumm, M. (2005). Audiology telepractice moves from theory to treatment. *ASHA Leader*, *10*(15), 22–25. Retrieved from http://www.asha.org/Publications/leader/2005/051108/051108f/

Krumm, M., Ribera, J., & Froelich, T. (2002, June 11). Bridging the service gap through audiology telepractice. *ASHA Leader*, 7(11), 6–7. Retrieved from http://www.asha.org/Publications/leader/2002/020611/f020611_2a/

Laerdal Medical. (n.d.). *Simulation & training.* Retrieved from https://www.laerdal.com/us/products/simulation-training/

LessonPix. (2011). [Computer software]. Retrieved from http://lessonpix.com/

Little Bee Speech. (2018). Articulation Station (2.6.2) [Mobile application software]. Retrieved from https://itunes.apple.com/us/app/articulation-station/id467415882?mt=8

Mashima, P. A. (2010). Using telehealth to treat combat-related traumatic brain injury. *ASHA Leader*, 15(13), 10–14. Retrieved from http://www.asha.org/Publications/leader/2010/101102/Using-Telehealth-to-Treat-Combat-RelatedTraumatic-Brain-Injury.htm

MED-EL. (2016). ADHEAR. Retrieved from https://www.medel.com/us/adhear/

Miller, J. F., & Nockerts, A. (n.d.). Systematic Analysis of Language Transcripts (SALT) [Computer software]. Retrieved from https://www.saltsoftware.com/

PCG Education. (n.d.). *IEP online.* Retrieved from https://xeponline.wa-k12.net/Account/LogOn?ReturnUrl=/

Pearson Education. (n.d.). *Speech and language.* Retrieved from https://www.pearsonclinical.com/language.html

Prensky, M. (2001). Digital natives, digital immigrants. *On the Horizon*, *9*(5). Retrieved from http://

www.marcprensky.com/writing/prensky%20-%20
digital%20natives,%20digital%20 immigrants%20
%20part1.pdf

Prentke Romich Company. (2019). LAMP Words
For Life (2.17.3) [Mobile application software].
Retrieved from https://itunes.apple.com/us/app/
lamp-words-for-life/id551215116?mt=8

Seaman, J., Allen, E., & Seaman, J. (2018). *Grade
increase: Tracking distance education in the United
States*, Babson Survey Research Group. Retrieved
from https://onlinelearningsurvey.com/reports/
gradeincrease.pdf

Seesaw Learning Inc. (2019). Seesaw: The Learning
Journal (6.2.1) [Mobile application software].
Retrieved from https://itunes.apple.com/us/app/
seesaw-the-learning-journal/id930565184?mt=8

Shah, D. (2018, November 21). *By the numbers:
MOOCS in 2017—Class central*. Retrieved
from https://www.class-central.com/report/
mooc-stats-2017/

Simucase. (2017). [Computer software]. Retrieved
from https://www.simucase.com/

Skype. (2003). [Computer software]. Retrieved from
https://www.skype.com/en/

Slack. (2013). [Computer software]. Retrieved from
https://slack.com/

SMART Board (n.d.) [Computer technology].
Retrieved from https://education.smarttech.com/

StoryMagic, Inc. (2017). Epic! (3.35) [Mobile application software]. Retrieved from https://itunes.apple
.com/us/app/epic/id719219382?mt=8

Tactus Therapy Solutions Ltd. (2012). Spaced
Retrieval Therapy (1.1) [Mobile application
software]. Retrieved from https://play.google
.com/store/apps/details?id=com.tactustherapy
.srt&hl=en_US

TheraSimplicity. (1998). [Computer software].
Retrieved from http://www.therasimplicity.com/
Default.aspx

United States. (2004). The Health Insurance
Portability and Accountability Act (HIPAA).
Washington, DC: U.S. Dept. of Labor, Employee
Benefits Security Administration.

Vayo, E., Ingram, S., Doyle, C., & Ingram, R. (2018,
November). *Augmented reality for at-home speech
and language intervention*. Presentation at the
American Speech-Language-Hearing Association
Conference; Boston, MA.

WaveSurfer. (2012). [Computer software]. Retrieved
from https://sourceforge.net/projects/wavesurfer/

WebEx. (1995). [Computer software]. Retrieved from
https://www.webex.com/

Wiig, E. H., Semel, E., & Secord, W. A. (2013).
*Clinical Evaluation of Language Fundamentals–Fifth
Edition* (CELF-5). Bloomington, MN: NCS
Pearson.

Williams, S. (2008, November 19). *WIRED for success:
Digital games, simulations and virtual worlds for
language and literacy instruction*. Paper presented at
the American Speech-Language-Hearing Association Convention, Chicago.

Resources

20 Great project management tools. (n.d.). http://www
.webdesignbooth.com/project-management-tools/

American Board of Audiology.
https://www.boardofaudiology.org/

American Speech-Language Hearing Association.
http://www.asha.org

American Speech-Language Hearing Association.
(n.d.). *Health information privacy: Frequently
asked questions*. https://www.asha.org/practice/
reimbursement/hipaa/privacy/

American Speech-Language-Hearing Association.
(n.d.). *Special Interest Group 18, Telepractice*. http://
www.asha.org/SIG/18/

American Speech-Language-Hearing Association.
(n.d.). *Telepractice for SLPs and audiologists*. http://
www.asha.org/practice/telepractice/

American Telemedicine Association. https://www
.americantelemed.org/about-us/

Boersma, P., & Weenink, D. (n.d.). *Praat: Doing
phonetics by computer*. http://www.fon.hum.uva.nl/
praat/

Cognitive Training Software. (2011). *BrainTrain*.
http://www.braintrain.com

Cohn, E., & Watzlaf, V. (2011). Privacy and internet-
based telepractice. *Perspectives on Telepractice, 1,*
26–37.

Copyright Clearance Center, Inc. (n.d.). Resource
Library http://www.copyright.com/learn/
resource-library/?topic-keywords=copyright-in-the-
classroom&media-type=&professional-area

Council of Academic Programs in Communication
Sciences and Disorders, Free Online Courses
in Clinical Education. http://www.capcsd.org/
clinical-education-courses/

George Lucas Educational Foundation. (n.d). http://
www.edutopia.org

SimuCase. (2011). http://www.simucase.com

Society for Information Technology & Teacher Education. http://site.aace.org/

28

Counseling

◇◇

Michael Flahive, PhD

Introduction

The addition of this chapter to *Professional Issues in Speech-Language Pathology and Audiology* is welcomed. Practitioners from the very earliest days of the professions have recognized that individuals who have a communication disorder and members of their families experience challenging emotional repercussions. Speech-language pathologists (SLPs) and audiologists (AuDs) need to be prepared to provide responses to these challenges with the same levels of skill and confidence as are applied to management of the disorders themselves. This chapter has a slightly different approach than some of the other chapters in this edition. It presents recommendations for optimizing information exchanges, building working relationships and advancing a conceptual framework for addressing emotional needs and functional procedures that support this essential service. The reason for this difference is intentional in that the methods for obtaining the knowledge and skills required for effective counseling are not necessarily well documented by academic programs to date. This situation will also be discussed later in the chapter.

The critical thinking section provides several exercises to challenge readers. These will underscore the importance of practical approaches to problem solving, addressing the "how to respond?" questions that follow diagnosis and accompany treatment.

Considering Your Personal Experiences

Before delving into counseling content, it is suggested that readers take a moment to consider personal experiences in working through "crises." These might include health conditions, growth and development concerns for ourselves or family members, or about relationships, personal or professional. The suggestion is being made because our learning will require introspection. Our objective will be to comprehend the scope and depth of a condition along with sensitivity to the consequences and human responses to them. This chapter seeks to prompt learning that goes beyond accumulation of facts—it will require calling on the emotional responses we have as humans. Be prepared to imagine!

Historical Context of Counseling in Audiology and Speech-Language Pathology

Let's place the provision of counseling services in context. The American Speech-Language-Hearing Association (ASHA) has identified counseling as a clinical service that SLPs and AuDs provide their clients. Specific charges are detailed in each profession's Scope of Professional Practice (ASHA, 2016, 2018). Scopes of practice and preferred practice documents seek to clarify the aspirations of professions to the general public,

support agencies, and members of other professions. Table 28–1 provides specific language included in each of the current Scope of Practice documents.

Bulleted points in the Audiology Scope of Practice distinguish between "informational counseling" and "adjustment counseling." This distinction will inform the model of counseling described in what follows.

History of the Scopes of Practice

Detail regarding the evolution of the Scope of Professional Practice is found in Chapter 2 of this text, "Professional Issues: A View from History." The reader is

Table 28–1. Scope of Practice Charges Related to Counseling

Audiologists engage in the following activities when counseling individuals and their families:

- Providing informational counseling regarding interpretation of assessment outcomes and treatment options
- Empowering individuals and their families to make informed decisions related to their plan of care
- Educating the individual, the family, and relevant community members
- Providing support and/or access to peer-to-peer groups for individuals and their families
- Providing individuals and their families with skills that enable them to become self-advocates
- Providing adjustment counseling related to the psychosocial impact on the individual
- Referring individuals to other professionals when counseling needs fall outside those related to auditory, balance, and other related disorders. (ASHA, 2018)

SLPs counsel by providing education, guidance, and support. Individuals, their families and their caregivers are counseled regarding acceptance, adaptation, and decision making about communication, feeding and swallowing, and related disorders. The role of the SLP in the counseling process includes interactions related to emotional reactions, thoughts, feelings, and behaviors that result from living with the communication disorder, feeding and swallowing disorder, or related disorders. SLPs engage in the following activities in counseling persons with communication and feeding and swallowing disorders and their families:

- Empower the individual and family to make informed decisions related to communication or feeding and swallowing issues.
- Educate the individual, family, and related community members about communication or feeding and swallowing disorders.
- Provide support and/or peer-to-peer groups for individuals with disorders and their families.
- Provide individuals and families with skills that enable them to become self-advocates.
- Discuss, evaluate, and address negative emotions and thoughts related to communication or feeding and swallowing disorders.
- Refer individuals with disorders to other professionals when counseling needs fall outside of those related to (a) communication and (b) feeding and swallowing. (ASHA, 2016)

advised to visit Chapter 2 because Scope of Practice statements are vital to contemporary professional function. Note, early versions of these statements spoke to professional activities by SLPs and AuDs in one voice. Individual statements for each profession then evolved as the professions grew and required specificity of roles and responsibilities. There are now two scope of practice statements, one for each profession.

Linking Counseling to Clinical Practice and Educational Training

Counseling has not always been an identified component of our skills list as a recognition of a need to value has taken time. One reason the evolution has experienced a slow trajectory may have been the long-standing reluctance to embrace counseling as a service SLPs and AuDs are sufficiently prepared to deliver. One explanation may simply be that there was not a perceived need to address feelings and emotions. Providers did not consider our background as essential in addressing the emotional aspects of treatment, as training efforts focused solely on remediation of mechanical or linguistic issues. Further, training programs were not directed toward learning how to foster emotional adjustment in clients in the clinical setting.

An associated explanation may reflect traditional roles served by other helping professions; psychology, social work and medical specialists. Each has a long track record in helping with individuals reacting to traumatic events and early providers may have been persuaded to avoid professional overlap. These disciplines may also have protected their perceived treatment territory, adversely influencing development of counseling skills in our professions. Over time, SLPs and AuDs have been successful in negotiating our rightful place among helpers as we are in the best position to counsel individuals regarding issues of communication dysfunction.

The extent to which counseling preparation can be identified in graduate program curricula varies. The Council on Academic Accreditation in Speech Pathology and Audiology (CAA) Accreditation Standard 3.0 (Council on Academic Accreditation, American Speech-Language-Hearing Association, 2019) requires educational experiences resulting in entry-level knowledge and skill. Experiences may take a variety of forms, including didactic coursework and/or clinical skill development. The CAA reviews preparation programs routinely and requires compliance with the requirement. Details regarding institutional methods of compliance are not routinely available, however.

Requisite Knowledge and Skill and Expectations

SLPs and AuDs frequently report being drawn to the professions by an interest in a helping career. There are different means to achieve this admirable objective. Several expectations are typically assigned to SLPs and AuDs. At the core is a genuine respect for the integrity of others, those who are the recipients of services. Accreditation standard vernacular discusses core attributes as "knowledge and skills" (Council on Academic Accreditation, American Speech-Language-Hearing Association, 2019). Holland and Nelson (2013) list the following as important knowledge areas:

- Maintain knowledge base
- Know time course
- Know patterns of change
- Problems that usually accompany
- Knowledge of resources

Each of these knowledge areas is covered in the sections below.

Maintain Knowledge Base

Clinicians enter the workplace with credentials and documents attesting to their preparation. Typically, this is an earned graduate degree, licensure and certification. The latter two are regulatory and vary by jurisdiction. Other considerations in obtaining a clinical position include experience with similar populations, special skills, and personal characteristics deemed important to the hiring agency. Various chapters in this volume provide detail regarding finding employment and building one's career. The bottom line is an expectation that entry-level service providers have sufficient background, skills, and temperament to be successful in the position they have secured.

There is a recognized need to have continuing educational experiences as SLPs and AuDs are in dynamic professions with ongoing research contributions that influence assessment, decision making, and provision of services. It is incumbent upon each provider to update their clinical knowledge on regular basis. National certification such as ASHA's Certificate of Clinical Competence (ASHA, 2019) and state-level regulatory agencies licensure requirements specify continuing education in an effort to assure consumers that practitioners are maintaining currency with respect to contemporary practices. Chapter 3 of this text addresses issues of licensure and certification.

After the initial hire, employers anticipate that SLPs and AuDs will increase their knowledge and skills, becoming focused on issues that impact the quality of service to the clientele being served. For example, school-based entry-level SLPs would likely be ready to assess children who have been identified as being at risk and that, as providers, they will have a variety of assessment plans alongside different approaches for addressing frequently occurring communication issues. This focused technical information can be obtained from first-hand practical experiences in training (e.g., practicum experience), mentors in new work settings, in-service training activities, professional conferences, etc.

In the context of informational counseling, the expectation is that clinicians are sufficiently knowledgeable to inform clients and families about issues being evaluated and, when appropriate, to discuss outcomes of evaluations and options in response to those outcomes. Inherent in the information exchanges is a general sensitivity to the potential impact the "news" may have on the individual and family members. If we engage in the suggested reflection activities ourselves, we will likely sense some of the emotional reactions that clients and their families may experience.

Knowing Time Course

It is important that clinicians have knowledge of the time course related to the condition being evaluated. For example, an SLP assessing a 3-year-old child who has been referred for a repaired bilateral, complete cleft of the lip and palate will need to fully appreciate the time window for this type of diagnosis. This background will certainly influence the kinds of questions to be asked regarding the child's birth-to-3 history, and the parents' knowledge of what the journey may look like to them. They will also serve to establish assessment procedures and treatment planning for the future. The information provided at this juncture will also be important to the family in making short-term and long-term decisions. And, yes, information to be shared has the potential to influence the overall mental well-being of both the client and the family.

Knowing Patterns of Change

One ongoing aspect of our engagement with clients is to monitor "current status" and to identify needs to adjust intervention activities. Over time, clinicians will build their experience base in concert with the accumulated knowledge of conditions, interventions and reactions. Observational experience, whether with familiar clients or from observing others, allows us to learn about patterns of change. Developing an understanding of patterns of change, typically with the assistance of mentors

early in your career, will provide you with a greater sense of what is working with regard to clinical judgments.

Problems That Often Accompany

Holland and Nelson (2013) caution that clinicians need to anticipate issues that may accompany the communication problem, the so-called "ripple effects." For example, the child with a variety of speech distortions may be difficult to understand and is subject to ridicule in school. Likewise, the adult with aphasia may no longer be capable of doing the family's finances and loses that role. The astute clinician will be sensitive to these related issues as they may have a negative effect on treatment outcomes over time.

Knowledge of Resources

Effective clinicians improve their professional credibility by building a list of local resources and revisiting the list on an ongoing basis. This topic is addressed later in this chapter.

In addition to knowledge expectations and use of appropriate resources, there are personal attributes that support skills critical to success in the counseling process, including: empathy, objectivity, humor, resourcefulness, integrity, ethics, and communication skills.

Optimizing Information Exchanges

As you have read, the section on our knowledge base ended with "Knowledge of Resources." It is sometimes assumed that counseling is "relaying and collecting information" and nothing more. However, nothing could be farther from reality for the experienced clinician. In this next section, there is a discussion of information exchanges in the context of counseling. This is followed by the consideration of personal strengths and their role in a model of personal adjustment counseling. You will observe that information-gathering and dissemination may appear more concrete than other areas of personal adjustment counseling. However, remaining patient and mindful as you practice as a new clinician will help you grow and develop your skills on a broader level.

Gathering and Giving Information

Information exchange refers to the activities of gathering and giving information and is a crucial, ongoing component of clinical care. It is assumed that professionals have developed competence in gathering information (e.g., interviewing, taking case histories) and giving information (e.g., sharing assessment outcomes, proposing treatment goals, reviewing prognosis, discussing therapy plans). Professional preparation in both academic courses such as "diagnostic methods" and "assessment" and in clinical training experiences are likely to have focused on techniques of interviewing and the efficient and effective provision of information. The value of information exchanges is valuable strategically as it represents an important opportunity for building our credibility. If successful in interviewing and informing our client and their family, we establish ourselves as a meaningful ally. It is important to recognize the exchanges of information with clients from different cultural backgrounds as well. Multicultural sensitivity and strategies in response to cultural differences are critical. See Chapter 25 for more information on cultural diversity in our practice.

Information exchange is guided by the need to develop a strong working relationship between the clinician, the person with the communication disorder, and the family. It is most helpful to know and value the family's view of the client's condition and how that is likely to change over time. While not typically evaluated, SLPs and AuDs should possess a minimal level of social engagement competence. This is not to suggest that all students should have similar temperaments, rather an acknowledgement that there is a place for consideration of engagement style as a measure of successful treatment.

Gathering Information

Gathering information is a routine component to clinical practice. In your own experience with health care providers, for example, you have likely been asked "How may I be of help to you?" or a similar question, providing an opportunity to state your concerns and symptoms. Investigating concerns regarding behavior involve gathering background detail, such as the case history interview. Experience suggests active dialogue and frank exchanges of specific information help inform the provider while fostering confidence in the clinician. Interviews, in this context, are directed conversations in which the clinician's personal engagement style can play an important role. Exchanges also prompt clients and family members to visit and revisit needs for sharing detail.

Texts in assessment are replete with sample case history forms. Case histories vary in design, some seeking general information, others may be specific to particular diagnoses. Implicit is the prospect of continued gathering of data as the working relationship progresses—as we move further along in "understanding" there is likely a need for additional detail, as the process is often a dynamic one.

Giving Information

One traditional component of counseling is providing information to clients and their families about the nature, causes, and prognosis of communication disorders, as well as about the goals and processes of therapy. Various workplace demands may result in limited attention to this responsibility. Be aware that time constraints may result in an inadvertent information "dump and run" in which the information is given in terms too technical for laypeople. It will be important to infuse measures of comprehension, such as active listening techniques, into the information sharing conversation to prevent this scenario.

There are numerous options for information exchanges including the internet. While the internet is a valuable tool, readers are cautioned that it is also home to misinformation. Clinicians should possess listings of dependable, comprehensive resource materials to share with clients when providing informational counseling. Sources of reliable information include professional organizations such as the American Speech-Language-Hearing Association (ASHA) and the American Academy of Audiology (AAA). Organizational membership invests in the development and provision of material that can be provided clients and their families to support better understanding of causes and treatments of conditions. Materials from national professional societies are vetted for their accuracy, important in learning and in maintaining our credibility. Other resources include written material in addition to various media.

It is suggested that listings of resources be provided early in the working relationship, perhaps as part of the evaluation process. Selected documents can then be recommended that will be helpful in educating clients and their families. There are also resource materials prepared by clinicians that have been developed over years of work with particular clinical groups, such as autism and cleft palate, Down syndrome, etc. A number of blogs currently exist that are maintained by clinicians in the field, frequently sharing provider "nuggets" of valuable information. The same cautions are posited as previously noted regarding the accuracy and quality of online material.

It is recommended that students begin to accumulate listings of reference and even handout materials to provide direction when there is call for expanding the knowledge base of new clients. These instructional exchanges will be part of the working relationship, as we ultimately want our clients and their families to become experts in the disorder being addressed. Be mindful of the fact that credibility may be enhanced or diminished as a function of the material recommended to clients.

Information Retention. The primary objective of information giving is for the client and family to benefit from our knowledge relative to their condition. Therefore, it is important that they comprehend the information we wish to share. It is easy to make assumptions about the extent of success in the back-and-forth of the information sharing process, but these assumptions may not be legitimate.

In a classic online review of study results on information retention, Margolis (2004) reported that, in many cases, patients immediately forget 50% of what they are told by clinicians and over time misunderstand most of what is retained. This may come as a surprise; however, consider one's own experience, perhaps with a familiar health care provider.

Table 28–2 summarizes Margolis' observations regarding information retention and our clients. It is note-worthy that a number of studies Margolis investigated suggested intelligence does not appear to play a role in retaining information. At the same time anxiety and denial appear to be important variables for clients.

Several ideas related to the manner of presentation and client retention are listed in Table 28–3. One suggests being conscious of the primacy effect, that which is presented first. Those are more likely to be recalled than other facts. Another useful suggestion is the use of explicit categorization. Margolis provides an example utilizing this principle when summarizing a hypothetical client audiological visit—reviewing specific diagnostic activities, repeating results of the evaluation and the recommendations, in a step-by-step fashion. This concept should be familiar as clinicians utilize it with diagnostic protocols and many cognitive remediation practices. A third useful suggestion is the utility of tangible materials

---

Table 28–2. Recall Depends on Clients

- Intelligence has not been shown to affect the proportion of information retained.
- General familiarity with information does increase retention.
- A finding that one expects is more likely to be retained.
- A finding that is more desirable is more likely to be retained.
- Anxiety affects recall—high anxiety negatively influences recall, moderate anxiety may increase the probability of remembering.
- Denial may contribute to poor recall—or in the process of accurately representing information accurately to family members.
- Look for indicators of denial as it will impede progress.

Source: Based on information from Margolis, 2004.

Table 28–3. Recall Depends on Presentation

- Information presented in a simple, easy-to-understand format is better remembered.
- The more information presented, the less is recalled.
- Categorizing information improves recall.
- Consider the *primacy effect*.
- Margolis recommends a "method of explicit categorization."
- Prompt questions in each category prior to moving forward.
- Written/graphic material supplement information giving and enhance recall.

Source: Based on information from Margolis, 2004.

to be given to clients and their families. While contemporary technological advances have provided numerous online resources, Margolis values materials that can be handed directly to individuals. These serve to prompt conversation and information exchanges in the moment, increasing odds for provision of clarifying detail and in reading the client and the family for comprehension.

Additional information related to clinical style and information retention is listed in Table 28–4. These suggestions focus on the engagement components of the back and forth of information exchanges. For example, simple sentence structure and clear language are logical and would seem obvious. However, clinicians may occasionally drift into linguistic habits that cause clients and their family members to get lost and lose focus. Likewise, the implied importance of content we may be delivering suggests that the listener pay attention, increasing odds that the material will be retained. Again, Margolis notes the importance of handout material.

In addition, it may be important for clinicians to pay attention to the amount of information being provided at any one time. All of the suggestions posited merit our consideration if our goal is a more well-informed client and/or family member,

Gauging Client Understanding. It is recommended to expand the perspective of understanding to include a focus on the explanatory processes used by individuals with communication disorders and their families. Sample questions can include: What do you think caused your problem? What do you think this problem does to you? How severe is it? What kind of treatment do you think you should receive? What are the chief difficulties your problem has caused for you? What do you fear most about your problem? Tactics for gauging the level of understanding will be important in maximizing the information exchange as well as in guiding the assembly of resources to promote additional learning.

Measuring Effectiveness in Information Exchange

After considering the provision of information in effective ways, another important concern is how we measure effectiveness in information sharing. Many listeners will smile and nod when provided content, whether understanding or not. Humans often find it difficult to admit to not comprehending. Where does this leave us? Should you directly quiz? Why or why not? What about specific assignments as checks?

One potential approach is the "teach-back" method (Dinh et al., 2016). This is a confirmation tactic used in health care and education to ensure individuals understand what is being explained to them. The premise is that if individuals understand, they are able to teach content back accurately. Perhaps readers can recall elementary school experiences when a teacher prompted a "tell me what this means?" or "what did I just say?" The approach should be employed when the working relationship allows for comfortable back-and-forth.

We shall also see that support groups can serve as additional sources for information sharing. One important function of support groups is to mediate challenges in receiving information comfortably, in circumstances not as intimidating as a one-to-one encounter where one may feel put on the spot. Support groups also afford opportunities for brainstorming possible solutions.

A Caution

Luterman (2017) cautions about the amount of information provided early in a working relationship, believing that an overabundance might foster a dependency on the clinician as a necessary source of direction. Being perceived this way may send a message about inadequacy of the client or family. Implicit in this consideration is

---

Table 28–4. Recall Depends on the Clinician

- Convey information with simple sentence structure and clear language.
- Determine what the individual or family member want to learn and their level of understanding—this requires LISTENING.
- Information presented as more important will more likely be recalled—style of delivery makes a difference.
- Written/graphic material supplement information giving and enhance recall.

Source: Based on information from Margolis, 2004.

skill at "reading" client and family understanding. This may require particular focus in preparation or early in a work career.

Building Working Relationships: Identifying Our Strengths and Developing Our Skills

Now that we have reviewed how information plays a role in counseling, it is reasonable to move forward and consider how personal strengths and other skills may assist the clinician in becoming even more effective in the clinical exchange. Although this area may appear less concrete than dealing with information, it is critical to the success of those we serve.

An important factor in the clinical dynamic is the relative strengths of the clinician, as noted by a number of authors, including Luterman (2017) and Holland and Nelson (2013). One method for examining personal strengths is the *Values in Action* survey, described as:

> The Values in Action (VIA) Survey of Character Strengths is a 240-item face-valued self-report questionnaire intended for use with adults. The measure uses 5-point Likert-style items to measure the degree to which respondents endorse items reflecting the 24 strengths of character that comprise the VIA Classification. The survey takes about 25 minutes to complete, although there is no time limit. It has been completed by over 5 million individuals world-wide. It is at no cost on the Positive Psychology website *Authentic Happiness.* (https://www.authentichappiness.sas.upenn.edu/)

This tool focuses on positive personality attributes and may prove valuable in organizing one's own personal conceptual framework. There is also great potential in employing survey results as a motivator with adult clients. One activity in the critical thinking section of this chapter involves working with the VIA survey.

We can also consider our strengths in the context of skills that we can develop within the context of counseling. Flasher and Fogle's text *Counseling Skills for Speech-Language Pathologists and Audiologists* (2012) includes an extensive chapter on interviewing and utilization of microskills. Their description of microskills, taken from Ivey (1998):

> Microskills is a term used in counseling psychology that refers to specific communication skills that help clinicians interact more intentionally with clients, that is, to thoughtfully but quickly choose

responses to the client from a wide range of possibilities. (p. 126)

Brammer and McDonald's classic text *The Helping Relationship: Process and Skills* (8th ed., 2003) was written to help caregivers' function more effectively by focusing on communication skills important in relationships. It emphasizes self-help and improved coping skills. They note that microskills training emphasizes learning individual skills. This is accomplished by observing good models of helping behavior followed by directed practice, during which a supervisor can reward or assist in modifying student performance. Skills are then employed in the "artful act of helping," moving from practice to real life. Ideally, improvement in microskill utilization should continue to develop throughout a career.

Microskills important to SLPs and AuDs include but are not limited to open-ended and close-ended questions, affirmation, reflection, clarification, reframing, paraphrasing, and silence. Microskills support these actions. Appendix 28–A contains detail regarding microskills.

Advancing a Conceptual Framework for Addressing Emotional Needs: Personal Adjustment Counseling

In addition to our responsibilities for providing information and using our microskills, we are also charged to discuss, evaluate, and address negative emotions and thoughts related to communication or feeding and swallowing disorders. (ASHA, 2016). Our goal in this chapter is to become sensitized to the probable impact of communication disorders on the lives of the client and members of their families and to react accordingly. Holland and Nelson (2013) note, "we help persons live productively- with the communication problem or despite them or around them." (p. 1). Attending, in detail, to the "what to do?" questions for specific disorders will be beyond our efforts here. Instead, we will review principles of helping with adjustment while addressing communication disorders.

At the outset of this chapter it was suggested that we imagine a challenging hypothetical scenario resulting in a communication disorder. While onset may be gradual or the result of an immediate crisis, the potential communication component would likely have a major impact on the ability to maintain essential life connections. Specialists in communication disorders arguably are in the strongest position to assist the individual clinically while simultaneously attending to reactions that accompany the condition. Holland and Nelson (2013) identify this responsibility as *communication counseling*. Flasher and Fogle (2012, p. 5) indicate that in the many and varied interactions, while not counseling per se, counseling behaviors may be utilized. It is imperative that we are prepared to address clinical and emotional needs, either in direct communication counseling or utilizing particular counseling behaviors. Emotional considerations addressed in the following areas are in the context of loss, and reaction to loss, with a focus on grieving and depression.

Loss and Reactions to Loss

Consider the concept of loss as it relates to your imagined catastrophe. You may experience shock having just received confirmation of an existing communication problem. Luterman (2017) discusses the typical mental balance between our emotional self and intellectual self. In reacting to a catastrophe, you are likely to experience a strong movement in one or another of these directions—a highly emotional reaction or a more focused attempt to understand what has occurred. In any case, confusion and disorientation may be paramount. As clinicians, we should ask ourselves if we fully appreciate the magnitude of information we share with clients and their families. In our imagined scenario, what responses should we be expecting from ourselves, our clients, and their family members?

In responding to the question of how humans react to these major life events, it is highly likely there is a sense of loss. Loss is defined as real or perceived deprivation of something deemed meaningful (Humphrey, 2009, p. 5). A natural consequence of loss is grief. It is essential that we accept the presence of grieving as it will be a consideration with the individuals we are serving.

Returning to reflection, it is likely that most of us have experienced the death of family members or other important people in our lives. In the immediate aftermath of such an event, there would be a range of reactions that one would typically experience. The death itself is considered a form of primary loss. A secondary loss would refer to other, associated outcomes related to the death. The person who died may have been a parent, representing a significant loss in our lives. With such a loss we may experience the loss of companionship, the source of advice and counsel, economic supports and any number of other connections that relate to the role the individual played in our personal constellation. There is another type of loss: symbolic. According to Flasher and Fogle (2012) symbolic loss involves the loss of self-esteem or professional standing. In the case of the loss of a parent, a symbolic dimension may well be status associated with being "Charlie's boy" or other relationships with the deceased.

Grieving

Life experiences afford many the opportunity to learn, first-hand, about the repercussions of catastrophic events. The aforementioned ideas related to loss lead to the process of grieving. Webster (1961) defines *grieving* as "to feel sorrow" (p. 364).

Elizabeth Kubler-Ross, author of the classic text *Death and Dying* (1969), wrote extensively on the experiences of the terminally ill. Her research resulted in the identification of five stages of the grieving process: denial, anger, bargaining, depression, and acceptance. These emotions do not necessarily occur in sequence or independently of one another. The result of her work is a general roadmap regarding the human emotional condition. We should consider these stages in our reflections on reactions to our hypothetical catastrophic life events.

Consider Kubler-Ross's stages in the scenario of the identification of significant hearing loss in a toddler. Although early identification of hearing loss has become standard practice as a result of legislation, it is still possible that a hearing loss may not be identified during infancy. Upon confirmation of the diagnosis of hearing loss there may be a strong reaction on the part of the parents and other family members.

Denial typically emerges first, as the diagnosis was not anticipated and may come as a shock. One can easily imagine, as evidence is gathered, that anger is not far behind. Anger may not be particularly focused, as parents may be angry with themselves, with those providing the diagnosis, or with any other conceivable entity, for that matter. Each of us has experienced anger at one time or another in our lives. If we reflect on how that time was resolved, it likely included a period of "cooling off" along with supports from those around us. The nature of the support will be most powerful if it acknowledges the anger and the disappointment that it brings. In those moments it is likely not productive to try to identify with what the individual is going through, as we are not personally experiencing their anger. This is where the technique of active listening makes an impact; where we acknowledge that we understand their anger and that we are there for them now and when they want to talk about moving forward.

Bargaining may emerge in a variety of forms or, perhaps, not at all. It would not be unusual for a client or family member to test the waters with attempts at minimizing the extent of an issue, perhaps in situations where there is not absolute clarity. An example of this might be a language delay. The primary clinical objective in this situation is for the client or family to come to the table and learn more about the condition and the prognostic potentials. That said, reliance on facts will be paramount as you help them understand the course of events. Conversation may evolve into a series of "if/then" discussions with the ultimate objective of acceptance.

Depression

Depression should be a concern in our professional practice. We continuously work with individuals who may be experiencing psychological reactions to their current state that result in feelings of sadness, lack of self-esteem, diminished focus and attention, and possible physical symptoms such as loss of appetite. It is important to recognize the association of communication disorders and depression and learned helplessness (Maier & Seligman, 1976). Communication disorders have the potential for resulting in reactive depression for both the affected person and his or her family members. We may also find concomitant depression among persons with acquired disorders, resulting from brain damage. And, yes, some individuals may come to their communication disorder already having depression (Holland & Nelson, 2013).

Depression is a diagnosis made by qualified mental health or medical personnel. Speech-language pathologists and audiologists are not trained to perform these evaluations nor provide specific treatment for this (*ICD-10 classification of mental and behavioural disorders: Clinical descriptions and diagnostic guidelines.* Geneva: World Health Organization, 1992). We are careful to practice within the boundaries of our license and Scopes of Practice. These boundaries do not limit the probability that we will encounter individuals who are suffering from depression and we need to be alert to behavioral signs that might require a referral for qualified professional help. It is recommended that one's list of professional resources include this category of information.

Your Role in Personal Adjustment Counseling

Luterman's (2017) disposition is that the role of counseling is to help individuals feel more empowered, <u>not</u> necessarily to make them happy. Instead we help them deal with the problem they are confronting, assisting in making better decisions. The ultimate objective of our client support is to reach a level of acceptance of the condition. This allows both the client and the family to move forward, exploring where they are currently and where the process of development or recovery is going. It opens the door to the important steps of building resilience and optimism.

It is Luterman's opinion that the traditional "medical model" does not appear appropriate for counseling in communication disorders. The approach is not collaborative, as the "expert" controls all aspects of assessment, diagnosis and treatment. His concern is that this approach creates a dependency on the clinician to make decisions for the client and family. This is in direct contrast with the belief that clinicians should be fostering less dependency as adjustment progresses.

An additional aim is to foster an appropriate locus of control, that is, in fostering adjustment, we must assist the client in becoming more congruent. The next section reviews congruence and provides the reader with more context for clinical service delivery, particularly in the context of emotional adjustment.

Congruence

Congruence is a core condition in building relationships and is fundamental to the person-centered approach taken by the eminent psychologist Carl Rogers. It is about the clinician being genuine which is critically important to developing the kind of relationship Rogers believes will ultimately allow the individual to vent his emotions and help process information. Rogers (1986):

> It is that the individual has within himself or herself vast resources for self-understanding, for altering his or her self-concept, attitudes and self-directed behavior—and that these resources can be tapped if only a definable climate of facilitative psychological attitudes can be provided.

Central to Rogers' (1959) original theory is the notion of "self" or "self-concept." This is defined as "the organized, consistent set of perceptions and beliefs about oneself." It consists of all the ideas and values that characterize "I" and "me" and includes perception and valuing of "what I am" and "what I can do."

Client-centered therapy operates according to three basic principles that reflect the attitude of the therapist to the client:

1. The therapist is with the client.

2. The therapist provides the client with unconditional positive regard.

3. The therapist shows empathic understanding to the client.

Congruence is also called "genuineness" and is the most important attribute in counseling, according to Rogers. This means that unlike the psychodynamic therapist who generally maintains a "blank screen" and reveals little of their own personality in therapy, clinicians following Rogers allow clients to experience them as they really are. The therapist does not utilize a façade but is authentic.

Luterman notes that our objective is to help the person gain access to his feelings, not telling him how to feel. He is confident in humans' ability to regain homeostasis, the psychological balance between intellect and emotions.

Putting It Together

In the sixth edition of his text *Counseling Persons with Communication Disorders and Their Families* (2017), Luterman provides a critique of clinical activities with attention to opportunities for support to foster adjustment. He cautions that a medical model or institutional practice in assessment may limit the clinician's ability to gather information from family members or to build working relationships. Rather, he recommends a collaborative approach which will afford opportunities for family members to contribute to a collective understanding. At this time, he cautions to respect the needs for processing time, appreciating the "shock value" with trauma. Similarly, the potency of the news we may bring with the results of our evaluations also needs to be appreciated. He also cautions about "information overload," the possibility that we may inundate the client and family with too much information. As a result, Luterman prefers to minimize what he shares with clients and waits until they ask.

It is important to appreciate that when persons feel more personal power, they feel they control their own destiny, feeling less controlled by others. This defines an inner locus of control. Luterman's discussion regarding "locus of control" is insightful as it underscores the need for sensitivity in working toward the client having a sense of ownership and empowerment.

Luterman maintains an existential perspective—bad things happen in life. As helpers we need to avoid projecting possible solutions to problems based on how we would like to see things unfold. The process is about the client—Luterman's continuous mantra is "it's not about us" (2017).

Advancing a Conceptual Framework for Addressing Emotional Needs: Positive Psychology Approaches to Personal Adjustment Counseling

Holland and Nelson (2013) have a different perspective on assisting with personal adjustment. They are advocates of the positive psychology point of view, focused on what is right with people, not what is wrong with them. Recall the earlier quotation: "we help persons live productively—with the communication problem or despite them or around them" (p. 1). Their objective is

to identify strengths to assist in fostering optimism and building resilience.

Similar to others, Holland and Nelson (2013) value listening as fundamental to helping, advocating for initial attempts that try to understand how the world looks to the client. They do so by encouraging expression of feelings, concerns, anxieties, etc. This, of course, includes family members along with the client themselves. An important element, in their view, is providing information all parties will need to understand what has happened, assisting them in figuring out how to get on with their lives and live in a productive way—helping them translate information into satisfying and productive actions. Ultimately, they are interested in clients moving to acceptance and resolving initial reactions to the crisis.

Positive Psychology

The work of Martin Seligman has prompted the development and emergence of "positive psychology" as an alternative to historical perspectives on human behavior. The movement evolved from his work on "learned helplessness" (Maier & Seligman, 1976) followed by "learned optimism" (Seligman, 2006). He and his followers challenged traditional psychology to focus energy on mental wellness. Proponents note that happiness is not the opposite of depression, and that "not depressed" is not necessarily being happy. Their view is that psychologists ought to focus on what is *right* with human behavior and on how happiness can be increased

Holland and Nelson (2013) have embraced principles of positive psychology as they may work for persons with communication disorders. They propose this rationale:

- We shouldn't assume that physical disability or the course of aging necessarily have negative consequences.

- Human strengths can be described and measured.

- It is possible to use personal strengths to increase life satisfaction and happiness.

- People can be helped to develop resilience and optimism.

- Positive psychology represents an alternative to thinking about communication disorders through a "disease model" lens.

In their view there should be equal focus on maximizing strength and modulating or compensating for weakness. There is extensive information regarding positive psychology at the Authentic Happiness website (http://www.authentichappiness.org).

Operationalizing Communication Counseling

Holland and Nelson (2013) suggest that communication counselors appreciate their personal attributes. This is a principle that is shared by others in communication disorders (Flasher & Fogle, 2012; Luterman, 2017). At this point readers should be considering perspectives to assist with the building of one's own conceptual framework. What are values and themes that reflect your view? How would you best describe your personal ideology? Specialists in communication disorders and even those outside the field identify *listening* as an essential skill in facilitating interactions between clients, their families, and the professional provider. Wolven and Coakley (1982) provide extensive detail on the topic in their text entitled "Listening." In reviewing the history of definitions of listening, the authors cite no fewer than 15 different renditions. Kenneth O. Johnson (1951) defines it simply as "the ability to respond effectively to oral communication."

Wolven and Coakley outline several forms of listening: therapeutic listening, appreciative listening, critical listening, and discriminative listening. They provide detailed descriptions of physiologic, linguistic, cognitive, and pragmatic elements of the process. In the Wolven and Coakley model the category "therapeutic listening" appears most applicable to our interests. They indicate that therapeutic listening "requires the listener to discriminate and to comprehend the sender's message while providing the sender with a 'sounding board' to talk through his or her problems" (p. 109). As we shall see, this is exactly what different authors refer to, although specific terminology varies.

Rogers (2016) is among clinicians who have advanced the importance of listening. He embraced the idea of "empathic listening" when he wrote:

It means entering the private perceptual world of the other and becoming thoroughly at home in it. It involves being sensitive, moment by moment, to the changing felt meanings which flow in this other person, to the fear or rage or tenderness or confusion or whatever it is that he or she is experiencing. It means temporarily living in the other's life, moving about in it delicately, without making judgments.

To be effective, clinicians need to have a clear enough understanding of clients' struggles to assist them in finding solutions. This is a central tenet of the client-centered approach utilized by many helping professionals. Numerous authors among SLPs and AuDs subscribe to the client-centered model as fundamental to their conceptual framework. The reader is reminded that attention is being paid to fundamental issues as we move toward crystallizing our own conceptual framework for practice.

Brammer and MacDonald (2003) provide a full chapter devoted to helping skills for understanding in which they examine behaviors that promote understanding of self and others. Skills are organized into seven clusters: listening skills, leading skills, reflecting skills, challenging skills, interpreting skills, informing skills, and summarizing skills. Detail is then provided for subcomponents of the identified skill sets. "Listening" subskills include attending, paraphrasing, clarifying, and perception checking. These action verbs suggest that active or deep listening is not at all passive. Authors among SLPs and AuDs identify listening as paramount in the development of the clinical relationship. It is critically important, although labeled in various ways. We will refer to "active listening" for consistency, moving forward.

Building Working Relationships

Luterman (2017) notes that the essence of our counseling is to establish a relationship wherein persons have permission to feel as they need to by our validation of their feelings. This may be hard to do, but clinicians must trust that people have what Luterman calls "a marvelous capacity to make themselves feel better." At the same time, it is a tendency of humans to try and make the victim or the family feel better when catastrophe occurs. Be mindful of the fact that your actions may be telling them, in one way or another, that they shouldn't feel that way, taking away their permission to grieve. We also need to avoid falling into the standard comparisons trap, suggesting "it could be worse." Luterman's position is that what a person in pain needs most is someone to listen and to validate the experience.

Holland and Nelson (2013) talk about the importance of using stories to begin to understand how the world looks to the client or the family. This reinforces Rogers' suggestion that we need to understand the "perceptual world" of the client. Listening is incumbent in this process. They elicit stories to assist in the process of coming to a more detailed understanding of their condition. In addition to the value focused listening provides, there is a therapeutic benefit to repetition of the story regarding the clinical issue. The intensity of emotions frequently begins to become better managed with repetition.

Barriers to Listening Effectively

Among considerations surrounding the process are several potential barriers to listening actively. From the environmental perspective, the signal-to-noise ratio of the immediate environment may provide contaminants that make speech processing challenging. The listener may have a conflicting agenda and be unable to focus. The speaker may have speech and language characteristics that reduce intelligibility. If we are the speaker, we need to be cognizant, early on, of any and all inhibiting elements relative to our communicative exchanges. This includes various pragmatic considerations such as eye contact, use of microskills including affirmation and the sharing of self, when appropriate. Clinicians may need to actively mediate issues that inhibit focus and intensity required to qualify as active listening. It is incumbent upon us as experts to ensure optimal dialogue.

The Effective Working Relationship

In our early engagement with clients we encourage expression of feelings, anxieties, etc. The process of relationship building begins with the initial contact. For example, assessment activities are often positively influenced by family member participation. Clinicians can advance the developing relationship through efforts in information gathering that are engaging and collaborative. Active listening validates clients' concerns with issues they are facing and provides family members with critical supports. The effective working relationship can then assist in meeting our objective to foster resilience.

Mindfulness. Mindfulness is the psychological process of bringing one's attention to experiences occurring in the present. This may be achieved through the practice of meditation and other training. The concept has gained popularity as various "wellness movements" have advanced.

Proponents indicate that mindfulness may help individuals connect with the speaker, improve memory of events, and reduce errors through increased self-awareness, wherein one will experience the environment more deeply.

Listening mindfully helps us receive information, both verbal and nonverbal, and assists with retention. A caveat, however, is that it requires being open to hearing a message that may differ from our own and eliminating our personal agenda from the interaction. Listening also includes nonverbal elements, as body language may provide important signals about conversational flow and effectiveness of our efforts at mindful listening.

Mindfulness has been cited in speech-language pathology literature. Boyle (2011) provides a mindfulness training program for fluency management. Beck and Verrichio (2018) report on the effects of mindfulness practice with graduate and undergraduate students in communication sciences and disorders. Mindfulness

is also the topic of a number of online programs for personal and professional development. Rogers (1986) reinforces the concept of mindfulness by stating:

> It is that the individual has within himself or herself vast resources for self-understanding, for altering his or her self-concept, attitudes and self-directed behavior—and that these resources can be tapped if only a definable climate of facilitative psychological attitudes can be provided.

Building Our Conceptual Framework

The chapter introduction indicated content would be provided for (1) optimizing information exchanges, (2) building working relationships, and (3) advancing a conceptual framework for addressing emotional needs and functional procedures that support this essential service.

It is now time to organize a conceptual framework to support actions to be taken in the counseling process. "Conceptual framework" has been our term for personal philosophy. Readers are directed to Appendix 28–B, which provides brief summaries of major psychological theories for review. These may be helpful in conceptual framework design. Elements of these perspectives are likely familiar to most readers as fundamental information concerning human behavior is readily available. Whether evolving from general psychology classes or more focused coursework, our present charge is to identify a model or components of models to support our clinical decision making: the "why" of what we do.

If the reader is already an experienced clinician, you are encouraged to review the perspective from which your clinical decisions are made. Early on in practice it may be helpful to rely on models of other practitioners to support position development. The short-term objective is a "working hypothesis" which understandably is subject to change. Moving forward in practice it should be anticipated that modifications will occur as experience is gained and perspectives adjusted. Note, one major rationale for continuing professional education is to support continued development and prevent intellectual rigor mortis. Our professions are respected because they are dynamic and respond to evidence suggesting better options. Expect that you will always be evaluating new evidence to inform actions and beliefs.

Following is a review of what we've learned of Luterman and Holland and Nelson's philosophical dispositions. While reading, actively consider elements that you may care to adopt in your own conceptual framework. Readers are encouraged to examine these authors and others in communication disorders beyond this chapter.

Luterman

Luterman (2017) advocates an approach that promotes listening and valuing which, in turn, fosters empowerment that will be important in assisting the client in making better decisions. Our assistance will enable the client to have a stronger sense of control, a shift in the locus of control regarding the communication issue.

Luterman (2017) noted that early in his career, his use of a content-based approach provided material with which he was most familiar, but was not in the best interest of his clients. When families would be seen for follow-up, he realized they had not heard what he had said; that they had missed what he thought was a good explanation of conditions. While the approach was serving his need to provide detailed information, he felt it fostered a dependence. The result was an overwhelmed client and family that had not had their basic needs addressed, including time to process and grieve, gradually leading to acceptance. Luterman's observation was that in delivering bad news, families would go into a "fight or flight" mode, as they were not prepared to process catastrophic detail. He argues that, in retrospect, his provision of extensive detail was not what was most needed at the time, and was, in fact, self-serving. He opted to place greater emphasis on listening.

Luterman's outlook raises questions regarding the importance of informational counseling, or at least the timing of informational exchanges. He notes the importance of knowing the "feeling state" of the individual and their family. His philosophical perspective is that in order to be effective he needed to give himself permission to enter the client's feeling state. This is not to diminish the importance of giving information, rather it is a caution about when it is most appropriate to do so. His perspective is that clients and families will ask for information when they need it. He asserts that our role is not to help make people feel better, it is to validate their experience and to allow them to react naturally.

Thus, the essence of our counseling is to establish a relationship wherein persons have permission to feel as they need to feel by our validation of their feelings. Counseling essences include: (1) accepting the emotions as they come about and (2) enabling people to be empowered—be in a position to make decisions independent of us. Our responsibility, according to Luterman, is to build relationships that allow for the expression of feelings in addition to the content exchange that needs to take place and empowers.

Holland and Nelson

Holland and Nelson focus is on individuals and their needs, with equal focus on maximizing strength and modulating or compensating for weakness. This is dis- tinctly different from more medical model approaches which typically focus on modulating or compensating for weakness.

They also suggest that communication counselors understand their personal attributes. In their text *Counseling in Communication Disorders: A Wellness Perspective* (2013) they note: "A cornerstone of this book is that the counselor-clinician needs to know themselves" (p. 35). An exercise proposed in the Critical Thinking section of this chapter focuses on the determination of various personal attributes, a function of better knowing oneself. Results provide a list of personal strengths that may be enlightening or affirming and can be utilized in building and maintaining the conceptual framework.

The authors are straightforward in specifying our responsibilities in providing counseling. They note: "we help persons live productively—with the communication problem or despite them or around them" (p. 1). In making this assertion the assumption is that persons whom we counsel will otherwise be moving through life, absent the catastrophe. Persons with mental illness issues prior to a communication disorder pose different challenges and would require services from professionals qualified to work with the mental health concerns. In those circumstances we might be involved in a collaborative role. Our focus in this chapter has been on individuals for whom life is otherwise moving along reasonably well.

Holland and Nelson view the listening process as the first task in trying understand how the world looks to the client. As previously noted, stories are vehicles used to support this ambition. They also encourage the expression of feelings, concerns, anxieties, etc. while building the working relationship. They use phrases such as: "tell me about," or "what do you think about?" or "please describe" to prompt reactions and reflection.

A third role that we serve is in advising, that is, providing information that people need as they work to understand what has happened. They will need to learn how to get on with their lives and live in a productive way. They will also need assistance in translating information into satisfying and successful actions. According to Holland and Nelson, this may be the most challenging objective we face in our counseling roles. Lastly, they indicate that we assist in development of a healthy resolution of "crisis"—the catastrophe. This runs parallel to steps others identify in moving from identification, to acknowledgement, to acceptance, and to moving on.

Coaching. Holland and Nelson speak to the idea of coaching, analogous to the sideline directional activities found in sports. In this case, the clinician is offering support by directing versus being personally involved in each step of a process. The term has different interpretations depending on your view. The construct is occasionally applied when working with adults as many may have had life experiences reflecting a coaching model.

Other Considerations for a Personal Conceptual Framework

The following variables represent potential issues that will have influence in building one's conceptual framework and clinical practice, and should be considered.

One variable to consider is the age of the client when it comes to treatment approaches. For instance, what about providing personal adjustment facilitation activities with children? You would need to answer questions including: When are children old enough? How do we broach "feelings"? Should we work alongside school counselors or other professionals? How do we gauge feelings and measure success?

As an example, consider utilization of play therapy techniques, prompting children to talk about reactions they may be experiencing with a communication issue. While we may not be prepared to provide extensive treatment in this kind of scenario, exploring the issue may be essential to our understanding of the child's view. It may also be important for children to spend time with an adult who truly appears to understand their problems. SLPs and AuDs possess the knowledge and skills to build relationships with children as well as adults.

Such conversations may also provide the basis for referral to individuals trained to provide more in-depth counseling support. We need to be mindful of our scopes of practice and to feel comfortable in informing families of our strengths, limitations, and boundaries. Foremost in our relationships will be the primary recipient. It may be that if one's work situation is exclusively child based, particular attention may need to be devoted in continuing education to improve our knowledge and skills in this category of service provision.

Going Forward and Putting It Together

Thus far this chapter content has reviewed Scope of Practice mandates and placed the provision of counseling services in context. A model identifying informational and personal adjustment components has been posited and sources of support in each category have been identified and referenced. The works of Luterman and Holland and Nelson have been reviewed. Each has made extensive contributions in communication sciences and disorders specific to responsibilities professionals in audiology and speech-language pathology have

to clients and their families. References in psychology and other helping disciplines have also been cited as additional sources of support for developing a conceptual framework. This construct will be central to our clinical practice and we are now ready to identify principles aligned with the framework.

If already a practicing clinician, it is suggested that you engage in an internal audit regarding how you make clinical decisions. Simply put, what are the theories that drive the way you do the things you do? Consider logging your responses for reflection and review at a later date.

For those preparing to enter practice, learning about the philosophical principles that drive decision making may be a meaningful exercise. The following items are general recommendations that you may consider as you move forward. In addition, the scenarios provided in the Critical Thinking section may serve as helpful prompts on which to begin. The idea is to make internal deliberation as authentic as possible. Perhaps ideas could be floated with a colleague or supervisor—a form of "what would you do?" The goal is to engage in a realistic and challenging exercise.

Checklist of To Dos

Proposing or prescribing should be appreciated for what they are—ideas that may contribute to your success. This is not about *having to*, but rather what *might work* for you in your practice.

Reflection. One of the most helpful practices clinicians can undertake is reflection. The term is used here to indicate conscious introspection, the process of deliberately reviewing what has taken place and how successful (or not) it has been relative to our clearly defined objectives. Our formal preparation has likely focused on building "plans" which are roadmaps for objectives. Developing clinicians may be hard pressed to accomplish the planning process easily, but that does not negate the necessity. Rather, take comfort, experience teaches all of us how to build and build efficiently. We will rely on the wisdom of those overseeing our activities to support the build. Do not hesitate to consult those supervising as you experience the ups and downs of clinical learning.

Feelings. This author has spent more than 40 years preparing students for clinical practice. One general take-away has been that students, and many times their supervising clinicians, did not broach the topic of their clients' feelings. The question "how do you feel?" was not often heard in clinical exchanges. We may be squeamish about asking, or afraid of the answer, but it does not diminish the importance of asking. It is true that once on the table it can't be ignored, that there may be answers to that question that necessitate responses. The question may invoke emotional reactions such as crying, and perhaps that may explain the general reluctance to ask the question in the first place. So, what will you do?

This is where a developing conceptual framework is put to the test. Are we more disposed to Luterman's existential thinking? What about Holland and Nelson's proposition that stories are helpful, both for our learning as well as in diminishing the pain of disappointment for the client or their family? At the core of either ideological approach or that of others is the fundamental requisite of listening. We will do well to practice active listening. The value and necessity of listening is the most important take-away from this chapter.

In addition to listening, it may be most helpful to engage with the client and/or family in discussing how they see the process of helping as they move forward. Luterman (2017) declared that humans have "the marvelous capacity to heal." If so, what may be highly emotionally charged in the moment will diminish as we acknowledge the issue and allow the individual and family to grieve. Our responses will give permission which will be essential to our developing relationship, build our credibility, and place our role as a helper into perspective.

The proposition that we discuss with the client and/or family assumes that we have developed a working relationship allowing for that candor. The request is an entrée to a partnership in decision making. This may challenge one's basic view of client–clinician relationships but may be a key to success in confronting the issue at hand while allowing for the issue of ownership to be addressed. In Luterman's view this addresses the essences of counseling: (1) accepting emotions as they come about, (2) enabling people to be empowered—be able to make decisions independently of us.

Continuing Education.   SLPs and AuDs have come to the issue of counseling later than many other helping professions. The professions will need to continue to evolve with respect to preparation of future professionals with greater focus on the emotional conditions of our clients. This may involve more extensive formal preparation. This may involve more attention in professional continuing education. This may involve initiated action by individual professionals when recognizing needs to increase their comfort level in raising the question "how do you feel?"

Summary

This chapter has addressed the responsibilities of SLPs and AuDs in providing counseling services to individuals with communication disorders and their families. The chapter began by referencing the Scopes of Professional Practice, documents that identify expectations, and parameters for clinical service provision. Readers have been prompted to begin identifying a conceptual framework for their service provision. "Conceptual framework" is synonymous with philosophy—the underlying beliefs that guide decision making. It is anticipated these positions will be "tentative" early on in one's career, subject to modification with experience.

An operational model was developed within the context of our conceptual framework. One component supports information exchanges, providing detail to clients and their families that will allow them to understand the nature, causes and treatments for the clinical issue. An additional function is to build relationships that effectively support treatment activities and emotional adjustment relative to the condition.

Work of Luterman and of Holland has served as our counseling gold standard in communication disorders. Both have had extensive clinical experience; Luterman in audiology and Holland in speech-language pathology. Each has written extensively, providing text material to assist students to prepare for careers in the professions with respect to counseling services. Their philosophical perspectives differ, although there are several principles each identifies as important in counseling with communication disorders. Foremost among these is listening. Both Luterman and Holland indicate listening to be the most important skill clinicians bring to the clinical process. This skill prompts growth in the developing working relationship, essential in both informational exchanges and personal adjustment facilitation. Our chapter has also noted the value of developing active listening skills

Luterman and Holland also note the importance of clinicians and what they bring to the counseling process. Personal style describes how our own values influence the relationship being fostered between us and our clients and families.

It is recommended that readers establish lists of local, regional, and online resources regarding treatment recommendations or other professional issues. It is important to verify all resources for quality and update as needed. Clinicians are held in high regard when they can be relied upon to have good ideas to support clinical questions. Experience will serve as a reasonable teacher—the good student will pay close attention to the lessons being provided—for the benefit of many.

Continuing education has been noted to be a requirement for maintenance of credentials and licensure. Readers are encouraged to have a proactive mindset regarding continuing education, that requirements provide opportunities to expand our knowledge base and broaden our personal range of competence. An "ideal" scenario would see practitioners near the end of their careers with similar enthusiasm to learning new information, as would be the case in their first few years of practice. It is true that research and development provides for the ongoing expansion of knowledge regarding communication disorders. Strong professionals will consume that knowledge across their time in practice.

Critical Thinking

1. Utilizing Personal Character Strengths
   Go to the Values in Action questionnaire at the Authentic Happiness site and complete the VIA (Values in Action) questionnaire. (http://www .authentichappiness.sas.upenn.edu/Default.aspx) Results include a list of the respondents' five strongest character strengths as measured by the instrument. Are these accurate for you? How do you employ them in your efforts to provide counseling services as outlined in the chapter?

   Reflect on one of the identified strengths. How do you believe you have developed it? Do you consciously "maintain" it? Choose one of the strengths that was not listed among your "top 5." How might you go about cultivating that strength?

2. "What's My Verb?"—Introspective thinking at its finest!
   Imagine a television game show host facing a group of contestants on stage in a fun exercise in labeling. What term would you use to describe what you do as a clinician providing remediation? Do you condition? Do you teach? Do you rehabilitate?

   At the core level, what is it you actually do? It is likely your conceptual framework description will reflect how you respond to this question. Make a note in your long-term record keeping to revisit your descriptor choice down the road—and, at that point, ask yourself again, what's my verb?

3. Reviewing Information Exchange Practices— Information Retention
   The chapter has provided detail regarding Robert Margolis' summary of articles examining information retention in clinical exchanges. Visit one of the online sources of the Margolis article. Reflect on practices he recommends to enhance information retention. How do your practices match the Margolis suggestions?

   http://www.audiologyonline.com/articles/ article_detail.asp?article_id=548

   Another version of this information appears as a pdf file online at: http://www .audiologyincorporated.com/PDF%20files/ RecallMSLongVersion.pdf

4. Considerations for Working with Older Clients
   The National Institute on Aging has a number of resources to support efforts at communication with older individuals—important if we serve these folks. Go to: https://www.nia.nih.gov/ health/understanding-older-patients

   Click the "Ensure Understanding" paragraph. It places the "teach back" idea in context. Next go to YouTube: https://www.youtube.com/ watch?v=pCNCqA5LqFo

   and watch the video which provides instruction in the "Teach Back" method, a strategy for providing a means to check on comprehension.

   Reflect on the extent to which your style incorporates requests for active response with clients when exchanging information—clients of any age! It may be particularly important to incorporate teach back when working with older individuals.

References

American Speech-Language-Hearing Association. (2016). *Scope of practice in speech-language pathology* [Scope of practice]. Retrieved from http://www .asha.org/policy/

American Speech-Language-Hearing Association. (2018). *Scope of practice in audiology* [Scope of practice]. Retrieved from http://www.asha.org/ policy/

American Speech-Language-Hearing Association. (2019). *Certification.* Retrieved from https://www .asha.org/certification/

Authentic Happiness. University of Pennsylvania Positive Psychology Center website. Access at: http://www.authentichappiness.org

Beck, A., & Verticchio, H. (2018). Effectiveness of a method for teaching self-compassion to communication sciences and disorders graduate students. *American Journal of Speech-Language Pathology, 27*(1), 291–206.

Boyle, M., (2011). Mindfulness training in stuttering therapy: A tutorial for speech-language pathologists. *Journal of Fluency Disorders, 36,* 122–129.

Brammer, L., & MacDonald, G. (2003). *The helping relationship: Process and skills* (8th ed.). Boston, MA: Allyn & Bacon.

Chial, M. R., & Flahive, M. J. (2011) *Simple counseling* (CD-ROM). San Diego, CA: Plural Publishing.

Council on Academic Accreditation, American Speech-Language-Hearing Association. (2019). *Standards for accreditation of graduate education programs in audiology and speech-language pathology.* Retrieved from: http://www.caa.asha.org/reporting/standards/

Dinh, H., Thuy, T., Bonner, A., Clark, R., Ramsbotham, J., & Hines, S. (2016). The effectiveness of the teach-back method on adherence and self-management in health education for people with chronic disease: A systematic review. *JBI Database of Systematic Reviews and Implementation Reports, 14*(1), 210–247.

Flahive, M., & Chial, M. (2008). SIMPLE: Aphasia Resources. Washington, DC; Fund for the Improvement of Postsecondary Education (FIPSE), Project P116B031062.

Flasher, L., & Fogle, P. (2012). *Counseling skills for speech-language pathologists and audiologists* (2nd ed.). Boston, MA: Cengage Learning.

Holland, A., & Nelson, R. (2013). *Counseling in communication disorders: A wellness perspective* (2nd ed.). San Diego, CA: Plural Publishing.

Humphrey, K., (2009). *Counseling strategies for loss and grief.* Alexandria, VA: American Counseling Association.

Ivey, A., Ivey, M. B., & Zalaquette, C. P. (2009). *Intentional interviewing and counseling: Facilitating client development in a multicultural society* (7th ed.). Clifton Park, NY: Cengage Learning.

Johnson, K. O., (1951). The effects of classroom training upon listening comprehension. *Journal of Communication, 1*(1), 57–62.

Kubler-Ross, E. (1969). *On death and dying.* New York, NY: Macmillan.

Luterman, D. (2013). *Sharpening counseling skills* [DVD]. No.9800. Memphis, TN: The Stuttering Foundation of America.

Luterman, D. (2017). *Counseling persons with communication disorders and their families* (6th ed.). Austin, TX: Pro-Ed.

Maier, S. F., & Seligman, M. E. P. (1976). Learned helplessness: Theory and evidence. *Journal of Experimental Psychology: General, 105*, 3–46. https://doi.org/10.1037/0096-3445.105.1.3

Margolis, R. (2004). *In one ear and out the other—what patients remember.* Retrieved from https://www.audiologyonline.com/articles/in-one-ear-and-out-1102

Orenstein, E., Basilakos, A., & Marshall, R. S. (2012). Effects of mindfulness meditation on three individuals with aphasia. *International Journal of Language and Communication Disorders, 47*(6), 673–684.

Rogers, C. R. (1986). Carl Rogers on the development of the person-centered approach. *Person-Centered Review, 1*(3), 257–259.

Rogers, C. (2016, July 16). *Empathic listening.* Audio recording available from https://www.youtube.com/watch?v=2dLsgpHw5x0

Seligman, M.E.P. (2006). *Learned optimism: How to change your mind and your life* [Audio-book]. Vintage eBook, Amazon.com eISBN: 978-0-307-80334-4

Spillers, C. (2007). An existential framework for understanding the counseling needs of clients. *American Journal of Speech-Language Pathology, 16*(3), 191–197.

Teach Back method. Available from https://www.youtube.com/watch?v=UBrFs0z55f0

Webster's New Collegiate Dictionary. (1961). Cambridge, MA: The Riverside Press.

Wolven, A., & Coakley, C., (1982). *Listening.* Dubuque, IA: Brown.

World Health Organization (1992). *International classification of diseases and related health problems* (10th rev., ICD-10). Geneva, Switzerland: Author.

Appendix 28–A

Conversational Counseling Tools: Microskills

The following microskills are commonly employed in informational and adjustment forms of counseling. Here is a limited skill list followed by bulleted idea expansion. Microskills are identified in literature in helping professions, including speech-language pathology and audiology (Brammer & MacDonald, 2012; Flasher & Fogle, 2012). Notes suggest advantages and disadvantages when being employed.

- open-ended questions
- closed-ended questions
- interlocking questions
- affirmation
- clarification
- paraphrasing
- reflection
- reframing
- silence

Open-Ended Questions

Open-ended questions encourage more complex or expansive answers. The person replying to the question has options of what to include. Open-Ended Questions have the following attributes:

- Do not restrict the client or family.
- Make it difficult for the client or family to respond using only one or two words.
- Increase the likelihood that the client will raise the issues that are most important to them.
- Encourage a more active exchange.
- Provide access to information that may not have been offered in a more restricted exchange.

Closed-Ended Questions

- Give one person control over the exchange.
- Are useful when used occasionally to gain specific information.

- Can be viewed by client as authoritative or patronizing.
- Often imply there is a "right" answer.

Paraphrase

Paraphrasing is restating what the individual has just said using different, but equivalent terms or images. Paraphrasing has several purposes:

- Assures patients that the clinician has accurately heard the central meaning of their message.
- Allows the patient to hear how someone else perceives them.
- Can keep the patient focused on a particular topic of discussion.
- Permits the client to reexamine the statement to make sure that is what they really meant.

Interlocking (or Crosshatching) Questions

Interlocking or crosshatching questions are useful when a clinician needs to elicit more detail about a topic that they believe has been glossed over. Interlocking Questions have the following attributes:

- The tactic involves asking the same thing in a different way and at different points during the interview.
- Interlocking questions are used when there are discrepancies that must be resolved

Affirmation

- "A conscious, positive gesture or thought that helps change a particular image or belief that a person has about him or herself" (Flasher & Fogle, p. 252).
- Affirmation has the following attributes:
  - ☐ Affirmation begins with first person, present tense and may be helpful in times of crisis or relative calm.

- □ Affirmations can serve as powerful forms of positive self-talk.
- □ Affirmation is a term also used more generally outside of the context of counseling to suggest words, phrases and gestures that are intended to reinforce.

Clarification

- Clarification seeks to confirm clinician understanding of what is said by a client or family member and to invite elaboration from the informant—encourages the client to consider the clinician's statement and modify or change the message to the clinician.
- Requesting clarification or checking for understanding involves continuing conversation based on the client's responses to earlier exchanges.
- Techniques include objectifying patient statements through repetition, paraphrasing, probing, sequencing or summarization.
- Direct or indirect requests can also be used for confirmation of the client's communicative intent. (See Open-Ended Questions and Closed-Ended Questions)

Reflection

- Shows the interviewee that they are being heard and understood—used the same way as summaries

- In reflection, the interviewer feeds back the interviewee's very words
  - □ e.g., Interviewee: "His teacher has told me that she finds him very difficult to understand."
  - □ Interviewer: "His teacher has said that he is difficult to understand?"

Reframing

- The process of reshaping a client's negative perception into a more positive perspective—provides the client with a new frame of reference from which to view the problem.
- Reframing has the following attributes:
  - □ Helps the client focus on strengths.
  - □ Suggests alternative more productive ways of thinking about a situation.
  - □ Must be used carefully to avoid appearing either unsympathetic or overly optimistic.

Silence

- Used to encourage the client to talk or to have time to reflect about what has just been discussed
- Silence frequently serves as a powerful stimulant, prompting additional content as the client may sense that the clinician is waiting for more detail

Source: Chial, M. R., & Flahive, M. J. (2011). *Simple counseling* [CD-ROM]. San Diego, CA: Plural Publishing.

Appendix 28–B

✕✕✕

Counseling and Scopes of Practice

Counseling is among the clinical services claimed for speech-language pathologists and audiologists by the American Speech-Language-Hearing Association (ASHA). The scope of practice for audiology makes several references to "psychosocial adjustment counseling" in the context of rehabilitation (Scope of Practice in Audiology, ASHA, 2018) while the entire reference to counseling in the scope of practice for speech-language pathology is as follows: "counseling individuals, families, coworkers, educators, and other persons in the community regarding acceptance, adaptation, and decision making about communication and swallowing" (Scope of Practice in Speech-Language Pathology, ASHA, 2016).

Scopes of practice and preferred practice documents seek to clarify the aspirations of professions to the general public and to members of other professions. Relative to counseling, differences among such statements suggest that a consistent definition of "counseling" has yet to emerge for the discipline of communication disorders.

Titles

In many states, the titles "professional counselor" and "mental health counselor" are legally reserved for licensed clinical social workers or clinical psychologists. These professions require considerable emphasis on the theories, methods, and skills required for the services they provide.

Major Therapy Traditions

For professional counselors and for others who have good reason to use counseling methods, there are several relevant therapy traditions.

Psychoanalytic and Psychodynamic Therapies

These therapies are based on the theories of ego and past conflict developed by Sigmund Freud, Carl Jung, Erich Fromm, Otto Rank, and Erik Erikson. See the American Psychoanalytic Association (APsaA, http://www.apsa.org).

Behavioral Therapies (John Watson and B. F. Skinner)

These therapies employ learning principles to manage responses to potentially upsetting experiences, reward desirable actions, gradually approximate challenging (but desirable) activities, and model desired behaviors. Some behavioral approaches employ biofeedback. See the Association for Behavioral and Cognitive Therapies (http://www.abct.org/Home/).

Humanistic Therapies

Humanistic therapies tend to avoid the medical (disease) model of psychoanalysis and emphasize opportunities for dialog between clients/patients and counselors. Founders include Abraham Maslow, Rollo May, and Carl Rogers. See the Association for Humanistic Psychology website (http://www.ahpweb.org). Major schools of thought in humanistic therapy include the following:

- Person-centered therapy (PCT) or client-centered therapy (CCT), developed by Carl Rogers, emphasizes the conditions required to achieve growth and therapeutic change, namely unconditional positive regard, empathy, and congruence on the part of the counselor. Over time, PCT evolved from non-directional to experiential. See: https://counsellingresource.com/therapy/types/person-centred/

- Existential therapy (Rollo May, Irvin Yalom) contends that death, freedom (and responsibility), isolation, and meaninglessness lie at the root of human experience and that these issues ultimately cannot be resolved. See the Wikipedia entry for existential therapy.

- Gestalt therapy (Fritz Perls, Laura Perls, and Paul Goodman) emphasizes setting aside preconceptions and biases, avoiding interpretation and evaluation, "dialogical relationship" between the client/patient, and therapist and experimentation directed by the counselor. See the Wikipedia entry for Gestalt therapy.

- Cognitive therapies include the rational-emotive therapy (RET) of Albert Ellis and cognitive behavior therapy (CBT). These schools focus on changing thoughts and beliefs that compromise emotional adjustment and behavior. See these links for more: RET and CBT.

■ Skilled helping is less a school of therapy than a method for helping people solve problems. Major contributors to this relatively new approach include Gerard Egan and Lawrence Brammer. Skilled helping heavily relies upon counseling micro skills and client/patient experimentation coached by counselors.

■ Positive psychology is another relatively new school of thought advocated by psychologist Martin Seligman that focuses on habits of thought and behavior that promote happiness. See the positive psychology website (http://www.authentichappiness.org).

Source: Chial, M. R., & Flahive, M. J. (2011). *Simple counseling* [CD-ROM]. San Diego, CA: Plural Publishing.

29

Stress, Conflict, and Coping in the Workplace

◇◇

Lisa A. Scott, PhD

Introduction

This chapter is all about stress. Fun! It is important to understand stress, though, because it can produce physical and emotional symptoms that inhibit our ability to accomplish work or personal goals. Stress can also interfere with our overall happiness. Stress is pervasive in everyday life, but it does not need to prevent us from enjoying our jobs and relationships.

One misconception is that stress is always a bad thing; in fact, we all need a low level of it to help drive us to accomplish tasks. In this chapter, we will examine what we know about stress, including its signs and symptoms, why it can be prevalent in helping professions, and how it differs from mental health diagnoses like anxiety or depression. Then, we will discuss workplace conflict which can be a major source of stress. This chapter offers some basic strategies that may help begin resolving workplace conflict or eliminate it entirely in less severe situations. Last, we will examine the importance of self-care in combating stress and conflict, and how self-care is a fundamental component of ethical behavior.

What Is Stress?

Stress is something that all individuals will experience at some point in their lives. A conceptual definition of stress is that it is a person's subjective reaction and vulnerability to a given situation. Subjective reactions to stressful situations are really your opinion of the situation, not actual fact. What the person is interpreting subjectively results in both emotional reactions like worry or anger, and physiological responses such as increased heart rate, headaches, or digestive disturbances. Vulnerability to stress means that we will probably only feel stressed about a situation if we are vulnerable to it in some way, such as being a person who has a hard time taking critical feedback. If you are sensitive to others critiquing your behavior, receiving critical feedback will cause you stress (Zurich, Alstötter-Gleich, Gerstenberg, & Schmitt, 2015).

Stress can be experienced short- or long-term and work-related stress is the leading cause of workplace health problems, even more so than obesity or inactivity (NIOSH, 2017). One-fourth to one-third of employees view their jobs as the number one stressor in their lives; at least 40% of individuals describe their jobs as "very stressful," and 75% of workers believe they have more on-the-job stress than previous generations (Centers for Disease Control and Prevention, 2017). Work problems are more strongly related to health complaints than are other life stressors such as financial or family problems (National Institute for Occupational Safety and Health, 1999).

A common misconception about stress is that it is always unhelpful. Some stress can be helpful, though, because it can motivate us to accomplish tasks or change our behavior. In many cases, however, prolonged stress can affect one physically in a negative way.

Symptoms of Stress

Acute, or short-term, stress can produce a fight-or-flight response, which is a physical change in body functions in response to a perceived threat. During a highly stressful moment, our body interprets this threat much in the same way that cavemen saw bears as threats to their safety. These days, most of us do not live where we might be chased by a bear. Instead, experiences that threaten our physical or emotional health can trigger the fight-or-flight response. Ross (2011) described the physiological changes experienced during fight-or-flight, presented in Table 29–1. It is important to note that these physiological reactions are normal and exactly the way your body is supposed to react when confronted with a perceived threat.

The downside to this appropriate and normal body response is that it can make us feel very uneasy and upset. Some people may even experience a panic attack, which feels similar to a heart attack with chest pain, shortness of breath, and dizziness.

Fortunately, our evolutionary response to threats has remained much the same as it was in prehistoric times and produces this physiological stress response. It is normal and tells us our bodies are working correctly when we are confronted with a stressful situation. What is different is that the kinds of stressors that cause this acute problem have evolved, however. Instead of bears, we might be faced with a stressor such as an unhappy patient or colleague expressing their anger at us, or being late to work when you have an important appointment scheduled first thing in the morning.

Causes of Stress

Many situations can cause a person to feel stressed. Sometimes, we are stressed by our personal factors, such as relationships with partners, family members, or friends. Other life circumstances, such as challenging work environments or unstable living situations, can contribute to stress. Some of these stressors might be temporary and addressable, such as car trouble, a disagreement with a friend, or being assigned a new project at work. Other

Table 29–1. Physiological and Physical Responses to Perceived Threats and Possible Impact

Physiological Response	Physical Result	Impact
Liver spills adrenaline and sugar into the bloodstream	Spikes in energy	Restlessness, increased feelings of tension can lead to feeling that something really bad is about to happen
Heart rate increases	Increases blood flow to muscles to facilitate quick responses	Feeling your heart racing can contribute to feeling shaky or unstable, which can increase our worry that something is seriously wrong
Respiration increases in frequency but becomes more shallow	Provides oxygen to muscles to facilitate quick responses	Feeling like you can't catch your breath; increases our worry that something is seriously wrong
Impulsive responses	Increases risk-taking	Rash judgments, i.e., "Act first, think later"
Experience a range of difficult emotions	Irritability, anger, fear, hostility	Acting short-tempered and aggressive toward others, less patience for ourselves and others

stressors can be continuous and less easily resolved: being in an unhealthy relationship, death of a family member, unemployment, or overwhelming student debt.

Sometimes, a stressor is more long-term in nature, such as a difficult colleague, a high caseload, unreasonable demands from administration, or problems at home that interfere with work and vice versa. These stressors may not be intense at any given moment yet cause problems because of their continuous nature. These long-term stressors also produce physiological changes like low energy, headaches, stomach upset that can include nausea and changes in bowel habits, sleeplessness, and/or aches and pains. Emotional symptoms of long-term stress can include being quicker to anger or get upset, not wanting to be around others, or difficulty thinking clearly when stress is at its peak (National Alliance for the Mentally Ill, 2018). It is not unusual for a person to first attribute these physical and emotional changes to a temporary illness such as the flu, yet the symptoms last longer than that of a common virus.

Stress in Helping Professions

People who work in helping professions may encounter stressors within the workplace. High caseloads, demanding employers, difficult clients and families, or unreasonable productivity expectations can all contribute to workplace stress. In a study examining occupational stress among audiologists (AuDs) in New Zealand, (Severn, Searchfield, & Huggard, 2012), six factors were identified as leading to occupational stress, burnout, and compassion fatigue: (1) time demands, (2) interactions with patients, (3) changing clinical protocols, (4) management of a clinical audiology practice, including paperwork, (5) maintaining equipment, and (6) patient accountability. Interestingly, increasing age of the audiologist was most related to the risk for burnout. In another study of AuD stress, sales pressure by employers was perceived as the most stressful aspect of clinical practice and could even result in unethical practice (Simpson, Phillips, Wong, Clarke, & Thornton, 2018). Similar findings to Severn et al. (2012) and Simpson et al. (2018) have been reported for both Swedish and Indian AuDs (Bränsström et al., 2016; Ravi, Gunjawate, & Moyas, 2015). SLPs are not immune to very similar stressors, but the literature examining stress specifically in SLPs is less rich (McLaughlin, Lincoln, & Adamson, 2008).

Another possible source of workplace stress comes from witnessing the stress of clients or the client's caregivers. Being diagnosed with a communication disorder disrupts family and work routines to the extent that the client and caregivers will become highly stressed. It is difficult for helping professionals to witness those they

care for experience difficult situations and know that as a professional, it is impossible to "fix" everything a client or family may need.

An individual's response to stress is just that, individual. Some of us have lots of experience dealing with stressful situations because of previous life experiences. As a result, we may have learned a variety of coping skills to combat stress. Coping skills can be more or less helpful, depending on the person and the situation. Regardless of your individualized response to stress, it is important to recognize that we can learn how to deal more effectively with it and increase our repertoire of helpful strategies for combating it. Ignoring stress can lead to negative consequences, such as burnout, which has been demonstrated to be a leading cause of leaving the field (McLaughlin et al., 2008).

Burnout and Compassion Fatigue

One possible consequence of unrelenting stress is burnout, a phenomenon that has been discussed in helping professions since the early 1970s (Cedoline, 1982). It was noticed that helping professionals occasionally presented as being exceptionally tired, uninterested in their work, and having difficulty coping with their work and home lives (Lyndon, 2016). When stress arises from a mismatch in workplace demands with employee capacities, it triggers even greater stress. Ross (2011) wrote that burnout results from prolonged stress over time, and should be considered the last stage of stress.

What Is Burnout?

Generally accepted as a psychological condition, an early and widely accepted definition of burnout identifies three essential parameters: (1) *exhaustion*, which can be emotional, physical, or both; (2) *cynicism*, described as indifference about the worker's own efforts and his or her colleagues; and (3) *professional inefficacy*, or a lack of confidence in being able to perform a job well (Maslach, 2007; Maslach & Jackson, 1982).

Exhaustion. If you are experiencing burnout-related exhaustion, you are probably feeling very drained, especially when thinking about going to work or performing work-related tasks. This exhaustion makes it difficult to cope with circumstances at work or with difficult colleagues, and you may have some physical symptoms as well, such stomach troubles, pain/achiness, or headaches.

Cynicism. When you are feeling cynical about work, you are likely experiencing feelings of bitterness and distrust. These feelings may be to do with the agency you work for; perhaps it expects too much of you in terms of caseload, workload, or productivity. You may also feel doubtful or pessimistic about the agency, your colleagues, or that your situation will ever improve.

Professional Inefficacy. The last major category of burnout is professional inefficacy, or feeling as though you do not have the skills to stay on top of your work expectations. You may feel too challenged in the environment because it feels impossible to be good at all things, or you might find yourself feeling underchallenged and therefore bored and disinterested. It can be difficult to overcome these feelings in the face of changing work expectations that occur frequently as new laws are passed or as insurance regulations change. An ever-expanding scope of practice can also lead to feelings that you may never "master" any of the assessments or treatments you are providing. These feelings are often symptomatic of professional inefficacy and make it difficult to concentrate or be creative in your approach to work tasks.

Is Compassion Fatigue the Same Thing as Burnout?

Compassion fatigue is similar to burnout in that it is work related, but is a special type of burnout that results from the stresses involved in caring for others. Merriam-Webster's (2016) definition of compassion fatigue is "the physical and mental exhaustion and emotional withdrawal experienced by those who care for sick or traumatized people over an extended period of time." Note that compassion fatigue focuses specifically on caregiving and the results of being responsible for others, whereas burnout applies more globally to all kinds of work stressors. Burnout and compassion fatigue share similar symptoms, however, so I will use burnout as the general term in discussing it as a potential consequence of stress.

What Are the Risks for Experiencing Burnout?

Risk for burnout is both individual and environmental. Individual factors that put you at risk for burnout include their ability to balance their work and personal life, having a highly demanding *or* underchallenging workload, and feeling that you have little control over your work or saying in workplace policies and procedures (Cendone, 1982; Mayo Clinic, 2018). Farber (1990, 2000) discussed three individual sub-types of

people who experience burnout. "Frenetic" workers tend to work harder until they reach exhaustion as they seek success and recognition for their efforts. "Underchallenged" workers do not perceive satisfaction from their work because the conditions do not stimulate them. "Worn-out" workers are those who, when faced with a level of stress, will give up easily. These sub-type categorizations focus on the worker's style as contributing significant risk for burnout.

Later theories of burnout, however, also focus on burnout as an environmental disorder (Montero et al., 2013), because the workplace places a unique set of demands on each worker. Environmental risk factors for burnout include lack of control over your schedule or work assignments, unclear job expectations, lack of feedback about your performance, unhealthy workplace dynamics and interpersonal relationships, isolation at work, and work over- or underload (Cendone, 1982; Mayo Clinic, 2018).

This interface between worker type and workplace demand will result in individualized responses to stress. That is, some workers will experience burnout more readily than others, and addressing burnout will require individualized interventions that take both the worker and the environment into consideration.

As researchers explored the concept of burnout, it was applied across professions, including health care workers, engineers, and others (cf. Brown, Schell, & Pashniak, 2017; Michalilidis & Banks, 2016; Montero-Marín et al., 2013; Severn, Searchfield, & Huggard, 2012). Despite the realization that burnout is universal to all work environments, Lubinski (2013) attributed causes of burnout for AuDs and speech-language pathologists (SLPs) as being related to helping complex clients; not always being able to evaluate "success" in a meaningful, measurable way; that others may have poor opinions of our help or relationships with them; and the difficulty in contributing to decision making in some helping agencies.

Am I Burnt Out, or Is It Something Else?

A challenge in identifying burnout is that its symptoms, such as fatigue and apathy, are often the same symptoms we observe in people diagnosed with anxiety disorders or depression. Teasing out whether you may be suffering from burnout versus a mental health condition can be a bit challenging, but typically involves assessing whether the symptoms you are having are related primarily to work as opposed to life in general. Corey (2016) provided guiding questions to help assess whether you might be experiencing burnout. A few include:

- Does the thought of getting up and going to work make you tired or anxious?

- Do you experience significant variations in your work productivity?

- Is it difficult to concentrate on work?

- Do you notice yourself being more impatient than normal with clients, colleagues, or your boss?

- Is it difficult to be creative and help identify possible positive outcomes when confronted with a work problem that needs to be solved?

- When someone compliments you on your work, do you find it difficult to accept her/his words as truthful or meaningful?

- Have you noticed changes in sleeping, eating, headaches, stomach problems, or other physical symptoms?

If your answers to these questions relate more to life in general, you may want to consult a counselor to determine whether you are experiencing a mental health condition such as anxiety or depression. Table 29–2 presents a list of general characteristics of stress, anxiety disorder, and depression.

Approximately 20% of the U.S. population experiences one or more of these mental health conditions (NAMI, 2018a), so thinking that you are alone in your excessive worry or unhappiness is inaccurate. Many of us have gone through episodes that may have been temporary; others may have a chronic mental health condition.

Regardless, help is available, and it works. More information on the kinds of help available will be discussed in the section on self-care.

Workplace Conflict

A common source of stress for SLPs and AuDs is workplace conflict. In fact, it is identified as a leading source of stress for any employee regardless of profession and is an inevitable occurrence when people with different professional roles, values, opinions, priorities, and goals interact. Therefore, having awareness of conflict, being able to pinpoint why it occurs, and having strategies for your own participation in de-escalation are critical components of your professional knowledge and skills.

Defining Workplace Conflict and Its Sources

Saltman, O'Dea, and Kidd (2006) defined workplace conflict as "a disagreement within oneself or between people individuals that causes harm or has the potential to cause harm" (p. 9). The authors also differentiate between disagreements, which they define as differences of opinion versus conflict, which has the added harm component. It is completely reasonable for us to express differences of opinion without harming the other or the situation in some way. The kinds of harm that can result from conflict at work include negative consequences on a provider's stress level, decreased workplace morale, increased employee turnover, and compromised client care. Some people even go so far as to leave their

Table 29–2. General Characteristics of Stress, Anxiety Disorder, and Depression

Stress	Anxiety Disorder	Depression
Affects everyone	Does not affect everyone	Does not affect everyone
Can produce changes in physical and mental health	Can produce changes in physical and mental health	Can produce changes in physical and mental health
Can be positive OR negative	Is generally only negative and unhelpful	Is generally only negative and unhelpful
Stressors can be short or long term	Typically lifelong, with some variation in intensity across time	Can be episodic or chronic
Can be managed without professional intervention	May need professional intervention to achieve functional living	Often requires professional intervention

professions when conflict is unable to be successfully resolved (Kfouri & Lee, 2019; Morrison, Lincoln, & Reed, 2011).

In 2006, Saltman et al. emphasized that many of us may expect that a harmonious workplace is the natural state of things, and that if conflict exists, something must be wrong and that it is most likely attributable to people with personality problems. Instead, they asserted that workplace conflict is the normal state of affairs and there are multiple reasons for it.

Saltman et al.'s (2006) description of conflict as a normal state of affairs is a more traditional view. In 2017, Currie, Gormley, Roche, and Teague stated that in the past, "conflict at work was commonly viewed as something similar to the arrival of bad weather, not particularly welcomed, but inevitable nonetheless" (p. 492). In their comprehensive review of human resources literature, they found that current theories and practices among human resource managers have shifted to a view that when workplace conflict exists, it represents managerial failure that should and could be avoided. The authors go on to assert that based on their review, there is a lack of even simple consensus on what the best methods are addressing workplace conflict that result in positive outcomes.

Sources of Workplace Conflict. When we consider sources of conflict at work, they can be divided into two main categories: interpersonal reasons and organiza-tional reasons. Table 29–3 provides a list of just some of the possible reasons for interpersonal and organizational sources of conflict (Currie et al., 2017; Kfouri & Lee, 2019; Saltman et al., 2006).

Although we might assume that our personal responsibility in resolving conflicts is only necessary when we have a role in the conflict at hand, that assumption is misleading. First, as an employee, your responsibilities are not just related to client care but also to being a "good citizen" and working to increase the success of the organization as a whole. Second, if you are effective at things like being organized, following policies and procedures, and maintaining positive interactions with co-workers and superiors, you may be promoted into a managerial role where you will have direct responsibility for resolving conflicts. Thus, becoming familiar with strategies for resolving both interpersonal and organizational conflicts is highly relevant to your working life.

Strategies for Addressing Workplace Conflict

In today's workplace, many professionals are required to work interprofessionally to serve clients. The increase in interprofessional practice also leads to the possibility for increased conflict. Cain, Frazer, and Kilaberia (2019) describe that a requirement for successful interprofessional teaming means the employee has developed both

Table 29–3. Possible Reasons for Workplace Conflict

Interpersonal Reasons	Organizational Reasons
Personality differences	Human resources managers may not be up-to-date with more recently identified methods for conflict resolution
Disrespectful or deceptive interactions	A change in conflict resolution policies and procedures may pose an overwhelming burden for the organization
Inability to solve differences of opinion regarding roles, goals, and desired outcomes for a situation	Diffusion of or unclear responsibility for conflict resolution: is it the job of the human resources office or immediate/intermediate supervisors?
Lack of needed information being shared	Lack of training on workplace conflict for immediate and intermediate supervisors
Competition for resources and/or recognition by superiors	Requirements for interprofessional practice or broader kinds of teamwork
Organizational stress that is inherent to the particular workplace in question	General lack of strategies for improving workplace morale

a professional identity and a team-based identity. How does my team interact to provide high-quality service delivery to our clients, and how do I fit into the team as the only SLP or AuD? What am I bringing to the table for my colleagues and our clients?

Our perception of our professional role in the team may conflict with other team members' perceptions of our role and lead to confusion and tension. This is just one way that we may experience conflict in the workplace in regard to teaming. Examining methods for resolving teaming issues in the health care environment is an increasing area of focus, but it seems less discussed for interprofessional teaming in educational settings (cf. Andre, 2018; Cain et al., 2019; Cooper-Duffy & Eaker, 2017; Marks, 2018).

Saltman et al. (2006) and Kfouri and Lee (2019) identified four typical ways people handle interpersonal conflicts. The first is avoidance: not addressing the problem as it is developing or denying that a problem even exists. In the immediate situation, this is often our go-to strategy. This can be useful, as having time to step away and consider the problem may lead to a satisfactory resolution at a later date. In one of my favorite books, *The Gift of Therapy*, Yalom (2002) describes this as "strike while the iron is cold" (p. 121) and describes its benefit as being able to share feedback when emotions are not so high. Trying to resolve a problem when it is in process or escalating often leads to defensiveness. If we are feeling stress in the moment, it also means we have fewer intrapersonal resources to draw from to facilitate de-escalation.

The second method we resort to is accommodation: giving up on our own needs and letting the other person get what he or she wants. This is another mostly immediate response to conflict. It can be effective in the short-term but have negative long-term impact. You might go home at the end of the day and struggle with how you handled the situation and be frustrated that you did not get what you wanted. This increases your overall stress and may contribute to buildup of a bad attitude about your colleague(s) or the workplace itself. It may also lead to your colleague(s) expecting that when you are in conflict, you should and will be the one to capitulate vs. their giving in to you. This can result in workplace bullying.

The third strategy that people may use when in interpersonal conflict is competition. I say "people" because of course, we would never engage in competition with our co-workers! Other people might do so, but not us! Competition has more of a time-delay in implementation because it requires being able to assess the situation, the other person's areas of vulnerability, and loopholes in the environment that can facilitate competition, e.g., supervisor favoritism toward certain employees. Using competition as a strategy is ineffective at best. If you

find yourself feeling like you need to compete with a co-worker regarding a conflict, you can ask yourself, "Why is it so important for me to be right," or "What is driving my need to win?" Carefully considering these needs is an important step toward your own successful contributions to problem solving. Another question that can be helpful is "What if the opposite were true?" (see the Box below for an example of this).

A colleague asks me to make a special accommodation for her that will directly affect her management of others. Her request is not outlandish, but will result in more work for me. I have a history of negative interactions with this colleague, as do most others in my workplace, so my immediate response is "Meeting your individual need through increased work for me is not going to happen. Besides, I have never known you to do any favors for me or others, so why should I do one for you?"

After considering the situation overnight (i.e., strike while the iron is cold), I asked myself, "What if the opposite were true?" That is, what if the colleague making such a request was my best work friend instead of this person I genuinely dislike?

I know that if my best work friend asked me to do this favor, I would do it in a heartbeat and not complain. My answer to the "opposite" question helped me realize that my initial reaction was a competitive one and would not facilitate any future positive interactions nor lead to a good outcome for our organization. I was only considering my perspective and my feelings about my colleague. I wanted to demonstrate my power to her instead of really considering whether her request might be best for our organization as a whole.

As a result of shifting my perspective in this way, I emailed her the next day and agreed to her request. I was able to feel good that I was contributing to our organization through this extra work, instead of creating more obstacles and tension.

The fourth strategy we implement is collaboration (Kfouri & Lee, 2019; Saltman et al., 2006). Collaboration means that when in conflict, we are able to balance our own interests with the interests of others. This requires objectivity, a belief in your own rationale in the situation, and a willingness to give up a part of your own goal so that others' goals can be met.

The Importance of Good Communication Skills in Resolving Interpersonal Conflicts. When considering the list of possible reasons for interpersonal conflict in Table 29–3, it seems clear that the underlying issues most likely relate to our ability to communicate with our co-workers. It is natural to think that when we say something to others, they understand what we mean and will behave in the way we have expressed. If we perceive that the other person or people are feeling slightly uncomfortable about what we are saying, we may feel uncomfortable or lack needed skills for directly and positively addressing a communication breakdown.

You are spending time in graduate school learning how to adapt your communication to perform professional tasks with clients, to deliver information to clients and caregivers, and to interact in a professional manner with your colleagues. Some of us receive more emphasis on these skills than others, and it may be unlikely that communication in times of workplace conflict is even addressed.

If you are interested in learning how to develop your communication skills in times of conflict, one of the most widely used resources is the book *Crucial Conversations: Tools for Talking When Stakes Are High* (Patterson, Grenny, MacMillan, & Switzler, 2011). It is widely available and written in a straightforward manner, and systematically discusses how to implement essential components to stressful interactions. If you read this book and are interested in learning more, the authors have published additional books on workplace topics and all share the excellent characteristics of the original volume.

Organizational Conflict Management Strategies. Despite agreement across many organizations that workplace conflict is unhelpful, examination of the literature in human resources reveals there is no standard method for addressing it at the organizational level (Currie et al., 2017). The authors observed, however, that there is an increasing trend for organizational conflict management to be handled by a direct or intermediate supervisor instead of someone from human resources. They attribute this to organizations' desires to use mentoring and coaching to help employees develop skills and competencies, and the preference for solving problems as close to their origins as is possible.

Further, Currie et al. (2017) identified several strategies organizations use to decrease workplace conflict from occurring. One is to create alternative dispute resolution (ADR) procedures, such as "workplace mediation, fact-finding, ombudsmen, arbitration, and review panels composed of managers or peer employees" (p. 496). Another is to develop procedures as conflict arises, which leads to inadequate organizational change.

Yet another organizational conflict resolution the authors suggested is to provide supervisors with training in workplace conflict management. Although this may seem logical and optimal, it does not typically happen in many organizational environments. Additionally, some supervisors may contribute to organizational conflicts because they see conflict management as secondary to their main job responsibilities and feel pressured for their employees' productivity.

In a survey of 303 hospital employees across all departments and levels of responsibility, Kfouri and Lee (2019) reported that 54% of respondents rated the opinion statement "there is a lot of conflict in my workplace" (p. 18) between 5 and 7 on a strength of agreement index where 7 equaled strong agreement.

With regard to training in conflict management, results revealed only 42% had had previous training, with 49% of these respondents indicating that it had taken place in their respective training programs. Despite possible previous education in conflict resolution, only 20% felt adequately trained, and 59% believed they needed to learn more. Interestingly, only 18% of the 303 participants had plans for enrolling in conflict resolution workshops in the future, despite 74% indicating that workplace conflict increased their stress.

Are there factors that can alleviate workplace conflict from occurring at the organizational level in the first place? Yes. Avgar, Kyung Lee, and Chung (2014) identified that organizations with strong organizational citizenship among employees and management exhibit fewer instances of organizational conflict. What are the characteristics of good organizational citizenship? In other words, how might you contribute directly to the prevention of conflict in your workplace? Currie et al. (2017) answered in terms of employees who see their own role and career development being intertwined with the success of an organization as a whole. Godard (2014) identified multiple qualities of good organizational citizenship behavior demonstrated by individual employees as including:

- Demonstrating willingness to help colleagues and go above and beyond when needed;
- Building tolerance of day-to-day stressors;
- Supporting the mission of the organization;
- Internalizing organizational policies and procedures and being willing to follow them; and
- Making an effort to build their individual skills and abilities

These citizenship strategies are part of ethical behavior and require the desire for lifelong learning.

Workplace Violence

Episodes of workplace violence are on the rise. It seems we hear of an episode almost weekly. The U.S. Department of Health's National Institute for Occupational

Safety and Health (NIOSH) defines workplace violence as "the act or threat of violence, ranging from verbal abuse to physical assaults directed toward persons at work or on duty" (NIOSH, 2018).

Many reputable online resources, including NIOSH, the U.S. Department of Labor's Occupational Safety and Health Administration (OSHA), the National Safety Council (NSC). and the Society for Human Resource Management (SHRM), all offer excellent resources for recognizing warning signs of workplace violence, how organizations can develop prevention plans, and how to respond both in immediate situations and in the aftermath of a workplace violence episode. Some of these organizations even offer online training for employees and managers.

When and Where Does Workplace Violence Happen? Although the workplace violence we read about in the news frequently involves a homicide or multiple injured employees (or both), it can also include threatening language or lesser forms of assault. There are four categories of workplace violence: (1) between co-workers; (2) between partners in personal relationships; (3) between service providers and clients/customers; and (4) criminal intent (NIOSH, 2018). According to the National Safety Council (NSC, 2019), health care, social assistance, and the education industries are most likely to have episodes of workplace violence, with NIOSH (2018) reporting that 70% of all workplace violence episodes occur in these industries. Episodes can occur as an act of revenge, an expression of one's ideology, or as part of a robbery. Perpetrators may or may not have mental illness. Further, Workplace Responds (n.d.) tells us that 24% of workplace violence episodes are the outcome of problematic personal relationships, and perpetrators are committing crimes targeting their current or previous partners.

Warning Signs. There is no way to predict when an attack may occur. You may observe behavior, though, that would be characteristic of warning signs. If you do observe single or multiple warning signs in a colleague, report him/her to management. A list of warning signs exhibited by a troubled employee is provided by the NSC (2019):

- Excessive use of alcohol or drugs

- Unexplained absenteeism, change in behavior, or decline in job performance

- Depression, withdrawal, or suicidal comments

- Resistance to changes at work or persistent complaining about unfair treatment

- Violation of company policies

- Emotional responses to criticism, mood swings

- Paranoia

- Termination

For you to notice these warning signs, you must listen well and carefully observe your colleagues' behaviors and conversations about their personal life, their mental health, and their attitudes toward work. Again, if you see/hear something, say something. It may result in your colleague getting much-needed help before escalation to violence happens.

Workplace Responsibility for Prevention and Response. The NSC (2019) and the Society for Human Resource Management (SHRM, 2019) emphasize that every organization needs to be concerned about the possibility of workplace violence. Both organizations describe methods for preventing it, including providing training to all employees, developing an emergency plan, being familiar with both individuals' warning signs and possible risky situations, encouraging reporting of these instances, and adopting a zero-tolerance policy for workplace violence. Additionally, if an episode occurs, the organization should consider how to respond in the aftermath, such as creating threat assessment teams who can be trained to evaluate the likelihood a person or situation is at increased risk.

In an active shooter situation, the Federal Bureau of Investigation (FBI, n.d.) provides recommendations for three different actions you can take to protect your own life. Knowing the three options and being able to determine the most reasonable way to protect yourself is critical.

1. Evacuation: Attempt to evacuate the building, leaving your belongings behind and regardless of whether others are going to go with you. Call 911 once you are out and prevent other individuals from entering the building.

2. Hide: Try to find a spot out of the shooter's view, and if possible, lock or blockade doors into the area where you are hiding. Make sure any cell phones are on silent and all other noise sources (e.g., radio or televisions, computers) are turned off. Remain as quiet as possible.

3. Take action against the shooter: Yell, throw things at the shooter that can distract or cause injury, and act as aggressively as possible toward him/her.

You should now be aware of the components and causes of stress, and your own role and responsibility in addressing workplace conflict at the interpersonal and organizational levels. Another important consideration is recognizing and responding to episodes of workplace violence, and you may refer to Chapter 22 for further discussion on workplace violence. After reading all of this stressful information, you're probably wondering how you can effectively cope with it all. Thankfully, there are multiple methods for doing so.

Coping with Stress: The Importance of Self-Care

Learning to cope with stress is a life skill. When we are feeling burnt out or in conflict with others at work, we may actually be in danger of committing ethical violations. The physical and emotional consequences of stress can lead to diminished decision-making abilities, lead to substance abuse, and interfere with forming harmonious working relationships. These factors put the practitioner at risk for compromised patient care. Therefore, coping with stress is not only important for your own personal health, but critical to the work that you do.

Because sources of stress are individualized, so are strategies for successful management. Where one strategy, i.e., exercise, might work well for your friend, it may not work as effectively for you. It is encouraging, however, to know that there is a wide array of strategies available, and it is highly likely that you will find one or more that are helpful to you.

First Steps to Coping

Before seeking specific methods for combating stress, it is important to know how it affects you and what kinds of situations are most likely to increase your stress level (NAMI, 2018b). Some people respond to stress with physical symptoms such as those listed in the first part of this chapter. Do you get headaches? Do you feel wiped out after a stressful encounter? Does stress interfere with your ability to sleep, or cause stomach/digestive symptoms? Others will experience emotional responses such as memory lapses or less patience with themselves and others.

Having an idea of the kinds of situations that will increase your stress level and cause you to feel physically or emotionally uncomfortable is essential in determining how best to cope. Some stressful situations are temporary and can be easily addressed by simply gathering information. For example, if you are traveling to a conference in an unfamiliar city and are unsure about transportation to the venue, you can utilize sources like the city's website or convention and visitors' bureau to learn more about what kinds of transportation are available and how much you can expect to pay. Many stressful situations require approaches, though, that are more consistent in their application and sophisticated in their implementation.

Ensuring Your Basic Needs Are Being Met

After you have been able to give some thought to what factors are causing your stress and how you respond to it, it is time to start taking first steps towards management. Meeting your basic needs, such as getting enough sleep, eating nutritious food, engaging in some simple relaxation exercises, and confiding in a good friend all have the ability to make a major impact on your daily stress management.

Sleep. One common effect of stress is insomnia. There are over-the-counter sleep aids that can be helpful for a temporary bout of insomnia, but it is important to monitor your usage of them because it is possible to become dependent. They can also have negative side effects, such as feeling groggy and nauseous when you wake up. Prescription sleep aids are available as well, but these too can have negative side effects and cause dependency.

One popular method for dealing with insomnia is practicing good sleep hygiene. Sleep hygiene is a set of practices that individuals engage in to prepare for bed and increase the likelihood that they will be able to fall and stay asleep, resulting in being more alert in the daytime. The options for creating a sleep routine are varied and should be individualized to each person, as the evidence for its effectiveness in the general population is equivocal (Irish, Kline, Gunn, Buysse, & Hall, 2015). Commonly recommended sleep hygiene strategies are described in Table 29–4.

Eating Well. Our bodies need adequate fuel to accomplish daily tasks and cope with excess demands such as stress. When we are undergoing a period of high stress, it is tempting to skip a meal or grab whatever food is closest/easiest, which is not typically as nutritious as what your body requires. Inconsistent meals can lead to a drop in your blood sugar, which will contribute to feeling shaky and confused. If you are working long hours or taking work home, it can be difficult to plan meals and prepare lunches and dinners that are better for you than fast- or frozen-food options.

Meal planning is one way to increase your nutritional intake. Using a meal plan to determine how to grocery shop and implement meal prep time can make a significant difference in how you eat, helping reduce your

Table 29–4. Commonly Recommended Sleep Hygiene Practices

Practice	Description
Exercise	Promotes release of muscle tension, increased oxygenation, and release of endorphins. Be cautious about vigorous exercise right before bed, however; it can interfere with your ability to relax.
Make environmental adjustments	Your mattress/pillows should be comfortable; the ideal room temperature for sleep is between 60 and 67 degrees (National Sleep Foundation, 2019). Limit light, especially from cell phones/computers/tablets. Using white noise machines or apps that provide calming sounds may also be useful.
Establish consistent bedtime and wake-up time	Having consistent bedtime and wake-up time both on weekdays and weekends helps establish a routine so that your body begins to expect when to go to sleep and when to wake up.
Limit certain types of foods just before bedtime	Foods that are likely to cause indigestion or reflux, such as fried, spicy, citrus-based foods and heavy meals can interfere with digestion.
Limit daytime naps	Napping can seem like a great way to rid yourself of tiredness, but it can interfere with your nighttime sleep. The National Sleep Foundation (2019) recommends limiting naps to 20–30 minutes.
Establish a relaxing bedtime routine	Light stretching, taking a warm bath or shower, or reading for a set period of time, e.g., 20 minutes, also helps your body recognize that it's bedtime.
Avoid stimulants a few hours before bedtime	Caffeine, nicotine, and some prescription drugs provide enough stimulation to your nervous system that it significantly interferes with your ability to fall and/or stay asleep.

stress. Fortunately, access to nutritious and convenient food is becoming increasingly available, although usually at an increased financial cost. Many grocery stores now offer convenience foods such as rotisserie chicken or prepared salads, and meal preparation kits that can be delivered to you are some of the different kinds of options available.

Relaxation Exercises. Our bodies' chemical responses to stress can lead to increases in muscle tension. This can result in headaches, stomach/digestive disturbances, or back or neck pain. Recognizing when you have excess muscle tension is not always intuitive, especially if you are enduring a period of prolonged stress. Some simple ways to check in with your body to investigate muscle tension include abdominal breathing; do you notice a change in where your shoulders are as you breathe in and out? Can you easily turn your neck from side to side? Do you feel relief in your lower back when you bend over and try to touch your toes?

There are a number of stretches easily discovered from multiple sources. If you are an SLP student, you may have taken a voice disorders class where you learned

specific relaxation exercises that you can apply to yourself, not just your clients!

A popular approach was first advocated by Herbert Benson and Miriam Klipper in 1976, *The Relaxation Response*. Originally designed for use with cardiac patients, the techniques outlined in the book have been adopted, modified, and researched, resulting in an evidence-based approach to relaxation. Practicing a relaxation routine can result in stress-reduction benefits such as lowered blood pressure and better sleep. An important advantage to learning relaxation techniques is that they often come at low or no cost and do not require assistance from another professional or coach.

Talking With Others

Our stress and worried thoughts can magnify when we keep silent about them. We tell ourselves that if we talk about our stressors, others will think we are overdramatizing what to them may seem a small problem. We discount the significance of our stressors, thinking that others have it worse off than we do, so we should not discuss our problems in case the listener has a bigger problem.

Here is a secret: it is not a competition. Being the most stressed person you know does not win you a prize, nor does being less stressed than someone else. If what you are going through is the most stressful thing you have ever encountered, then it is the most stressful thing.

You can experience significant relief from your worries just by talking about them to someone else. Friends, colleagues, family members, and religious advisors are all examples of people you might seek out to help you think about a problem that has you stressed. Not every one of the people around you are best suited to listen to you, however. Follette and Pistorello (2007) describe making a list of the people you are close to across all environments. Then, write down the kinds of things you typically confide in them about. Sometimes making an explicit list like this can be helpful in determining who the best person might be for you to talk to about a given stressful situation.

Employee Assistance Programs

Another more formal option for talking with someone about your stress is seeking out help through an Employee Assistance Program (EAP). EAPs are a benefit offered by many employers; check with your human resources department about whether they have an arrangement with an EAP provider. EAP is designed to be a short series (often fewer than eight sessions) of free, confidential counseling appointments that deal with a focused issue (OPM, n.d.). These issues can range from helping you figure out how to reduce or cope with workplace conflict, with stress in general, or even with financial issues, relationships, and parenting. The rationale behind EAPs is that happier workers make for more productive working environments. Services are confidential, and if after completing the available number of EAP visits it is determined that you may need additional assistance, EAP counselors can help make referrals to other providers who are better able to support you long term.

Mindfulness Practices for Stress Reduction

One of the hottest topics in mental health and stress reduction today is the implementation of mindfulness practices into everyday life. When I first learned about the concept of mindfulness in 1999 via a workshop, I had to actively seek out more information about it because it just wasn't something people readily discussed. Now, it seems like you can find information about mindfulness and its variations almost anywhere you look. Enter "mindfulness" into Google and you will return more than 10 pages of listings that include definitions, articles on the benefits of mindfulness, mindfulness mediation practices, etc. The list goes on and on. For our purposes, we will use a general definition amalgamated from multiple sources, and then discuss how some researchers have implemented mindfulness practices to facilitate stress reduction.

Defining Mindfulness. There are many definitions available for mindfulness, depending on whether you are accessing them via general sources like dictionary .com, Merriam Webster's Dictionary, or Wikipedia. Other sources are more specific depending on the individual offering the definition and his or her orientation to mindfulness practice (e.g., yoga, meditation).

A conceptual definition of mindfulness is being aware and present with your thoughts, feelings, and physical experiences at any given moment. Another component used in some definitions but not others is that your awareness of these thoughts, feelings, and physical experiences is nonjudgmental. Thoughts or feelings are not good or bad, they are just what you are thinking or feeling in the moment.

If you are mindful, it means that you take a moment, or more than one, to notice what is around you. Are you feeling hot or cold? Tense or relaxed? What are you thinking about right now? Do you notice any particular noise in the environment? What about your breathing? When was the last time you took a deep breath and really noticed how great it feels to breathe in and out? When we are stressed, it is not uncommon to hold our breaths and not take nice, deep breaths in and out. The oxygenation a deep breath provides can relieve muscle tension almost right away.

Kabat-Zinn (2005) described being nonjudgmental about our thoughts by imagining that we were sitting by a stream and watching the leaves float by. Each leaf has one of our ideas on it. Some leaves get caught up against a rock and spin for a bit. This is like when we have a thought that we cannot let go of, and we turn it over and over in our heads. Turning thoughts over and over is one kind of stress response. Kabat-Zinn discusses observing that leaf being caught and trying not to do anything about it to urge it down the stream, instead being patient and noticing that the "stuck" aspect will eventually allow the leaf to work itself out. The same can be true of our thoughts. Judging our thoughts as good or bad, immature, helpful or unhelpful can lead us to try to push them away, resulting in feeling even more stressed.

Strategies for Increasing Mindfulness in Everyday Life. There are many ways to begin increasing your mindfulness, whether it is through formal practice such as yoga or meditation or through informal means such as reading the works of well-known practitioners such as Jon Kabat-Zinn, Thich Nhat Hanh, and Pema Chodron and then trying to implement their suggestions. You can also find mindfulness workshops around the country that will help you get started.

Is There Evidence for Mindfulness in Reducing Stress? A number of research centers around the country focus on researching and acquiring evidence for mindfulness practice. Kabat-Zinn's (2005) book was borne out of his research at a university hospital with cardiac patients, where he found that blood pressure and patient-reported experiences of stress were reduced when they engaged in brief daily mindfulness sessions. Other research centers include the Mindful Awareness Research Center at the University of California–Los Angeles and the Greater Good Science Center at the University of California–Berkeley.

When examining the use of mindfulness in our own professions, Beck and Verticchio (2014) described a pilot study where six yoga sessions were used with a small group of first-semester graduate students as a method for increasing mindfulness and reducing stress. A control group of students were offered instruction in traditional stress-management techniques. Students who participated in traditional stress-management instruction reported no meaningful reduction in their feelings of stress, whereas students who participated in at least five of the six yoga sessions reported feeling lower levels of perceived stress.

Regardless of how you choose to learn about and implement mindfulness into your everyday life, whether it be through reading more about mindfulness, taking a workshop, or starting regular yoga or meditation classes, it is well worth exploring as a stress management tool.

Summary

In this chapter, you learned about stress: what it is, what contributes to personal stress, why workplace conflicts occur and your own role in their resolutions, and a variety of strategies for self-care to increase your coping skills when you feel stressed. As you move forward with your career, remember that stress is inevitable and some level of stress helps us accomplish our goals. Overwhelming levels of stress can lead to damaged mental and physical health, though, and it is important to ask for help when you need it. Last, learning strategies for reducing workplace stress and your own stress level is an essential component to ethical behavior.

Critical Thinking

1. When you are feeling stress, what reactions do you notice in your body? Have you found any strategies that are helpful in alleviating those reactions?

2. When you think about your most frequently caused stressors, can you identify any commonalities across personal and professional situations?

3. Consider your own most frequently used conflict management strategy. What percentage of your conflict management behaviors would you attribute to avoidance, accommodation, competition, and collaboration?

4. How might you work on improving your strategies when confronted with workplace conflict?

5. What would others describe about your abilities regarding workplace conflict management?

6. On a scale of 1 to 10 with 10 representing highly skilled, how would you rate your basic-level stress management skills (e.g., adequate sleep and nutrition, willingness to talk to others about your stress/worries)?

References

Andre, S. (2018). Embracing generational diversity: Reducing and managing workplace conflict. *Operating Room Nurses Association of Canada (ORNAC) Journal, 36*, 13–35. https://doi.org/10.1310/hpj 4807-537

Avgar, A. C., Kyung Lee, E., & Chung, W. (2014). Conflict in context: Conflict, employee outcomes, and the moderating role of social capital and discretion. *International Journal of Conflict Management, 25*, 276–303. https://doi.org/10.1108/ IJCMA-03-2012-0030

Beck, A. R., & Verticchio, H. (2014). Facilitating speech-language pathology graduate students' ability to manage stress: A pilot study. *Contemporary Issues in Communication Sciences and Disorders, 41*, 24–38. https://doi. org/1092-5171/14/4101-0024

Benson, H., & Klipper, M. Z. (1976). *The relaxation response*. New York, NY: Harper Collins Publishing.

Brännström, K. J., Holm, L., Larsson, J., Lood, S., Notsten, M., & Turunen Taheri, S. (2016). Occupational stress among Swedish audiologists in clinical practice: Reasons for being stressed. *International Journal of Audiology, 55*, 447–453. https://doi.org/10.3109.14992027.2016.1172119

Brown, C. A., Schell, J., & Pashniak, L. M. (2017). Occupational therapists' experience of workplace fatigue: Issues and action. *Work, 57*, 517–527. https://doi.org/10.3233/WOR-172576.

Cain, C. L., Frazer, M., & Kiolaberia, T. R. (2019). Identity work within attempts to transform health care: Invisible team processes. *Human Relations, 72*, 370–396. https://doi.org/10.1177/00187267.187 64277

Cedoline, A. J. (1982). *Job burnout in public education: Symptoms, causes, and survival skills.* New York, NY: Teachers College Press.

Centers for Disease Control and Prevention. (2017). *Tip Sheet: Stress at work.* Retrieved from https://www.cdc.gov/healthcommunication/toolstemplates/entertainmented/tips/StressWork.html

Clark, D. A., & Beck, A. T. (2011). *The anxiety and worry workbook: The cognitive behavioral solution.* New York, NY: Guilford Press.

Cooper-Duffy, K., & Eaker, K. (2017). Effective team practices: Interprofessional contributions to communication issues with a parent's perspective. *American Journal of Speech-Language Pathology, 26*, 181–192. https://doi.org/10.1044/2016_AJSLP-15-0069

Corey, G. (2016). *Theory and practice of counseling and psychotherapy* (10th ed.). Independence, KY: Cengage Learning.

Currie, D., Gormley, T., Roche, B., & Teague, P. (2017). The management of workplace conflict: Contrasting pathways in the HRM literature. *International Journal of Management Reviews, 19*, 492–509. https://doi.org/10.1111/ijmr.12107

Farber, B. A. (1990). Burnout in psychotherapists: Incidence, types, and trends. *Psychotherapy in Private Practice, 8*, 35–44. https://doi.org/10.1300/J294v08n01_07

Farber, B. A. (2000). Introduction: Understanding and treating burnout in a changing culture. *Psychotherapy in Private Practice, 56*, 675–689. https://doi.org/10.1002/(SICI)1097-4679(200005)56:5<589::AID-JCLP1>3.0.CO;2-S

Follette, V. M., & Pistorello, J. (2007). *Finding life beyond trauma: Using Acceptance and Commitment Therapy to heal from post-traumatic stress and trauma-related problems.* Oakland, CA: New Harbinger Publications.

Federal Bureau of Investigation. (n. d.) *Responding to an active shooter crisis situation.* Retrieved from https://www.fbi.gov/about/partnerships/office-of-partner-engagement/active-shooter-resources/responding-to-an-active-shooter-crisis-situation

Godard, J., (2014). The psychologisation of employment relations? *Human Resources Management Journal, 24*, 1–18. https://doi.org/10.1111/1748-8583.12030

Harris, S. F., Prater, M. A., Dyches, T. T., & Heath, M. A. (2009). Job stress of school-based speech-language pathologists. *Communication Disorders Quarterly, 30*, 103–111. https://doi.org/10.1177/1525740108323856

Informed Health Online [2017]. *Depression: What is burnout?* Retrieved from https://www.ncbi.nlm.nih.gov/books/NBK279286/

Irish, L. A., Kline, C. E., Gunn, H. E., Buysse, D. J., & Hall, M. H. (2015). The role of sleep hygiene in promoting public health: A review of empirical evidence. *Sleep Medicine Reviews, 22*, 23–36. https://doi.org/10.1016/j.smrv.2014.10.001

Kabat-Zinn, J. (2005). *Wherever you go, there you are: Mindfulness meditation in everyday life.* New York, NY: Hachette Book Group.

Kfouri, J., & Lee, P. E. (2019). Conflict among colleagues: Health care providers feel undertrained and unprepared to manage inevitable workplace conflict. *Journal of Obstetrics and Gynaecology Canada, 41*, 15–20. https://doi.org/10.1016/j.jogc.2018.03.132

Lubinski, R. (2013). Stress, conflict, and coping in the workplace. In, M. Hudson & R. Lubinski, (Eds.), *Professional issues in speech-language pathology and audiology* (4th ed.). Clifton Park, NY: Delmar.

Lyndon, A. (2016). Burnout among health professionals and its effect on patient safety. *Perspectives on Safety/PSNet, Feb. 2016.* Retrieved from https://psnet.ahrq.gov/perspectives/perspective/190/burnout-among-health-professionals-and-its-effect-on-patient-safety

Marks, A. K. (2018). Interprofessionalism on the augmentative and alternative communication team: Mending the divide. *Perspectives of the ASHA Special Interest Groups, 3*, 70–79. https://doi.org/10.1044/persp3.SIG12.70

Maslach, C. (2007). Burnout in health professionals. In S. Ayers, A. Baum, C. McManus, S. Newman, K. Wallston, J. Weinman, & R. West (Eds.), *Cambridge handbook of psychology, health and medicine* (2nd ed., pp. 427–430). Cambridge, UK: Cambridge University Press.

Maslach, C., & Jackson, S. E. (1982). Burnout in health professions: A social psychological analysis.

In Sanders, G. & Suls, J. (Eds.), *Social psychology of health and illness.* Hillsdale, NJ: Erlbaum.

Mayo Clinic. (2018). *Job burnout: How to spot it and take action.* Retrieved from https://www.mayo clinic.org/healthy-lifestyle/adult-health/in-depth/burnout/art-20046642

McLaughlin, E., Lincoln, M., & Adamson, B. (2008). Speech-language pathologists' views on attrition from the profession. *International Journal of Speech-Language Pathology, 10,* 156–168. https://doi.org/10.1080/17549500801923310.

Michailidis, E., & Banks, A. P. (2016). The relationship between burnout and risk-taking in workplace decision-making and decision-making style. *Work & Stress, 30,* 278–292. https://doi.org/10.1080/02678373.2016.1213773.

Montero-Marín, J., Prado-Abril, J., Carrasco, J. M., Asensio-Martinez, A., Gascon, S., & Garcia-Campayo, J. (2013). Causes of discomfort in the academic workplace and their associations with the different burnout types: A mixed-methodology study. *BMC Public Health, 13,* 1–24. https://doi.org/10.1186/1471-2458-13-1240

Morrison, S. C., Lincoln, M. A., & Reed, V. A. (2011). How experienced speech-language pathologists learn to work on teams. *International Journal of Speech-Language Pathology, 13,* 369–377. https://doi.org/10.3109/17549507.2011.529941

National Alliance on Mental Illness. (2018a). *Mental health facts in America.* Retrieved from https://nami.org/NAMI/media/NAMI-Media/Infographics/GeneralMHFacts.pdf

National Alliance on Mental Illness. (2018b). *Taking care of yourself.* Retrieved from https://www.nami.org/Find-Support/Family-Members-and-Caregivers/Taking-Care-of-Yourself

National Institute for Occupational Safety and Health. (2017, August). *New frontiers in workplace health* (webcast). Retrieved from https://www.cdc.gov/grand-rounds/pp/2017/20170815-workplace-health.html.

National Institute for Occupational Safety and Health. (2018). *Occupational violence.* Retrieved from https://www.cdc.gov/niosh/topics/violence/default.html

National Safety Council. (2019). *Assaults fourth-leading cause of workplace deaths.* Retrieved from https://www.nsc.org/work-safety/safety-topics/workplace-violence

National Sleep Foundation. (2019). *Sleep hygiene.* Retrieved from https://www.sleepfoundation.org/articles/sleep-hygiene

Office of Personnel Management. (OPM). (n.d.). *What is an Employee Assistance Program (EAP)?* Retrieved from https://www.opm.gov/faqs/QA.aspx?fid=4313c618-a96e-4c8e-b078-1f76912a10d9&pid=2c2b1e5b-6ff1-4940-b478-34039a1e1174

Patterson, K., Grenny, J., MacMillan, R., & Switzler, A. (2011). *Crucial conversations: Tools for talking when stakes are high* (2nd ed.). New York, NY: McGraw-Hill Education.

Patterson, K., Grenny, J., MacMillan, R., Switzler, A., & Maxfield, D. (2011). *Crucial accountability: Tools for resolving violated expectations, broken commitments and bad behavior* (2nd ed.). New York, NY: McGraw-Hill Education.

Ravi, R., Gunjawate, D., & Ayas, M. (2015). Audiology occupational stress experienced by audiologists practicing in India. *International Journal of Audiology, 54,* pp 131–135. https://doi.org/10.3109/14992027.2014.975371

Ross, E. (2011). Burnout and self-care in the practice of speech pathology and audiology. In R. J. Fourie (Ed.), *Therapeutic processes for communication disorders: A guide for clinicians and students* (pp. 213–228). New York, NY: Psychology Press.

Saltman, D. C., O'Dea, N. A., & Kidd, M. R. (2006). Conflict management: A primer for doctors in training. *Postgraduate Medical Journal, 82,* 9–12. https://doi.org/10.1136/pgmj.2005.034306

Severn, M. S., Searchfield, G. D., & Huggard, P. (2012). Occupational stress amongst audiologists: Compassion satisfaction, compassion fatigue, and burnout. *International Journal of Audiology, 51,* 3–9. https://doi.org/10.3109/14992027.2011.602366

Simpson, A., Phillips, K., Wong, D., Clarke, S., & Thornton, M. (2018). Factors influencing audiologists' perceptions or moral climate in the workplace. *International Journal of Audiology, 57,* 385–394. https://doi.org/10.1080/14992027.2018.1426892

Society for Human Resource Management. (2019). *Understanding workplace violence prevention and response.* Retrieved from https://www.shrm.org/resourcesandtools/tools-and-samples/toolkits/pages/workplace-violence-prevention-and-response.aspx

Workplaces Respond. (n.d.) *The facts on gender-based workplace violence*. Retrieved from https://www.workplacesrespond.org/resource-library/facts-gender-based-workplace-violence/

Yalom, I. D. (2002). *The gift of therapy: An open letter to a new generation of therapists and their patients*. New York, NY: HarperCollins.

Zurich, E., Alstötter-Gleich, C., Gerstenberg, F. X. R., & Schmitt, M., (2015). Perfectionism in the Trans-actional Stress Model. *Personality and Individual Differences*, *83*, 18–23. https://doi.org/10.1016/j.paid.2015.03.029

Resources

There are many resources available to you on the internet and apps for increasing mindfulness/stress reduction. Given that these sources of information change frequently, I'm going to instead provide you a list of my most favorite books that address many of the concepts covered in this chapter. Here are a just a few. The reference list contains complete indexing information for each.

■ Clark & Beck (2011), *The Anxiety And Worry Workbook: The Cognitive Behavioral Solution*. Cognitive behavioral therapy is an evidence-based approach for treating anxiety. This workbook is just that: it contains exercises that help you to decrease worry. The exercises are explained in easy-to-understand terms, include example charts or worksheets, and provide a rationale for when a particular exercise is helpful to you. I have used the exercises for myself, with clients, and with family and friends and found it to be helpful to all.

■ Kabat Zinn (2005), *Wherever You Go, There You Are*. Kabat-Zinn helps beginners seeking to develop their mindfulness through practical strategies and essays to guide mindfulness practice. This book has been an invaluable part of my personal and professional life, and I will open it across the year to read the mindfulness essay prompts that help me focus. He also dispels myths about mindfulness, such as you must have a quiet mind or spend long periods of time in mindfulness practice in order to experience benefits. One of my favorite essay prompts addresses how simple it can be to be mindful during daily activities like washing dishes. His writings improved the quality of my life and continue to do so.

■ Patterson, Grenny, MacMillan, and Switzler (2011). *Crucial Conversations: Tools for Talking When Stakes are High*. Before reading this book, I considered myself to be an expert in communicating. After all, I have a PhD in speech-language pathology, engage in therapy with clients, and teach courses! I will admit, though, that my most frequent approach to conflict management was to be accommodating to others. I wanted my colleagues to appreciate my work. When I began working as an administrator, I quickly realized I needed to improve my conflict management skills and it should start with improving my skills for engaging in challenging conversations. This book saved my professional life!

■ Patterson, Grenny, MacMillan, Switzler, and Maxfield (2013), *Crucial Accountability: Tools for Resolving Violated Expectations, Broken Commitments, and Bad Behavior*. This book builds on the concepts *from Crucial Conversations* and is so useful in increasing your ability to navigate and resolve conflicts.

■ Yalom (2002), *The Gift of Therapy*. Yalom retired as a faculty psychiatrist from Stanford Medical School, and also maintained a private practice. Different from today's version of psychiatrists who mainly administer and monitor drugs for mental health disorders, Yalom spent time counseling his patients. This book was written as his reflections on his long career and is addressed to psychiatry students, but I find much of the information just as applicable to our work. It is written in very short chapters – there are 85 in just 259 pages. It is possible to read only the chapters that interest you and not have to read the entire text. Reading this book was a gift to myself. I hope you will feel the same.

30

Advocacy

Tommie L. Robinson, Jr., PhD and Janet Deppe, MS

Introduction

The role of advocacy has been a part of our society from the beginning of time. Clearly, in order to accomplish a variety of things, one has to advocate in order to obtain them. Difficulty abounds when attempting to imagine any aspect of our lives where there is no advocacy for self or each other. As we think about childhood, advocacy becomes a part of us very early on in development. "Mrs. Smith, can Johnny come out and play with us? We promise to stay in the yard." This is an example of an advocacy activity. In this example, Johnny was likely grounded or could not go out. But his friend came over and advocated for him. Let's think of another example: "Mom and Dad, I have been thinking. My allowance is not enough. I have done my budget and it seems that I will not have enough money to do those things that I am obligated to do. Is it possible that I might have an additional $30 a week?" This is an example of advocating for one's self. What about Dr. Martin Luther King, Jr.? He worked on behalf of individuals who were treated unfairly and fought to have the laws changed. He is a well-known example of an advocate who worked for others and his work impacted change. Finally, the American Civil Liberties Union (ACLU) is an example of an organization that advocates and fights for the rights of all individuals.

As we move into the professional arena, advocacy becomes extremely important. We find that advocacy work affects every aspect of our professional lives and every work setting. No one is untouched by the need for advocacy. It is seen from mandating funding for the schools to demanding coverage of services for senior citizens. Advocacy is also viewed as a venue for individuals, organizations, and groups to intervene and achieve system-wide change (Gardner & Brindis, 2017). While the results of advocacy can be rewarding, it is also challenging to undertake such tasks. It can also be a slow process. Understanding the steps in the process is very important and can often save time and resources.

Advocacy may also be a political process by an individual or a large group which normally aims to influence public policy. All members of the speech, language, and hearing community have the right to engage in advocacy activities. Advocacy is important because of the following:

A. **It empowers and accomplishes goals.** This means that any member of the community has the authority to participate in advocacy activities. It allows individuals to be confident and strong, especially in controlling their rights;

579

B. **It provides the opportunity to participate in government and local decision making.** As speech-language pathologists (SLPs) and audiologists (AuDs), we each have the opportunity to be a "citizen advocate" and meet with the legislators who work for us as citizens. Our presence aids in educating legislators on the impact of the public policy for those we serve; and

C. **It is a part of the ASHA Code of Ethics.** While the notion of advocacy is implied throughout the ASHA Code of Ethics, it is specifically expressed in the Principle of Ethics III, which states, "Individuals shall honor their responsibility to the public when advocating for the unmet communication and swallowing needs of the public and shall provide accurate information involving any aspect of the professions" (ASHA, 2016).

This chapter will focus on the nomenclature used in helping to understand advocacy. It will also address the benefits of being an advocate. The majority of the chapter will be devoted to developing a practical approach to the advocacy process, and will include: how to develop a plan of action; establish a grassroots advocacy network; work with the legislature; negotiate; and leverage the media. Finally, this chapter will focus on available resources to aid in the advocacy process.

Definitions

Table 30–1 is a list of terms that are used in the advocacy process.

Recognizing the Benefits of Being an Advocate

Advocates are in a unique position to make changes to or lend support for issues that impact the well-being of communities. There are many benefits associated with being an advocate as well as the individuals for whom the action was directed. The advocate receives self-satisfaction and a sense of purpose, while the individuals for whom the advocate acts receive the benefits of the advocacy efforts.

There are other benefits that are more global and impactful. Policymakers or decision makers carry a lot of weight and power; so the role of the advocate is to ensure that the decisions being made are completed in the best interest of those whose lives are impacted by the decisions. The global benefits are as follows:

Educate Decision Makers about Issues of Concern

We cannot be so naïve as to think that decision makers have all of the answers. It is helpful if we assume that there is always an opportunity for educating the policymakers on the issues relative to communication sciences and disorders. This opens the door to opportunities to educate decision makers about the concern regarding the policies being considered. Oftentimes, decisions are made relying on the advice of the trusted aides. If these aides have not had experiences with a communication or a related disorder, then the decision will likely reflect that perspective and may not serve in the best interest of the individuals being affected. Our role as advocates

Table 30–1. Advocacy Nomenclature

Terms	Definitions
Advocate	A person who works effectively to bring about positive change by influencing public policy.
Self-advocacy	An act in which people speak out for themselves to express their own needs and interests. This type of advocacy is often seen with people with disabilities.
Group advocacy	A group coming together to support a cause or an issue to work in a concerted manner to call for change.
Citizen advocacy	When actively involved and engaged citizens provide long-term advocacy to individuals with a disability.
Professional advocacy	When professionals advocate to provide their services for the benefit of their patients/clients/students. In this case the SLP or audiologists are advocating for prevention, assessment, and treatment that would benefit those receiving the services.
Grassroots advocacy	An organized way to achieve change that benefits a group (professionals and consumers).

is to teach them as much information as we can about every aspect of the issue.

Share Knowledge on an Issue's Impact in the Local Area. The impact of a decision can be negative or positive. Our role as advocates is to emphasize a positive outcome based on the decision of the policy under consideration. It is crucial that the advocate points out all aspects of the policy and the effect that it might have on the local area. Moreover, the importance of understanding policy changes at the "bigger level" might have an exorbitant adverse effect at the local level. For example, let's say there is a change to the clinical or academic standards at the national level. This does not mean that the requirements for licensure at the state level will change and yet there might be some conflict. It is important to educate the policymakers about this potential conflict and what it means to the constituents.

Help Legislators, Regulators, and Other Decision Makers Understand How Audiology and Speech-Language Pathology Services Improve the Quality of Life for Their Constituents. Our highest calling in the advocacy process is to make legislators, regulators, and other decision makers understand how audiology and speech-language pathology services work. As advocates, we need to educate them about the services that we offer and the impact they have on the lives of their constituents. A rule of thumb is to help them connect the dots. Often, if they have had a personal experience along these lines, they understand things better. Sometimes we have to share the process and help them become cognizant of the fact that there are adverse communication results if preventative measures are not in place. The advocate's role is to make the decision makers fully aware of who we are and what our roles and responsibilities are, particularly along the lines of assessment, prevention, and treatment. As SLP and AuD advocates we need to help those in power understand the impact their actions have on the patients/students/clients and families that we serve.

As one can see there are many benefits to both patients and communication sciences disorders (CSD) professionals as a result of advocacy activities. Additionally, lawmakers are now able to make decisions based on factual and pragmatic information.

Advocacy Case Examples

Advocacy for Patients/Students/Clients

Case: Robert is a middle school student who does excellent work in the classroom. He is a straight A student in all of his classes. However, he stutters. The school system indicates that he is not eligible for speech therapy

for his stuttering because there is no "academic impact." The speech-language pathologist works with the school's administration and other team members to make a case for the adverse "educational" impact the stuttering has on Robert's everyday communicative and social-pragmatic interactions as well as on his general performance. Robert typically does not participate in classroom discussions, raise his hand to answer questions, and/or partner with others on projects in or outside the classroom despite his ability to earn all A's. He gets the services that he needs because the speech-language pathologist advocates for him.

Advocacy for Professions

Case: The District of Columbia Speech-Language-Hearing Association (DCSHA) discovered that a bill was being considered by the city council to require licensure for all speech-language pathologists and audiologists practicing in Washington, DC. The association leaders were totally unaware of this initiative at a time when licensure did not exist for SLPs or audiologists. The speech-language pathologists and audiologists in the area requested a meeting with city council leaders to obtain a better understanding of how and why this bill was created. The DCSHA leaders communicated with ASHA and established a meeting with the council leaders and Department of Health Administration to shape the bill in accordance with the ASHA recommended scope of practice requirements. It was determined that the bill originated from the otolaryngologists (ENT) association American Academy of Otolaryngology–Head and Neck Surgery (AAOHNS). The ENTs included themselves in the bill to have two seats on the Speech-Language Pathology and Audiology Licensure Board. Most boards are small (six to eight members) and consist of a majority of practitioners within the discipline and members of the public. Typically, a physician is included who may or may not be an ENT. One physician or less, a consumer, and practitioners is a typical composition for a licensure board.

DCSHA leaders met individually and collectively with the city council members to help them understand the roles and responsibilities of SLPs and audiologists in communication processes. It was determined that a few of the aides and members had experiences with speech-language pathologists and audiologists through family members and personal accounts. This helped in the process. Through their lobbying efforts, the DCSHA leaders advocated with the city council and were able to achieve council approval to reduce the number of ENTs on the board to one and increase public participation. This is an example of how professionals can advocate together to have a public policy changed. It took dedication, time, and grassroots efforts, but the mission was accomplished.

Advocacy for Changes to Public Policy at the National Level

Case: There was once a $1500 Medicare cap on outpatient rehabilitation therapy services originally instituted under the Balanced Budget Act of 1997 (BBA-97) (GovTrack.US, 2019). The original bill required speech-language pathology and physical therapy (PT) combined services to be capped at $1500. Occupational therapy services had their own separate cap. The shared speech-language pathology and PT services were secondary to a misplaced comma. For years, ASHA members representing every U.S. state lobbied on Capitol Hill after receiving training from the association's advocacy administrators, to have the cap repealed. It was always met with temporary relief. This process continued for 21 years and was finally permanently repealed in 2018. This was due to the efforts of the national ASHA headquarters aiding members in grassroots and organized lobbying efforts (ASHA, 2018; Jones-McNamara, 2001).

When each of these situations ended, the necessary individuals were educated, the local impact was minimized, and the legislators, regulators, and policymakers had a new-found appreciation for SLPs and AuDs.

Developing a Game Plan for Advocacy

The aforementioned cases, though few, reveal how service providers are implementing advocacy efforts daily and are getting results. In order to meet with success, one has to develop a game plan. Below are elements used in creating a successful game plan for approaching advocacy activities. The process includes: developing an action plan; establishing a grassroots advocacy network; working with the legislature; negotiating; and leveraging the media.

The first act of advocacy is to *Develop an Action Plan.* There are three steps in the action plan development process: (1) identify issues and set priorities, (2) identify the factors necessary for change, and (3) identify the key decision makers. Each step is detailed below:

1. Identifying issues and setting priorities is the first action item as it creates the roadmap. It starts with the advocate or the advocacy administrator identifying the constituency groups. The groups must be surveyed in order to assess and identify issues. This can be done via traditional survey methods or with a series of focus groups. After completing the survey, advocacy goals are established. These goals are prioritized by the group. The final step in this process is to develop a timeframe for implementing and achieving the goals.

2. Step two is to identify the factors necessary for change. The advocacy group determines what the realistic factors are to begin developing the action plan. In order to achieve this, there are several questions that may be asked. Question 1. Is your issue a priority for the leadership? This is important because there must be leadership buy-in in order to implement or push forward the action plan. This positions the leaders to champion the cause and to serve as advocates for the plan. Question 2. Are there sufficient financial resources available to achieve the plan? This, too, goes back to leadership. In order to move the plan forward, there must be adequate financial support and that rests in the hands of leadership. Question 3. Is there significant opposition to the plan? This gives the creators of the plan use of a straw poll to determine support for the plan. If there is significant opposition, then it is evident that the plan will likely not move forward and will adversely affect funding or financial resources.

3. The final step of developing the action plan is to identify the key decision makers. Decision makers come in a number of different forms. They may be legislators on committees of the jurisdiction, state or local Department of Health and Education officials, regulators or insurers, school officials, superintendents, special education directors, employee unions, and so forth. Sometimes it is important to rely on connections. This can be done by determining who in the group knows or has a connection to one of the key decision makers. It is imperative that advocates determine the level of support or opposition of these different key decision makers. It is also important that the political climate be evaluated, as there are times when the situation may not be conducive for certain policy decisions. Finally, the activities/actions need to be determined to garner support from the key decision makers.

Example

A group of SLPs in a school district have met and agree that their caseloads are too high, there is too much paperwork and no time for planning, and their salaries are not commensurate with other local school districts. In accordance with the game plan, the group meets to prioritize the issues and agrees to address caseload/paperwork issues. They rule out salary negotiations as the district has already indicated that there will be some layoffs and no additional pay raises in the coming year. They understand that reducing caseload size will necessitate additional hires but learn about a service delivery model (3:1) that will help lessen the impact of the large caseloads and help reduce the paperwork burden. They identify the decision makers and determine who will support and oppose this effort. They develop advocacy tools such as fact sheets, survey results from similar districts, examples of districts where the 3:1 model is used successfully, a PowerPoint presentation, and appoint a spokesperson for the group. They identify a decision-making timeline to ensure their best chance for success and begin the process of advocating for the new model. Successful advocacy takes patience and persistence and they recognize that they may need to compromise to eventually achieve their goal. The result of their negotiation is an agreement to pilot a 3:1 model for one year and reevaluate. This example reflects a successful negotiated outcome.

NOTE: In the 3:1 model, the SLP provides direct services to children on the caseload for three consecutive weeks each month, followed by a week of paperwork, testing, and meetings with parents, teachers and staff, including individualized educational plan (IEP) and eligibility meetings. This model helps the SLP achieve a more productive balance between caseload and workload requirements.

Legislative advocacy and *establishing a grassroots advocacy network* are among the most important parts of the advocacy process. In order to establish the network, one must recruit like-minded individuals who will become key contacts in the legislative districts. It is important that the key leaders establish a database to keep track of those contacts and develop a system to connect and communicate within the network of members. Remember, there is power in grassroots advocacy networks! These are the individuals who will walk the halls and meet with the key decision makers or write letters and make telephone calls. They are often described as the ones on the ground or the ones who have their fingers on the pulse of the issues.

Working with the legislature can be intimidating but it is important to remember that the legislators work for us, their constituents. It is their job and responsibility to meet with advocates and listen to concerns. Having said this, there are a few things that one might consider when working with the legislature:

1. Understand your audience. Prior to meeting with legislators, it is important to know their political views and the policy interests. Learn about their constituent base and who these individuals are and what might be appealing to them. Identify the committee to which the legislator is assigned. Read their biographies and identify personal interests. It is also advantageous to know the legislators' own political agenda. The bottom line is, do the necessary homework.

2. Learn the best way to "influence" decision makers. Find out what works best for them. Are they individuals who enjoy face-to-face conversations? Would letters be appropriate? If so, letters need to be original. Are they individuals who will respond to telephone calls? If so, find the best time to call and who to call. Also, learn email addresses because email is effective. In addition, follow their social media sites (for example, Facebook, Twitter, Instagram, or blogs).

3. Plan a visit to the legislators' offices and attend a legislative session. Prepare a fact sheet with talking points that provide background information, data, and facts to support your position. Invite a consumer or plan to share a personal story during the visit. And finally, create a handout or other "leave behind" information sheet with contact information to share with them.

4. Deliver the message. Make an appointment and be on time. When delivering the message, please be sure to do the following:

   - Be accurate and concise, and do not get off message
   - Use facts and data to support your position
   - Eliminate jargon
   - Ask for support and wait for a reply
   - Share a personal story
   - Be courteous and polite even if your positions differ
   - Promise to follow up with answers to questions you do not know
   - Do not overstay your welcome

5. After the meeting, write a personal thank you note. Then inform your group of the results. Please remember to get back to the legislator with answers to questions you did not know.

Negotiation is the life blood of politics (Shell & Moussa, 2007). If the advocate does not understand this fact, then the outcome is likely not going to be successful. Negotiating is nothing more than the ability to win others over; it is also about compromising, or meeting in the middle. If an advocate thinks 100% of a request is going to be granted, then the loss is going to be particularly disappointing. Negotiating involves trust and understanding in addition to an element of education that aids in the process. Each of the heretofore ideas and strategies turns on negotiation. The passion that the advocate brings to the process helps in selling the idea. It therefore is imperative and important to speak from the heart. Tell a story, personalize it, and make the listeners a part of it. Bring it to life by making it vivid and forcing them to think and start questioning the obvious. This could result in a reversal from the legislators' initial perspective. When this happens, the advocate has found the correct formula and process.

Leveraging the media to your advantage is also an excellent way to implement advocacy work. The easiest way to begin this process is to locate a reporter who covers issues focusing on health care, education, or whatever area that meets your advocacy needs. Determine what the reporter wants and what the reporter is looking for and create a spin on the issues based on your need. It is important to develop a "tip sheet" with the issues at hand. Develop a reciprocal, long-term relationship with the reporter, one that is based on trust, where you become the most valuable "go-to" resource for information.

The media is your biggest friend in the advocacy process. Building exposure tells the story that needs to be told. Contacting the media to gain or maintain visibility is crucial to this process. It is important to develop a media plan that includes a calendar of events, a list of potential sources and contacts, as well as a newsworthy story. Some key factors to consider when developing the story is "the angle," the timing, the uniqueness, and the broad audience appeal.

Resources

Finally, advocates do not need to feel as if they do not know where to start. *Utilize ASHA resources* (ASHA, 2019a). ASHA has a team of government affairs and public policy professionals who can assist with advocacy planning and advocacy needs. In addition, examine the following:

Use of ASHA's E-advocacy tool (ASHA, 2015, 2019b):

- Helps with developing advocacy messages and sending an email blast

- Helps with getting assistance from ASHA state liaisons to create legislative and regulatory messages to member advocates

Apply for a grant: State grant applications are available in the first quarter of each year to assist state associations in advocacy activity. The application is available online via the ASHA website (ASHA, 2019c).

Summary

Politics, policy, and advocacy shape our daily lives and future in fundamental ways. Without it, our professions would not be positioned where they are today. This chapter addressed the nomenclature used in helping to understand advocacy and the benefits of being an advocate. It presented a practical approach to the advocacy process including how to develop a plan of action; establish a grassroots advocacy network; work with the legislature; negotiate; and leverage the media, and offered some available resources to aid in the advocacy process.

There are many advocacy opportunities. It takes work, but the knowledge that your efforts may have contributed to positive changes for the patients/clients/students and families you serve can be extremely rewarding. The number of members in the speech-language pathology and audiology professions along with those entering our fields can make a difference when their collective voices are heard. Examples noted in the chapter prove there is power in numbers and thereby power in advocacy.

Critical Thinking

1. What types of advocacy activities have you done in your personal life, and using the advocacy nomenclature from Table 30–1, how would you classify those activities?

2. What types of advocacy activities have you done in your professional life, even as a student, and using the advocacy nomenclature from Table 30–1, how would you classify those activities?

3. How would you expand the global benefits of advocacy in communication sciences and disorders?

4. How would you create and design an advocacy project on a specific issue in communication sciences and disorders?

5. How would you write a story that might be used in negotiation on a specific topic in the advocacy process?

References

American Speech Language-Hearing Association. (2015). *ASHA state-by-state.* Retrieved from: http://www.asha.org/Advocacy/state/

American Speech-Language-Hearing Association. (2016). *Code of ethics.* Retrieved from http://www.asha.org/policy

American Speech-Language-Hearing Association. (2018). *Congress permanently repeals the medicare therapy caps and ensures payment for speech-generating devices.* Retrieved from https://www.asha.org/news/2018/congress-permanently-repeals-the-medicare-therapy-caps-and-ensures-payment-for-speech-generating-devices/

American Speech-Language-Hearing Association. (2019a). *Advocacy.* Retrieved from https://www.asha.org/advocacy/

American Speech-Language-Hearing Association. (2019b). *Access to email blasts and e-advocacy system: Benefit of ASHA recognized state associations.* Retrieved from https://www.youtube.com/watch?v=9ilrIzwoBfY

American Speech-Language-Hearing Association. (2019c). *ASHA state grants: Procedures and guidelines.* Retrieved from https://www.asha.org/Advocacy/stateleaders/ASHA-State-Grants--Procedures-and-Guidelines/

Gardner, A., & Brindis, C. (2017). *Advocacy and policy change evaluation: Theory and practice.* Stanford, CA: Stanford Business Books.

GovTrack.us. (2019). *H. R. 2015—105th Congress: Balanced Budget Act of 1997.* Retrieved from https://www.govtrack.us/congress/bills/105/hr2015

Jones-McNamara (2001). Legislation to create SLP Medicare independent practitioner status introduced in Senate. *Perspectives in Administration and Supervision, 11*(3), 25.

Shell, R., & Moussa, M. (2007). *The art of woo: Using strategic persuasion to sell your ideas.* London, UK: Penguin Books.

Index

Salaries, 6, 205–207
in academia, 207
of audiologists, 6, 206
considerations for, 224
in health care settings, 206
hourly rate breakdown for, 224
in school settings, 206–207
of speech-language pathologists,
6, 206–207
Scheduling, 237
flex, 237
nontraditional, 394
in school settings, 323
of speech-language pathology
services, 394
Scholarly journal, 194
Scholars, 153–155
Scholarships, for graduate
education programs, 91, **92**
School(s). *See also* Public education
access to records of, **406**,
406–407
Americans with Disabilities Act,
313
bilingual education in, 494–495,
495
discrimination in, 313
English Language Learners in,
313, 323–324
Every Student Succeeds Act,
313–314
funding of, 315–316
general education in
definition of, 316
services within, 316–317
high-poverty, 312
indirect services, 321–322
interprofessional practice
collaborations in, 326
legislation and laws that affect,
313–315, **314**
literacy in, 326
Medicaid in, 316
Response to Intervention in,
324–325
safety in, issues regarding, 6
special education in
classroom-based services, 321
curriculum-relevant services,
321
definition of, 316
eligibility for, 319–320, 325,
408, **409**
evaluation for, 319

evidence-based practice uses
in, 322–323
individualized education plan
for, 320
progress monitoring in, 412
pull-out services, 321
reevaluation for, 322
referral for, 319
services within, 317–318
transition services, 322
speech-language pathologists in
comprehensive assessments
performed by, 326
general education services
from, 316–317
indirect services, 321–322
intern supervision by, 318
interprofessional practice
collaborations by, 326
performance appraisal of, 327
roles and responsibilities of,
316, 318
service delivery models used
by, 321
special education services
from, 317–318
specialized areas for, 318
statistics regarding, 311
student diversity in, 312–313
technology in, 327, 528, 530
telepractice in, 327
3:1 model, 322
School settings
assessment report used in, 408,
410
audiologists in, 311, 328
audiology reports, 410
certification for, 63
communication in, 324
disabilities in, 312, **312**
documentation in, 324,
402–417, **403–405**
dysphagia in, 326–327
English Language Learners in,
313, 323–324
errors in, **455–456**
evidence-based practice in,
322–323
high-poverty schools, 312
language learning disorders in,
72
privacy issues in, 324
salaries in, 206–207
scheduling in, 323

speech-language pathology
assistants in, 251–252
statistics regarding, 312–313
student diversity in, 312–313
types of, 311
workload model used in, 323
Science
public awareness and
expectations of, 192–193
technology and, 193–194
tensions, pressures, and
opportunities for, 191–192
Scope of practice
for audiology, 9–38
counseling, 542–543, 561–562
nomenclature committee, 65
for speech-language pathology,
39–56
Seashore, Carl, 59, 61, 69
Second interviews, 222–223
Second opinions, 112–113
Section 504, 313, **403–404**,
415–416
Seesaw, 534
Selective outcome reporting, 178
Self-advocacy, **580**
Self-assessment performance
reviews, 243
Self-concept, 550
Self-neglect, 470, **474**
Self-supervision, 510, 512
Seligman, Martin, 551, 562
Sensitivity, **172**, 172–173
Service coordinator, for early
intervention services,
349–350, **350**
Service-learning alliances, 141, 153
Sexual abuse
of child, **463**
of elder, **473**
Short-term limited duration plans,
283–284
Signage, for workplace safety,
442–443, **443**
Silence, **342**, 560
SimuCase, 304
Simulations
clinical, 304
virtual, 529, 533
Skilled helping, 562
Skilled nursing facilities, 5, **292**,
293, 419
Skype™, 530
Sleep, 572, **573**